The Royal Marsden Manual of
Cancer Nursing Procedures

The Royal Marsden Manual of
Cancer Nursing Procedures

Edited by

Sara Lister

RN, PGDAE, BSc(Hons), MSC, Dip, Counselling, MA, MBACP
Head of Psychological Support and Pastoral Care
The Royal Marsden NHS Foundation Trust

and

Lisa Dougherty

OBE, RN, MSc, DClinP
Formerly Nurse Consultant
The Royal Marsden NHS Foundation Trust

Assistant Editor

Louise McNamara

RN, BN, MSc
Independent Consultant

The ROYAL MARSDEN
NHS Foundation Trust

WILEY Blackwell

Registered Office(s)
John Wiley & Sons, Inc., 111 River Street, Hoboken, NJ 07030, USA
John Wiley & Sons Ltd, The Atrium, Southern Gate, Chichester, West Sussex, PO19 8SQ, UK

Editorial Office
9600 Garsington Road, Oxford, OX4 2DQ, UK

For details of our global editorial offices, customer services, and more information about Wiley products visit us at www.wiley.com.

Wiley also publishes its books in a variety of electronic formats and by print-on-demand. Some content that appears in standard print versions of this book may not be available in other formats.

Library of Congress Cataloging-in-Publication Data

Names: Lister, Sara, editor. | Dougherty, Lisa, author. | Dougherty, Lisa, editor. | McNamara, Louise, editor. | Royal Marsden NHS Foundation Trust, issuing body.
Title: The Royal Marsden manual of cancer nursing procedures / edited by Sara Lister and Lisa Dougherty; assistant editor, Louise McNamara.
Other titles: Manual of cancer nursing procedures | Cancer nursing procedures | Complemented by (expression): The Royal Marsden manual of clinical nursing procedures. Ninth edition.
Description: Hoboken, NJ : Wiley ; [London] : Royal Marsden NHS Foundation Trust, 2018. | Companion to: The Royal Marsden manual of clinical nursing procedures / edited by Lisa Dougherty and Sara Lister. Professional edition. 9th ed. 2015. | Includes bibliographical references and index. | Identifiers: LCCN 2018013210 (print) | LCCN 2018013546 (ebook) | ISBN 9781119245179 (pdf) | ISBN 9781119245209 (epub) | ISBN 9781119245186 (paperback)
Subjects: | MESH: Oncology Nursing—methods | Evidence-Based Nursing | Nursing Process | Patient Care Planning | Neoplasms—nursing
Classification: LCC RT42 (ebook) | LCC RT42 (print) | NLM WY 156 | DDC 610.73—dc23
LC record available at https://lccn.loc.gov/2018013210

Cover image: Labor Omnia Vincit Crest is a registered Trademark of The Royal Marsden NHS Foundation Trust
Inside cover images: Courtesy of The Royal Marsden NHS Foundation Trust
Cover design by Wiley

Set in Lexia 9/10 by Aptara
Printed and bound in Singapore by Markono Print Media Pte Ltd

1   2019

Brief table of contents

Detailed table of contents

Foreword

As the Chief Nurse of the Royal Marsden Hospital NHS Foundation Trust and a contributor and clinical user for many years, it is a special pleasure and honour to be asked to introduce the very first edition of *The Royal Marsden Manual of Cancer Nursing Procedures*. This companion textbook to the internationally renowned *Royal Marsden Manual of Clinical Nursing Procedures* has been written with the same commitment to ensuring that practice can be underpinned by evidence and is effective.

With an increase in the number of cancers diagnosed year on year set against considerable improvements in survival, most nurses working in acute care will at some point find themselves involved in the care of individuals with a cancer diagnosis. This *Royal Marsden Manual of Cancer Nursing Procedures* brings together the key aspects of care and the related procedures. With chapters ranging from *Acute oncology* to *Living with and beyond cancer* this unique and comprehensive textbook will, I hope, prove invaluable to nurses in all settings delivering care to those whose lives have been impacted by cancer.

Finally, I would like to pay a warm tribute to the excellent work undertaken by the nurses and allied health professionals at the Royal Marsden Hospital who have worked so hard on this exciting new textbook

Eamonn Sullivan
Chief Nurse
The Royal Marsden Hospital NHS
Foundation Trust

Acknowledgements

Based on the success of previous manuals, for the 9th edition in 2015, it was felt necessary to remove the chapters specific to cancer care in order to expand on the general procedures required in acute care.

At the same time, the number of procedures being undertaken by nurses in cancer care were increasing and we felt it was time to write and publish a complete manual devoted to the procedures required within cancer nursing.

As with previous manuals, the authors of each chapter were selected for their expertise and included are nurses and other allied healthcare professionals.

Some of the chapters, for example, *Haematology* and *Cytotoxic therapy* (now *Systemic anticancer therapy*) have been reviewed and updated, others are similar to those in the current 9th edition but have been edited to be more specific to cancer care. There are also a number of new chapters such as *Acute oncology* and *Living with and beyond cancer*.

We would like to thank all the lead authors and contributors to the chapters for their time and effort on this new publication. We would also like to thank other key people:

YiWen Hon and Neil Pearson, David Adams Library at the Royal Marsden School for their help and support of the authors searching and obtaining the necessary references to support the content.

Stephen Millward and the medical photography team for all the new photographs.

Our families and friends who continue to encourage us in this momentous task.

Finally our thanks go to Louise McNamara, Alison Nick, Aileen Castell and the staff of Wiley for their advice and support in all aspects of the publishing process.

Sara Lister
Lisa Dougherty

List of contributors

Kate Ashforth MSc Cert MRCSLT
Joint Head of Speech and Language Therapy
(Chapter 8: Living with and beyond cancer)

Janet Baker RN, BSc, MSc
CNS/Lecturer Practitioner
Apheresis Nurse Specialist
(Chapter 2: Haematological procedures)

Sue Broom RN
Sister Day Surgery and Surgical Admissions
(Chapter 8: Living with and beyond cancer)

Louise Causer RN, Onc cert, MBA
Clinical Nurse Specialist for Radioisotope Therapy
(Chapter 1: Diagnostic investigations; Chapter 5: Radionuclide therapy)

Suzanne Chapman MSc, BSc, RN
Clinical Nurse Specialist, Pain Management
(Chapter 3: Cancer pain assessment and management)

Jill Cooper MSc
Head Occupational Therapist
(Chapter 8: Living with and beyond cancer)

Andrew Dimech RN, BN, MSc ICU, Dip Onc
Divisional Clinical Nurse Director, Clinical Services and Lead Cancer Nurse
(Chapter 1: Diagnostic investigations)

Dr Lisa Dougherty OBE, DClinP, RN, MSc
Independent Nurse Consultant (Intravenous Therapy)
(Chapter 4: Administration of systemic anticancer therapies)

Dr Natalie Doyle RN Dnurs MSc BSc
Nurse Consultant, Living with and beyond cancer
(Chapter 8: Living with and beyond cancer)

Andreia Fernandes RN, BSc, MSc
Clinical Nurse Specialist in Gynae Oncology
(Chapter 1: Diagnostic investigations)

Denise Flett RN, MSc, BSc, DepHE
Advanced Nurse Practitioner, Breast/Nursing Research Fellow
(Chapter 8: Living with and beyond cancer)

Alyson Foyle RN
Ward Sister
(Chapter 2: Haematological procedures)

Martin Galligan PGCert, BSc, RN
Clinical Nurse Specialist, Pain Management
(Chapter 3: Cancer pain assessment and management)

Jane Gauld BSc (Hons)
Macmillan Specialist Lymphoedema Practitioner
(Chapter 8: Living with and beyond cancer)

Ali Hodge Post Grad Dip Advanced Nurse Practitioner, MSc, PCGE, BSc (Hons)
Advanced Nurse Practitioner Acute Oncology
(Chapter 7: Acute oncology)

Nikki Holloway RN
Prostate and Testes Cancer Clinical Nurse Specialist
(Chapter 8: Living with and beyond cancer)

Sonja Hoy PGDip, BSc (Hons), RN
Clinical Nurse Specialist in Head, Neck, Thyroid Oncology and Radiation Protection
(Chapter 5: Radionuclide therapy)

Lorraine Hyde RN, Dip Nursing, ONC, BSc (Hons)
Matron-Lead Nurse Medical Day Units
(Chapter 4: Administration of systemic anticancer therapies)

Kate Jones Grad Dip Phys; MSc
Clinical Specialist Physiotherapist
(Chapter 8: Living with and beyond cancer)

Louisa Jones BA, BSc, RN, Dep HE
Ward Sister
(Chapter 2: Haematological procedures)

Netty Kinsella RN, BSc, MSc
Uro-Oncology Nurse Consultant
(Chapter 1: Diagnostic investigations)

Hayley Leonard BSc (Hons), Dip, RN
Anthony Nolan Post Transplant Clinical Nurse Specialist
(Chapter 6: Wound management)

Sara Lister MA, MSc, PGDAE, BSc (Hons), RN, Dip, Counselling, MBACP
Head of Pastoral Care and Psychological Support/Nurse Counsellor
(Chapter 8: Living with and beyond cancer)

Angela Little BSc, RN
Matron Drug Development Unit
(Chapter 4: Administration of systemic anticancer therapies)

Rebecca Martin MSc, BSc (Hons), RN, NIP
Advanced Nurse Practitioner – Urology
(Chapter 1: Diagnostic investigations)

Louise McNamara MSc, BN, RN
Assistant Editor
(Chapter 8: Living with and beyond cancer)

Jessica Pealing MPharm, PGDipGPP
Specialist Lung Cancer and Clinical Commissioning Pharmacist
(Chapter 4: Administration of systemic anticancer therapies)

Justin Roe BA (Hons), PG Dip, MSc, PhD
Joint Head of Speech and Language Therapy
(Chapter 8: Living with and beyond cancer)

Cathy Sandsund MSc, Dip Grad Pys, MCSP
(Chapter 8: Living with and beyond cancer)

Dr Clare Shaw PhD RD
Consultant Dietitian
(Chapter 8: Living with and beyond cancer)

Nikki Snuggs RN, BSc (Hons)
Matron, Breast and Plastics CBU
(Chapter 1: Diagnostic investigations; Chapter 6: Wound management)

Dr Anna-Marie Stevens RN, DcP, MSC, BSc (Hons) onc cert
Nurse Consultant Palliative Care
(Chapter 3: Cancer pain assessment and management; Chapter 9: End of life care)

Samantha Wigfall MSc, BSc (Hons), Dep HE, RN, NIP
Matron/Lead Nurse Haematology
(Chapter 2: Haematological procedures)

Jennifer Wiggins MSc, GCRB registered
Senior Genetic Counsellor
(Chapter 1: Diagnostic investigations)

Mary Wilkins DCR (T)
Radiotherapy Superintendent
(Chapter 6: Wound management)

Pauline Doran Williams BSc, RN
Clinical Nurse Specialist Plastic Surgery
(Chapter 6: Wound management)

Lynn Worley BSc (Hons) RGN RMN
Clinical Nurse Specialist Plastic Surgery
(Chapter 6: Wound management)

List of abbreviations

AA	Attendance Allowance
ABPI	ankle to brachial pressure index
ACB	Association of Clinical Biochemistry and Laboratory Medicine
ACDA	anticoagulant citrate dextrose
ACE	angiotensin-converting enzyme
ACH	acetylcholine
ADLs	activities of daily living
AE	adverse event
AFP	alpha-fetoprotein
AKI	acute kidney injury
ALARP	as low as reasonably practicable
ANC	absolute neutrophil count
ANDI	aberration of normal development and involution
AOS	acute oncology service
APC	argon plasma coagulation
ARSAC	Administration of Radioactive Substances Advisory Committee
AVPU	alert, voice, pain, unresponsive
B_2M	beta$_2$-microglobulin
BCG	bacille Calmette–Guérin
BD	twice a day
BIS	Body Image Scale
BMAS	British Medical Acupuncture Society
BMI	body mass index
BP	blood pressure
BPE	benign prostate enlargement
BTCP	breakthrough cancer pain
Bx	biopsy
CA	carbohydrate/cancer antigen
CA	Carer's Allowance
CAR	carotid artery rupture
CBT	cognitive behavioural therapy
CCaT	Consequences of Cancer and its Treatment collaborative group
CCU	critical care unit
CD	cluster of differentiation
CDT	*Clostridium difficile* toxin
CEA	carcinoembryonic antigen
CHD	congenital heart disease
CID	chemotherapy-induced diarrhoea
CINV	chemotherapy-induced nausea and vomiting
CIPN	chemotherapy-induced peripheral neuropathy
CIS	carcinoma *in situ*
CML	chronic myeloid leukaemia
CNS	central nervous system
COPD	chronic obstructive pulmonary disease
COSHH	Control of Substances Hazardous to Health
COX	cyclo-oxygenase
CPNB	continuous peripheral nerve block
CRF	cancer-related fatigue
CRP	C-reactive protein
CRT	catheter-related thrombus
CSAS	chemotherapy symptom assessment scale
CSF	cerebrospinal fluid/colony-stimulating factor
CSS	Clinical Sterile Services
CT	computed tomography
CTZ	chemoreceptor trigger zone
CVAD	central venous access device
CVC	central vascular/venous catheter
CYFRA	cytokeratin fragment
DLA	Disability Living Allowance
DMSA	dimercaptosuccinic acid
DMSO	dimethyl sulfoxide
DNA	deoxyribonucleic acid
DRE	digital rectal examination
DTPA	diethylenetriamine penta-acetic acid
DVLA	Driving and Vehicle Licensing Agency
DVT	deep vein thrombosis
DWP	Department for Work and Pensions
EBRT	external beam radiotherapy
ECG	electrocardiogram
ECOG	Eastern Cooperative Oncology Group
ECP	extracorporeal photopheresis
EDTA	ethylenediamine tetra-acetic acid
EGFR	epidermal growth factor receptor
EPO	erythropoietin
ESA	Employment and Support Allowance
ESR	erythrocyte sedimentation rate
EWS	Early Warning Score
FACIT	Functional Assessment of Chronic Illness Therapy
FBC	full blood count
FDG	fluorodeoxyglucose
FFP	fresh frozen plasma/filtering facepiece
FSFI	Female Sexual Functioning Index
FSS	Fatigue Severity Scale
GABA	gamma-aminobutyric acid
G-CSF	granulocyte colony stimulating factor
GFR	glomerular filtration rate
GM-CSF	granulocyte-macrophage colony stimulating factor
GvHD	graft-versus-host disease
HAMA	human anti-mouse antibodies
hCG	human chorionic gonadotrophin
HDP	hydroxymethylene diphosphonate
HE4	human epididymis protein 4
HER-2/neu	human epidermal growth factor receptor
HG	high-grade
HIV	human immunodeficiency virus
HLA	human leucocyte antigen/hyaluronic acid
HME	heat–moisture exchange system
HNA	holistic needs assessment
HPA	Health Protection Agency
HPCT	haematopoietic progenitor cell transplant
HPV	human papillomavirus
HRT	hormone replacement therapy
IBM	interactive biopsychosocial model
ICP	intracranial pressure
IIEF	International Index of Erectile Function
IIF	indirect immunofluorescence
IL	interleukin
IM	intramuscular
IMP	investigational medicinal product
INR	international normalized ratio
ITC	intrathecal cytotoxic chemotherapy
ITDD	intrathecal drug delivery
ITP	immune thrombocytopenic purpura

IV	intravenous(ly)
IVC	inferior vena cava
IVF	*in vitro* fertilization
JVP	jugular venous pressure
LBC	liquid-based cytology
LCA	London Cancer Alliance
LDH	lactate dehydrogenase
LDL	low density lipoprotein
LFT	liver function test
LG	low-grade
LMWH	low molecular weight heparin
MAA	macroaggregated albumin
MB	methylene blue
MBO	malignant bowel obstruction
MC&S	microscopy, culture and sensitivity
M-CSF	macrophage colony stimulating factor
MDP	methylene diphosphonate
MDT	multidisciplinary team
MHRA	Medicines and Healthcare products Regulatory Agency
mIBG	meta-iodobenzylguanidine
MLD	manual lymphatic drainage
MMPs	matrix metalloproteinases
MRI	magnetic resonance imaging
MRSA	methicillin-resistant *Staphylococcus aureus*
MSCC	metastatic spinal cord compression
MSU	midstream urine
mTOR	mammalian target of rapamycin
MTT	molecular targeted therapy
MUAC	mid upper arm circumference
MUO	malignancy of undefined primary origin
NAC	nipple–areola complex
NCSI	National Cancer Survivorship Initiative
ND	nasoduodenal
NEWS	National Early Warning Score
NG	nasogastric
NGF	nerve growth factor
NICE	National Institute for Health and Care Excellence (previously National Institute for Health and Clinical Excellence)
NJ	nasojejunal
NMC	Nursing & Midwifery Council
NPA	nasopharyngeal aspirate
NPSA	National Patient Safety Agency
NRS	numerical rating scale
NSAID	non-steroidal anti-inflammatory drug
NSCLC	non-small cell lung cancer
NSE	neuron-specific enolase
OTFC	oral transmucosal fentanyl citrate
P	pulse
PCA	patient-controlled analgesia
PCEA	patient-controlled epidural analgesia
PEG	percutaneous endoscopic gastrostomy
PEJ	percutaneous endoscopic jejunostomy
PET	positron emission tomography
PG-SGA	patient generated subjective global assessment
PICC	peripherally inserted central catheter
PIP	Personal Independence Payment
PLAP	placental alkaline phosphatase

PO	*per os*, by mouth
POMs	prescription-only medicines
PPE	personal protective equipment
PRES	posterior reversible encephalopathy syndrome
PSA	prostate-specific antigen
PTH	parathyroid hormone
QDS	four times a day
RA	right atrium
RCN	Royal College of Nursing
RCT	randomized controlled trial
RMNST	the Royal Marsden Nutrition Screening Tool
RR	respiratory rate
RSV	respiratory syncytial virus
SACT	systemic anticancer therapy
SAE	serious adverse event
SAQ	Sexual Activity Questionnaire
SC	subcutaneous(ly)
SCC	squamous cell carcinoma
SCCA	squamous cell carcinoma antigen
SCLC	small cell lung cancer
SDF	stromal cell-derived factor
SGA	subjective global assessment
SHIM	Sexual Health Inventory for Men
SLD	simple lymphatic drainage
SLT	speech and language therapist
SOL	space-occupying lesion
SPICT	Supportive and Palliative Care Indicator Tool
SSI	static stiffness index
SSRI	selective serotonin reuptake inhibitor
SVC	superior vena cava
SVCO	superior vena cava obstruction
SVR	surgical voice restoration
TCC	transitional cell carcinoma
TDS	three times a day
TED	thromboembolic deterrent
TENS	transcutaneous electrical nerve stimulation
TEP	tracheoesophageal puncture
TKI	tyrosine kinase inhibitor
TLD	thermoluminescent dosimeter
TLS	tumour lysis syndrome
TNF	tumour necrosis factor
TPN	total parenteral nutrition
TPS	tissue polypeptide specific antigen
TRUS	transrectal ultrasound
TTO	to take out
TTP	thrombotic thrombocytopenia purpura
TURP	transurethral resection of the prostate
U&Es	urea and electrolytes
UC	Universal Credit
US	ultrasound
UTI	urinary tract infection
VAS	visual analogue scale
VC	vomiting centre
VEGF	vascular endothelial growth factor
VPF	vascular permeability factor
VTE	venous thromboembolism
VUS	variation of uncertain significance
WHO	World Health Organization

Quick reference to the procedure guidelines

How to use your manual

Features contained within your manual

Every chapter begins with a **list of procedures** found within the chapter.

The Royal Marsden Manual of Cancer Nursing Procedures

Your manual is full of **photographs, illustrations and tables**

The Royal Marsden Manual of Cancer Nursing Procedures

Post-procedural considerations

Once a sequential circumference measurement of both limbs has been recorded, a few formulas may be used to calculate the limb volume of each limb (Williams and Whitaker 2015).

The formula for the volume of a cylinder (Box 8.8) considers the limb as a series of cylinders, each with a height of 4 cm.

To calculate the volume of the limb, each measurement needs to be converted into a volume for that segment of the cylinder and then totalled. This is illustrated in Table 8.11.

The volume difference between the limbs is then usually expressed as a percentage. The calculation for this is shown in Table 8.12.

Compression bandaging

Definition

Short-stretch, inelastic bandages are used during the intensive or reduction phase of treatment for lymphoedema.

Related theory

The bandages used in compression therapy are termed 'short-stretch bandages'. They have a high resistance to stretch. When applied to a limb, they provide it with a firm external encasement. During joint movement and muscular contraction of the limb, pressure against the firm external encasement leads to a temporary increase in pressure within the tissues (working pressure), providing a massaging effect on the lymphatics as well as the

Box 8.8 Procedure for calculating volume from circumferences

The formula for calculating the volume of a cylinder is $\frac{\text{circumference}^2}{\pi}$. The formula must be applied to each circumference measurement ($circ_1$, $circ_2$, …, $circ_n$) in order to calculate the volume of each segment; the volumes are then totalled to give the total limb volume.

So $\left(\frac{circ_1 \times circ_1}{3.1415} \right) + \left(\frac{circ_2 \times circ_2}{3.1415} \right) + \left(\frac{circ_3 \times circ_3}{3.1415} \right) + \ldots$ etc.

Using a programmable calculator to calculate the volume of a cylinder will speed up the process of calculation.

Table 8.11 Example calculation of the total volume of a limb using the formula in Box 8.8

Circumference measurement (cm)	C^2/π (3.14)	Volume of each cylinder (mL)
18.4	=	107.7
19.1	=	116.1
21	=	140.3
23.2	=	171.3
24.9	=	197.3
25.7	=	210.2
26.6	=	225.2
29.6	=	278.8
30.3	=	292.2
31.7	=	319.8
32.7	=	340.3
33.5	=	357.2
Total volume	**=**	**2757**

Table 8.12 Calculating the volume difference between the limbs as a percentage

Formula for calculation

Divide 100 by unaffected limb volume and multiply by the volume difference between the limbs

Worked example

Swollen limb volume	Unaffected limb volume	Difference between the limbs
2757	Minus 2459	Equals 298
100 divided by 2459 (unaffected limb volume)	Multiplied by 298 (volume difference between the limbs)	Equals 12.11

The swollen limb is 12% bigger than the normal limb

venous system to stimulate lymph drainage (Partsch and Mortimer 2015, Williams 2012b). Conversely, when the muscle is inactive during rest, short-stretch bandages support the tissues and provide a relatively low resting pressure. This ensures that the patient remains comfortable and encourages compliance with the planned course of treatment (Williams 2012b).

Long-stretch bandages with a high degree of elasticity are unsuitable for the management of lymphoedema. These bandages exert a high working and high resting pressure on the tissues of the limb and can be uncomfortable when left in place for long periods of time.

The pressure exerted by the short-stretch bandage on the limb is influenced by a number of factors:

- *The circumference of the limb*: the highest pressure is achieved where the limb is narrowest (Partsch 2012). When a bandage is applied to a limb of normal proportions, therefore, the highest pressure will be achieved at the ankle or wrist, with graduated, reducing pressure along the length of the limb as the circumference increases (Quéré and Sneddon 2012). Limbs that are thin and areas where there are bony prominences will need careful protection to avoid high pressure on these exposed areas which can lead to skin or tissue damage (Linnitt 2011).
- *The number of layers*: every bandage is applied with a degree of overlap. Several layers applied over each other increase the stiffness and pressure applied to the limb (Partsch and Mortimer 2015).
- *The components of the bandage system*: the use of padding and foam beneath the bandages increases the sub-bandage pressure and stiffness of the assembled bandage (Partsch and Mortimer 2015).

Evidence-based approaches

Rationale

Indications
- *Large limbs*. Elastic compression garments used on large swollen limbs may be ineffective due to the difficulties of applying sufficient tension to compress the limb (Linnitt 2011).
- *Mis-shapen limbs*. Elastic compression garments cannot accommodate extreme shape distortion (Linnitt 2011). Elastic compression garments can tourniquet in skin folds if the limb is awkwardly shaped, and can cause discomfort or skin damage (Todd 2013). Foam or soft padding placed under short-stretch bandages will smooth out the folds and restore normal shape to the limb. (See Figures 8.15 and 8.16 for examples of a misshapen limb before and after bandaging.)

Chapter 8 Living with and beyond cancer

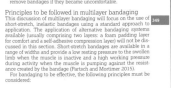
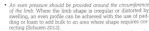
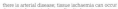

Figure 8.15 Example of a misshapen limb before bandaging. *Source*: Dougherty and Lister (2011).

- *Severe lymphoedema*. Large limbs with long-standing oedema require high pressures to break down tissue fibrosis. Short-stretch bandages provide a low resting and high working pressure which promotes a softening of hardened tissues (Partsch and Moffatt 2012).
- *Lymphorrhoea*. The leakage of lymph fluid from the skin responds readily to external pressure provided by short-stretch bandages (Board and Anderson 2013).
- *Damaged or fragile skin*. Elastic compression garments can cause damage to fragile skin. Short-stretch bandages should be used until the skin condition improves (Linnitt 2011).

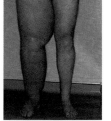

Figure 8.16 Example of a misshapen limb after bandaging. *Source*: Dougherty and Lister (2011).

Contraindications

Short-stretch bandages should not be used if (Todd 2013):
- there is arterial disease; tissue ischaemia can occur
- there is infection in the swollen limb; pain may occur
- there is uncontrolled cardiac failure; fluid overload can occur
- there is deep vein thrombosis; anticoagulation therapy should be commenced prior to the use of bandages
- the patient lacks manual dexterity and would be unable to remove bandages if they became uncomfortable.

Principles to be followed in multilayer bandaging

This discussion of multilayer bandaging will focus on the use of short-stretch, inelastic bandages using a standard approach to application. The application of alternative bandaging systems available (usually comprising two layers: a foam padding layer for comfort and a self-adhesive compression layer) will not be discussed in this section. Short-stretch bandages are available in a range of widths and provide a low resting and high working pressure to the swollen limb when the muscle is inactive and a high working pressure during activity when the muscle is pumping against the resistance created by the bandage (Partsch and Mortimer 2015).

For bandaging to be effective, the following principles must be considered:

- *An even pressure should be provided around the circumference of the limb*. Where the limb shape is irregular or distorted by swelling, an even profile can be achieved with the use of padding or foam to add bulk to an area where shape requires correcting (Schuren 2012).
- *The pressure from the bandages must be graduated along the length of the limb to ensure that the greatest pressure is achieved distally and the least proximally*. Graduated pressure will be achieved naturally in a regularly shaped limb where the circumference of the wrist or ankle is smaller than the circumference of the root of the limb. Graduated pressure can also be achieved by selecting the correct bandage width for the size of the limb and controlling the amount of bandage tension and overlap used (Hegarty-Craver et al. 2014). Moderate tension only should be used and the bandages should never be stretched to their maximum length.
- *The pressure applied to the limb should be adequate to counter the limb circumference*. Greater pressure is required when the circumference of the limb is large. This can be achieved by using more than one layer of bandages and selecting the correct width of bandage for the circumference of the limb (Hegarty-Craver et al. 2014).
- *The bandages should be left in place day and night and removed once every 24 hours*. This enables skin hygiene to be attended to and the condition of the skin to be checked. Reapplication of the bandages then ensures that effective compression is maintained on the changing limb shape (Quéré and Sneddon 2012).
- *The bandages should be comfortable for the patient and removed at any time if they cause any pain, numbness or discoloration (blueness) in the fingers or toes*. This may indicate a variety of causes, including too great a compression on the limb. A satisfactory outcome of treatment should be achieved within 2–3 weeks. More advanced stages of lymphoedema may require up to 4–6 weeks of treatment. The patient may then begin the maintenance phase of treatment in which containment compression garments are fitted.

Palliative care

Compression bandaging can be versatile and extremely useful in the palliative care setting when volume reduction may be unrealistic or not indicated and the emphasis is on optimizing the patient's quality of life.

The burden of treatment should not exceed the benefit to be gained from providing support and comfort to a limb with a

Introduction

Overview

This introductory chapter gives an overview of the purpose and structure of the book.

This is the first edition of the Royal Marsden Manual of Clinical Cancer Nursing Procedures and brings together the specific procedures that are applicable in the care of the individual with cancer from diagnosis to either living with and beyond cancer or dying. The Manual is informed by the day-to-day practice in the care of cancer patients in the hospital; however it does not cover aspects of acute nursing practice that are included in the Royal Marsden Manual of Nursing Procedures, Ninth Edition. Core to nursing, wherever it takes place, is the commitment to care for individuals and to keep them safe so that when and wherever the procedures are used, they are to be carried out within the framework of the Nursing and Midwifery Code, (NMC 2015). In respect of clinical competency, the NMC Code states that you must:

- have the knowledge and skills for safe and effective practice without direct supervision
- keep your knowledge and skills up to date throughout your working life
- recognize and work within the limits of your competence (NMC 2015).

This book has been written following the familiar and tested structure of the Royal Marsden Manual. This structure is designed to enable nurses to develop competence, recognizing that competence is not just about knowing how to do something but also about understanding the rationale for doing it and the impact it may have on the patient.

Evidence-based practice

Nursing exists in a healthcare arena that routinely uses evidence to support decisions and nurses must justify their rationales for practice. Where historically, nursing and specifically clinical procedures were based on rituals rather than research (Ford and Walsh 1994, Walsh and Ford 1989), evidence-based practice (EBP) now forms an integral part of practice, education, management, strategy and policy. Nursing care must be appropriate, timely and based on the best available evidence.

What is evidence-based practice?

Evidence-based practice has been described by Sackett, a pioneer in introducing EBP in UK healthcare, as:

the conscientious, explicit and judicious use of current best evidence in making decisions about the care of the individual patients. The practice of evidence-based medicine means integrating individual clinical expertise with the best available external clinical evidence from systematic research. (Sackett et al. 1996, p. 72)

Despite the emphasis on research in EBP, it is important to note that where research is lacking, other forms of evidence can be equally informative when making decisions about practice. Evidence-based practice goes much wider than research-based practice and encompasses clinical expertise as well as other forms of knowing, such as those outlined in Carper's seminal work (1978) in nursing. These include:

- empirical evidence
- aesthetic evidence
- ethical evidence
- personal evidence.

This book continues to use clinical expertise and guidelines to inform the actions and rationale of the procedures in addition to research evidence. This type of evidence continues to be important as long as it is used with care and critical consideration.

Porter (2010) describes a wider empirical base upon which nurses make decisions and argues for nurses to take into account and be transparent about other forms of knowledge such as ethical, personal and aesthetic knowing, echoing Carper (1978). By doing this, and through acknowledging limitations to these less empirical forms of knowledge, nurses can justify their use of them to some extent. Furthermore, in response to Paley's (2006) critique of EBP as a failure to holistically assess a situation, nursing needs to guard against cherry-picking, ensure EBP is not brandished ubiquitously and indiscriminately and know when judicious use of, for example, experiential knowledge (as a form of personal knowing) might be more appropriate.

Evidence-based nursing (EBN) and EBP are differentiated by Scott and McSherry (2009) in that EBN involves additional elements in its implementation. Evidence-based nursing is regarded as an ongoing process by which evidence is integrated into practice and clinical expertise is critically evaluated against patient involvement and optimal care (Scott and McSherry 2009). For nurses to implement EBN, four key requirements are outlined (Scott and McSherry 2009):

1 To be aware of what EBN means.
2 To know what constitutes evidence.
3 To understand how EBN differs from evidence-based medicine and EBP.
4 To understand the process of engaging with and applying the evidence.

We contextualize information and the decisions to be made to choose the best possible practice for the patient. This includes understanding and using research evidence, alongside the preferences of the patient (Guyatt et al. 2004).

Knowledge can be gained that is both propositional, that is from research and generalizable, and non-propositional, that is implicit knowledge derived from practice (Rycroft-Malone et al. 2004). In more tangible, practical terms, evidence bases can be drawn from a number of different sources, and this pluralistic

The Royal Marsden Manual of Cancer Nursing Procedures. Edited by Sara Lister and Lisa Dougherty, with Assistant Editor Louise McNamara.
© 2019 The Royal Marsden NHS Foundation Trust. Published 2019 by John Wiley & Sons, Ltd.

approach needs to be set in the context of the complex clinical environment in which nurses work in today's NHS (Pearson et al. 2007, Rycroft-Malone et al. 2004). The evidence bases can be summarized under four main areas.

1 Research
2 Clinical experience/expertise/tradition
3 Patient, clients and carers
4 The local context and environment (Pearson et al. 2007, Rycroft-Malone et al. 2004)

Grading evidence in *The Royal Marsden Manual of Clinical Cancer Nursing Procedures*

The type of evidence that underpins procedures is made explicit by using a system to categorize the evidence which is broader than that generally used. It has been developed from the types of evidence described by Rycroft-Malone et al. (2004) in an attempt to acknowledge that 'in reality practitioners draw on multiple sources of knowledge in the course of their practice and interaction with patients' (Rycroft-Malone et al. 2004, p. 88).

The sources of evidence, along with examples, are identified as follows.

1 *Clinical experience (E)*
   • Encompasses expert practical know-how, gained through working with others and reflecting on best practice.
   • *Example*: (Dougherty 2008: E). This is drawn from the following article that gives expert clinical opinion: Dougherty, L. (2008) Obtaining peripheral vascular access. In: Dougherty, L. & Lamb, J. (eds) *Intravenous Therapy in Nursing Practice*, 2nd edn. Oxford: Blackwell Publishing.
2 *Patient (P)*
   • Gained through expert patient feedback and extensive experience of working with patients.
   • *Example*: (Diamond 1998: P). This has been gained from a personal account of care written by a patient: Diamond, J. (1998) *C: Because Cowards Get Cancer Too*. London: Vermilion.
3 *Context (C)*
   • Can include audit and performance data, social and professional networks, local and national policy, guidelines from professional bodies (e.g. Royal College of Nursing [RCN]) and manufacturer's recommendations.
   • *Example*: (DH 2001: C). This document gives guidelines for good practice: DH (2001) *National Service Framework for Older People*. London: Department of Health.
4 *Research (R)*
   • Evidence gained through research.
   • *Example*: (Fellowes et al. 2004: R). This has been drawn from the following evidence: Fellowes, D., Wilkinson, S. & Moore, P. (2004) Communication skills training for healthcare professionals working with cancer patients, their families and/or carers. *Cochrane Database of Systematic Reviews*, 2, CD003751. DOI: 10.10002/14651858.CD003571.pub2.

The levels that have been chosen are adapted from Sackett et al. (2000) as follows.

1 **a.** Systematic reviews of randomized controlled trials (RCTs)
   b. Individual RCTs with narrow confidence limits
2 **a.** Systematic reviews of cohort studies
   b. Individual cohort studies and low-quality RCTs
3 **a.** Systematic reviews of case–control studies
   b. Case–control studies

4 Case series and poor-quality cohort and case–control studies
5 Expert opinion

The evidence underpinning all the procedures has been reviewed and updated. To reflect the current trends in EBP, the evidence presented to support the procedures within the current edition of the Manual has been graded, with this grading made explicit to the reader. The rationale for the system adopted in this edition will now be outlined.

As we have seen, there are many sources of evidence and ways of grading evidence, and this has led us to a decision to consider both of these factors when referencing the procedures. You will therefore see that references identify if the source of the evidence was from:

• clinical experience and guidelines (Dougherty 2008: E)
• patient (Diamond 1998: P)
• context (DH 2001: C)
• research (Fellowes et al. 2004: R).

If there is no written evidence to support a clinical experience or guidelines as a justification for undertaking a procedure, the text will be referenced as an 'E' but will not be preceded by an author's name.

For the evidence that comes from research, this referencing system will be taken one step further and the research will be graded using a hierarchy of evidence. The levels that have been chosen are adapted from Sackett et al. (2000) and can be found in Box 1.1.

Taking the example above of Fellowes et al. (2004) 'Communication skills training for healthcare professionals working with cancer patients, their families or carer', this is a systematic review of RCTs from the Cochrane Centre and so would be identified in the references as: Fellowes et al. (2004: R 1a).

Through this process, we hope that the reader will be able to more clearly identify the nature of the evidence upon which the care of patients is based and that this will assist when using these procedures in practice. You may also like to consider the evidence base for other procedures and policies in use in your own organization.

Structure of chapters

The structure of each chapter is consistent throughout the book.

• *Overview*: as the chapters are larger and have considerably more content, each one begins with an overview to guide the reader, informing them of the scope and the sections included in the chapter.
• *Definition*: each section begins with a definition of the terms and explanation of the aspects of care, with any technical or difficult concepts explained.
• *Anatomy and physiology*: each section includes a discussion of the anatomy and physiology relating to the aspects of nursing care in the chapter. If appropriate, this is illustrated with diagrams so the context of the procedure can be fully understood by the reader.
• *Related theory*: if an understanding of theoretical principles is necessary to understand the procedure then this has been included.
• *Evidence-based approaches:* this provides background and presents the research and expert opinion in this area. If appropriate, the indications and contraindications are included as well as any principles of care.
• *Legal and professional issues:* this outlines any professional guidance, law or other national policy that may be relevant to the procedures. If necessary, this includes any professional competences or qualifications required in order to perform

the procedures. Any risk management considerations are also included in this section.

- *Pre-procedural considerations:* when carrying out any procedure, there are certain actions that may need to be completed, equipment prepared or medication given before the procedure begins. These are made explicit under this heading.
- *Procedure:* each chapter includes the current procedures that are used in the acute hospital setting. They have been drawn from the daily nursing practice at The Royal Marsden NHS Foundation Trust. Only procedures about which the authors have knowledge and expertise have been included. Each procedure gives detailed step-by-step actions, supported by rationale, and where available the known evidence underpinning this rationale has been indicated.
- *Problem solving and resolution:* if relevant, each procedure will be followed by a table of potential problems that may be encountered while carrying out the procedure as well as suggestions as to the cause, prevention and any action that may help resolve the problem.
- *Post-procedural considerations:* care for the patient does not end with the procedure. This section details any documentation the nurse may need to complete, education/information that needs to be given to the patient, ongoing observations or referrals to other members of the multiprofessional team.
- *Complications:* any ongoing problems or potential complications are discussed in a final section which includes evidence-based suggestions for resolution.
- *Illustrations:* colour illustrations have been used to demonstrate the steps of some procedures. This will enable the nurse to see in greater detail, for example, the correct position of hands or the angle of a needle.
- *References and reading list:* the chapter finishes with a combined reference and reading list. Only recent texts from the last 10 years have been included unless they are seminal texts. A list of websites has also been included.

This book is intended as a reference and a resource, not as a replacement for practice-based education. None of the procedures in this book should be undertaken without prior instruction and subsequent supervision from an appropriately qualified and experienced professional. We hope that *The Royal Marsden Hospital Manual of Clinical Cancer Nursing Procedures* will be a resource to deliver high-quality care that maximizes the well-being and improves the health outcomes of individuals impacted by cancer.

Conclusion

It is important to remember that even if a procedure is very familiar to us and we are very confident in carrying it out, it may be new to the patient, so time must be taken to explain it and gain consent, even if this is only verbal consent. The diverse range of technical procedures that patients may be subjected to should act as a reminder not to lose sight of the unique person undergoing such procedures and the importance of individualized patient assessment in achieving this.

When a nurse
Encounters another
What occurs is never a neutral event
A pulse taken
Words exchanged
A touch
A healing moment
Two persons
Are never the same
(Anon in Dossey et al. 2005)

Box 1.1 Levels of evidence

1 a. Systematic reviews of RCTs
  b. Individual RCTs with narrow confidence limits
2 a. Systematic reviews of cohort studies
  b. Individual cohort studies and low-quality RCTs
3 a. Systematic reviews of case–control studies
  b. Case–control studies
4 Case series and poor-quality cohort and case–control studies
5 Expert opinion

RCTs, randomized controlled trials.
Source: Adapted from Sackett et al. (2000). Reproduced with permission from Elsevier.

Nurses have a central role to play in helping patients to manage the demands of the procedures described in this Manual. It must not be forgotten that for the patient, the clinical procedure is part of a larger picture, which encompasses an appreciation of the unique experience of illness. Alongside this, we need to be mindful of the evidence upon which we are basing the care we deliver. We hope that through increasing the clarity with which the evidence for the procedures in this edition is presented, you will be better able to underpin the care you deliver to your patients in your day-to-day practice.

References

Carper, B. (1978) Fundamental patterns of knowing in nursing. *ANS Advances in Nursing Science*, 1(1), 13–23.

DH (2001) *National Service Framework for Older People.* London:.

Diamond, J. (1998) *C: Because Cowards Get Cancer Too.* London: Vermilion.

Dossey, B.M., Keegan, L. & Guzzetta, C.E. (2005) *Holistic Nursing: A Handbook for Practice*, 4th edn. Sudbury, MA: Jones and Bartlett.

Dougherty, L. (2008) Obtaining peripheral vascular access. In: Dougherty, L. & Lamb, J. (eds) *Intravenous Therapy in Nursing Practice*, 2nd edn. Oxford: Blackwell Publishing.

Fellowes, D., Wilkinson, S. & Moore, P. (2004) Communication skills training for health care professionals working with cancer patients, their families and/or carers. *Cochrane Database of Systematic Reviews*, 2, CD003751.

Ford, P. & Walsh, M. (1994) *New Rituals for Old: Nursing Through the Looking Glass.* Oxford: Butterworth-Heinemann.

Guyatt, G., Cook, D. & Haynes, B. (2004) Evidence based medicine has come a long way. *BMJ*, 329 (7473), 990–991.

NMC (2015) *The Code: Standards of Conduct, Performance and Ethics for Nurses and Midwives.* London: Nursing and Midwifery Council.

Paley, J. (2006) Evidence and expertise. *Nursing Enquiry*, 13(2), 82–93.

Pearson, A., Field, J. & Jordan, Z. (2007) *Evidence-Based Clinical Practice in Nursing and Health Care: Assimilating Research, Experience, and Expertise.* Oxford: Blackwell Publishing.

Porter, S. (2010) Fundamental patterns of knowing in nursing: the challenge of evidence-based practice. *ANS Advances in Nursing Science*, 33(1), 3–14.

Rycroft-Malone, J., Seers, K., Titchen, A., Harvey, G., Kitson, A. & McCormack, B. (2004) What counts as evidence in evidence-based practice? *Journal of Advanced Nursing*, 47(1), 81–90.

Sackett, D.L., Rosenberg, W.M., Gray, J.A., Haynes, R.B. & Richardson, W.S. (1996) Evidence based medicine: what it is and what it isn't. *BMJ*, 312(7023), 71–72.

Sackett, D.L., Strauss, S.E. & Richardson, W.S. (2000) *Evidence-Based Medicine: How to Practice and Teach EBM*, 2nd edn. Edinburgh: Churchill Livingstone.

Scott, K. & McSherry, R. (2009) Evidence-based nursing: clarifying the concepts for nurses in practice. *Journal of Clinical Nursing*, 18(8), 1085–1095.

Walsh, M. & Ford, P. (1989) *Nursing Rituals, Research and Rational Actions.* Oxford: Heinemann Nursing.

Chapter 1
Diagnostic investigations

Procedure guidelines

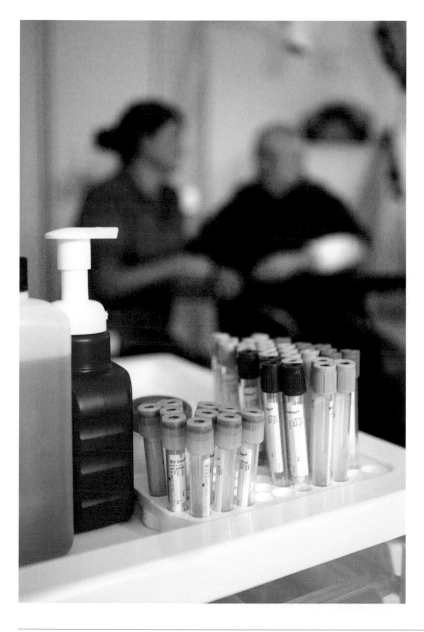

The Royal Marsden Manual of Cancer Nursing Procedures. Edited by Sara Lister and Lisa Dougherty, with Assistant Editor Louise McNamara.
© 2019 The Royal Marsden NHS Foundation Trust. Published 2019 by John Wiley & Sons, Ltd.

Overview

In clinical practice, cancer nurses or other nurses are required to instigate, participate or assist in diagnostic tests and the collection of body fluids and/or specimens for varying diagnostic purposes. This chapter will discuss various diagnostic tests encountered in clinical practice that are used during the diagnostic process, to support ongoing treatment decisions and surveillance of cancer. These include:

- tumour markers
- cervical smears
- diagnostic radioisotope procedures (nuclear medicine)
- transrectal prostate biopsy
- flexible cystoscopy
- breast diagnostics
- genetic testing.

Diagnostic tests and investigations

Definition

A diagnostic test is a procedure that is used to aid in the detection and/or diagnosis of disease (Chernecky and Berger 2013, Higgins 2013).

Related theory

Diagnostic tests and investigations are undertaken to aid in diagnosis and treatment of various conditions. The investigations are used to identify diseases from their characteristics, signs and symptoms and to identify changes or abnormalities. Diagnostic tests include the collection of blood, tissue or body fluids.

Evidence-based approaches

Rationale

Diagnostic tests and investigations are essential in cancer care, however their selection and use must be considered carefully. The overuse of diagnostic tests is a contributor to needless healthcare costs. This leads to poor quality services and continuing financial pressure on departments and organizations (Korenstein et al. 2012), hence it is essential that healthcare providers and professionals ensure that the tests used are of adequate benefit to the patient's health (Qaseem et al. 2012).

Indications

Conducting a diagnostic test or collecting a specimen is often the first crucial step in determining diagnosis and subsequent mode of treatment for patients with suspected infections or to aid in the diagnosis of specific conditions. In other aspects the collection or test may help determine variation from normal values such as blood sampling or endoscopic findings (Box 1.1).

Box 1.1 Good practice in specimen collection

- Appropriate to the patient's clinical presentation.
- Collected at the right time.
- Collected in a way that minimizes the risk of contamination.
- Collected in a manner that minimizes the health and safety risk to all staff handling the sample.
- Collected using the correct technique, with the correct equipment and in the correct container.
- Documented clearly, informatively and accurately on the request forms.
- Stored/transported appropriately.

Source: Adapted from NHS Pathology (2014), WHO (2015).

Principles of care

Cancer nurses and nursing staff play a key role within the diagnostic testing process because they often identify the need for diagnostic investigations, initiate the collection of specimens and assume responsibility for timely and safe transportation to the laboratory (Higgins 2013). Nurses are vital in the screening and surveillance of disease progression and may undertake ongoing surveillance procedures.

Methods of investigation

Initial examination

The initial assessment of the patient will determine the potential diagnostic tests or samples that are required. The patient's clinical history and/or symptom progression will determine the need for further diagnostic or surveillance tests.

Cytology

Cytology is the study of the cell, its structure, structural transformations, molecular biology and cell physiology. The specimen can be a fine-needle aspiration, a sample of body fluid or a scrape/brush. The specimen is placed onto a glass slide and examined for the presence of abnormal cells. This includes benign, pre-cancerous or cancer cells. The test can also be used to diagnose infective processes (Chernecky and Berger 2013).

Histology

Histology is the study of cells and tissues within the body. It also studies how the tissues are arranged to form organs. The histological focus is on the structure of individual cells and how they are arranged to form the individual organs. The types of tissues that are recognized are epithelial, connective, muscular and nervous (Kierszenbaum and Tres 2016, Mescher 2016).

The tissues are examined under a light microscope where light passes through the tissue components after they have been stained. As most tissues are colourless, they are stained with dyes to enable visualization. An alternative is the electron microscope in which the cells and tissue can be viewed at magnifications of about 120,000 times (Kierszenbaum and Tres 2016, Mescher 2016).

Legal and professional issues

An organization providing diagnostic services must have clear identifiable policies and procedures in regards to diagnostic tests. Bidirectional communication must be open between the department, organizational board and national bodies such as the Medicines and Healthcare products Regulatory Agency (MHRA) to ensure appropriate care is delivered. Internal monitoring processes must be in place to identify potential clinical or organizational risks.

Competencies

In accordance with the Nursing and Midwifery Council (NMC)'s *The Code: Professional Standards of Practice and Behaviour for Nurses and Midwives* (NMC 2015), the collection of specimens should be undertaken by professionals who are competent and feel confident that they have the knowledge, skill and understanding to do so, following a period of appropriate training and assessment.

Consent

It is essential that healthcare practitioners gain consent before beginning any treatment or care; this includes the collection of samples or conducting a diagnostic test. Consent is continuous throughout any patient episode and the practitioner must ensure that the patient is kept informed at every stage (RCN 2016a, 2017b). For specimen collection this includes:

- informing the patient of the reason for specimen collection
- what the procedure will involve
- ascertaining their level of understanding
- how long the results may take to be processed

- how the results will be made available
- information about the implications this may have for their care or treatment plan.

Risk management

New research and evidence continue to be produced. It is essential that any risk or change in practice is communicated to clinicians. Alerts from the MHRA and changes in practice should be acted upon. Several agencies such as the Health Protection Agency (HPA) also contribute new guidance and best practice using the the latest available evidence.

Accurate record keeping and documentation

Good record keeping is an integral part of nursing practice, and it is essential to the provision of safe and effective care (NMC 2010a). Accurate, specific and timely documentation of specimen collection or diagnostic tests should be recorded in the patient electronic or paper notes, care plan or designated record charts/forms. This assists in the communication and dissemination of information between members of the inter-professional healthcare team.

Pre-procedural considerations

Equipment

There is a variety of equipment/tools designed for the collection of specimens such as blood bottles, specimen pots and other receptacles (Figure 1.1 and Figure 1.2). It is essential that the specimen and its transport container are appropriate for the type of specimen or sample. Failure to utilize the correct collection method leads to inaccurate results so it is vital that an adequate quantity of material is obtained to allow complete examination.

Equipment used for transportation

Within healthcare institutions, specimens should be transported in deep-sided trays that are not used for any other purpose and are disinfected weekly and whenever contaminated (HSE 2003), or robust, leak-proof containers that conform to 'Biological Substances, Category B – UN3373' regulations (HSE 2005). Specimens that need to be moved outside the hospital must be transported using a triple-packaging system dependent on the infectious status of the sample (HSE 2005, WHO 2015). This consists of a watertight, leak-proof, absorbent primary container, a durable, watertight, leak-proof secondary container and an outer container that complies with 'Biological Substances, Category B – UN 3373' standards (HSE 2005). A box for transportation is essential and should carry a warning label for hazardous material. It must be made of smooth impervious material, such as plastic or metal, which will retain liquid and can be easily disinfected and cleaned in the event of a spillage (HSE 2003, WHO 2015).

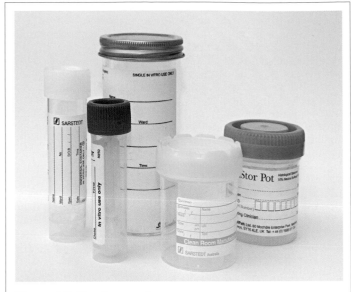

Figure 1.2 Specimen pots.

Handling specimens

Specimens should be obtained using safe techniques and practices and practitioners should be aware of the potential physical and infection hazards associated with the collection of diagnostic specimens within the healthcare environment. Standard (universal) infection control precautions should be adopted by healthcare workers who have direct contact or exposure to the blood, bodily fluids, secretions and excretions of patients (Gould and Brooker 2008). In addition to personal protection, the person collecting the specimen should also be mindful of the collective health and safety of other people involved in the handling of samples. Every health authority must ensure that medical, nursing, phlebotomy, portering and any other staff involved in handling specimens are trained to do so (RCN 2017a, WHO 2015).

In relation to specimen collection, standard (universal) infection control precautions should include the following (RCN 2017a):

- hand hygiene
- the use of personal protection equipment (PPE)
- safe sharps management
- safe handling, storage and transportation of specimens
- waste management
- clean environment management
- personal and collective management of exposure to body fluids and blood.

Selection of PPE should be based upon an assessment of risk of exposure to body fluids. As minimum precautions, gloves and aprons should be worn when handling all body fluids. Protective face wear (e.g. goggles, masks and visors) should be worn during any procedure where there is risk of blood, body fluid, secretions or excretions splashing into the eyes or face (RCN 2017a).

Specimens should be placed in a double, self-sealing bag with one compartment containing the specimen and the other containing the request form. The specimen container used should be appropriate for the purpose and the lid should be securely closed immediately to avoid spillage and contamination. The specimen should not be overfilled and not be externally contaminated by the contents. Any accidental spillages must be cleaned up immediately by staff wearing appropriate protective equipment (HSE 2003, RCN 2017a, WHO 2015).

If a specimen is suspected or known to present an infectious hazard, particularly Hazard Group 3 pathogens (such as hepatitis B or C virus, human immunodeficiency virus [HIV],

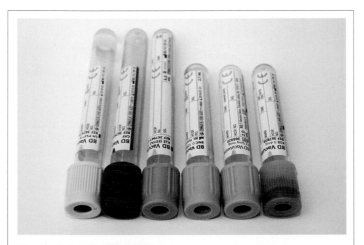

Figure 1.1 Blood bottles.

Mycobacterium tuberculosis), this must be clearly indicated with a 'danger of infection' label on the specimen and the request form to enable those handling the specimen to take appropriate precautions (HSE 2003, WHO 2015).

Specimens from patients who have recently been treated with toxic therapy such as gene therapy, cytotoxic drugs, radioactivity or active metabolites need to be handled with caution. Local guidelines on the labelling, bagging and transportation of such samples to the laboratory should be followed. For example, in the case of gene therapy, the specimen must be labelled with a 'biohazard' label, double bagged and transported to the laboratory in a secure box with a fastenable lid (HSE 2003, WHO 2015).

Selecting specimens

Selecting a specimen that is representative of the disease process is critical to the ability of the laboratory to provide information that is accurate, significant and clinically relevant. Incorrect specimen selection or technique can be life threatening to patients (Wegerhoff 2006). Specimens should only be taken when indicated.

Assessment and recording tools

Request forms

The form should include as much information as possible as this allows the laboratory or department conducting the investigation to select the most appropriate equipment and/or media examination (NHS Pathology 2014).

Request forms should include the following information:

- patient's name, date of birth, ward and/or department
- hospital number
- investigation required so as to avoid indiscriminate specimen analysis which wastes time and money
- date and time of specimen collection
- type and site of specimen; this should specify the actual anatomical site
- diagnosis and relevant clinical information which can help in the interpretation of a sample (Higgins 2013)
- relevant signs and symptoms
- relevant history, for example recent foreign travel
- present or recent antimicrobial therapy
- whether the patient is immunocompromised as these patients are highly susceptible to opportunistic infections and non-pathogenic organisms (Weston 2008)
- consultant's name
- name and contact details of the doctor requesting the investigation, as it may be necessary to telephone the result before the report is dispatched.
- labelled with 'danger of infection' if the specimen is high risk (HSE 2003, WHO 2015).

Communication

For certain specimens that have specific collection techniques or require prompt processing, communication with the laboratory before the sample collection is essential. Providing specimen arrival time to the laboratory can improve efficiency of processing and accuracy of results. Where a diagnostic test is to be undertaken, it is essential that the patient is prepared appropriately with consideration of fasting times, the cessation of certain medications and post-procedural care. A patient information leaflet explaining the test can be given to prepare the patient for pre- and post-procedural care. Communication with the department where the test will be conducted is essential.

Collecting specimens

The production of high-quality, accurate results which are clinically useful is very much dependent upon the quality of the specimen collection (Higgins 2013, Wegerhoff 2006). The greater the quantity of material sent for laboratory examination, the greater the chance of isolating a causative organism. Specimens should

be taken as soon as possible after the manifestation of clinical signs and symptoms.

Specimens are readily contaminated by poor technique, and analysis of such specimens could lead to adverse outcomes such as misdiagnosis, misleading results, extended length of stay, inappropriate therapy or potentially disastrous consequences for the patient (Wegerhoff 2006). Therefore, care must be taken to avoid inadvertent contamination of the site of the sample or the specimen itself.

Post-procedural considerations

Immediate care

Clinical waste

It is essential that all clinical waste is disposed of appropriately. This ensures that healthcare activities do not go on to pose further infection risks and that waste is securely managed. There are various regulatory regimes that pertain to the destruction of healthcare waste, which include environment and waste, controlled drugs, infection control, health and safety and transport. Specialist disposal of cytotoxic and radioactive waste must also be considered. Due to variation in product availability and local waste arrangements it is important to follow local policy and guidelines (DH 2013).

Transporting specimens

An awareness of the type of organism being investigated and its growth requirements gives the healthcare professional an insight into the correct collection, storage and transportation methods. Delays in transporting a specimen to the laboratory can compromise the specimen's integrity, leading to false-negative or -positive results, because the sample is no longer representative of the disease process (Higgins 2013). If delays are anticipated, samples need to be stored appropriately, depending on the nature of the specimen, until they can be processed. This could be in a specimen fridge, freezer or another storage unit (HSE 2003, WHO 2015).

The transport of clinical specimens must conform to health and safety legislation and regulations, and there are more specific guidelines on the labelling, transport and reception of specimens within clinical laboratories and similar facilities (HSE 2003, WHO 2015).

Documentation

Labelling specimens

Prompt specimen analysis is only possible if specimens and their accompanying request forms are sent with specific, accurate and complete patient information. Incorrectly labelled or unlabelled specimens will be discarded (HSE 2003, NHS Pathology 2014).

Samples should include the following information:

- patient's name, date of birth, ward and/or department
- hospital number
- date and time of specimen collection
- type and site of specimen. This should specify the actual anatomical site
- labelled with 'danger of infection' if a specimen is high-risk (HSE 2003, WHO 2015).

Tumour markers

Definition

Tumour markers are molecules of wildly divergent characteristics that may indicate the presence of cancer or a malignancy. They are laboratory based tests that are also able to indicate the likely future behaviour of a cancer. Although generally not diagnostic they can provide information that may contribute to the diagnostic process. A tumour marker can be obtained from serum and tissue with other tests undertaken on body fluids (Duffy 2013, European Group on Tumour Markers (EGTM) 2018).

Related theory

The diagnostic value of the tumour marker is dependent on its specificity and sensitivity and the prevalence of cancer in the population. The specificity is the percentage of persons with benign conditions where a negative result is obtained; the greater the specificity, the fewer the false positives. The sensitivity is the number of test results that are positive in the presence of a tumour; the greater the sensitivity, the fewer the false negatives. The limitations of tumour markers for cancer screening particularly are associated with the lack of sensitivity for early invasive disease or pre-malignant lesions and the lack of specificity for malignancy (Association for Clinical Biochemistry and Laboratory Medicine (ACB) 2013, Duffy 2013, EGTM 2018). The low prevalence of cancer in the general population prohibits most biomarkers being used in cancer screening. Some markers or tests have been evaluated or are undergoing evaluation for asymptomatic cancer screening such as prostate-specific antigen (PSA) and carbohydrate antigen 125 (CA 125) (Duffy 2013) (Table 1.1).

There are no tumour markers that are specific for malignancy. An elevated tumour marker may be due to another malignancy or benign disease. A normal tumour marker result does not exclude the presence of a malignancy or recurrence, and in general serum tumour markers are rarely elevated in patients with early malignancy (EGTM 2018). The tumour marker results should always be interpreted in context of laboratory and clinical information, particularly serial results. The results obtained

Table 1.1 Common tumour markers and clinical application

Tumour marker or test	Sample source	Normal ranges	Purpose/findings
AFP (alpha-fetoprotein)	Serum	<14 µg/L	**Indication:** screening (high-risk groups) and monitoring hepatic carcinoma, diagnosis hepatoblastoma, diagnosis and monitoring germ cell tumours **Elevated levels:** hepatocellular carcinoma, germ cell, hepatoblastoma, lung and pancreatic with metastasis, gastric with liver metastasis **Potential false positives:** autoimmune disease, hepatobiliary disease, pregnancy
B$_2$M (beta$_2$-microglobulin)	Serum	1.2–2.4 mg/L	**Indication:** monitoring haematological malignancy, multiple myeloma, lymphoma **Potential false positives:** chronic liver disease, infection, autoimmune diseases, renal failure
CA 15-3 (carbohydrate antigen 15-3/cancer antigen 15-3)	Serum	<32 KU/L	**Indication:** monitoring treatment for advanced breast cancer, detecting recurrence in breast cancer **Elevated levels:** advanced breast cancer (80% of patients), may also be elevated in adenocarcinoma with distant metastasis, lung, liver, pancreas, colon, ovarian, cervix and endometrium, prostate **Potential false positives:** treatment with colony-stimulating factor of granulocytes, lung infection diseases, autoimmune diseases, ovarian cysts, renal failure, pregnancy
CA 19-9 (carbohydrate antigen 19-9/cancer antigen 19-9)	Serum	<37 KU/L	**Indication:** diagnosis, pre-operative marker for resectability, surveillance and monitoring in pancreatic carcinoma. Diagnostic aid in cholangiocarcinoma **Elevated levels:** pancreatic, colorectal, gastrointestinal, hepatobiliary, lung, testicular carcinoma and cholangiocarcinoma **Potential false positives:** benign lung diseases, gastrointestinal pathology, renal failure, ovarian cysts, liver diseases, pancreatitis, cholestasis, bronchiectasis
CA 125 (carbohydrate antigen 125/cancer antigen 125)	Serum	0–35 KU/L	**Indication:** monitoring ovarian and breast carcinoma, monitoring response to chemotherapy, pre-operatively, post-operatively and during first three treatments of chemotherapy, annually in women with hereditary ovarian cancer syndrome **Elevated levels:** stage I epithelial ovarian (50% of women), stage II epithelial ovarian (90% of women), stage III and IV epithelial ovarian (90% of women), breast, cervix, colon, endometrial, gastrointestinal, liver, lung, lymphoma, non-Hodgkin's lymphoma, ovarian, pancreatic **Potential false positives:** ovulation, menstruation, COPD, lung infections, nephritic syndrome, endometriosis, liver failure, kidney failure, pregnancy, fluid retention
Calcitonin	Serum	Male: <11.8 ng/L Female: <4.8 ng/L	**Indication:** diagnosis and monitoring medullary thyroid cancer, multiple endocrine carcinoma screening, lung cancer, neuroendocrine tumours
CEA (carcinoembryonic antigen)	Serum	<5 µg/L	**Indication:** determining prognosis pre-operatively, surveillance post curative resection, monitoring advanced colorectal carcinoma **Elevated levels:** colorectal carcinoma (60% of patients and 80–100% with hepatic metastasis), may also be elevated in advanced adenocarcinomas of the lung, breast, pancreas, liver, stomach, ovary, prostate, rectum **Potential false positives:** smokers, benign diseases, liver failure, kidney failure, Crohn's disease, ulcerative colitis
Chromogranin A	Serum (EDTA)	0–60 pmol/L	**Indication:** monitoring and detecting recurrence of neuroendocrine tumours, neuroblastomas **Potential false positives:** hypertension, sepsis, cardiac failure, cardiomyopathy

(continued)

Table 1.1 Common tumour markers and clinical application *(continued)*

Tumour marker or test	Sample source	Normal ranges	Purpose/findings
CYFRA 21-1 (cytokeratin fragment)	Serum	<3.3 ng/mL	**Indication:** differential diagnosis lung cancer, prognosis non-small cell lung cancer (NSCLC), treatment monitoring NSCLC, detection or recurrence in squamous cell lung cancer
			Potential false positives: effusions, psoriasis, liver diseases, cirrhosis of the liver, renal failure
hCG (human chorionic gonadotrophin)	Serum Urine CSF	<5 IU/L <25 IU/L <2 IU/L	**Indication:** diagnosis, prognosis and monitoring of germ cell tumour and gestational trophoblastic disease, metastatic spread to brain (CSF)
			Elevated levels: testicular seminoma, gestational trophoblastic disease, non-seminomatous germ cell of testis and ovary
			Potential false positives: autoimmune diseases, marijuana use, renal failure, pregnancy
HER-2/neu (human epidermal growth factor receptor)	Tissue	IHC test: 0–1+ FISH test: negative	**Indication:** breast cancer
			Elevated levels: prostate, lung cancer
			Potential false positives: renal failure, liver diseases
HE4 (human epididymis protein 4)	Serum	<150 pmol/L	**Indication:** ovarian, endometrial, lung, adenocarcinoma
			Potential false positives: liver disease, effusions, renal failure
NSE (neuron-specific enolase)	Serum	<13 ng/mL	**Indication:** diagnosis in lung cancer, support diagnosis in small cell lung cancer (SCLC), differential diagnosis in lung cancer of unknown origin, pre-treatment and follow-up in SCLC, prognosis in SCLC and NSCLC, treatment and follow-up of neuroblastoma, differential diagnosis between Wilms' tumour and neuroblastoma in paediatrics
			Elevated levels: adrenocortical carcinoma, medullary carcinoma of the thyroid, neuroblastoma, pancreatic islet cell tumour
			Potential false positives: liver disease, lung disease, renal failure, cerebral haemorrhage and ischaemia, haemolysis
PLAP (placental alkaline phosphatase)	Serum	<100 mlU/L	**Indication:** aid in germ cell tumour diagnosis, monitoring progression, testicular seminoma, ovarian carcinomas
			Potential false positives: smokers
PSA (total) (prostate-specific antigen)	Serum	<4 µg/L	**Indication:** aid diagnosis, determine prognosis, monitoring and early detection of recurrence in patients with prostate cancer
			Elevated levels: prostate cancer
SCCA (squamous cell carcinoma antigen)	Serum	0–150 ng/dL	**Indication:** squamous cancers, cervical cancer, lung cancer
			Potential false positives: liver or lung diseases, renal failure
S-100	Serum	<0.2 ng/mL	**Indication:** malignant melanoma
			Potential false positives: liver disease, autoimmune disease, renal failure

Source: Adapted from Chernecky and Berger (2013), Duffy (2013), EGTM (2018).
COPD, chronic obstructive pulmonary disease; CSF, cerebrospinal fluid; EDTA, ethylenediaminetetraacetic acid; FISH, fluorescence *in situ* hybridization; IHC, immunohistochemistry.

using different methods are not necessarily comparable (ACB 2013).

A tumour marker should have the following characteristics (Duffy 2013):

- a high positive and negative predictive value
- an inexpensive, standardized and automated assay
- clearly defined reference limits
- acceptable to patients undergoing the test
- a large prospective trial to validate its clinical value.

Evidence-based approaches

As there are over 200 cancer types with each having different but sometimes overlapping features, there is a variation in referral and testing for possible cancers. The National Institute for Health and Care Excellence (NICE 2015b) has produced evidence-based guidance (NG12) for suspected cancers and their recognition and referral in children, young people and adults. Recommendations are presented by the site

of the cancer. Further NICE (2010) guidance (CG104) has been produced for malignancy of undefined primary origin (MUO) and metastatic malignant disease of unknown primary origin in adults.

In 2013, the ACB made the following recommendations as a result of the ACB national audit on tumour marker service provision. Laboratories should:

- adopt local guidelines for non-specialist laboratories informing them of the most appropriate use of tumour markers that are based on nationally or internationally developed evidence-based guidelines
- provide guidance on frequency of tumour marker measurement
- regularly audit their tumour marker service to review the requesting patterns and use
- review their tumour marker requests, in particular those sent to another laboratory assay
- state on reports for tumour markers measured on fluids that these results have not been validated

- state the relevant reference range on the report and that the results are not well defined and are to be only used for guidance
- state that a result out of the reference range does not imply tumour presence or exclude tumour presence
- state that benign conditions may cause elevated serum results that can lead to misinterpretation
- state that medication, medical intervention and lifestyle can influence results
- advise users that factors such as urinary tract infection (UTI), catheterization prior to serum PSA and correct time of serum PSA after digital rectal examination may affect the result (ACB 2013).

Rationale

Tumour markers are used in cancer detection and management. The tests are potentially useful in cancer screening, aiding diagnosis, determining prognosis, surveillance post curative surgery, predicting drug response or resistance and monitoring therapy in advanced disease (ACB 2013, Duffy 2013). Tumour markers should only be requested where the results can influence clinical practice and have a favourable outcome for patients (ACB 2013).

Indications

The main indication for serum tumour marker testing is the monitoring of patients diagnosed with cancer.

- *Primary care* – the only tests that should be performed are PSA in males, CA 125 in females, and where the GP is following up a patient being cared for by a secondary physician.
- *Asymptomatic patients* – potentially used for screening in early malignancy.
- *Symptomatic patients* – to assist in differential diagnosis of benign and malignant disease, following diagnosis and surgical

removal of a cancer to assess prognosis, post-operative surveillance, therapy prediction, and monitoring the systemic therapy response (ACB 2013, Duffy 2013; EGTM 2018).

- *Metastatic malignant disease of unknown primary origin in adults: second diagnostic phase* – only in the following:
  - alpha-fetoprotein (AFP) and human chorionic gonadotrophin (hCG) in patients with germ cell tumours, particularly in young men with mediastinal and/or retroperitoneal masses
  - AFP in patients with hepatocellular cancer
  - PSA in men with prostate cancer
  - CA 125 in women with ovarian cancer including inguinal node, chest, pleural, peritoneal or retroperitoneal presentations (NICE 2010).

Contraindications

There are certain circumstances where tumour markers should not be used. These include:

- metastatic malignant disease of unknown primary origin in adults: second diagnostic phase (NICE 2010)
- patients with vague symptoms when likelihood of cancer is low (ACB 2013)
- multiple tumour marker requests in the attempt to identify a primary cancer or the presence of secondary cancers; this is rarely valuable (ACB 2013).

Pre-procedural considerations

There are various pre-procedural considerations such as timing of specimen collection, other current treatment or medications, the patient's renal function, possible contamination of samples, type of specimen and the stability of the specimen during storage (Table 1.2).

Table 1.2 Pre-analytical/pre-procedural considerations

Consideration	Potential tumour markers affected
Timing of specimen collection	• **Pre-treatment:** specimen desirable for all markers • **Time of day variation:** specimens can be taken any time for most markers • **Post-operatively:** CA 125 may be increased in peritoneal trauma • **Menses:** avoid sampling during menses, especially CA 125 for high-risk patients • **Urology:** prostate biopsy/transurethral resection of the prostate (TURP), catheterization and acute painful urinary retention may increase serum PSA • **Prostatitis/UTI:** may increase serum PSA. Sampling should occur several weeks after resolution of symptoms/infection • **Digital rectal examination (DRE):** transient elevation of serum PSA • **Ejaculation:** potential increase post ejaculation, note time post ejaculation • **Chemotherapy:** hCG specimen: post chemotherapy timings need to be checked to avoid misleading elevated results
Effects of other treatment/medication	• **Immunometric methods:** vulnerable to human anti-mouse antibodies (HAMA) • **Monoclonal antibodies:** previous treatment to be noted on request form • **Radioisotopes:** invalid CA 19-9 results if patient received radioisotopes within past 30 days • **Radioactive dyes:** invalidates B$_2$M results if taken within one week of the test
Effect of renal failure/impairment	• **Potential elevation:** in PSA, tissue polypeptide specific antigen (TPS) and other cytokeratins
Effect of cholestasis	• **Potential marked increase:** carbohydrate antigen 19-9 (CA 19-9)
Contamination with saliva	• **Potential marked increase:** CA 19-9, squamous cell carcinoma antigen (SCCA), carcinoembryonic antigen (CEA) and TPS
Type of specimen	• **Serum or plasma:** generally most appropriate and suited to most commercial assays • **Serum and EDTA plasma:** difference in results may be due to complement effects, however little evidence available on effect of gel tubes
Stability of specimen on storage	• **Serum:** stable. Separation of serum from clot and storage +4°C (short term) or −30°C (long term) preferably within 3 hours or as soon as possible • **Heating:** usually undesirable, e.g. PSA, human chorionic gonadotrophin (hCG) • **PSA:** separation of serum from clot and storage +4°C (short term) or −30°C (long term) preferably within 3 hours or as soon as possible. Refrigerate specimens up to 24 hours; beyond 24 hours specimens should be frozen at at least −20°C. Longer term storage −70°C

Source: Adapted from Chernecky and Berger (2013), EGTM (2018).
B$_2$M, beta-2 microglobulin; PSA, prostate-specific antigen; UTI, urinary tract infection.

Equipment

The equipment required will vary depending on the type of specimen to be collected such as serum, urine or cerebrospinal fluid (CSF). Please refer to Dougherty and Lister (2015) *The Royal Marsden Manual of Clinical Nursing Procedures, Ninth Edition*: Chapter 10 Interpreting Diagnostic Tests for the various types of equipment and method required, for example blood test, urine collection, CSF collection. The collection vessels or containers may vary according to each organization or laboratory. It is therefore essential to identify the required collection vessels or containers.

Post-procedural considerations

Ongoing care

It is important to ensure that the patient is informed in regards to the significance of the tumour marker results in the context of other clinical examinations and investigations. Refer to Chapter 4, Communication, in *The Royal Marsden Manual of Clinical Nursing Procedures, Ninth Edition*.

Cervical uterine smear

Definition

The cervical smear is a test in which a specimen of cellular material is scraped from the cervix. The specimen is then examined under a microscope by a cytologist to identify early cellular changes (Kumar and Clark 2016).

Anatomy and physiology

The cervix is the narrow neck of the uterus and is located between the vagina and the uterus. It projects into the vagina and the cavity of the cervix is known as the cervical canal. The cervical canal's glands secrete a mucus that blocks the entry of sperm except in the midcycle when a reduction in viscosity allows sperm to pass (Marieb and Hoehn 2015) (Figure 1.3).

Related theory

The intention of a smear test is to collect squamous epithelial cells and some endocervical cells from the transformation zone (see Figure 1.3) and squamocolumnar junction of the cervix where most cervical cancers arise. The sampling technique must take into consideration that the position of the squamocolumnar junction changes with age, contraception and parity (Higgins 2013, WHO 2014).

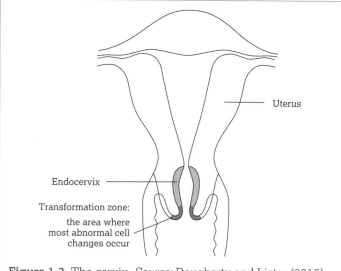

Figure 1.3 The cervix. *Source:* Dougherty and Lister (2015).

Evidence-based approaches

Rationale

The ideal time for obtaining a cervical smear is midcycle if the woman is premenopausal; this prevents contamination from menstrual flow and allows for accuracy of results (Higgins 2013, WHO 2014). It is not ideal to take a cervical smear if a woman is pregnant or immediately post partum as results obtained can be misleading. The WHO suggests that if a woman is in the target age group and there are concerns about access to screening post-partum, then a cervical smear should be taken following childbirth after consent is obtained (WHO 2014).

In the UK, 80% of cervical smears are taken in the primary care setting and most are taken by practice nurses. Screening is recommended in the UK for all women between the ages of 25 and 64 years and is an investigation to confirm that the cervix is healthy and there are no abnormal changes to the cells; it is not a test for diagnosing cervical cancer (Higgins 2013, NHSCSP 2004). Human papillomavirus (HPV) testing was included in the current NHS cervical screening programme in April 2011. HPV testing does not require any other additional procedures in addition to the regular smear test. In practice, the residual smear sample is used to test for HPV and this is conducted in a laboratory (NHSCSP 2013).

Indications
- Women between the age of 25 and 64.

Contraindications
- During pregnancy.
- Immediately post-partum.

Method for cervical smears: liquid-based cytology

Liquid-based cytology (LBC) is the established method for cervical smears in Europe and the USA. Other countries may still use the conventional cytology methods depending on human, infrastructure and financial resources. The sample used to test for human papillomavirus deoxyribonucleic acid (HPV DNA) can also be used to test for sexually transmitted diseases such as chlamydia and gonorrhoea (Schuiling and Likis 2013).

Legal and professional issues

It is advised that the practitioner offers the patient the option of having a chaperone. The chaperone may be a person of the patient's choice who will accompany them throughout the procedure. The decision of the patient in regard to a chaperone should be documented (RCN 2106b). Healthcare professionals conducting cervical smears should also be familiar with national guidance (NHSCSP 2015).

Governance

Smear tests are often performed by doctors and nurses. Training for cervical sample takers is designed to support the education and training of competent practitioners (NHSCSP 2017). Training should reflect current trends, developments and understanding of the cervical screening process in light of new recommendations (RCN 2013).

Risk management

It is essential that women are informed that the likelihood of an inadequate test is about 1–2% for LBC and 9% for conventional cytology (NHSCSP 2017).

Pre-procedural considerations

Equipment

There are several devices that are used in sampling the uterine cervix (Figure 1.4).

- *Vaginal speculum*: this is an instrument used during gynaecological examination to facilitate the visualization of the vagina

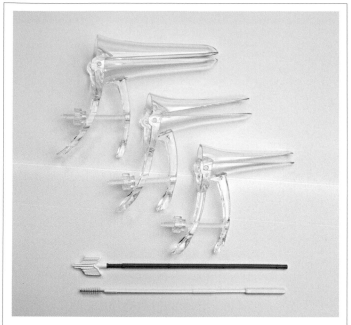

Figure 1.4 Vaginal specula and cervical broom.

os with the lower bristles remaining visible, and rotated between a half and a whole turn to reduce trauma (Insinga et al. 2004).

LBC is the current standard method of screening in the NHS cervical screening programme (NHSCSP 2015). The National Institute for Health and Clinical Excellence (2003) recommended that LBC be used as the primary means of processing samples in the cervical screening programme in England and Wales. It achieves 'cleaner' preparations, which are generally easier to read. Its advantage is a reduction in inadequate samples and there may be gains in reducing borderline results and increasing sensitivity (NHSCSP 2004).

Whichever device is used, once the sample is taken it is vital that the cells collected are transferred onto a glass slide and preserved immediately or placed into the correct vial containing liquid preservative and fixative. Slides must not be placed in a refrigerator (Higgins 2013, NHSCSP 2017).

The environment is also important, with the following equipment required:

- height-adjustable couch
- angle-positioned light source which is ideally free standing for manoeuvrability (RCN 2013).

Specific patient preparation

The examination must be undertaken in a private room which cannot be entered during the examination. Adequate private changing facilities that are warm and comfortable should also be available. Where possible, face the examination couch away from the door to enhance privacy and dignity for the patient (RCN 2013).

The patient should be given the opportunity to empty her bladder prior to the examination. Ask the patient to undress and explain the position required on the couch. The most common position is prone or alternatively left lateral as it is comfortable and aids in the visualization of the cervix. Once the patient is ready, she should inform the practitioner. A modesty towel or covering should be supplied to enable the patient to partially cover herself (RCN 2013).

Education

Explain the procedure to the patient prior to commencing. It is good practice to offer the patient a demonstration of the speculum and to explain what part will be inserted into the vagina. Any possible side-effects such as spotting post examination should also be discussed prior to commencing the examination (RCN 2013).

and cervix. The speculum is introduced via the vagina, and its cylinder with a rounded end shape allows easy passage. Once *in situ*, the speculum is opened, holding the vagina open and allowing the healthcare professional to have access to the cervix and perform the cervical smear. Most speculums are now made of plastic and are single use, replacing those formerly made of metal and requiring sterilization after use. There are two categories of speculum: virgin and non-virgin. The latter is available in four sizes: small, medium, large and long. Special attention should be paid when selecting a speculum for use in women previously treated with pelvic radiotherapy or who are postmenopausal (Singh et al. 2013).

- *Cervical broom*: these are plastic broom-shaped tools with a pyramidal arrangement of flexible flat 'teeth'. The longer 'central' tuft fits into the cervical os and must be rotated clockwise through a full circle five times. When used to take a conventional smear, this brush is an adequate and effective sampling device (NHSCSP 2017). The brush should be inserted into the cervical

---

Procedure guideline 1.1   Cervical uterine smear using liquid-based cytology

Essential equipment
- Alcoholic handrub
- Light source
- An examination couch
- Disposable clean paper couch covers
- Various sized specula (disposable or reusable)
- Disposable clean gloves
- Cervix brush
- LBC container
- Black ballpoint pen for labelling LBC container
- Specimen form and plastic specimen bag
- A container of warm water
- Box of tissue paper
- Clinical waste container
- Trolley
- Disposable apron
- Lubricant

Optional equipment
- A collecting container for Clinical Sterile Services (CSS) if reusable instruments are used

(continued)

Procedure guideline 1.1 Cervical uterine smear using liquid-based cytology *(continued)*

Pre-procedure

Action	Rationale
1 Discuss benefits and limitations of screening and significance of smear results. Explain the purpose of the procedure and explain what will occur at each step.	To ensure that the patient/client understands that the procedure involves removing underwear and that the speculum will be inserted into her vagina, and consents to the procedure (NHSCSP 2017, **C**; RCN 2017b, **C**). Allows the woman time to ask any questions. **E**
2 Document the woman's clinical and screening history, specifically: • date of last menstruation • any abnormal bleeding • any unusual vaginal discharge • contraception • date of last cervical smear • any abnormal smear results • any treatment to the cervix.	To ensure relevant history is recorded (NHSCSP 2017, **C**).
3 Place all the equipment required for the procedure on the trolley.	To facilitate the efficient taking of the smear. **E**
4 Close room door or curtains and ask the patient/client to remove her underwear.	To provide privacy and comfort for the patient/client. **E**

Procedure

5 Turn the light source on and position at end of examination table.	To provide illumination of the cervix and increase the accuracy of the smear taking (NHSCSP 2004, **C**; NHSCSP 2017, **C**; RCN 2013, **C**).
6 Assist the patient/client into a supine position on the couch, with knees drawn up and legs parted. Keep her as covered as possible.	To facilitate easy access of the vaginal speculum and the taking of the cervical smear (NHSCSP 2004, **C**; NHSCSP 2017, **C**; WHO 2014, **C**).
7 Wash hands with antibacterial detergent and running hand-hot water. Ensure hands are dried with disposable paper hand towels.	To reduce the risk of contamination and cross-infection (Fraise and Bradley 2009, **E**; RCN 2017a, **C**).
8 Apply gloves and apron.	To reduce the risk of contamination and cross-infection (Fraise and Bradley 2009, **E**; RCN 2017a, **C**).
9 Select the appropriate size speculum, from very small, small, medium, large including a long-bladed narrow speculum if the vagina is long or the cervix is lying posterior. If a reusable sterilized speculum is used it can be warmed or cooled using clean tap water.	To promote patient comfort and reduce anxiety (NHSCSP 2017, **C**). If removed from a sterilizer, speculum may need to be cooled down, if cold then warmed up to reduce patient discomfort. It must be explained to the patient that the speculum has been sterilized but the water will not contaminate it. **E**
10 Apply lubricant to the speculum. Part the labia and, holding the speculum blades together sideways, slip the speculum into the vagina.	To insert the speculum and reduce patient discomfort (Fraise and Bradley 2009, **E**; WHO 2014, **C**; RCN 2013, **C**).
11 When the speculum is halfway into the vagina, turn it so that the handle is facing down.	To promote patient comfort and reduce contamination of the cervix with lubricants (NHSCSP 2017, **C**).
12 Gently open the blades of the speculum and look for the cervix. It may be necessary to move the speculum up or down until the entire cervix is visible.	To reduce patient discomfort and visualize the cervix (WHO 2014, **C**).
13 Using the cervix brush, insert the central bristles into the endocervical canal so that the shorter, outer bristles fully contact the ectocervix.	To ensure accuracy of site sampled (NHSCSP 2004, **C**; NHSCSP 2017, **C**; Singh et al. 2013, **R5**).
14 Using pencil pressure, rotate the brush in a clockwise direction five times and then remove the brush. *Note*: the plastic fronds of the brush are bevelled for rotation in a clockwise direction only.	To ensure good contact with the ectocervix and gather a high cellular yield (NHSCSP 2004, **C**; NHSCSP 2017, **C**). Firm pressure is required to ensure the cells cling to the brush (NHSCSP 2004, **C**; NHSCSP 2017, **C**).

Either:

Using Thinprep, using a swirling motion, rinse the brush into the fixative vial; then push the brush into the base of the vial at least 10 times, forcing the bristles apart.	To ensure a usable amount of cellular material is collected (NHSCSP 2004, **C**; NHSCSP 2017, **C**).

	Inspect the brush for any residual material and remove any remaining material by passing the brush over the edge of the fixative vial.	To ensure the cellular material reaches the preservative solution (NHSCSP 2004, **C**; NHSCSP 2017, **C**).
	Ensure that the material reaches the liquid. Then tighten the cap so that the material passes the torque line on the vial and give the vial a shake.	To ensure that the cells do not cling to the device (NHSCSP 2004, **C**; NHSCSP 2017, **C**).
	Or:	
	Using SurePath, remove head of the brush from the stem and place into the vial of fixative. Then screw lid on tightly and shake the vial. *Note*: it is essential that the sample is placed into the vial immediately in order to achieve fixation.	To ensure accurate preservation of cervical material (NHSCSP 2004, **C**; NHSCSP 2017, **C**).
15	Gently pull the speculum out until the blades are clear of the cervix, then close blades and remove speculum, placing in clinical waste bin if disposable or into CSS container if reusable.	To prevent pinching cervix or vaginal walls and ensure safe disposal of contaminated equipment (NHSCSP 2017, **C**; WHO 2014, **C**).
16	Cover the patient/client and offer tissue paper to wipe away any excess vaginal discharge.	To ensure dignity and privacy while promoting hygiene and comfort. **E**
Post-procedure		
17	Remove gloves and dispose of waste in clinical waste receiver.	Safe disposal of clinical waste (DH 2013, **C**).
18	Assist the patient/client off the examination table and allow her to dress.	To ensure safety and promote dignity and privacy. **E**
19	Using a black ballpoint pen, label the vial with patient/client name, clinic number and date of birth.	To ensure patient details are documented correctly. **E**
20	Place the vial into plastic specimen bag with the correctly labelled specimen form and send to laboratory.	To ensure safe handling and transportation of a biohazard (HSE 2003, **C**; DH 2013, **C**; WHO 2015, **C**).
21	Document the procedure in the patient's records.	To ensure timely and accurate record keeping (NMC 2010a, **C**).

Problem-solving table 1.1 Prevention and resolution (Procedure guideline 1.1)

Problem	Cause	Prevention	Action
Inadequate sample.	Cervix has not been scraped firmly enough to obtain adequate epithelial cells (WHO 2014).	Ensure adequate pressure to obtain sample.	Repeat cervical smear.
	Brush not rinsed immediately, allowing the sample to dry and causing the cells to become misshapen (NHSCSP 2015).	Ensure brush is rinsed immediately after scraping the cervix.	Repeat cervical smear.
	Sample contaminated with lubricants, spermicide or blood (Higgins 2013).	Ensure sample is not contaminated by educating the patient not to use lubricants or spermicide 24 hours prior to test.	Repeat cervical smear.
Unable to visualize the cervix.	Position of the patient or anatomical position of the cervix.	Adequate positioning of the patient.	Reposition the patient from the prone to the lateral position. Place a pillow under the buttocks or turn the speculum. Consider assistance from another sample taker or refer to colposcopy clinic if unable to visualize.

Post-procedural considerations

Immediate care
Ensure patient modesty is maintained throughout and directly after the examination. To maintain privacy and dignity, the nurse should leave the room while the patient gets undressed and dressed, and advise them to call when ready (RCN 2013).

Ongoing care
The results should be communicated to the patient and appropriate follow-up and/or referral to secondary services arranged where necessary. It is important that the healthcare professional considers how the patient may react if abnormal results are to be delivered and ensures necessary support (RCN 2013).

Documentation
The nurse should ensure that the request form has been adequately completed and that the samples are also labelled correctly and accurately. If other microbiological tests are conducted, ensure the correct forms are completed and the samples are labelled and document any findings and resulting actions (RCN 2013).

Education of patient and relevant others

It is not unusual for the patient to experience some spotting after the cervical smear. This must be explained to the patient to ensure she is aware and will not be worried. The healthcare professional should promote health education providing advice in the prevention of cervical cancer and encouraging screening to those who are eligible such as accurate information and advice in the prevention of cervical cancer. Patient information leaflets are offered to patients to ensure they have the appropriate information (RCN 2013).

Diagnostic radioisotope procedures (nuclear medicine)

Definition

Nuclear medicine involves the administration of radioactive material in the form of a radiopharmaceutical to patients for diagnosis or therapy (DH 2016, HPA 2016). In both cases, the radioactive material is attached to a pharmaceutical chosen according to the organ or system to be investigated or treated. For example, radioactively labelled phosphates will be concentrated in the bone and are therefore used for bone scans, whereas radioactive iodine (given in the form of sodium iodide) concentrates in the thyroid and is used for both imaging and treating various thyroid conditions, forming a radiopharmaceutical (DH 2016, HPA 2016).

A radionuclide investigation involves administration of the appropriate radiopharmaceutical and using dynamic imaging or waiting a predetermined time to allow the radiopharmaceutical to be taken up in the organ to be investigated (Table 1.3). The patient is then positioned on the camera table, usually lying flat, and is required to keep still during the scan. Movement causes artefacts which reduce diagnostic accuracy. The scan may last 15–60 minutes (DH 2016).

Evidence-based approaches

Rationale

The important properties that make the radiopharmaceutical useful for diagnostic purposes include:

- the physical half-life
- decay characteristics
- ease of incorporation into radiopharmaceuticals
- availability of radionuclide.

A desirable radionuclide should have a half-life just long enough to allow for preparation, administration and concentration in the region of interest, but short enough for radiation to effectively disappear after the test (Cherry et al. 2003). Imaging studies commonly performed in a nuclear medicine department include:

- assessment of structures and/or function of organs
- sites of infection
- presence of tumours.

Table 1.3 Radionuclide investigations

Investigation/target organ	Radiopharmaceutical	Procedures and clinical interventions
Imaging studies		
Bone scan		
Used to assess bone function in which malignancy, fractures and diseases such as osteomalacia and Paget's disease can be diagnosed	Technetium (^{99m}Tc) phosphate and phosphonate compounds, including methylene diphosphonate (MDP) and hydroxymethylene diphosphonate (HDP)	Patient to drink 5–6 cups of fluid and to empty bladder regularly while waiting for scan. This is to enhance soft tissue clearance and minimize absorbed radiation dose to the bladder
Renogram (dynamic renal study)		
Used to assess renal function by monitoring clearance of radiopharmaceutical via kidneys	^{99m}Tc MAG$_3$ Benzoylmercaptoacetyltriglycine ^{99m}Tc DTPA (diethylenetriamine penta-acetic acid)	Patients to drink approximately 600 mL of fluid and to empty bladder prior to scan, which takes approximately 1 hour. Intravenous diuretic is to be administered to patient during the scan to diagnose obstructive uropathy (Russell 1998)
Static renal study		
Used to assess size, shape, position and function of kidneys. Used to diagnose renal scarring in children	^{99m}Tc DMSA (dimercaptosuccinic acid)	No preparation
Perfusion lung scan		
Used to assess blood supply to alveolar tree. Provides complementary information to a ventilation lung scan. Used to diagnose pulmonary embolism	^{99m}Tc MAA (macroaggregated albumin)	Radiopharmaceutical is administered as a slow bolus intravenous injection. Patient to lie supine and breathe deeply while injection is being given. This is to enhance even distribution of MAA through the lung capillary bed. If the patient is pregnant, administered activity or dose needs to be reduced
Ventilation lung scan		
Provides complementary information to a perfusion lung scan in diagnosis of pulmonary embolism. Used to assess patency of airways	^{99m}Tc Technegas, ^{99m}Tc aerosol, ^{81m}Kr gas, ^{133}Xe gas	A chest X-ray performed within the preceding 24 hours is required prior to scan, to assist with interpretation of lung scan. Patient breathes the radiopharmaceutical through a special mouthpiece while scan is being performed

Investigation/target organ	Radiopharmaceutical	Procedures and clinical interventions
Cardiac studies: perfusion imaging		
Used to assess areas of viable perfused myocardium. This is a two-part test with myocardial perfusion monitored under stress and subsequently at rest. Stress may be exercise or pharmacologically induced. Often performed on patients with suspected coronary artery disease, recent myocardial infarction or those who have undergone coronary artery bypass surgery	^{99m}Tc MIBI (methoxyisobutyl isonitrile), ^{99m}Tc tetrafosmin, ^{201}Tl thallous chloride	Patient vital signs need to be closely monitored during post-exercise period because there is the potential risk of triggering a myocardial infarction after stress This test is usually performed within a cardiology unit with appropriately trained personnel and equipment. Patient is usually kept in the department until they have been assessed by a clinician
Cardiac studies: left ventricular ejection fraction/multiple gated acquisition scan		
Used to evaluate cardiac function in patients prior to and during courses of chemotherapy containing cardiotoxic agents such as epirubicin	^{99m}Tc-labelled red blood cells	Current weight of patient is required for calculation of dose of a red blood cell labelling agent, which ensures red blood cells are labelled with required radioactivity. The volume calculated is then administered intravenously 20–30 minutes prior to scan. Patient lies supine for 30–40 minutes
Thyroid scan		
May be used to confirm presence of one or more nodules within the thyroid, or to identify functional characteristics of nodule(s)	^{99m}Tc pertechnetate, ^{123}I/^{124}I/^{131}I sodium iodide	Patient to avoid foods containing iodine (including sea salt, seafood, cod liver oil, mineral tablets and kelp) for 3 days prior to test. These foods decrease uptake of radiopharmaceutical within thyroid bed. Patient to discontinue thyroid medication for between 3 days and 3 weeks prior to test, depending on specific instructions given by clinician
Parathyroid scan		
Used to diagnose parathyroid adenomas in patients with primary hyperparathyroidism	^{99m}Tc pertechnetate, ^{201}Tl thallous chloride	This is a two-part test, comprising a thyroid scan which is completed prior to the parathyroid scan. Patient should follow instructions for thyroid test
Tumour imaging		
Used to differentiate between metabolically active tumours and space-occupying lesions, or for the diagnosis of unknown primary tumours	^{18}F 2-fluorodeoxyglucose (FDG)	Patient to fast for up to 6 hours prior to injection, with only water to be taken. Patients may experience a metallic taste in the mouth immediately after administration. Waiting interval between injection and scan is 30 minutes, scan being performed with a positron emission tomography (PET) camera
Used to diagnose infection and diagnose and stage cancers such as lung, Hodgkin disease lymphomas and neuroendocrine tumours	^{67}Ga gallium citrate	Due to excretion of gallium citrate via the gastrointestinal tract, patients should be given laxatives or encouraged to increase fibre and fluid intake to avoid constipation
Used to diagnose and assess patients with neuroectodermal tumours including phaeochromocytomas, neuroblastomas, carcinoid, medullary thyroid cancers and paragangliomas	^{123}I mIBG (meta-iodobenzylguanidine)	Patient must take Lugol's iodine or potassium iodide for 2 days prior to and 3 days after day of administration. mIBG may cause hypertension and is administered slowly over a 10-minute period. On occasions, patients may experience some discomfort at the injection site. This may be relieved by applying heat to the area of discomfort and reducing rate of infusion. For paediatric patients, it is preferable to administer mIBG via a central venous catheter. Some drugs that act on the adrenergic system may interfere with uptake of mIBG
Often used in conjunction with mIBG scans to assist with localization of the primary tumour and sites of metastatic spread in the aforementioned diseases, e.g. neuroendocrine tumours	^{111}In octreotide DTPA-d-Phe-1-octreotide	Patients with insulinoma should have their blood sugar levels monitored before and after injection. An intravenous solution containing glucose should be available in case of hypoglycaemia. Patients should be encouraged to increase fluid and fibre intake to avoid constipation
Sites of infection		
To identify areas of lymphocyte localization in patients with either acute or chronic inflammatory infections	Labelled white blood cells	50 mL of blood is taken from patient using a 19 G needle. Labelled blood is reinjected after approximately 2 hours, following which patient is scanned later the same day and/or the following day

(continued)

Table 1.3 Radionuclide investigations *(continued)*

Investigation/target organ	Radiopharmaceutical	Procedures and clinical interventions
Gastrointestinal tract		
To determine cause of gastrointestinal bleeding, including Meckel's diverticulum	^{99m}Tc pertechnetate	Patients (usually children) need to fast for 4–6 hours before scan; adults to fast from midnight
Non-imaging studies		
Kidney function		
Measurement of glomerular filtration rate (GFR) provides an assessment of renal function. Often used in renal transplant patients, in compromised renal function due to long-term use of certain drugs (e.g. ciclosporin) or in patients with systemic lupus erythematosus. Oncology patients often have renal function assessed prior to chemotherapy, particularly if regimen includes platinum-based cytotoxic agents	^{51}Cr EDTA (ethylenediamine tetra-acetic acid)	Renal clearance of administered radiopharmaceutical is assessed from residual radioactivity in blood samples taken from patient at either 3 hours, or at 2, 3 and 4 hours post injection. Patient's height and weight are required to enable GFR to be calculated accurately. It is important that no hydration or blood products are commenced during the test as this may alter results of test
Red cell mass/plasma volume		
Often used to diagnose polycythaemia vera in patients with cardiovascular disease	^{125}I human serum albumin, ^{51}Cr or ^{99m}Tc-labelled red blood cells	10 mL of blood is taken from patient using a 19 G needle. Labelled blood is re-injected after approximately 1.5 hours, following which patient's blood is taken at 10-minute intervals for 40 minutes. Patient's height and weight are recorded
Sentinel node localization. Sentinel lymph nodes receive drainage from the breasts (Luini et al. 2005). By undertaking biopsies of these nodes, the surgeon can predict the cancer status of all nodes in the axillary region. This procedure allows for accurate diagnosis of the patient's cancer status, avoiding unnecessary axillary dissection (Schrenk et al. 2005)	^{99m}Tc colloid	0.1–0.2 mL is injected intradermally into the designated area on the breast for location of main sentinel node. Minimum of 1 hour (up to 24 hours) prior to surgical procedure
		During the procedure all staff must wear their film badges and those handling the specimen must wear finger dosimeters. The theatre door should be labelled with a warning controlled area sign and disposable drapes and gowns should be used. The specimen should be placed in a screw-top container, which is labelled with the radioactive symbol and the details recorded in the log book. The specimen is then stored for 48 hours in a temperature monitored fridge, after which time it is sent to histopathology in the normal way. The radioactive label is removed in histology after 1 week when the specimen is then considered non-radioactive
		On completion of the procedure, the used drapes, gown and gloves should be placed in a hospital approved clinical waste bag and the environment and waste monitored to ensure no contamination is present. Any contaminated items should be marked radioactive and stored in a secure store until sufficient radioactive decay has occurred. Only then should the warning symbols be removed by the physics department and the waste disposed of as clinical waste

Source: Adapted from Henkin (2006), Peter and Gambhir (2004), Ziessman et al. (2006).

Common non-imaging studies include investigations into red cell mass and plasma volume, and gastrointestinal tract and renal function (DH 2016).

Principles of care

Radiation protection is more complex than for X-ray procedures because, in addition to the external hazard, there is an internal hazard from contamination arising from contact with the radiopharmaceutical itself or with the patient's body fluids.

Once a patient has been given a radioactive material, they become radioactive themselves; how much and for how long depend on the type and amount of radioactive material used. In the case of diagnostic nuclear medicine, the safety of ward staff nursing these patients can be assured by following very simple advice. The advice regarding therapeutic procedures is more detailed and the nuclear medicine department, Radiation Protection Adviser or Supervisor should always discuss procedures with the ward before the patient is treated (IRMER 2000).

Legal and professional issues

Radiopharmaceuticals are legally categorized as prescription-only medicines (POMs), and, in addition to the standard legislation surrounding the administration of such drugs, are subject to regulations related to their radioactive content. In the UK, a statutory committee called the Administration of Radioactive Substances Advisory Committee (ARSAC) was established to give ionizing radiation advice to health ministers and to manage the certification process for administration of radiopharmaceuticals. This committee issues certificates which authorize individuals to administer radiopharmaceuticals to patients. It also lists the maximum permissible doses of radioactivity that may be administered to adult patients, and appropriately reduced adult doses for children, according to a child's bodyweight or body surface area (HPA 2016).

Pre-procedural considerations

The patient should be physically and psychologically prepared for the procedure so they understand the procedure and give their informed consent (O'Dwyer et al. 2003). The following aspects should be considered prior to the procedure.

Patient considerations

- Pregnant women will generally not be scanned. When essential tests must be undertaken, the patient must sign a consent form and receive a reduced dose of radionuclide. This is to avoid unnecessary irradiation to the abdominal/pelvic region which will include the embryo or fetus (Ionizing Radiation Regulations 1999).
- The person accompanying the patient should not be pregnant, or bring young children or babies with them, so that unnecessary exposure in the time period immediately after the radionuclide administration can be avoided (DH 2016, HPA 2016).
- In women of reproductive age, the possibility of pregnancy must be excluded routinely via a urine test and the patient asked if her menstrual period is late. Patients receiving iodine-131 or any other radioactive agent with a long half-life should not become pregnant for a minimum of 3 months after the procedure (Sharp et al. 1998) to ensure that unnecessary irradiation to the abdomen of a woman who may be pregnant is avoided (HPA 2016).
- If mothers are breastfeeding, then advice from the Radiation Protection Adviser should be sought. Radioactivity can be excreted in breast milk. Therefore, breastfeeding may need to be suspended (HPA 2016) and the mother encouraged to avoid unnecessary cuddling of the child during this time (DH 2016).
- Patients with pain should be provided with effective pain control to ensure they are pain free so that immobility during scan time can be maintained.
- If the patient is incontinent, the test may not go ahead; however, if a decision is made to do so, proceed with caution. Incontinence pads should be worn and universal precautions are to be adopted, to limit the spread of contamination. Disposable gloves and apron should be worn and hand washing performed following patient contact, as these will prevent contamination of staff in close contact with the patient (DH 2016). Urine bags must be emptied regularly to remove the radioactivity from the patient area. Items must be disposed of in hospital approved body fluid and clinical waste.
- Debilitated patients may require prolonged close contact. Nursing staff should share the care of these patients, by regular rotation of staff. This will keep doses to staff as low as possible and avoid prolonged exposure to any one member of staff (DH 2016).
- Patients should keep to a minimum prolonged close contact (less than 1 metre) with anyone who is pregnant.
- Patients should keep to a minimum prolonged close contact (less than 1 metre) with any child under the age of 5 years.
- Patients should pay extra attention to their own personal hygiene, washing their hands thoroughly after each visit to the lavatory.
- Drink plenty of fluids and empty their bladder frequently, as this will hasten the removal of the radioactive tracer from the body (DH 2016, HPA 2016, Sharp et al. 1998).

Ward considerations

Although the amount of radioactivity administered is low, the patient will emit a small amount of radiation for some time after the radioactive tracer has been given. The amount of radioactivity within the patient decreases in two ways. The first way is by the natural physical decay of the radioisotope used, which we cannot change. The second way is by excretion of the radioactive tracer from the patient's body, usually via the urine and occasionally the faeces (HSE 2014, HPA 2016, Vialard-Miguel et al. 2005).

All patients who have been administered a radiopharmaceutical will be issued a yellow wrist or ankle band. The purpose of the yellow band is to act as a visual, easily recognized indicator of the fact that a patient has attended for a nuclear medicine investigation. The band should only be worn on the day of the scan unless the patient is specifically instructed to the contrary and has been given clear radiation protection instructions. Patients wearing a yellow band will also have been issued with a card outlining basic precautions and listing contact telephone numbers if they (or a ward/department) have any queries. When nursing patients who have received a radiopharmaceutical, nurses and other healthcare providers should adhere to the following guidelines.

Patient care

- Nurse in an appropriate controlled area of the hospital designed to manage patients with radioactive sources.
- Encourage their patient to take in plenty of fluid and empty their bladder frequently.
- Wear gloves when emptying catheter bags or bedpans, but dispose of the urine/faeces in the usual way.
- Try to empty catheter bags (if in use) frequently and not allow them to get too full.
- Minimize time spent in close proximity of patients.
- All emergency procedures such as cardiac arrest or deterioration must continue to be provided with adequate safeguards in place such as healthcare professional monitoring, rotation of emergency responders and the ability to manage patients in other settings such as critical care or operating theatres (HPA 2016, Resuscitation Council 2015).

Blood samples and further tests

- Where possible, all blood tests should be performed prior to administration of the radiopharmaceutical.
- Only clinically urgent blood tests may be performed on patients with yellow wrist bands.
- If samples are to be taken from patients with yellow bands, then both the sample and the form *must* have a radioactive sticker placed on them. The pathology department must contact radiation protection to collect and dispose of the sample after testing has been performed.
- Further examinations such as X-ray or CT may be carried out on patients; however it is best practice for the patient to inform the nuclear medicine team of their appointments prior to administration of the radiopharmaceutical (Larkin et al. 2011).

Contaminated sharps or dressings

When removing inserted devices from patients wearing yellow bands, the waste items should be placed in an orange bag or sharps bin (radioactive specific) and taken to the nuclear medicine department.

- These items can then be handed to a member of staff for disposal.
- When handing the item over, please ensure the receiving staff member is told of the patient's details so that it may be disposed of correctly (DH 2013, HSE 2003).

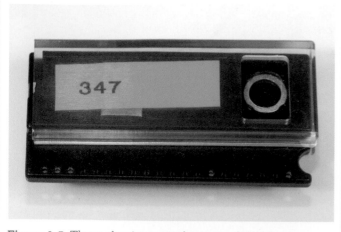

Figure 1.5 Thermoluminescent dosimeter (TLD) badge.

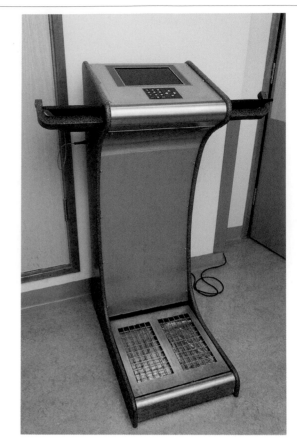

Figure 1.6 Hand and foot radiation monitor.
Source: Dougherty and Lister (2011).

Body fluid and body fluid spillage management

In the event of a patient's incontinence or a spill from a bedpan, catheter bag or other body fluid:

- The soiled linen should be placed in an orange clinical waste bag, and clearly labelled 'Radioactive – Do not dispose'.
- Contact the department of nuclear medicine or Radiation Protection Service to arrange for collection or further advice. It is important to follow local hospital guidelines as local variation may occur (DH 2013, HSE 2003).

Equipment

There are various additional pieces of equipment that are required to safely undertake the procedure. These include lead-lined receptacles and monitoring devices.

Lead-lined equipment

Lead-lined equipment is required to protect the clinician or operator and the environment from radioactive sources.

- *Lead shields.* All syringes containing radiopharmaceuticals should be in a shielded compartment. This is a lead shield to protect the fingers of the operator.
- *Lead-lined disposal bins.* All clinical waste should be disposed of in lead-lined clinical waste and sharps bins. The disposal of this waste must be followed as per hospital policy (DH 2016, HPA 2016).

Monitoring equipment

- *Staff radiation protection.* All staff administering radiopharmaceuticals should be provided with body thermoluminescent dosimeter (TLD) film badges (Figure 1.5).
- *Contamination monitors* to check hands and feet of staff (Figure 1.6). The contamination monitors are required to check the environment at the end of each day or more frequently if a spill occurs. Local hospital guidelines must be followed in the event of a spill of a radiopharmaceutical or contaminated body fluid (HPA 2016).

Procedure guideline 1.2   Unsealed radioactive sources for diagnostic investigations

Essential equipment

- Selection of needles (safety needles may not be appropriate therefore use needles as per local guidelines and specific procedures) and syringes (sizes dependent on volume required)
- Various gauge sizes of cannula
- Alcohol wipes
- Syringe shield
- Lead shield
- Tape and gauze
- Documentation regarding the isotope to be administered
- Radioactive isotope
- Disposable apron and non-sterile gloves
- Thermoluminescent dose (TLD) finger meter
- Film badge
- Sharps bin (radioactive specific)

Pre-procedure

Action	Rationale
1 Explain and discuss the procedure with the patient, and, if relevant, with the relative/significant other accompanying the patient.	To ensure the patient is physically and psychologically prepared for the procedure and understands the procedure and gives their informed consent (O'Dwyer et al. 2003, **E**).
2 Before administering, look at the patient's prescription chart or protocol and confirm patient's identity.	To ensure the correct patient is given the correct radioactive source (NMC 2010b, **C**). To protect the patient from harm (NMC 2010b, **C**).
3 Apply the relevant TLD meter and film badge.	To measure radiation doses received by member of staff (Ionizing Radiation Regulations 1999, **C**).
4 Wash hands with liquid soap and warm water.	To reduce the risk of contamination (DH 2016, **C**).
5 Apply disposable gloves and plastic apron.	To reduce the risk of contamination (DH 2016, **C**).

Procedure

Action	Rationale
6 Cannulate patient as per 'Procedure guideline 14.4 Peripheral cannula insertion' in *The Royal Marsden Manual of Clinical Nursing Procedures, Ninth Edition*.	To ensure venous access is obtained. **E**
7 Place the empty syringe in a lead syringe shield and attach needle. Place behind the lead body shield.	To reduce exposure to radiation (DH 2016, **C**; IRMER 2000, **C**).
8 Stand behind lead body shield and draw up the prescribed dose of the radiopharmaceutical.	To reduce exposure to radiation (DH 2016, **C**).
9 Administer the radionuclide intravenously via cannula with cap. There is no evidence to support the use of central venous access devices (CVADs). Please refer to local guidelines.	To administer the radionuclide. **E**
10 Remove cannula, apply pressure and cover the exit site with gauze and secure with tape.	Prevent any blood loss from skin exit site and possible contamination. **E**
11 Dispose of all used syringes, needles, and cannula in a designated radioactive sharps disposal bin which is stored within a lead shield.	To contain radioactivity and allow safe disposal (Ionizing Radiation Regulations 1999, **C**).
12 Remove disposable gloves and wash hands at end of procedure.	To remove any possible radioactive contamination (DH 2005, **C**; DH 2000, **C**).

Post-procedure

Action	Rationale
13 Place a yellow identity bracelet on the wrists of all inpatients and complete information card with the details of when precautions can be discontinued. Give the completed information card to the patient or the nurse accompanying the patient.	The yellow wristband will provide visual warning to inform all healthcare workers of the patient's recent diagnostic investigation. The information card will inform ward staff of restrictions related to managing a patient, as well as when measures that have to be adopted in the event of the patient vomiting or being incontinent can be discontinued (DH 2000, **C**). The card also states where to obtain help and advice related to the patient's diagnostic investigation. **E**
14 Sign and complete administration documentation.	To ensure timely and accurate record keeping (NMC 2010a, **C**).
15 Monitor hands at end of procedure and before leaving the room by using the hand and foot monitor.	To check for possible radioactive contamination (DH 2000, **C**).
16 Monitor the room for radioactive contamination at the end of each day or if contamination may have occurred.	To establish whether contamination has occurred (DH 2000, **C**).

Post-procedural considerations

Immediate care

As the patient will excrete the radioactive substance, avoid urine, faecal and blood sample collection for laboratories other than nuclear medicine for the first 24 hours. If collection is unavoidable, a radiation warning sticker must be attached to the specimen and request card, and the specimen taken to the laboratory under the supervision of the physics departmental staff. This is to prevent contamination of the laboratory and its staff, as specimens taken within 24 hours of some scans may contain radioactivity (HPA 2016, HSE 2003, Vialard-Miguel et al. 2005). If an outpatient or inpatient has an acute deterioration and requires additional inpatient or critical care, follow the 'ward considerations' discussed earlier in this chapter with guidance from the physics department (HPA 2016).

Ongoing care

Bone marrow and stem cell harvests should be avoided for 24 hours. Advice should be sought from the physics department as cells may contain radioactivity (HSE 2003, Vialard-Miguel et al. 2005). Seek advice from physics staff if the patient is to undergo a procedure in the operating theatre within 24 hours of a scan in order to prevent theatre equipment from becoming contaminated with radioactivity. Place soiled bed linen used within the first 24 hours of certain scans, for example bone scan, within an orange plastic bag (radioactive specific) and inform the physics departmental staff for collection (HPA 2016). Other issues concerning the management of patients undergoing radionuclide therapy are discussed in Chapter 5.

Education of patient and relevant others

Patients and relevant others should be provided with education and information leaflets prior to leaving the department. Patient care, considerations and information should also be provided for healthcare professionals from referring hospitals prior to the patient's discharge or transfer (HSE 2006, SNMMI 2016).

Transrectal ultrasound (TRUS) prostate biopsy

Definition

A transrectal ultrasound and prostate biopsy (TRUS Bx) uses an ultrasound probe to visualize the prostate. Once the prostate can be seen, a fine biopsy needle is passed down a probe guide to take small tissue samples from the prostate. The number of tissue samples taken ranges from 2 to 12 depending on local policy and degree of clarification required (Turner et al. 2011).

Anatomy and physiology

The prostate gland has an average volume of 25 mL. It is approximately 3.5 cm long, 4.0 cm wide and 2.5 cm deep from posterior to anterior – about the same size as a walnut (Tortora and Derrickson 2014).

The prostate is an extraperitoneal structure, lying anterior to the rectum and sitting around the neck of the bladder encircling the urethra. It comprises three distinct areas/zones: the central, peripheral and the transition zones, which conform to a cone or inverted pyramid. The base of the prostate lies against the bladder and the apex on the urogenital diaphragm, which is a fibrous supporting ring that also contains the urethra. The gland is surrounded by the prostate capsule and beyond that smooth muscle and connective tissue. Between the prostate gland and the rectum

lies Denonvilliers' fascia – a peritoneal plane or space (Turner and Pati 2010, Turner et al. 2011) (Figure 1.7).

Related theory

As a man ages, the transition zone increases in size due to benign prostate enlargement (BPE) while the central zone atrophies and the peripheral zone remains the same. It is the peripheral zone, however, in which the majority of prostate cancers are found and therefore clinically this is the most important region to target during prostate biopsy.

Transrectal biopsy of the prostate is most commonly undertaken in an outpatient setting. Many thousands of prostate biopsies are undertaken every year throughout the UK. First described by Astraldi in 1937, it remains the gold standard investigation for diagnosing prostate cancer (Turner et al. 2011).

Prostate biopsy specimens

The number of specimens to be collected and the location will depend on the patient's clinical condition. The following should be considered when determining specimen collection:

- Ultrasound does not detect areas of prostate cancer with adequate reliability and therefore targeted prostate biopsies on the basis of ultrasound alone are unproductive. However, occasionally additional biopsies of abnormal areas identified on magnetic resonance imaging (MRI) can be useful (Heidenreich et al. 2014, Siddiqui et al. 2015). On the first biopsy (baseline biopsy) the sample sites should be as far posterior and lateral in the peripheral zone as possible.
- When cancer is suspected a 12 core biopsy protocol should be observed (Heidenreich et al. 2014). However, if the patient has proven or strongly suspected advanced prostate cancer or is part of a clinical trial, limited cores should be taken (2–4 being optimal).
- The 12 core biopsy protocol is as follows (Figure 1.8):
  - right apex lateral × 2
  - right mid lateral × 2
  - right base lateral × 2
  - left apex lateral × 2
  - left mid lateral × 2
  - left base lateral × 2.

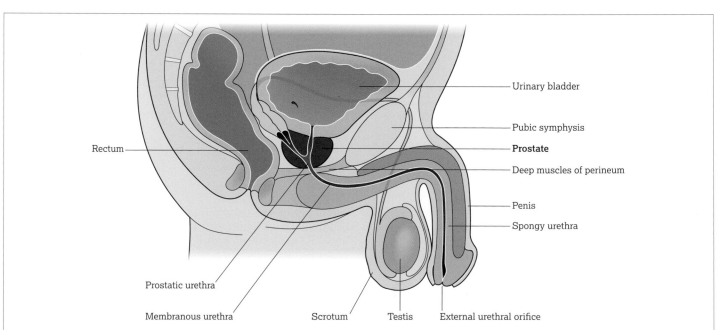

Figure 1.7 The prostate and its zones. *Source:* Adapted from Tortora and Derrickson (2011). Reproduced with permission of John Wiley & Sons.

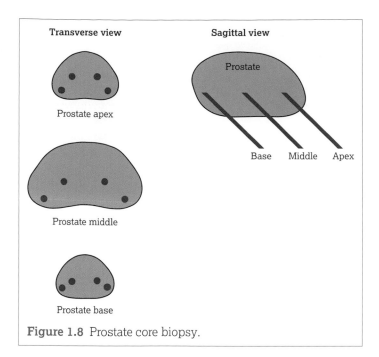

Figure 1.8 Prostate core biopsy.

Evidence-based approaches

Rationale
A prostate biopsy should only be considered and undertaken if it influences the management of the patient. It should be determined on the basis of the PSA level and/or a suspicious digital rectal examination (DRE) and/or suspicious prostate MRI. Factors such as patient age and co-morbidities should also be considered (Batura and Gopal Rao 2013).

Indications
There are many indications for prostate biopsy which include:

- raised PSA level in the absence of urinary tract infection, acute urinary retention or acute prostatitis
- abnormalities identified through DRE or MRI of the prostate
- patients being assessed for radiation failure (i.e. PSA increases post radiotherapy)
- patients on an active surveillance protocol requiring repeat biopsies
- patients with previous histology requiring repeat biopsy (e.g. high-grade prostatic intra-epithelial neoplasia or suspicious but not diagnostic for carcinoma)
- patients on an ethically approved clinical trial (NICE 2014, Turner et al. 2011).

Contraindications
It is important to note that patients with the following risk factors may require special preparation:

- patients on anticoagulation therapy or with coagulation disorders that may interfere with haemostasis and increase the risk of haemorrhage. Low-dose aspirin (75–150 mg) is not a contraindication but discontinuation should be discussed with the medical team
- patients with an identified urinary tract infection as the risk of septicaemia may be increased
- patients with an allergy to latex, antibiotics or local anaesthetic
- patients with diabetes mellitus who may be at increased risk of infection
- patients on steroid medication which may increase the risk of infection

- patients who are immunocompromised. It may be necessary to seek advice from other healthcare professionals on complex medical conditions
- patients with urinary obstruction (Giannarini et al. 2007, Lange et al. 2009, Loeb et al. 2013).

There is a lack of agreement in the literature specifying those with an absolute increased risk of complications. It is therefore at the discretion of the person performing the procedure to proceed to biopsy based on local policy and/or professional judgement. However, it has been suggested that certain patient groups should undergo biopsy by a transperineal approach only (Miller et al. 2005). This includes those with:

- prosthetic cardiac valve or prosthetic material used for cardiac valve repair
- congenital heart disease (CHD)
- completely repaired congenital heart defect with prosthetic material or device, whether placed by surgery or by catheter intervention, during the first 6 months after the procedure
- repaired CHD with residual defects at the site or adjacent to the site of a prosthetic patch or prosthetic device (which inhibit endothelialization)
- cardiac transplantation recipients who develop cardiac valvulopathy.

Some patients should be considered for exclusion from biopsy altogether and managed conservatively. This will require local agreement. Such patients are those with:

- previous infective endocarditis
- CHD (dependent on clinical assessment and review)
- unrepaired cyanotic CHD, including palliative shunts and conduits.

Legal and professional issues
The nurse is required to have an intimate understanding of the anatomy and physiology of the male urinary system, factors that affect PSA measurement and other conditions of the urinary system and their management. In addition, the nurse must be competent in DRE and have a thorough understanding of the role of TRUS and possible ultrasound findings as well as familiarization with the possible complications of TRUS and their management (Greene et al. 2015).

For nurse specialists a minimum of 20 cases should be performed under supervision (Greene et al. 2015, Turner et al. 2011, Turner and Pati 2010). The nurse could be trained by any competent healthcare professional but ultimately competence should be assessed by an experienced practitioner, usually a urologist or radiologist. Each practitioner should regularly audit the outcome and management of complications. Examples and guidance for how this can be achieved exist within the published literature (Greene et al. 2015, Turner and Pati 2010).

Consent
At the appointment at which the biopsy is requested, the patient should be counselled about the procedure and a transrectal prostate biopsy information sheet should be given, for example the British Association of Urology Surgeons' Prostate Biopsy patient information leaflet' (BAUS 2017). This information leaflet outlines the procedure in detail including benefits, risks, potential complications and emergency contacts. Patients should be warned of the possible side-effects (Table 1.4) as part of the informed consent process.

It is imperative that the procedure, potential complications, potential outcomes and discomfort to the patient are explained to the patient. Answer questions at a level and pace appropriate to the patient's understanding, culture and background, preferred way of communicating and needs. Both verbal and written consent must be obtained from the patient (DH 2009). The signed consent should be scanned to the patient's electronic records or kept in their clinical notes as a hard copy.

Table 1.4 Possible side-effects of transrectal ultrasound and prostate biopsy

Frequency	Side-effect
Common (greater than 1 in 10)	Blood in urine
	Blood in semen for up to 6 weeks
	Blood in stools
	Urinary infection (up to a 10% risk)
	Discomfort from the prostate due to bruising
	Haemorrhage (bleeding) causing inability to pass urine (2% risk)
Occasional (between 1 in 10 and 1 in 50)	Blood infection (septicaemia) needing admission to hospital (2% risk)
	Haemorrhage (bleeding) needing admission (1% risk)
	Failure to detect a significant cancer of the prostate
Rare (less than 1 in 50)	Inability to pass urine (retention of urine)
Hospital-acquired infection	Colonization with MRSA (0.9% – 1 in 110 patients)
	MRSA bloodstream infection (0.02% – 1 in 5000 patients)
	Clostridium difficile bowel infection (0.01% –1 in 10,000 patients)

Source: Adapted from BAUS (2017).
MRSA, meticillin-resistant *Staphylococcus aureus*.

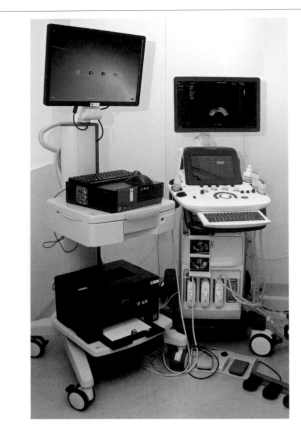

Figure 1.9 Ultrasound machine and probe.

It is a legal requirement to seek written consent for transrectal biopsy. The healthcare professional responsible for carrying out the procedure is ultimately responsible for the patient consent for the examination (DH 2009, Turner and Pati 2010).

Consent should be taken using a dedicated consent form in which the following should be discussed with the patient:

- how the biopsy is taken
- the risks and benefits of the procedure
- potential complications of the procedure and whether the risk is major or minor
- the number of cores that will be taken
- if any additional cores will be taken using MRI fusion.

It is also important that the patient is made aware of the potential outcome of the prostate biopsy, which may include:

- false negative result
- need for repeat biopsy
- cancer diagnosis.

Pre-procedural considerations

General assessment
A general assessment of the patient's fitness for the procedure is required. This is to include the ability to use local anaesthesia, including previous allergies to local anaesthetics. Identify any risk factors for which special precautions may be required. Determine the need for the biopsy and decide whether or not to proceed. If not already done, take a comprehensive health history including presenting complaint, health history, medication, family and social history.

Voiding studies
Before biopsy, the patient should undergo uroflowmetry with post urinary residual measurement. This should be recorded in the patient's notes and annotated in the post biopsy letter. If the post void residual urine is >150 mL, an alpha-blocker should be considered (Bozlu et al. 2003).

Equipment
It is important that the environment is suitably prepared and all the required equipment is available and checked to be in working order before commencing the procedure. All staff should be familiar with their expected roles and emergency procedures, the location of any emergency equipment and the ability to contact a senior clinician should the need arise. An ultrasound machine and probe must be available and in working order and used as per manufacturer's guidelines (Figure 1.9). Various needles and biopsy guns are available (Figure 1.10) and should be used as per manufacturer's guidelines.

Emergency equipment
Emergency equipment should be easily accessible in the rare event of a major complication such as uncontrollable bleeding per rectum or per urethra, retention of urine, anaphylaxis or vasovagal syncope.

Pharmacological support
Aerobic or anaerobic organisms may be introduced when performing TRUSBx, the more common being *Escherichia coli*, *Streptococcus faecalis* and *Bacteroides*. Thus, the use of broad-spectrum antibiotics is common practice but guidelines should be made locally in consultation with microbiology advice taking into consideration regional antibiotic resistance (Kapoor et al. 1998, Sieber et al. 1997, Zani et al. 2011).

Currently fluoroquinolones are the antibiotics of choice in transrectal US-guided prostate biopsy. Fluoroquinolones are well absorbed orally and have good prostate tissue levels (Hori et al. 2010, Lange et al. 2009). Evidence suggests that one dose is as effective as multiple-dose prophylaxis (Aron et al. 2000). The

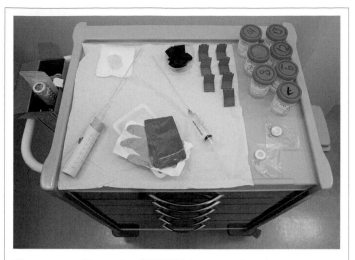

Figure 1.10 Example of TRUS biopsy equipment.

addition of gentamicin or metronidazole is optional (Bootsma et al. 2008).

As a standard, all patients should have a negative midstream urine (MSU) previous to the biopsy. If a negative MSU was obtained more than 4 weeks before the biopsy, a confirmatory dipstick test should be done on the day of the procedure.

There is a clear trend towards an increase in the rates of infectious complications after TRUS biopsy in the past few decades (Loeb et al. 2013, Nam et al. 2013). Accordingly, many authors

reported rising rates of antimicrobial, particularly quinolone, resistance (Feliciano et al. 2008, Williamson et al. 2013). It is therefore important to consider risk factors for pre-biopsy quinolone resistance (Challacombe et al. 2011, Patel et al. 2012, Taylor et al. 2012) such as:

- travel to Asia/Africa/Latin America in the previous 8 weeks
- use of quinolone in the previous 6 weeks
- chronic immunosuppression – chronic obstructive pulmonary disease (COPD), diabetes mellitus or long-term steroids use
- indwelling urinary catheter
- history of recurrent urinary tract infections.

If a patient has one of these risk factors a rectal swab should be considered to screen for quinolone resistance (Liss et al. 2015, Taylor et al. 2012). If this is not available, consider adding intravenous gentamicin 5 mg/kg (based on ideal bodyweight if the patient is obese, i.e. actual bodyweight is 20% higher than ideal bodyweight), 60 minutes before the procedure in this high-risk group of patients (Ho et al. 2009).

Lidocaine 1% is the standard agent for an ultrasound-guided peri-prostatic block. In addition, an intrarectal instillation of local anaesthetic can be done (Raber et al. 2008, Yun et al. 2007) at the discretion of the examiner. However, it should not be used as an isolated method, as it is inferior to the peri-prostatic block (Lee and Woo 2014).

Special recommendations

A cleansing enema before biopsy provides no clinically significant outcome advantage and potentially increases patient cost and discomfort. It is therefore not recommended (Carey and Korman 2001).

Procedure guideline 1.3   Transrectal ultrasound (TRUS) prostate biopsy

Essential equipment

- Biopsy gun
- Long spinal needles (to administer anaesthetic) – 20 cm
- Ultrasound probe cover (condom)
- Specimen pots – pre-labelled
- Lubricating jelly
- Wipes/gauze
- Non-sterile gloves
- Needle guide to accommodate biopsy gun gauge
- Sharps bin

- Pathology sponges
- Pathology cassettes
- Sterile gloves
- Sterile gown

Medicinal products

- Antibiotic prophylaxis – patient specific (if not previously administered)
- Local anaesthetic – lidocaine 1% (10 mL)

Pre-procedure

Action	Rationale
1 Check the environment, equipment and medication to ensure that everything is present for the procedure, including access to relevant personnel and emergency equipment.	To ensure the procedure will take place without delay for the patient and to ensure that the safety of the patient is addressed (Turner et al. 2011, **E**).
2 Ask assistant to set up trolley with sterile urology pack and in date sterile equipment.	To maintain infection control standards and minimize cross-infection and contamination (RCN 2017a, **C**).
3 Prepare the ultrasound machine by ensuring it is clean and prepare the probe by inserting some ultrasound gel into the end of the condom then roll the condom over the probe and carefully attach the needle guide without splitting the condom.	To ensure the equipment is functioning and ready for use (Turner et al. 2011, **E**).
4 Read the patient's record, referral letter and the results of any relevant investigations and identify any special instructions, investigations or items for which you need to seek advice or clarification.	To ensure correct identification of the patient and to identify details that might require an adaptation of the procedure (Turner et al. 2011, **E**).
5 Greet and accurately identify the patient and introduce yourself and any colleagues present.	To reduce patient anxiety and to ensure correct identification of the patient (Turner et al. 2011, **E**).

(continued)

Procedure guideline 1.3   Transrectal ultrasound (TRUS) prostate biopsy *(continued)*

Action	Rationale
6 Take a written consent using a dedicated consent form in which the following should be discussed with the patient: • how the biopsy is taken • the risks and benefits of the procedure, potential complications of the procedure and whether the risk is major or minor • the number of cores that will be taken • if any additional cores will be taken using MRI fusion.	The healthcare professional responsible for carrying out the procedure is ultimately responsible for the patient consent for the examination (BAUS 2017, **C**; DH 2009, **C**; Turner and Pati 2010, **E**).
7 Ensure the patient has removed clothing below the waist and offer a gown.	To provide privacy and comfort for the patient. **E**. To minimize the risk of a hospital acquired infection (BAUS and BAUN 2012b, **C**).
8 Ensure the patient has taken antibiotic prophylaxis as prescribed locally.	To ensure appropriate steps have been taken to prevent infection (Kapoor et al. 1998, **1b**; Sieber et al. 1997, **C**; Zani et al. 2011, **R1a**).
9 Position the patient correctly for the procedure (left lateral position ensuring that the knees are bent up towards the chest) and ensure their comfort within the constraints of the procedure, taking appropriate action to protect the patient's privacy and dignity throughout.	The left lateral position is preferred, particularly with an end firing probe, as imaging of the apex is easier and more comfortable for the patient (Vassalos and Rooney 2013, **C**).
10 Wash and dry hands using a bactericidal soap and apply non-sterile gloves.	To minimize the risk of infection (Loveday et al. 2014, **C**).
11 Undertake a digital rectal examination to identify symmetry, size, the presence of nodules, and tenderness and pain associated with the prostate. Careful attention should also be paid to exclude the presence of anal pathology or any other anomalies that may influence the procedure.	Any abnormality in shape of the prostate may necessitate additional biopsies to the standard biopsy protocol that is used. However, if the rectum is full of faeces and/or anal pathology is identified, transrectal biopsy is contraindicated (Greene et al. 2015, **C**).
12 Remove gloves and dispose of them. Wash and dry hands.	To minimize the risk of cross-infection (Loveday et al. 2014, **C**). To dispose of clinical waste (DH 2013, **C**; HSE 2003, **C**).
13 Apply non-sterile gloves and check the local anaesthetic agent to be used then draw up required volume into a syringe and attach the spinal needle ready for administration (the use of intrarectal lidocaine gel is optional).	To minimize the risk of cross-infection (Loveday et al. 2014, **C**), To ensure patient is comfortable. **E**.

Procedure

Action	Rationale
14 Apply lubricating gel to the covered TRUS probe and insert the probe gently into the patient's rectum, whilst monitoring progress on the ultrasound image.	To promote patient comfort and enhance the quality of the scan (Turner et al. 2011, **E**).
15 Scan and identify the prostate gland, seminal vesicles and surrounding structures, locating the apex and base of the prostate on the ultrasound image. The prostate volume should be measured in three dimensions. In the transverse view: • anterior to posterior (width) • height and, in the longitudinal plane, • from the bladder neck to the apex (length). Final volume can be calculated using the formula: $H \times W \times L \times 0.52$.	To orientate the operator and to identify areas to biopsy (Greene et al. 2015, **C**).
16 Take volume measurements and make note of any abnormalities detected on ultrasound and either print images or store them on the ultrasound machine for future reference.	To provide information that may be useful when discussing treatment options with the patient in the future. **E**.
17 Inform the patient that the local anaesthetic is about to be administered.	To reduce patient anxiety (Greene et al. 2015, **C**).
18 Introduce the local anaesthetic needle through the biopsy channel of the ultrasound probe until the needle tip can be visualized on the screen in the peri-prostatic tissue.	To promote patient comfort. To reduce pain (Turner et al. 2011, **E**).
19 Commence infiltration of the local anaesthetic observing the passage of the fluid throughout the peri-prostatic area.	Ultrasound-guided peri-prostatic block is standard. It does not make any difference whether the depot is apical or basal as long as it is given into Denonvilliers' fascia. In addition, an intrarectal instillation of local anaesthetic can be done (Raber et al. 2008, **R1b**; Yun et al. 2007, **R1b**) at the discretion of the examiner. However, it should not be used as an isolated method as it is inferior to the peri-prostatic block (Lee and Woo 2014, **R1a**).

20	Withdraw the needle and discard into a large 5 litre sharps bin.	To prevent sharps injury (DH 2013, **C**; HSE 2003, **C**).
21	Identify the appropriate locations for the biopsy samples according to clinical need, e.g. MRI findings, DRE findings or confidence in diagnosis of cancer.	To ensure the correct areas are biopsied and minimum number of cores taken to ensure a diagnosis is made (Greene et al. 2015, **C**).
22	Introduce the biopsy needle along the biopsy channel until the needle tip can be visualized on the screen in the peri-prostatic tissue, adjacent to the target area.	To ensure the correct areas are biopsied and minimum number of cores taken to ensure a diagnosis is made (Greene et al. 2015, **C**).
23	Inform the patient that the biopsy is about to be taken and warn them of the sound of the biopsy gun (sounds like a staple gun) and commence taking tissue samples.	To ensure patient comfort and to reduce anxiety (Greene et al. 2015, **C**).
24	Fire the biopsy gun and then withdraw it after firing on each occasion, in order to lay each tissue sample onto a sponge (a maximum of two per sponge). Repeat process. Lay a second sponge on top of the first after two samples have been taken.	Prostate biopsy cores taken from different sites should be sent to the laboratory with the use of sponges and cartridges in separate pots. This ensures that the cores do not become fragmented during transportation to the lab (Heidenreich et al. 2014, **C**).
25	Ensure that the samples taken are adequate for histopathology by comparing the length of the core with the length of the needle notch.	To ensure the correct length is taken and there is consistency of sampling (Greene et al. 2015, **C**).
26	Take additional samples only where there is clinical concern, e.g. abnormality found on DRE or seen on ultrasound or MRI.	To ensure the correct areas are biopsied and minimum number of cores taken to ensure a diagnosis is made (Greene et al. 2015, **C**).
27	Assess the patient's tolerance throughout the procedure and ensure they are happy to continue.	To ensure patient comfort. **E**.
28	Direct the assisting nurse to place each sponge sandwich into a cassette before inserting into a correctly and accurately pre-labelled sample container containing 10% formalin.	To ensure specimen is labelled correctly (NMC 2010a, **C**; WHO 2015, **C**).
29	Remove the TRUS probe from the patient's rectum and insert prophylactic antibiotic if indicated by local policy.	To minimize the risk of infection (Kapoor et al. 1998, **R1b**; Sieber et al. 1997, **C**; Zani et al. 2011, **R1a**).

Post-procedure

30	Wipe rectum, offer a surgical pad to protect the patients underwear and remove and discard gloves	To promote patient comfort. **E**.
31	Assist the patient into a sitting position.	To promote patient comfort. **E**.
32	Assess the patient for any complications and take appropriate action.	To ensure patient safety and comfort. (Greene et al. 2015, **C**).
33	Recognize the need for immediate management of acute emergencies associated with the procedure and respond appropriately.	To ensure patient safety and comfort (Greene et al. 2015, **C**).
34	Assess the patient's needs following the procedure and offer any verbal support, as required.	To promote patient comfort. **E**.
35	Ensure the patient has all required information and medication. Reiterate the possible complications and how they should be managed.	To ensure patient safety and reduce the risk of serious side-effects following the procedure (Greene et al. 2015, **C**).
36	Assess the patient's fitness for discharge by ensuring patient has voided and there are no other adverse events.	To ensure patient safety (Greene et al. 2015, **C**).
37	Ensure the ultrasound probe is cleaned in line with local infection control policy.	To ensure the safety of staff and patients. **E**.
38	Ensure that single-use items and sharps are disposed of and that non-disposable equipment is cleaned and/or sterilized.	To minimize the risk of cross-contamination and infection risks (DH 2013, **C**; HSE 2003, **C**).
39	Complete the histopathology request form ensuring it matches patient identity and includes all relevant clinical details, particularly relevant previous treatment, procedures and biopsies.	To ensure the correct results go to the correct patient (NMC 2010a, **C**; WHO 2015, **C**).
40	Record the details of the procedure in the patient's record, including details of the local anaesthetic and any medication given.	To ensure patient safety and accurate records for other practitioners who may see the patient (NMC 2010a, **C**; WHO 2015, **C**).

(continued)

Procedure guideline 1.3   Transrectal ultrasound (TRUS) prostate biopsy *(continued)*

Action	Rationale
41 Ensure that steps are taken to inform any other relevant practitioners of the procedure and plan, e.g. GP.	To ensure all relevant healthcare providers are informed of the procedure and its outcome. **E**.
42 Make the patient a follow-up appointment to discuss the results of the biopsy (usually 1–2 weeks).	To ensure adequate post-procedure follow-up (Greene et al. 2015, **C**).
43 Recognize when you need help and/or seek advice from appropriate sources.	To ensure patient safety (Greene et al. 2015, **C**).

Post-procedural considerations

Immediate care

Management of acute post-biopsy complications

Patients should be discharged with clear instructions on recognizing post-biopsy complications. Depending on the indication, patients with a severe complication (fever, urinary tract infection, acute bacterial prostatitis) after TRUS-guided prostate biopsy should have a course of antibiotic treatment (i.e. not just antibiotic prophylaxis for the prevention of surgical site infections). Some patients may require admission to hospital, such as those requiring intravenous antibiotics (urosepsis), or require catheter insertion (clot retention). Prompt recognition and initiation of antibiotic and support measures can save lives (Vassalos and Rooney 2013).

Biopsy complications

Acute bleeding – rectum (<2 days 1.3–45%, >2 days 0.7–2.5%)

A small volume of per-rectal bleeding is expected after the procedure. In the instance of abnormal significant bleeding the procedure should be stopped and transrectal direct finger pressure must be applied. The insertion of a balloon tamponade with a large-bore Foley catheter (50 mL saline in the balloon) is the next step (Challacombe et al. 2011). In the case of continuous bleeding, the patient should be admitted for observation and the consultant/urology specialist registrar should be informed.

Acute bleeding – urethra

Spontaneous urethral bleeding is not common but can occur during TRUS biopsy. If the bleeding does not subside, the patient should be admitted and the consultant/urology specialist registrar should be informed. A three-way 18 Fr Foley catheter should be inserted, with gentle traction applied over the bladder neck (Rodriguez and Terris 1998).

Haematospermia (1.1–93%)

A small volume of blood in the semen is known as haematospermia. Prostate biopsy is the most common cause of blood in the semen. In the case of very vascular prostates it can take up to 6 weeks for haematospermia to clear up. There is no treatment.

Haematuria

Some degree of haematuria is very common. If the patient has severe haematuria with clot retention, he should be admitted. A 22 Fr three-way silicone Foley catheter should be inserted, followed by bladder washout and continuous bladder irrigation with normal saline. In case of severe bleeding, formal washout in theatre may be required (Challacombe et al. 2011).

Urinary retention (0.2–1.7%)

All patients must spontaneously void before being discharged. If a patient complains of abdominal pain with inability to void or has no pain but a full bladder (confirmed on ultrasound), an 18 Fr Foley catheter should be inserted. An alpha-blocker, e.g. tamsulosin 400 µg, should be prescribed, and a trial of voiding without catheter should be booked to take place 7–10 days later (Batura and Gopal Rao 2013, Challacombe et al. 2011, Feliciano et al. 2008).

Vasovagal syncope

If the patient enters a pre-syncope state, the procedure should be immediately stopped. The probe should be removed from the rectum and the patient should be positioned in dorsal decubitus with a 30° Trendelenburg (on back, head down) position. Vital signs should be recorded. In case of complete loss of consciousness or sustained instability, the resuscitation or emergency team should be informed (Aydin et al. 2010).

Ongoing care

Post prostate biopsy review appointment

It is good practice to organize a return appointment for the patient to discuss the results of their biopsy before they have left the department. This will reduce the patient's anxiety caused by waiting for an appointment in the post. Usually this appointment is made 7–14 days after the biopsy to ensure the results are acted on expediently.

Audit

It is essential that the practitioner maintains a record of all procedures undertaken. This includes the review of histology results. This enables the practitioner to provide evidence of good practice and areas for improvement and development (Turner and Pati 2010).

Flexible cystoscopy

Definition

Flexible cystoscopy is a camera examination used to visualize the lower urinary tract including the urethra (including prostatic urethra), sphincter, bladder and ureteric orifices. Cystoscopy can assist in identifying problems with the urinary tract, such as early signs of bladder cancer, surveillance of bladder cancer, infection, strictures, obstruction, bleeding and other abnormalities. It is also an effective method for removing ureteric stents when they are no longer therapeutically indicated and in some cases treating some bladder abnormalities. The procedure is performed under local anaesthetic with the patient awake and takes place in a dedicated outpatient facility (Kumar and Clark 2016, Tortora and Derrickson 2014).

Anatomy and physiology

The urinary bladder is a muscular, expandable organ, hollow in nature, that is used as a storage and emptying structure for urine. It collects urine excreted by the kidneys, which enters the bladder from the ureters before disposal by urination, the urine exiting the body through the urethra (Marieb and Hoehn 2015) (Figure 1.11).

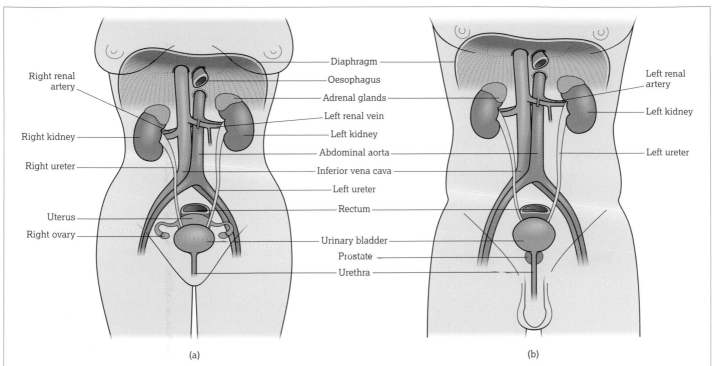

Figure 1.11 (a) Female urinary system. (b) Male urinary system. *Source:* Adapted from Tortora and Derrickson (2011). Reproduced with permission of John Wiley & Sons.

Related theory

Abnormalities of the lower urinary tract

Abnormalities of the lower urinary tract can be identified and in some cases biopsied/treated through flexible cystoscopy. These include:

- bladder cancer
- urinary tract infection
- interstitial cystitis/painful bladder syndrome
- bladder neck/urethral stricture
- prostatic enlargement/occlusion
- bladder stone.

Urinary stents can also be removed using a flexible cystoscope.

Bladder cancer

Most bladder cancers are transitional cell carcinomas (TCC). A minority of bladder tumours are squamous cell carcinomas (SCC). They are broadly categorized into non-muscle invasive (superficial), muscle invasive and metastatic, depending on the extent to which the cancer is invading into the bladder wall (NICE 2015a). Superficial tumours are largely confined to the bladder lining and superficial layers and do not penetrate the muscle layer of the bladder. Deep tumours penetrate the muscular wall of the bladder, and metastatic tumours are present beyond the primary organ (BAUS 2013).

Cancers are graded by their microscopic appearance. The cells of superficial cancers are similar in appearance to normal bladder cells and the tumours are generally slow growing (low grade). High-grade cancers often behave aggressively. Other factors of prognostic importance are: the number of tumours present, the size of the tumours, and their physical characteristics (EAU 2015).

The biopsy information will enable the *staging* and *grading* of the bladder cancer. The grade (Box 1.2) is in accordance with the cells' appearance and rate of growth. The TNM classification of malignant tumours (Table 1.5) describes the stage of a solid tumour according to its tissue involvement. *T* is the size of the original *tumour*, *N* is the nearby lymph *nodes* and *M* is the presence of distant *metastasis* (Brierley et al. 2017)

Box 1.2 WHO grading of bladder cancers

Grading of non-muscle-invasive bladder urothelial cancer

Papillary urothelial neoplasm of low malignant potential (PUNLMP)
Low-grade (LG) papillary urothelial carcinoma
High-grade (HG) papillary urothelial carcinoma

Histological classification for flat lesions

Hyperplasia (flat lesion without atypia or papillary aspects)
Reactive atypia (flat lesion with atypia)
Atypia of unknown significance
Urothelial dysplasia
Urothelial CIS is always high-grade

Source: Adapted from Eble et al. (2004).
CIS, carcinoma *in situ*.

Evidence-based approaches

Rationale

Flexible cystoscopy is undertaken to diagnose or conduct surveillance of cancer. Patient selection is based on locally agreed referral pathways. Commonly this would be through consultant referral or through diagnostic clinics.

Indications

- Referral from outpatient/inpatient clinics.
- Suspicion of a bladder abnormality based on clinical assessment in the outpatient department.
- Abnormal urine cytology.
- Routine bladder surveillance for bladder cancer based on national and local guidelines.
- Diagnostic referral pathways (e.g. for haematuria).
- Consultant referrals.
- Removal of ureteric stents.

Table 1.5 TNM classification of bladder cancer

Stage	Description

T – primary tumour	TX Primary tumour cannot be assessed
	T0 No evidence of primary tumour
	Ta Non-invasive papillary carcinoma
	Tis Carcinoma *in situ*: 'flat tumour'
	T1 Tumour invades subepithelial connective tissue
	T2 Tumour invades muscle
	  T2a Tumour invades superficial muscle (inner half)
	  T2b Tumour invades deep muscle (outer half)
	T3 Tumour invades perivesical tissue
	  T3a Microscopically
	  T3b Macroscopically (extravesical mass)
	T4 Tumour invades any of the following: prostate, uterus, vagina, pelvic wall, abdominal wall
	  T4a Tumour invades prostate, uterus or vagina
	  T4b Tumour invades pelvic wall or abdominal wall

N – lymph nodes	NX Regional lymph nodes cannot be assessed N0 No regional lymph node metastasis N1 Metastasis in a single lymph node in the true pelvis (hypogastric, obturator, external iliac, or presacral) N2 Metastasis in multiple lymph nodes in the true pelvis (hypogastric, obturator, external iliac, or presacral) N3 Metastasis in common iliac lymph node(s)
M – distant metastasis	MX Distant metastasis cannot be assessed M0 No distant metastasis M1 Distant metastasis

Source: Brierley et al. (2017). Reproduced with permission of John Wiley & Sons.

Contraindications

- If the information can be obtained using an alternative non-invasive approach such as an imaging scan to confirm or refute a diagnosis.
- Acute urinary tract infection – treat infection and reschedule the procedure.
- Warfarin or other anticoagulant therapy (if biopsies or cystodiathermy are required) – these should be discontinued according to patient risk/benefit profile and local guidelines.
- Allergy/intolerance to local anaesthetic agent – the examination should then be performed under general anaesthetic.
- High anxiety/phobia of the procedure – in this circumstance a general anaesthetic would be more appropriate (BAUS 2013).

Legal and professional issues

Flexible cystoscopy is the most commonly performed urological procedure. Nurses with specialist training have been performing this advanced role for several years. In 2000, the British Association of Urological Surgeons set up a working party and first published recommendations in support of nurse cystoscopy for surveillance of bladder cancer (Ellis et al. 2000). In the late 1990s nurse specialists began training to undertake flexible cystoscopy. The role of nurse cystoscopy has developed to encompass surveillance of superficial bladder cancer, diagnostic bladder biopsy, cytodiathermy and the removal of stents (BAUS and BAUN 2012a, b, Skills for Health 2010a, b, c, d).

Patients should expect that a nurse performing a flexible cystoscopy should be performing at a level of competence equivalent to that of a competent urologist (Cox 2010). Evidence from several UK studies suggests that nurse-led flexible cystoscopy is as effective as doctor-led services in correctly reporting abnormalities (Smith et al. 2015, Taylor et al. 2002). Although some studies suggest that nurse-led services have a greater tendency to over-report abnormalities, other studies suggest that doctors and nurses equally over-report abnormalities (Smith et al. 2015). However it is accepted that experience improves both abnormalities detected and over-reporting of abnormalities (Radhakrishnan et al. 2006).

The nurse cystoscopist

Nurse cystoscopy is increasingly common and several training courses are available in the UK. Training has also been extended to include diagnostic procedures such as biopsy, treatment with cystodiathermy and ureteric stent removal, as well as surveillance. Services are also being developed overseas following the UK model (Osborne 2007). The joint British Association of Urological Surgeons and British Association of Urology Nurses (BAUS and BAUN) guidelines were published in 2012 to guide training and practice.

Training should include all elements of practice as agreed by senior management and consultants and should always include consent training. Continuing professional development for the nurse cystoscopist should include regular updates on this element of practice. The nurse cystoscopist should also participate in regular clinical audit including comparison of accuracy of findings, patient satisfaction and service capacity/waiting times (BAUN and BAUS 2012a, b) to ensure the highest standards of clinical care are being met. It is also important for the nurse to perform regular audit. The audit data are required to reflect on the nurse's own practice and maintenance of competence in accordance with national and local policies and guidelines (BAUS and BAUN 2012a, b, Skills for Health 2010a, b, c, d).

A competent nurse cystoscopist must continue to have access to an experienced, designated urologist for clinical advice and support, and immediate access to a hospital urology team for technical or diagnostic advice (BAUN and BAUS 2012a, b).

Consent

Written consent must be obtained prior to the procedure (NMC 2013). The patient must be informed of the procedure, its risks and potential side-effects. Accurate and legible documentation should be recorded immediately after the procedure, including all the observations and decisions made before, during and after the procedure (NMC 2010a).

Pre-procedural considerations

To prevent an unnecessary invasive procedure, ensure that flexible cystoscopy is indicated and that the results required cannot be achieved by diagnostic imaging. In most cases appropriate diagnostic imaging will precede flexible cystoscopy.

Consideration of concurrent treatment such as chemotherapy, anticoagulants or other medications is required. A confirmation of allergy status must be obtained. In order to exclude a urinary tract infection a dipstick test should be performed prior to a flexible cystoscopy and/or MSU at least one week prior to the procedure. If the patient has an artificial urinary sphincter implanted, this must be deactivated prior to the procedure (BAUN and BAUS 2012a, b).

Equipment

Flexible cystoscopes and stack

As there are several different types of flexible cystoscope (Figure 1.12), it is essential that the practitioner familiarizes

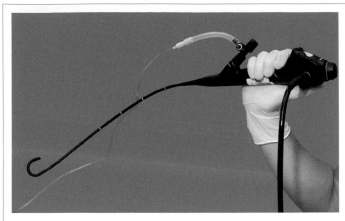

Figure 1.12 Flexible cystoscope.

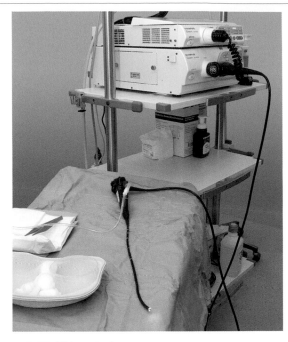

Figure 1.13 Video stack.

themselves with the equipment prior to use. A video stack is required to enable visualization and recording (Figure 1.13). Equipment familiarization should include:

- the function, specification and performance characteristics of the equipment to be used in cystoscopy, including how to record and store images
- the impact of equipment controls on the visual image
- the safe operation of cystoscopy equipment
- the importance of timely equipment fault recognition and local procedures for dealing with these
- equipment capabilities, limitations and routine maintenance.

Emergency equipment

Emergency equipment should be easily accessible in the rare event of a major complication. In addition, equipment required for urethral catheterization should be available in the event of a complication such as urinary retention.

Pharmacological support

A local analgesic such as a 2% lidocaine gel is inserted topically into the urethra 5–10 minutes prior to the procedure commencing. In males up to 11 mL and in females up to 6 mL are normally prescribed and applied (Peyronnet et al. 2016). If washings are required during the procedure, intravesical sodium chloride 0.9% is used to irrigate the bladder rather than sterile water to improve cell preservation during storage and transfer to the lab (BAUN and BAUS 2012a, b).

Procedure guideline 1.4   Flexible cystoscopy

Essential equipment
- Patient trolley
- Incontinence sheet
- Flexible cystoscope (optical/video)
- Urology sterile pack as determined by local practice, including sterile gauze and sterile forceps
- Procedure trolley
- Non-sterile gloves
- Apron
- Sterile gloves
- Sterile gown

- Sterile drapes
- Chlorhexidine cleansing solution or similar according to local guidelines
- Fluid administration set

Medicinal products
- 2% lidocaine gel (topically into urethra)
- Intravesical sterile water, or sodium chloride 0.9% if washings are required

Pre-procedure

Action	Rationale
1 Check the environment and equipment to ensure that everything is properly prepared for the procedure, including that the irrigation is attached and run through the scope, and awareness of the location and availability of emergency equipment.	To ensure the procedure will take place without delay for the patient and to ensure that the safety of the patient is addressed (BAUS and BAUN 2012a, b, **C**; Skills for Health 2010a, b, c, d, **C**).
2 Ask assistant to set up trolley with sterile urology pack and prepare scope.	To ensure that the safety of the patient is addressed (BAUS and BAUN 2012a, b, **C**; Skills for Health 2010a, b, c, d, **C**). To maintain infection control standards and minimize cross-infection and contamination (Fraise and Bradley 2009, **E**; RCN 2017a, **C**).

(continued)

Action	Rationale
3 Read the patient's notes, referral letter, patient history and relevant investigation results and identify any special instructions, investigations or items for which you need to seek advice prior to the procedure.	To ensure that the safety of the patient is addressed (BAUS and BAUN 2012a, b, **C**; Skills for Health 2010a, b, c, d, **C**).
4 Ensure that pre-procedure criteria have been met: • urine sample tested for infection, the results interpreted and a sample sent for further analysis if required • urine cytology obtained if required • pre-procedure medication has been taken as required such as prophylactic antibiotic • patient has emptied bladder • observations within normal limits • check medications and anticoagulation have been reviewed or withheld.	Requisite pre-procedure tests are performed to ensure patient safety is addressed (BAUS and BAUN 2012a, b, **C**; Skills for Health 2010a, b, c, d, **C**) and timely sampling of urine. **E**
5 Accurately identify the patient and introduce yourself and any colleagues present to the patient.	To ensure that the safety of the patient is addressed (BAUS and BAUN 2012a, b, **C**; Skills for Health 2010a, b, c, d, **C**). To ensure the patient is aware who is present during the procedure. **E**
6 Assess the patient's suitability for the procedure, including any changes to health since referral, medication or allergy status and seek advice or refer if necessary.	To ensure that the safety of the patient is addressed and to ensure relevant history is recorded (BAUS and BAUN 2012a, b, **C**; Skills for Health 2010a, b, c, d, **C**).
7 Explain the procedure and potential complications to the patient and accurately answer any questions at a level and pace that is appropriate to: • their level of understanding • their culture and background • their preferred way of communicating their needs.	To ensure informed consent has been obtained and also that patient's needs are appropriately addressed during procedure (DH 2009, **C**).
8 Ensure the patient's informed consent to the procedure has been given and, if not, obtain it.	To ensure informed consent has been obtained and also that patient's needs are appropriately addressed during procedure (DH 2009, **C**; NMC 2015, **C**).
9 Ask the patient to remove clothing below the waist. Offer a gown to cover the patient.	To provide privacy and comfort for the patient. **E**. To minimize the risk of a hospital acquired infection (BAUS and BAUN 2012b, **C**).
10 Assist the patient to position themselves onto an incontinence sheet on the trolley correctly for the procedure (supine), respecting their dignity and ensuring their comfort within the constraints of the procedure. Males lay flat and females with legs apart.	To enable easy passage of the cystoscope (BAUS and BAUN 2012a, b, **C**; Skills for Health 2010a, b, c, d, **C**) and maintain patient comfort and dignity. **E**.
11 Wash hands with soap and water and dry, followed by alcohol rub, and apply non-sterile gloves and apron.	To maintain infection control standards and minimize cross-infection and contamination (Fraise and Bradley 2009, **E**; RCN 2017a, **C**).
12 Identify, clean with cleansing solution such as chlorhexidine solution and examine the urethral orifice and surrounding area. In females open the labia, and in males retract the foreskin.	Initial examination of the patient and first findings, appropriate cleansing to minimize cross-infection/contamination (Reynard et al. 2013, **E**).
13 Insert local anaesthetic gel topically into the urethra, leaving for 5–10 minutes.	To maintain patient comfort **E** and allow smooth passage of the cystoscope (BAUS and BAUN 2012b, **C**). Appropriately applied lidocaine gel reduces pain in males during flexible cystoscopy (Aaronson et al. 2009, **R1a**).
14 Remove gloves and apron and discard in clinical waste.	To ensure correct disposal of clinical waste (DH 2013, **C**; HSE 2003, **C**).
15 Wash hands with soap and water, followed by alcohol rub, and apply sterile gloves and gown.	To maintain infection control standards and minimize cross-infection and contamination (Fraise and Bradley 2009, **E**; RCN 2017a, **C**).
16 Apply sterile drape over patient's lower body.	To maintain infection control standards and minimize cross-infection and contamination (Fraise and Bradley 2009, **E**; RCN 2017a, **C**).

Procedure

17	Maintain communication with the patient throughout the procedure, monitor and respond to any questions or needs.	To ensure ongoing informed consent (DH 2009, **C**; NMC 2015, **C**); patient comfort, safety and dignity maintained. **E**
18	Ensure the labia are held open in females or the foreskin is retracted in males. This should be done either by an assistant or with your non-dominant hand.	To ensure thorough and accurate examination (Reynard et al. 2008, **E**).
19	Introduce the cystoscope into the urethra and advance it gently under direct vision using deflection (**Action figure 19a**) and inflection (**Action figure 19b**) (change in angle) of the tip to avoid trauma to the urethral wall and ensure that the correct irrigation fluid is running (sterile water in most cases, normal saline if washings are required to preserve the cells).	To maintain patient safety and comfort. To ensure thorough and accurate examination (Reynard et al. 2008, **E**).
20	If insertion is difficult, or problems occur, seek advice or decide to terminate the procedure and record your findings.	To maintain patient safety. **E**
21	Fill bladder sufficiently with irrigation fluid to facilitate systematic examination of the internal structure of the bladder and to identify anatomical landmarks using tip deflection and inflection, instrument rotation and gentle advancement and withdrawal of the cystoscope.	To ensure a thorough and accurate examination (Smith et al. 2012, **E**) of the bladder (Figure 1.14).
22	Identify all abnormal lesions or structures observed throughout the examination. Record images throughout procedure using the video stack, external printer or software connected to the stack and scope.	To ensure a thorough and accurate examination (Smith et al. 2012, **E**).
23	Improve visualization, if necessary, by aspirating fluids from the bladder.	To ensure a thorough and accurate examination (Smith et al. 2012, **E**).
24	Once complete, fully withdraw cystoscope, maintaining irrigation until withdrawal of cystoscope is almost complete.	To ensure cystoscope is completely removed (BAUS and BAUN 2012a, b, **C**; Skills for Health 2010a, b, c, d, **C**). To maintain patient comfort and safety. **E**

Post-procedure

25	Reassure patient that the examination has been completed.	To maintain patient comfort and safety. **E**
26	Assist the patient to reposition, wipe surplus lubricant and dry.	To maintain patient comfort and safety. **E**
27	Remove gloves and dispose of all used single-use equipment. Return cystoscope for washing according to local guidelines.	To maintain infection control standards and minimize cross-infection and contamination (BAUS and BAUN 2012a, b, **C**; Fraise and Bradley 2009, **E**; RCN 2017a, **C**; Skills for Health 2010a, b, c, d, **C**).
28	Ask the patient to pass urine before leaving the department.	To ensure the patient is able to pass urine (BAUS and BAUN 2012b, **C**).

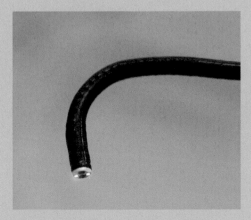

Action Figure 19a Cystoscope deflection.

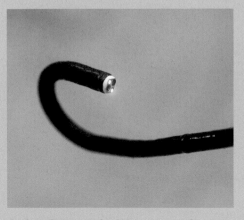

Action Figure 19b Cystoscope inflection.

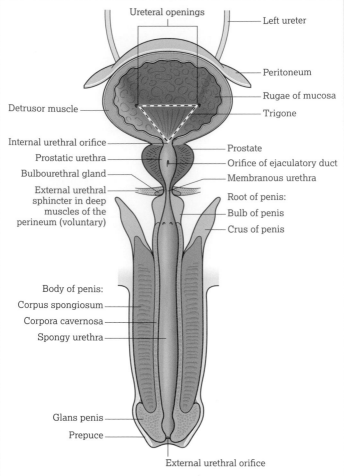

Ureteral openings —
Left ureter

Peritoneum

Rugae of mucosa

Detrusor muscle —
Trigone

Internal urethral orifice —
Prostatic urethra —
Bulbourethral gland —
External urethral sphincter in deep muscles of the perineum (voluntary) —

Prostate
Orifice of ejaculatory duct
Membranous urethra
Root of penis:
Bulb of penis
Crus of penis

Body of penis:
Corpus spongiosum —
Corpora cavernosa —
Spongy urethra —

Glans penis —
Prepuce —

External urethral orifice

Figure 1.14 Male internal bladder structure. *Source:* Adapted from Tortora and Derrickson (2011). Reproduced with permission of John Wiley & Sons.

Procedure guideline 1.5   Flexible cystoscopy with stent removal

Essential equipment
- Patient trolley
- Incontinence sheet
- Flexible cystoscope (optical/video)
- Urology sterile pack as determined by local practice, including sterile gauze and sterile forceps
- Procedure trolley
- Non-sterile gloves
- Apron
- Sterile gloves
- Sterile gown
- Sterile drapes
- Chlorhexidine cleansing solution or similar according to local guidelines

- Fluid giving set
- Stent grasping forceps

Optional equipment
- Fluid giving set
- 1 litre bag of sterile water/1 litre bag of sodium chloride (if washings required)

Medicinal products
- 2% lidocaine gel (topically into urethra)
- Intravesical sterile water or sodium chloride 0.9% if washings are required

Pre-procedure

Action	Rationale
Repeat steps 1–16 from Procedure guideline 1.4 Flexible cystoscopy	

Procedure

17 Maintain communication with the patient throughout the procedure, monitor and respond to any questions or needs.	To ensure ongoing informed consent (DH 2009, **C**; NMC 2015, **C**); patient comfort, safety and dignity maintained. **E**

18	Ensure the labia are held open in females or the foreskin is retracted in males. This should be done either by an assistant or with your non-dominant hand.	To ensure thorough and accurate examination (Reynard et al. 2008, **E**).
19	Introduce the cystoscope into the urethra and advance it gently under direct vision using deflection (**Action figure 19a**) and inflection (**Action figure 19b**) (change in angle) of the tip to avoid trauma to the urethral wall and ensure that the correct irrigation fluid is running (sterile water in most cases, normal saline if washings are required to preserve the cells).	To maintain patient safety and comfort. To ensure thorough and accurate examination (Reynard et al. 2008, **E**).
20	If insertion is difficult, or problems occur, seek advice or decide to terminate the procedure and record your findings.	To maintain patient safety. **E**
21	Fill bladder sufficiently with irrigation fluid to facilitate systematic examination of the internal structure of the bladder and to identify anatomical landmarks using tip deflection and inflection, instrument rotation and gentle advancement and withdrawal of the cystoscope.	To ensure a thorough and accurate examination (Smith et al. 2012, **E**) of the bladder (Figure 1.14).
22	Identify all abnormal lesions or structures observed throughout the examination. Record images throughout procedure using the video stack, external printer or software connected to the stack and scope.	To ensure a thorough and accurate examination (Smith et al. 2012, **E**).
23	Improve visualization, if necessary, by aspirating fluids from the bladder.	To ensure a thorough and accurate examination (Smith et al. 2012, **E**).
24	Select the grasping forceps and ensure they are working.	To ensure the correct device is selected and avoid adverse events during the procedure (BAUS and BAUN 2012b, **C**).
25	Visualize and locate the ureteric stent to be removed.	To ensure the correct stent is identified for removal and avoid removal of the wrong ureteric stent if bilateral ureteric stents are *in situ* (BAUS and BAUN 2012b, **C**).
26	Insert grasping forceps through the channel of the cystoscope using dominant hand while keeping the cystoscope tip in the straight position.	To ensure damage to the cystoscope does not occur (BAUS and BAUN 2012b, **C**).
27	Visualize the grasping forceps as they enter the bladder and field of vision.	To ensure the grasping forceps are in the correct position and not opened while within the cystoscope to avoid damage to both devices (BAUS and BAUN 2012b, **C**).
28	Use the cystoscope controls to orientate the grasping forceps over the ureteric stent.	To ensure the grasping forceps are in the correct position (BAUS and BAUN 2012b, **C**).
29	Open the jaws of the grasping forceps or instruct an assistant to operate the grasping forceps.	To ensure grasping forceps are operated correctly and safely. **E**
30	Grasp the stent firmly, ensuring that no mucosa or tissue has been inadvertently gripped.	To enable removal of ureteric stent and avoid damaging bladder (BAUS and BAUN 2012b, **C**).
31	Withdraw the cystoscope and grasping forceps together from the bladder and urethra under direct vision.	To enable removal of the ureteric stent while minimizing patient discomfort (BAUS and BAUN 2012b, **C**).
32	If resistance is encountered from the stent, stop the procedure and seek appropriate advice from a senior colleague.	To avoid damage to ureter, bladder and urethra (BAUS and BAUN 2012b, **C**).
33	Inspect the removed ureteric stent to ensure it is complete.	To ensure the device is completely removed and intact (BAUS and BAUN 2012b, **C**).

Post-procedure

34	Reassure patient that the examination has been completed.	To maintain patient comfort and safety. **E**
35	Assist the patient to reposition, wipe surplus lubricant and dry.	To maintain patient comfort and safety. **E**
36	Remove gloves and dispose of all used single-use equipment. Return cystoscope for washing according to local guidelines.	To maintain infection control standards and minimize cross-infection and contamination (BAUS and BAUN 2012a, b, **C**; Fraise and Bradley 2009, **E**; RCN 2017a, **C**; Skills for Health 2010a, b, c, d, **C**).
37	Ask the patient to pass urine before leaving the department.	To ensure the patient is able to pass urine (BAUS and BAUN 2012b, **C**).

32 | **Procedure guideline 1.6** Flexible cystoscopy with bladder biopsy

Essential equipment

- Patient trolley
- Incontinence sheet
- Flexible cystoscope (optical/video)
- Urology sterile pack as determined by local practice, including sterile gauze and sterile forceps
- Procedure trolley
- Non-sterile gloves
- Apron
- Sterile gloves
- Sterile gown
- Sterile drapes
- Chlorhexidine cleansing solution or similar according to local guidelines
- 1 litre bag of sterile water
- Fluid giving set
- Biopsy forceps
- Specimen container with formalin
- Cystodiathermy checked and in working order

Medicinal products

- 2% lidocaine gel (topically into urethra)
- Intravesical sodium chloride 0.9%

Pre-procedure

Action	Rationale
1 Check the environment and equipment to ensure that everything is properly prepared for the procedure, including that the irrigation is attached and run through the scope, and awareness of the location and availability of emergency equipment.	To ensure the procedure will take place without delay for the patient and to ensure that the safety of the patient is addressed (BAUS and BAUN 2012a, b, **C**; Skills for Health 2010a, b, c, d, **C**).
2 Ask assistant to set up trolley with sterile urology pack and prepare scope.	To ensure that the safety of the patient is addressed (BAUS and BAUN 2012a, b, **C**; Skills for Health 2010a, b, c, d, **C**). To maintain infection control standards and minimize cross-infection and contamination (Fraise and Bradley 2009, **E**; RCN 2017a, **C**).
3 Read the patient's notes, referral letter, patient history and relevant investigation results and identify any special instructions, investigations or items for which you need to seek advice prior to the procedure, including any metal prosthesis.	To ensure that the safety of the patient is addressed (BAUS and BAUN 2012a, b, **C**; Skills for Health 2010a, b, c, d, **C**).
4 Ensure that pre-procedure criteria have been met: • urine sample tested for infection, the results interpreted and a sample sent for further analysis if required • urine cytology obtained if required • pre-procedure medication has been taken as required, such as prophylactic antibiotic • patient has emptied bladder • observations within normal limits • check medications and anticoagulation have been reviewed or withheld.	Requisite pre-procedure tests are performed to ensure patient safety addressed (BAUS and BAUN 2012a, b, **C**; Skills for Health 2010a, b, c, d, **C**) and timely sampling of urine. **E**
5 Accurately identify the patient and introduce yourself and any colleagues present to the patient.	To ensure that the safety of the patient is addressed (BAUS and BAUN 2012a, b, **C**; Skills for Health 2010a, b, c, d, **C**). To ensure the patient is aware who is present during the procedure. **E**
6 Assess the patient's suitability for the procedure, including any changes to health since referral, medication or allergy status, and seek advice or refer if necessary.	To ensure that the safety of the patient is addressed and to ensure relevant history is recorded (BAUS and BAUN 2012a, b, **C**; Skills for Health 2010a, b, c, d, **C**).
7 Explain the procedure and potential complications to the patient and accurately answer any questions at a level and pace that is appropriate to: • their level of understanding • their culture and background • their preferred way of communicating their needs.	To ensure informed consent has been obtained and also that patient's needs are appropriately addressed during procedure (DH 2009, **C**).
8 Ensure the patient's informed consent to the procedure has been given and, if not, obtain it.	To ensure informed consent has been obtained and also that patient's needs are appropriately addressed during procedure (DH 2009, **C**; NMC 2015, **C**).
9 Ensure that the cystoscope is diathermy compatible.	To ensure cystodiathermy is undertaken safely (BAUS and BAUN 2012b, **C**).
10 Ensure that irrigation fluid is diathermy compatible, for example 1.5% glycine or normal saline.	To ensure cystodiathermy is undertaken safely (BAUS and BAUN 2012b, **C**).
11 Ask the patient to remove any metal jewellery or to cover with non-conductive tape.	To ensure that the safety of the patient is addressed (BAUS and BAUN 2012b, **C**).

12	Ask the patient to remove clothing below the waist. Offer a gown to cover the patient.	To provide privacy and comfort for the patient. **E**. To minimize the risk of a hospital acquired infection (BAUS and BAUN 2012b, **C**).
13	Assist the patient to position themselves onto an incontinence sheet on the trolley correctly for the procedure (supine), respecting their dignity and ensuring their comfort within the constraints of the procedure. Males lay flat and females with legs apart.	To enable easy passage of the cystoscope (BAUS and BAUN 2012a, b, **C**; Skills for Health 2010a, b, c, d, **C**) and maintain patient comfort and dignity. **E**
14	Ensure the patient is not in contact with any metal surface.	To ensure no adverse events occur with subsequent burns while using cystodiathermy (BAUS and BAUN 2012b, **C**).
15	Prepare the area for the diathermy plate by shaving excessive hair (usually the patient's thigh) while avoiding bony prominences, wet skin, scar tissue, metal prosthesis or tattoos.	To ensure no adverse events occur with subsequent burns while using cystodiathermy (BAUS and BAUN 2012b, **C**).
16	Wash hands with soap and water and dry, followed by alcohol rub, and apply non-sterile gloves and apron.	To maintain infection control standards and minimize cross-infection and contamination (Fraise and Bradley 2009, **E**; RCN 2017a, **C**).
17	Identify, clean with cleansing solution such as chlorhexidine solution and examine the urethral orifice and surrounding area. In females open the labia, and in males retract the foreskin.	Initial examination of the patient and first findings, appropriate cleansing to minimize cross-infection/contamination (Reynard et al. 2013, **E**).
18	Insert local anaesthetic gel topically into the urethra, leaving for 5–10 minutes.	To maintain patient comfort **E** and allow smooth passage of the cystoscope (BAUS and BAUN 2012b, **C**). Appropriately applied lidocaine gel reduces pain in males during flexible cystoscopy (Aaronson et al. 2009, **R1a**).
19	Remove gloves and apron and discard in clinical waste.	To ensure correct disposal of clinical waste (DH 2013, **C**; HSE 2003, **C**).
20	Wash hands with soap and water, followed by alcohol rub, and apply sterile gloves and gown.	To maintain infection control standards and minimize cross-infection and contamination (Fraise and Bradley 2009, **E**; RCN 2017a, **C**).
21	Apply sterile drape over patient's lower body.	To maintain infection control standards and minimize cross-infection and contamination (Fraise and Bradley 2009, **E**; RCN 2017a, **C**).

Procedure

22	Maintain communication with the patient throughout the procedure, monitor and respond to any questions or needs.	To ensure ongoing informed consent (DH 2009, **C**; NMC 2015, **C**); patient comfort, safety and dignity maintained. **E**
23	Ensure the labia are held open in females or the foreskin is retracted in males. This should be done either by an assistant or with your non-dominant hand.	To ensure thorough and accurate examination (Reynard et al. 2008, **E**).
24	Introduce the cystoscope into the urethra and advance it gently under direct vision using deflection (**Action figure 19a**) and inflection (**Action figure 19b**) (change in angle) of the tip to avoid trauma to the urethral wall and ensure that the correct irrigation fluid is running (normal saline if washings are required to preserve the cells).	To maintain patient safety and comfort. To ensure thorough and accurate examination (Reynard et al. 2008, **E**).
25	If insertion is difficult, or problems occur, seek advice or decide to terminate the procedure and record your findings.	To maintain patient safety. **E**
26	Fill bladder sufficiently with irrigation fluid to facilitate systematic examination of the internal structure of the bladder and to identify anatomical landmarks using tip deflection and inflection, instrument rotation and gentle advancement and withdrawal of the cystoscope.	To ensure a thorough and accurate examination (Smith et al. 2012, **C**) of the bladder (Figure 1.14).
27	Identify all abnormal lesions or bleeding areas throughout the examination. Record images throughout procedure using the video stack, external printer or software connected to the stack and scope.	To ensure a thorough and accurate examination (Smith et al. 2012, **E**).
28	Improve visualization, if necessary, by aspirating fluids from the bladder.	To ensure a thorough and accurate examination (Smith et al. 2012, **E**).

(continued)

Action	Rationale
29 Select the diathermy compatible biopsy forceps and ensure they are in working order.	To avoid an adverse event if cystodiathermy is required during the procedure and biopsy forceps are functional (BAUS and BAUN 2012b, **C**).
30 Insert biopsy forceps through the channel of the cystoscope using dominant hand while keeping the cystoscope tip in the straight position.	To ensure damage to the cystoscope does not occur (BAUS and BAUN 2012b, **C**).
31 Visualize the biopsy forceps as they enter the bladder and field of vision.	To ensure the biopsy forceps are in the correct position and not opened while within the cystoscope to avoid damage to both devices (BAUS and BAUN 2012b, **C**).
32 Use the cystoscope controls to orientate the biopsy forceps over the tissue to be sampled.	To ensure the biopsy forceps are in the correct position and not opened while within the cystoscope to avoid damage to both devices (BAUS and BAUN 2012b, **C**).
33 Open the jaws of the biopsy forceps or instruct an assistant to operate the biopsy forceps.	To ensure grasping forceps are operated correctly and safely. **E**
34 Close the biopsy forceps jaws, taking an adequate tissue sample.	To provide an adequate specimen for histopathological analysis while minimizing patient discomfort (BAUS and BAUN 2012b, **C**).
35 While biopsy forceps are closed, pull sharply from the bladder tissue.	To provide an adequate specimen for histopathological analysis while minimizing patient discomfort (BAUS and BAUN 2012b, **C**).
36 Withdraw the biopsy forceps via the cystoscope channel while keeping the jaws closed, or instruct the assistant to do so.	To ensure the sample is removed (BAUS and BAUN 2012b, **C**).
37 Deposit all of the tissue sample into the specimen pot or instruct the assistant, making sure the biopsy forceps do not touch the sterile pot.	To ensure the sample is maintained for histopathological analysis (BAUS and BAUN 2012b, **C**).
38 Clean the forceps between each sample in sodium chloride 0.9%.	To ensure biopsy forceps are clean and ready for additional sampling. **E**
39 Visualize biopsy sites for excessive bleeding and perform cystodiathermy if required (see Procedure guideline 1.7 Cystoscopy with APC/cystodiathermy.	To minimize the risk of clot retention of urine and haemorrhage (BAUS and BAUN 2012b, **C**).
40 Repeat steps 32–39 for subsequent samples.	
41 Once complete, fully withdraw cystoscope, maintaining irrigation until withdrawal of cystoscope is almost complete.	To ensure cystoscope is fully withdrawn. **E**

Post-procedure

Action	Rationale
42 Reassure patient that the examination has been completed.	To maintain patient comfort and safety. **E**
43 Assist the patient to reposition, wipe surplus lubricant and dry.	To maintain patient comfort and safety. **E**
44 Remove gloves and dispose of all used single-use equipment. Return cystoscope for washing according to local guidelines.	To maintain infection control standards and minimize cross-infection and contamination (BAUS and BAUN 2012a, b, **C**; Fraise and Bradley 2009, **E**; RCN 2017a, **C**; Skills for Health 2010a, b, c, d, **C**).
45 Label specimens and send to laboratory for histopathological analysis.	To ensure correct identification and correct analysis is undertaken (BAUS and BAUN 2012b, **C**).
46 Ask the patient to pass urine before leaving the department.	To ensure the patient is able to pass urine (BAUS and BAUN 2012b, **C**).

Procedure guideline 1.7   Flexible cystoscopy with argon plasma coagulation (APC)/cystodiathermy   35

Essential equipment
- Patient trolley
- Incontinence sheet
- Flexible cystoscope (optical/video)
- Urology sterile pack as determined by local practice, including sterile gauze and sterile forceps
- Procedure trolley
- Non-sterile gloves
- Apron
- Sterile gloves
- Sterile gown
- Sterile drapes

- Fluid giving set
- Chlorhexidine cleansing solution or similar according to local guidelines
- Argon plasma coagulation (APC)/cystodiathermy generator: APC/cystodiathermy probe and equipment stack loaded with correct settings and diathermy insulation coating intact (as determined by local practice and manufacturer's guidelines)

Medicinal products
- 2% lidocaine gel (topically into urethra)
- Intravesical sodium chloride 0.9%

Pre-procedure

Action	Rationale
Repeat steps 1–21 from Procedure guideline 1.6 Flexible cystoscopy with bladder biopsy	

Procedure

Repeat steps 22–28 from Procedure guideline 1.6 Flexible cystoscopy with bladder biopsy, then:	
29 Ask the assistant to apply the diathermy plate (patient return electrode).	To ensure no adverse events occur with subsequent burns while using cystodiathermy (BAUS and BAUN 2012b, **C**).
30 Ask the assistant to move the foot pedals into position for easy use.	To ensure diathermy controls are in safe working reach. **E**
31 Ask the assistant to connect the wire to the diathermy lead.	To ensure no adverse events occur with subsequent burns while using cystodiathermy (BAUS and BAUN 2012b, **C**).
32 Insert diathermy wire through the channel of the cystoscope using dominant hand while keeping the cystoscope tip in the straight position.	To ensure damage to the cystoscope does not occur (BAUS and BAUN 2012b, **C**).
33 Visualize the diathermy wire as it enters the bladder and field of vision advancing past the tip of the cystoscope.	To ensure diathermy is delivered only to the area required (BAUS and BAUN 2012b, **C**).
34 Position the diathermy wire gently at the area to be treated.	To ensure diathermy is delivered only to the area required (BAUS and BAUN 2012b, **C**).
35 Push the foot pedals in short bursts until bleeding has ceased or the abnormality is destroyed.	To ensure bleeding is ceased or abnormality is destroyed (BAUS and BAUN 2012b, **C**).
36 Remove the diathermy wire and hand to the assistant while maintaining asepsis.	To ensure all areas to be treated have been treated successfully (BAUS and BAUN 2012b, **C**).
37 Repeat steps 34–36 as required.	
38 Ensure all areas have been treated and if complete, remove the cystoscope.	To ensure all areas to be treated have been treated successfully (BAUS and BAUN 2012b, **C**).

Post-procedure

39 Reassure patient that the examination has been completed.	To maintain patient comfort and safety. **E**
40 Ensure the diathermy controls are moved away and the device is switched off.	To ensure safety of the patient and staff. **E**
41 Remove the diathermy plate and inspect area, ensuring there are no adverse events such as burns.	To ensure any damage to the skin is identified, treated and documented (BAUS and BAUN 2012b, **C**).
42 Assist the patient to reposition, wipe surplus lubricant and dry.	To maintain patient comfort and safety. **E**
43 Remove gloves and dispose of all used single-use equipment. Return cystoscope for washing according to local guidelines.	To maintain infection control standards and minimize cross-infection and contamination (BAUS and BAUN 2012a, b, **C**; Fraise and Bradley 2009, **E**; RCN 2017a, **C**; Skills for Health 2010a, b, c, d, **C**).
44 Label specimens and send to laboratory for histopathological analysis.	To ensure correct identification and correct analysis is undertaken (BAUS and BAUN 2012b, **C**).
45 Ask the patient to pass urine before leaving the department.	To ensure the patient is able to pass urine (BAUS and BAUN 2012b, **C**).

Problem-solving table 1.2 Prevention and resolution (Procedure guidelines 1.4, 1.5, 1.6, 1.7) (BAUS and BAUN 2012a, b; Skills for Health 2010a, b, c, d)

Problem	Cause	Prevention	Action
Urethral bleeding.	Urethral trauma.	Careful advancement of the cystoscope under direct vision during the procedure.	The procedure should be stopped and direct finger pressure must be applied to clamp the urethra. In the case of continuous bleeding, the patient should be transferred to the recovery area and escalated to the senior clinician (usually the responsible consultant). A three-way 18 Fr Foley catheter should be inserted, with gentle traction applied over the bladder neck.
Haematuria.	Underlying abnormality, intra-procedure bladder trauma, bladder biopsy.	Careful advancement of the cystoscope under direct vision during the procedure.	A 22 Fr three-way silicone Foley catheter should be inserted, followed by bladder washout and continuous bladder irrigation with normal saline. In case of severe bleeding, formal washout in theatre may be required.
Urinary retention.	Underlying abnormality.	All patients must spontaneously void before being discharged.	If a patient complains of abdominal pain with inability to void or has no pain but a full bladder (confirmed on ultrasound) a 12–18 Fr Foley catheter should be inserted on free drainage. A trial of voiding without catheter should be booked to take place in 7–10 days.
Vasovagal syncope.	Acute anxiety/fear.	Addressing patient anxiety pre-procedure, informing patient of what to expect. Recognizing acute anxiety pre-procedure.	Immediately stop the procedure. Remove the scope and position the patient in dorsal decubitus with a 30° Trendelenburg (on back, head down) position. Vital signs should be recorded. In case of complete loss of consciousness or sustained instability, escalate to the emergency response team and inform the lead clinician.
Urinary tract infection.	Contamination or cross-infection.	Adherence to infection control guidelines.	Recognize symptoms and treat according to local guidelines or microbiology result.
Pain.	Urethral trauma.	Use of 2% lidocaine gel.	In case of acute pain, the procedure should be discontinued and if incomplete it should be re-booked under a general anaesthetic. Pain should stop within a short period of the scope being withdrawn. If it does not, systemic analgesia should be administered and further investigations should be requested in discussion with the lead clinician.

Post-procedural considerations

Immediate care
It is imperative that the practitioner recognizes onset of any acute emergencies associated with the procedure and responds appropriately. Ensure the patient is aware of possible post-procedural complications such as infection and the possibility of expected urinary discomfort. Encourage the patient to maintain adequate fluid hydration. Give a full explanation of the results to the patient, allowing time for them to ask questions regarding the preliminary findings, and where appropriate offer support. Prescribe (non-medical prescriber), or supply under a Patient Group Direction, antibiotics or other follow-up therapy if required and provide the patient with information on their administration.

Remind the patient of the information and advice they have already been given with regard to lifestyle and side-effects and who to contact if problems arise. Respond to any questions or requests for further information. It is also important to confirm the details of how the full outcome of the examination will be communicated and of any future appointments and/or referrals (BAUS and BAUN 2012a, b, Skills for Health 2010a, b, c, d).

Documentation
Document the observations and outcomes of the procedure and record all decisions made in the patient record. Ensure that any specimens are labelled with the correct accompanying request forms (NMC 2010a).

Breast diagnostics

Definition
Reliable assessment of breast symptoms and diagnostics is expected to be a rapid, triple-modality approach comprised of clinical (or physical), radiological and histological components. Established good practice dictates that breast diagnosis is completed by a multidisciplinary team. The aim of triple assessment in a rapid setting is to ensure quick referral to oncological teams for treatment, if cancer is diagnosed, but also to promptly reassure patients when they do not have cancer (ABS 2010, Aebi et al. 2011, NICE 2002, NICE 2016).

Anatomy and physiology
The breast is a glandular and secretory organ which has the primary purpose of lactation. It is also a prominent secondary sexual feature. Prior to puberty there is no difference between the male and female breast bud. Commencement of female sex hormones at puberty causes significant development of the female breast tissue (Tortora and Derrikson 2014).

Breast tissue comprises 10–15% epithelial parenchyma, or functional tissue. The remaining tissue is the stroma, or framework tissue, to give it and maintain its form. Breast cancer arises within the functional parenchyma or epithelial cells. Differences in breast size and shape are generally due to the difference in stroma rather than parenchyma.

Breast parenchyma is composed of 15–20 lobes which can each sub-divide into smaller lobules. The lobules are made up of branched tubuloalveolar glands. Each lobe drains into a lactiferous

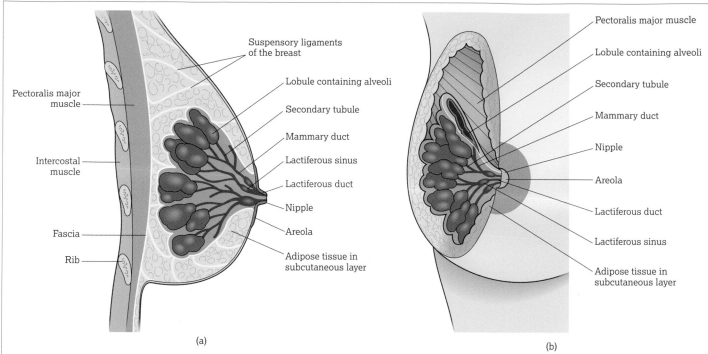

Figure 1.15 (a) Female breast (sagittal section). (b) Female breast (anterior view, partially sectioned). *Source:* Adapted from Tortora and Derrickson (2011). Reproduced with permission of John Wiley & Sons.

duct which runs toward the nipple (Figure 1.15). The lactiferous ducts dilate and coalesce into a lactiferous sinus beneath the areola and then open through a constricted orifice onto the nipple. Breast milk is secreted by the lobular tissue and transported toward the nipple by the breast ducts (Pandya and Moore 2011).

Oestrogen and progesterone both stimulate breast parenchyma during a normal menstrual cycle. Rising oestrogen levels in weeks 1–2 cause proliferation of the ductal system and, following ovulation, the rise in progesterone, synergistically with oestrogen, stimulates the lobular units. These changes give rise to the common breast changes which many women equate with their pre-period state. If no pregnancy ensues, decreasing hormone levels cause regression of this stimulated tissue (Ellis and Mahadevan 2013).

With the onset of menopause, as ovarian tissue ceases to produce high cyclical levels of oestrogen and progesterone, the majority of breast glandular tissue involutes or ceases to be active. Usually more adipose tissue is deposited and the postmenopausal breast is less dense on imaging. Due to this, mammography is more sensitive and specific in the postmenopausal breast.

Related theory

Benign breast disease is a term used to describe a variety of breast changes that are prevalent in the population. This is unsurprising when the stimulatory nature of the menstrual cycle on breast tissue is considered. Benign changes are hugely varied and can be developmental, inflammatory, fibrocystic or neoplastic in nature. They are often proliferative but not atypical in nature. Most can be safely left without intervention once biopsy proven (Guray and Sahin 2006). The most common benign presentations are listed in Table 1.6, related to age. Breast cancer is, however, the most commonly diagnosed cancer amongst women in the UK with 54,800 cases diagnosed per year (Cancer Research UK 2014) and has a high media and social profile (Xu et al. 2016).

Evidence-based approaches

The assessment of breast symptoms is heavily rationalized and covered by the need to ensure that the reported symptom or change is not breast cancer. Local, national and international guidance is clear; in the UK it is produced by the Association of Breast Surgery (ABS 2010) and National Institute for Health and Care Excellence (NICE 2013). Guidance used in other countries may show some variation in age of screening or follow-up pathways. However there is also a high degree of concordance noted, strengthening the evidence-based approach.

Rationale

The type of diagnostic procedure will vary depending on the clinical presentation of the patient. This may require a patient assessment and clinical breast examination, core biopsy, fine-needle aspiration, punch biopsy or nipple cytology.

Indications

Breast diagnostics are indicated for diagnosis and surveillance of breast changes or disease. The type of diagnostic procedure will vary depending on the clinical presentation of the patient.

Contraindications

The type of contraindication will vary depending on the diagnostic procedure, such as bleeding post biopsy.

Legal and professional issues

Breast diagnostics are increasingly undertaken by advanced nurse practitioners within breast teams. They routinely act as clinicians alongside radiologists, sonographers and pathologists. They will undertake clinical breast examination, instigate appropriate radiological investigations and may obtain tissue or cell specimens. Breast diagnostic techniques include:

- clinical breast examination
- core biopsy
- fine-needle aspiration
- punch biopsy
- nipple cytology.

Where any of these are undertaken by a nurse practitioner or advanced clinical nurse, that nurse should be acting within the scope of his or her professional practice (RCN 2012). Agreement should have been obtained by the employing trust or authority that he or she is competent through local assessment. Clinical assessment, prescription of ionizing radiation in the requesting

Table 1.6 Benign breast changes across ages

Age	Normal process	Aberration of normal development and involution (ANDI)		
		Clinical presentation	Underlying condition	Disease
15–24	Duct and lobule formation	Discrete lump	Fibroadenoma	Giant or multiple fibroadenoma
	Stroma formation	Uneven or excessive breast development	Juvenile hypertrophy	Uni- or bilateral macromastia
			Asymmetrical development	Poland's syndrome
25–34	Cyclical hormonal effects causing mild breast pain and alterations in size which fluctuate	Exaggerated hormonal effects causing moderate breast pain, nodularity and tenderness	None	Severe breast pain and tenderness interfering with normal activities
		Generally cyclical		Cyclical or non-cyclical in nature
				Continued nodularity
		Discrete lump	Fibroadenoma or macrocysts	Malignancy (uncommon in absence of family history)
35 onwards	Cyclical hormonal effects causing mild breast pain		Multiple microcysts	
			Sclerosing adenosis	
			Lobular hyperplasia	
	Lobular involution – microcysts, apocrine change, fibrosis, adenosis	Discrete lumps	Isolated macrocysts	Malignancy
		Nipple discharge	Duct ectasia	Multiple macrocysts
		Nipple retraction	Ductal hyperplasia	Periductal mastitis
	Ductal involution		Nipple discharge	Atypical ductal hyperplasia
				Multiple papillomata
	Normal		Periductal fibrosis	Discrete lumps requiring biopsy
			Nipple retraction	

Source: Adapted from Hughes (1991). Reproduced with permission of OUP; permission conveyed through Copyright Clearance Center, Inc.

of mammograms and undertaking tissue sampling all represent advanced nursing competencies.

Clinical breast examination

A clinical breast examination is required to gain information regarding the presenting symptom and patient background. It is also required to visually and palpably assess the breast and axilla in order to inform diagnostic tests required. It is indicated for any patient, male or female with a breast or axillary change, who is referred to a diagnostic breast clinic by a GP or other healthcare professional.

Rationale

A clinical breast examination is required to gain information regarding presenting symptoms and the patient's background to inform the potential diagnostic tests required.

Indication
Presentation with breast symptom or change including:

- lump
- thickening
- change in shape or appearance
- nipple discharge
- focal breast pain.

Contraindication
There are no contraindications to breast examination although inability to lie in the supine position or perform arm manoeuvres will limit the sensitivity of the examination and should be noted in the examination notes.

Procedure guideline 1.8   Clinical breast examination

Essential equipment

- Couch
- Gown
- Screen

Pre-procedure

Action	Rationale
1 Greet patient and introduce self and role and gain consent for procedure.	To put patient at ease and inform of process **E** and gain consent (RCN 2017b, **C**).
2 Offer chaperone.	Breast examination can be difficult for some women as it is considered intimate (RCN 2016b, **C**).

3 Review history of presenting symptom in patient's own words, noting when first noticed, triggering factors, alterations to symptom since first noting, intervening factors.	To establish duration of problem, constancy of symptoms. Breast cancer does not fluctuate but hormonal changes do (ABS 2010, **C**).
4 Assess menstrual history including: a. age periods started b. number of pregnancies – successful or not c. age of first pregnancy d. use of *in vitro* fertilization (IVF) e. experience of breastfeeding f. use of contraception g. regularity of periods h. age of menopause i. use of hormone replacement therapy (HRT) j. oophorectomy and/or hysterectomy.	Breast tissue is regulated by female hormones both over a lifetime and in each menstrual cycle. Information regarding oestrogen exposure is important to overall risk and may be pertinent to presenting symptom (ABS 2010, **C**).
5 Assess family history of breast and/or ovarian cancer.	Family history is a significant risk factor for breast cancer if present and may affect screening recommendations for current assessment and going forward (NICE 2013, **C**).
6 Assess previous medical history.	Relevant medical and surgical history as well as prescription drugs can be relevant (ABS 2010, **C**).
7 Assess lifestyle factors – weight, smoking history, alcohol intake.	To establish overall risk of breast cancer as well as other possible causes for symptom (ABS 2010, **C**).
8 Ask patient to remove upper clothes, including bra, behind curtain or screen. Provide a gown for use.	To enable ease of visible inspection and palpation. **E** Provide gown to maintain personal dignity (RCN 2008, **C**).
9 Wash hands with soap and warm water and dry, followed by alcohol rub.	To maintain infection control standards and minimize cross-infection and contamination (Fraise and Bradley 2009, **E**; RCN 2017a, **C**).

Procedure

10 Ask patient to open gown.	To allow for visual inspection. **E**
11 While patient is in sitting position with arms relaxed at sides, observe both breasts for contour, regularity, size, skin changes, nipple position and direction.	Malignant changes may attach internally and cause visible skin or shape changes such as tethering, dimpling and in-pulling (Pandya and Moore 2011, **E**).
12 Ask patient to raise arms together above head and observe movement of breast over chest wall. Check for symmetry and regular contour.	This allows inspection of the lower half of the breast (Pandya and Moore 2011, **E**).
13 Ask patient to bring hands together in prayer-like stance and push palms together or to put hands on hips and push down and in. Observe for any changes to breast outlines.	Contraction of muscles beneath breast tissue may exacerbate visible changes (Pandya and Moore 2011, **E**).
14 Ask patient to lie back on couch in supine position.	Breast examination is completed in supine position. **E**
15 Using the flat of 3 middle fingers, palpate the breast tissue firmly downwards toward the chest wall to assess texture of breast tissue.	Downward pressure should be constant and firm enough to cover superficial, middle and deep layers. **E**
16 Ensure that the entire breast is covered in a systematic fashion including the tail of tissue toward axilla. It is advised that either a vertical stripe (**Action figure 16a**), radial spoke (**Action figure 16b**) or concentric circular pattern (**Action figure 16c**) is followed. A consistent approach should be employed by the clinician.	A consistent approach increases the likelihood that breast examination is systematic and thorough (Pandya and Moore 2011, **E**).
17 Examine both breasts equally, starting with the 'normal' breast and finishing by specifically examining the area where a lesion is reported (if applicable).	To ensure an appreciation of what is normal and to allow comparison. To prevent concentrating on reported symptom at risk of missing a further change in a different area. **E**
18 Inform patient they can get dressed.	To maintain privacy and dignity. **E**

(continued)

40 | **Procedure guideline 1.8** Clinical breast examination *(continued)*

Post-procedure

Action	Rationale
19 Annotate findings and assessment on record sheet using the accepted and agreed grading system: a. clinically normal=P1 b. abnormal but no concern=P2 c. uncertain=P3 d. suspicious=P4 e. clinically malignant=P5. Note position of any palpated symptom by clock face and distance from nipple. Supplement with clinical picture.	Being required to describe findings and indicate need for investigation focuses the clinician to produce a result. This has been found to optimize clinical breast examination (Goodson et al. 2010, **E**; NMC 2010a, **C**).
20 Explain findings to patient and need for further radiological tests (as necessary).	To ensure that patient understands what the tests will involve and what to expect. This reduces anxiety and manages expectations realistically. **E**
21 Accurately complete request forms for mammography and/or breast ultrasound including patient demographics, history of symptoms and result of examination.	To ensure that only required tests are requested depending on patient history and symptoms (RCR 2008, **C**). To prevent unnecessary radiation exposure (RCR 2008, **C**).
22 Arrange to see patient with the results of radiological investigations or clearly arrange future follow-up.	To ensure that results are acted upon and patient informed of any decision. **E**

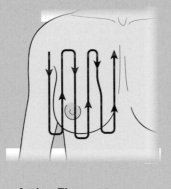

Action Figure 16a
Vertical pattern.

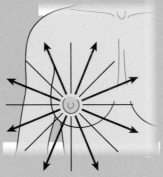

Action Figure 16b Radial
spoke pattern.

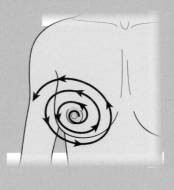

Action Figure 16c
Concentric circular pattern.

Core biopsy

Rationale

The aim of obtaining a core biopsy is to provide an intact histological sample of an area of clinical or radiological concern. Histological assessment of an intact lesion gives the most sensitive and complete result (Chou and Corder 2003) and should be the procedure of choice. In the case of a malignant result it will provide more detailed information to help guide the initial treatment options. It will be undertaken within the breast assessment clinic following clinical and radiological investigation. Clinical and radiological assessment should be completed prior to intervention to gain a tissue sample as this intervention itself may alter the outcome of the radiological and clinical assessment.

Breast biopsies should be guided by radiological imaging (mammogram, ultrasound or MRI) to reduce the need for repeat samples and to increase accuracy of the sample. In this case the procedure is carried out by a radiological consultant, junior doctor or appropriately trained sonographer. It is appropriate to carry out clinical biopsies, without radiological guidance, in cases of locally advanced lesions and clinically palpably lesions that are not visualized on imaging (Chou and Corder 2003).

Indication

A defined area within the breast or axilla that by clinical or radiological criteria is abnormal.

Contraindication

There is little agreement in research on the absolute need to stop anticoagulants prior to biopsy (Chetlen et al. 2013). Stopping anticoagulant therapy will cause delay and may increase the risk to the patient, depending on the reason for treatment. The latest guidance states that a recent international normalized ratio (INR) check (within the last 5 days or longer if stable) should be available.

- For a core biopsy it is suggested the INR must be <4 although there is little evidence (BSBR 2012).

- If the INR is > 4 then warfarin should be stopped for 3 days and restarted on the day of the biopsy.
- Patients on aspirin or clopidogrel do not need to stop treatment (BSBR 2012).

Equipment

Biopsy devices/needles

The biopsy device is a cutting needle with a hollow central cavity that is either integral to a disposable single-use firing apparatus or can be attached to a reusable firing apparatus or 'gun'. The apparatus is pulled back to hold the needle in a cocked position prior to introducing it into the patient. Releasing the firing mechanism launches or throws the needle forward to a specified penetration depth, typically 22 or 15 mm. As the needle moves forward through the anterior tissue it cuts and holds the sample within the hollow central needle space. An example is shown in Figure 1.16.

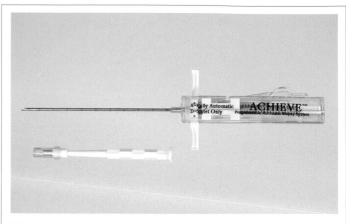

Figure 1.16 Biopsy device and needle.

Procedure guideline 1.9   Core breast biopsy

Essential equipment

- Procedure trolley
- Sterile dressing pack
- Sterile gloves
- Plastic apron
- Swab saturated with chlorhexidine in 70% alcohol (Chlora-Prep), or isopropyl alcohol 70% (ChloraPrep)
- Sterile syringe (2 mL)
- Sterile needles (23 G/25 G)
- 14 G biopsy needle and biopsy gun/apparatus
- Scalpel blade (size 11)
- Sterile iris scissors

- Histology pot
- Histology form
- Sterile gauze
- Steri-Strips™
- Sterile dressing, e.g. Mepore

Additional staff

- This procedure requires an assistant and should not be attempted by a solo practitioner

Medicinal products

- Lidocaine 1% for local anaesthetic

Pre-procedure

Action	Rationale
1 Explain the procedure to the patient.	To ensure that the patient understands the procedure and gives his/her valid consent (RCN 2017b, **C**).
2 Check that the identity of the patient matches the details on the patient notes.	To ensure that the sample is correctly labelled (RCN 2017b, **C**).
3 Ascertain whether the patient is allergic to skin cleanser, adhesive plaster or local anaesthetic.	To prevent an allergic skin reaction (NMC 2010b, **C**).
4 Check patient's medications. The patient should be asked if they are taking anticoagulants.	To ensure any contraindications are considered and appropriate management is in place regarding anticoagulants (BSBR 2012, **C**; Chetlen et al. 2013, **E**).
5 Ask the patient to change into the gown and position the patient on the couch in a position that facilitates access to the site requiring biopsy.	To ensure the patient is comfortable and to ensure safety should the patient feel faint during the procedure. **E**
6 Carefully wash hands using bactericidal soap and water, dry before commencement. Or decontaminate physically clean hands with alcohol-based handrub.	To minimize risk of infection (RCN 2017a, **C**).
7 Check all packaging for use-by date. Open and prepare the equipment on the procedure trolley.	To maintain asepsis throughout and check that no equipment is damaged. **E**
8 Isolate the palpable lesion between fingers.	To enable clinician to localize lesion and assess depth and position. **E**
9 Apply alcohol handrub and apply sterile gloves.	Sterile gloves form part of aseptic technique. Aseptic technique should be followed for any procedure that breaches the body's natural defences (Loveday et al. 2014, **C**).

Procedure

Action	Rationale
10 Clean the area of patient's skin to be anaesthetized with the locally agreed cleansing solution.	To reduce risk of contamination from skin flora (Gould 2012, **E**; Scales 2009, **E**).

(continued)

Procedure guideline 1.9   Core breast biopsy *(continued)*

Action	Rationale
11 Inform the patient that a local anaesthetic will be administered intradermally and subcutaneously and that it can result in a 'stinging' sensation.	To inform patient and manage anxiety (Rocha et al. 2013, **C**).
12 Draw up and then inject lidocaine 1% 2–3 cm from lesion.	The local anaesthetic should be injected up to the lesion and backwards along the path of the needle to reduce discomfort (Rocha et al. 2013, **C**).
13 Check that the area to be incised is numb by asking patient if any pain is felt by touching the skin with a sterile needle prior to the procedure.	To reassure patient that the local anaesthetic works (Rocha et al. 2013, **C**).
14 Pick up sterile scalpel blade with dominant hand.	Ensure that dominant hand is free and practitioner is in the best position to make incision (Rocha et al. 2013, **C**).
15 Localize the lesion by holding a small area of skin taut between thumb and forefinger of the non-dominant hand. Then, using the scalpel blade, break the integrity of the dermal layers. Incise scalpel blade to a depth of 5 mm maximum (**Action figure 15**).	To allow entry of biopsy needle into breast tissue beneath dermal layers (Rocha et al. 2013, **C**).
16 Withdraw scalpel blade and release skin.	To allow entry of biopsy needle into breast tissue beneath dermal layers (Rocha et al. 2013, **C**).
17 Pick up 14 G biopsy device with dominant hand and draw back into 'cocked' position.	14 G biopsy needle obtains greater sensitivity than 16 G or 18 G without increasing cost (Rocha et al. 2013, **C**; Wallis et al. 2006 **C**).
18 Introduce the biopsy needle through the puncture site in the dermis and advance toward the palpable lesion while isolating the lesion and fixing between the thumb and finger of the non-dominant hand.	Isolating the lesion with non-dominant hand enables the practitioner to map the position of the lesion and to gauge where the biopsy needle is in relation to it (Rocha et al. 2013, **C**).
19 Once the biopsy needle is appropriately positioned, at least 2–3 cm away from the lesion but directed at it, release the mechanism which propels the needle forward into the lesion. Ensure that the path of the biopsy needle is running parallel or oblique to deeper structures.	The biopsy apparatus allows for the hollow biopsy needle to be 'fired' into the lesion. If the needle is too close before the apparatus is deployed, the core may be taken from tissue beyond the target lesion. The practitioner must be aware of the length of throw of the biopsy needle. (Rocha et al. 2013, **C**).
20 Withdraw the needle and ask assistant to apply pressure to wound until no signs of bleeding.	Withdraw the needle in order to access the sample (Rocha et al. 2013, **C**). Applying pressure helps to stop bleeding. **E**
21 Move the biopsy needle above the sample pot containing formalin and draw back the cocking apparatus once to expose the core biopsy. Use sterile needle to move biopsy from needle into the sample pot.	Formalin fixes the tissue and preserves cellular architecture and composition ready for subsequent examination (Fox et al. 1985, **E**). Avoid crush artefact of biopsy core. **E**
22 Repeat steps 19–21 to obtain minimum of 4 cores if possible. Angle the biopsy needle through the lesion in different planes to increase representativeness of sample.	The number of cores obtained may vary as lesions are not always uniform and a higher number of samples increases the accuracy of the result (Wallis et al. 2006, **C**).
23 Once the required number of samples is obtained discard the biopsy device/needle in a sharps bin.	To reduce risk of sharps injury (RCN 2013, **C**).
24 Ensure pressure is correctly being applied by assistant and there is no active bleeding.	To reduce incidence of haematoma post procedure (Rocha et al. 2013, **C**).

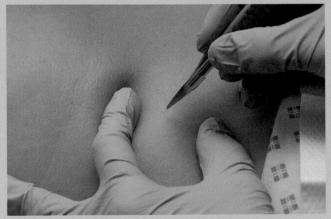

Action Figure 15 Biopsy site skin stretched.

Post-procedure

25	Close sample pot and ensure lid is on securely.	To ensure that sample remains in pot and is uncontaminated (WHO 2015, **C**).
26	Ensure correct patient identifier label is on the sample pot.	To ensure that the result is ascribed to correct patient. This should be done immediately and by the practitioner (NMC 2010a, **C**).
27	Inspect the puncture site before applying the dressing.	To ensure that the puncture point has sealed and that bleeding has stopped (Rocha et al. 2013, **C**).
28	Steri-Strips should be applied to close the wound.	To aid healing of the wound and minimize the risk of infection (Rocha et al. 2013, **C**).
29	Apply a sterile dressing over the Steri-Strips with pressure to continue compression.	To aid healing of the wound and minimize the risk of infection (Rocha et al. 2013, **C**).
30	Remove gloves and discard waste in the correct containers, for example sharps into a designated receptacle.	To ensure safe disposal and avoid injury to other members of staff or the public (DH 2013, **C**; HSE 2003 **C**).
31	Complete request form and place sample pot together with form.	To ensure that the result is ascribed to the correct patient. Ensure correct side of body is recorded and that clinical details are correct as this may help pathological interpretation (NMC 2010a, **C**; WHO 2015, **C**).
32	Ask the patient to re-dress.	To ensure dignity and privacy. **E**
33	Ensure that the patient is comfortable and arrange to be observed for swelling at biopsy site, bleeding through dressing or systematic symptoms such as dizziness or nausea for 30 minutes following injection of local anaesthetic.	To monitor for signs that may indicate adverse reaction to the local anaesthetic such as confusion, respiratory depression and hypersensitivity (Rocha et al. 2013, **C**).
34	Assess covered biopsy site after 30 minutes for signs of bleeding.	To ensure that the puncture point has sealed and that bleeding has stopped (Rocha et al. 2013, **C**).

Breast fine-needle aspiration (FNA)

Rationale

Fine-needle aspiration will provide cells for cytological assessment rather than a block of tissue. As the information available from cytology is less detailed, a biopsy is considered the best approach. However, FNA is performed if the lesion is positioned in such a way that a biopsy may be more hazardous to the patient. An FNA is also the standard pathological investigation for initial assessment of a lymph node. Standard cytological assessment will confirm whether cells are benign or malignant and this is satisfactory for benign outcomes.

Indications

FNA is the second choice for obtaining a pathological sample. It is indicated in the following situations:

- Where the presenting lesion is considered to be a lymph node rather than a breast lesion.
- Where the index lesion is located in a technically difficult area to biopsy.
- Where the biopsy may carry more risk.
- Where the area to be assessed is below the size suitable for a core biopsy.
- If the patient is on anticoagulant therapy with INR outside of range (>4) and said therapy cannot be stopped (BSBR 2012). Patients undergoing an FNA do not need to have INR checked or therapy stopped.

Contraindications

- Position and location of lesion that is inaccessible with FNA.

Procedure guideline 1.10   Breast fine-needle aspiration (FNA)

Essential equipment

- Procedure trolley
- Sterile dressing pack
- Sterile gloves
- Plastic apron
- Swab saturated with chlorhexidine in 70% alcohol (ChloraPrep), or isopropyl alcohol 70% (ChloraPrep)
- Sterile syringe (10 mL)
- Sterile needles (23 G/25 G)
- 4 glass slides
- Pencil

- Slide container
- Fixative
- Universal container with normal saline
- Cytology request form
- Sterile gauze
- Sterile dressing, e.g. Mepore

Medicinal products

- 10 mL sodium chloride 0.9% ampoule

Pre-procedure

Action	Rationale
1 Explain the procedure to the patient.	To ensure that the patient understands the procedure and gives his/her valid consent (RCN 2017b, **C**).
2 Check that the identity of the patient matches the details on the patient notes.	To ensure that the sample is correctly labelled (RCN 2017b, **C**).

(continued)

44 | **Procedure guideline 1.10** Breast fine-needle aspiration (FNA) *(continued)*

Action	Rationale
3 Ascertain whether the patient is allergic to skin cleanser, adhesive plaster or local anaesthetic.	To prevent an allergic skin reaction (NMC 2010b, **C**).
4 Check patient's medications. The patient should be asked if they are taking anticoagulants.	To ensure any contraindications are considered and appropriate management is in place regarding anticoagulants (BSBR 2012, **C**; Chetlen et al. 2013, **E**).
5 Ask the patient to change into the gown and position the patient on the couch in a position that facilitates access to the site requiring biopsy.	To ensure the patient is comfortable and to ensure safety should the patient feel faint during the procedure. **E**
6 Carefully wash hands using bactericidal soap and water, and dry before commencement. Or decontaminate physically clean hands with alcohol-based handrub.	To minimize risk of infection (RCN 2017a, **C**).
7 Check all packaging for use-by date. Open and prepare the equipment on the procedure trolley.	To maintain asepsis throughout and check that no equipment is damaged. **E**
8 Use alcohol handrub once again and put on sterile gloves.	Sterile gloves form part of aseptic technique. Aseptic technique should be followed for any procedure that breaches the body's natural defences (Loveday et al. 2014, **C**).
9 Attach the 10mL syringe to the sterile 14G needle and replace onto sterile area.	The syringe is to enable the practitioner to create a vacuum effect. **E**

Procedure

Action	Rationale
10 Clean the area of patient's skin to be anaesthetized with the locally agreed cleansing solution.	To reduce risk of contamination from skin flora (Gould 2012, **E**; Scales 2009, **E**).
11 Palpate and fix the clinical lesion between the fingers of your non-dominant hand.	To enable practitioner to map lesion and better position the needle. **E**
12 Warn the patient that the needle aspiration is about to be performed.	To manage patient anxiety and expectation. **E**
13 Introduce the needle into the approximate area of the lesion.	To ensure that cells are retrieved from the correct area (Wright 2012, **E**; Fornage et al. 2014, **E**).
14 Once the needle is inserted, pull back on the syringe approximately 3–4mL in order to create a vacuum.	The vacuum ensures that cells cut from the lesion by the needle are pulled back into the hollow core of the needle (Wright 2012, **E**; Fornage et al. 2014, **E**).
15 Keeping the vacuum in place, move the needle backwards and forwards through the lesion without removing the needle from the breast entirely.	Repeated passes through the target lesion ensure a higher chance of obtaining representative cells (Wright 2012, **E**; Fornage et al. 2014, **C**).
16 Release the vacuum gently by allowing the syringe to return to normal state.	Vacuum should be released while the needle is still within the breast to stop the obtained cells from being pulled up into the barrel of the syringe. Cells within the barrel of the syringe cannot be transferred to the slide (Wright 2012, **E**; Fornage et al. 2014, **C**).
17 Withdraw needle from breast once vacuum fully released and release skin being held by non-dominant hand.	Withdraw needle in order to release cells onto slide (Wright 2012, **E**; Fornage et al. 2014, **C**).
18 Ensure gauze and pressure are applied to the puncture site by an assistant while you are able to complete procedure away from patient.	To minimize bleeding and bruising (Wright 2012, **E**; Fornage et al. 2014, **C**).
19 In order to get cellular material from needle onto slide, disconnect needle from syringe and fill syringe with air by pulling the plunger back.	To gain air into syringe, which will expel cells from barrel of needle onto slide (Wright 2012, **E**; Fornage et al. 2014, **C**).
20 Reconnect syringe to the needle while ensuring the sharp is facing away from you and you are steadying the needle by the plastic cuff.	To gain air into syringe, which will expel cells from barrel of needle onto slide (Wright 2012, **E**; Fornage et al. 2014, **C**).
21 Push air from syringe back through the needle with needle directed at slide.	To expel cells onto slide (Wright 2012, **E**; Fornage et al. 2014, **C**).
22 Repeat steps 19 and 21 onto 4 slides if there is enough material.	

Post-procedure

Action	Rationale
23 Spread cell sample on each slide nusing a clean slide to apply gentle downward pressure and glide along the stained slide.	To spread cellular material out and achieve a monolayer. Clumping of cells will mask results (Wright 2012, **E**; Fornage et al. 2014, **C**).

24	If 4 good samples appear to have been obtained, 2 should be air dried and 2 should be fixed with formalin.	To achieve clear slides with intact cells for assessment. **E**
25	Label all slides with patient identifying details, procedure description and date using a pencil.	To ensure results are ascribed to correct patient. Pen will wash off in laboratory work-up so pencil must be used, **E** (NMC 2010a, **C**).
26	Place slides into slide container and label the outside of this with patient ID label.	To ensure results ascribed to correct patient (WHO 2015, **C**).
27	Use needles to draw up sodium chloride 0.9% into the syringe and then to push out sodium chloride into the universal container.	To obtain any cellular material that has been pulled up into barrel of syringe and to clean all material from needle barrel. **E**
28	Label universal container with patient identifying details, procedure description, location and date/time.	To ensure results are ascribed to correct patient (NMC 2010a, **C**).
29	Inspect skin wound and apply small sterile plaster.	To ensure that bleeding has stopped and that pressure can be released (Wright 2012, **E**; Fornage et al. 2014, **C**).
30	Remove gloves and discard waste in the correct containers, for example sharps into a designated receptacle.	To ensure safe disposal and avoid injury to other members of staff or the public (DH 2013, **C**; HSE 2003, **C**).
31	Advise patient to remove plaster later that day or the following day.	To manage anxiety and reassure patient. **E**
32	Ensure arrangements are made for patient to come back for or receive results as per local guidelines.	To manage anxiety and expectations. **E**
33	Ensure patient has an awareness of possible results expected.	To ensure good communication and manage expectations (ABS 2010, **C**).
34	Ensure patient can contact appropriate person if they experience any difficulties following the fine-needle aspiration.	To manage anxiety. **E**

Breast punch biopsy

A punch biopsy is a less invasive method in comparison to a core biopsy. It enables the nurse to take a specimen where the cutaneous (skin) layers are involved.

Indication
- Where the index lesion is involving cutaneous tissue.
- Locally advanced fungating lesions.

Contraindications
- Known sensitivity to local anaesthetic agents.
- Evidence of active infection may delay timing of biopsy unless the area is a fungating lesion which is chronically infected.

Procedure guideline 1.11   Breast punch biopsy

Essential equipment
- Procedure trolley
- Sterile dressing pack
- Non-sterile gloves
- Plastic apron
- Swab saturated with chlorhexidine in 70% alcohol (Chlora-Prep), or isopropyl alcohol 70%
- Sterile syringe (2 mL)
- Sterile needles (23 G/25 G)
- Punch biopsy instrument (3 or 4 mm)
- Sterile iris scissors
- Histology pot
- Histology form
- Sterile gauze
- Steri-Strips
- Sterile dressing

Medicinal products
- Lidocaine hydrochloride injection BP 1% w/v

Procedure

Action	Rationale
1 Explain the procedure to the patient.	To ensure that the patient understands the procedure and gives his/her valid consent (RCN 2017b, **C**).
2 Check that the identity of the patient matches the details on the patient notes.	To ensure that the sample is correctly labelled (RCN 2017b, **C**).
3 Ascertain whether the patient is allergic to skin cleanser, adhesive plaster or local anaesthetic.	To prevent an allergic skin reaction (NMC 2010b, **C**).
4 Check patient's medications. The patient should be asked if they are taking anticoagulants.	To ensure any contraindications are considered and appropriate management is in place regarding anticoagulants (BSBR 2012, **C**; Chetlen et al. 2013, **E**).
5 Ask the patient to change into the gown and position the patient on the couch in a position that facilitates access to the site requiring biopsy.	To ensure the patient is comfortable and to ensure safety should the patient feel faint during the procedure. **E**

(continued)

46 | **Procedure guideline 1.11**   Breast punch biopsy *(continued)*

Action	Rationale
6 Carefully wash hands using bactericidal soap and water; dry before commencement. Or decontaminate physically clean hands with alcohol-based handrub.	To minimize risk of infection (RCN 2017a, **C**).
7 Check all packaging for use-by date. Open and prepare the equipment on the procedure trolley.	To maintain asepsis throughout and check that no equipment is damaged. **E**
8 Position the patient on the couch in a position that facilitates access to the site requiring biopsy.	To ensure the patient is comfortable and to ensure safety should the patient feel faint during the procedure. **E**
9 Select the area to be biopsied. Commonly selected sites are the most abnormal-appearing site within a lesion or the edge of an actively growing lesion. Position of resultant scar should also be borne in mind.	To obtain a good representative tissue sample and minimize scar effect (Zuber 2002, **E**).
10 Select the appropriate size punch biopsy instrument. Punch biopsy needles range from 2 to 10 mm. 3–4 mm is usually sufficient for a good sample size.	To ensure that an adequate sample is taken (Zuber 2002, **E**).
11 Wash hands and put on non-sterile gloves.	To minimize risk of infection (RCN 2017a, **C**).

Procedure

Action	Rationale
12 Clean the area of patient's skin to be anaesthetized with the locally agreed cleansing solution.	To reduce risk of contamination from skin flora (Gould 2012, **E**; Scales 2009, **E**).
13 Inform the patient that a local anaesthetic will be administered and that it can result in a 'stinging' sensation.	To ensure the patient is fully informed and is aware of what to expect (Rocha et al. 2013, **C**).
14 Draw up lidocaine 1% in 5 mL syringe through 14 G needle.	To ensure the correct preparation. **E**
15 Inject lidocaine slowly into subdermal tissues.	To minimize pain or discomfort for the patient undergoing a punch biopsy of the nipple or cutaneous breast lesion (Zuber 2002, **E**).
16 Check that the area to be biopsied is numb by asking patient if any pain is felt when touching the skin with a sterile needle prior to the procedure.	To assess the effectiveness of the local anaesthetic prior to making the incision, to ensure that the procedure is pain free (Rocha et al. 2013, **E**).
17 When satisfied that the area to be biopsied is anaesthetized, the skin surrounding the biopsy site is stretched with the thumb and index finger of the non-dominant hand.	To stabilize the area before performing the punch biopsy. When the skin relaxes after the biopsy is performed, an elliptical-shaped wound remains. **E**
18 Warn the patient that the punch biopsy instrument is about to be placed on the skin of the breast/nipple and that they may feel a pushing sensation.	To reduce the risk of the patient moving, and to prepare them for what to expect. **E**
19 The punch biopsy needle should be held vertically over the skin by the dominant hand and rotated downward using a twirling motion created by the first two fingers on the dominant hand (**Action figure 19**). Once the instrument has penetrated the dermis into the subcutaneous fat, or once the instrument reaches the hub, it can be removed carefully and removed from the patient. The sample does not come away with the biopsy needle.	To obtain an adequate specimen from the appropriate area (Zuber 2002, **E**).

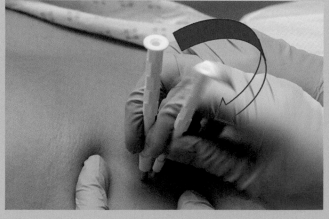

Action Figure 19 Punch biopsy technique.

| 20 | Ensure safe disposal of biopsy needle into sharps container. | To ensure safe disposal and avoid injury to other members of staff or the public (DH 2013, **C**; HSE 2003, **C**). |
| 21 | Using the local anaesthetic needle held in the non-dominant hand, raise the cylindrical skin specimen from the biopsy site. The use of forceps is discouraged. Iris scissors held in the dominant hand can be used to cut the specimen free from the subcutaneous tissues. The cut should be made below the level of the dermis. | To retrieve a good, intact sample and to avoid crush artefact or damage to the sample (Zuber 2002, **E**). |

Post-procedure

22	Place sterile gauze onto the biopsy site and apply digital pressure until bleeding has ceased.	To reduce the risk of leakage and to allow the puncture site to close (Rocha et al. 2013, **C**).
23	The specimen should then be placed into an appropriate formalin container, and labelled with the patient details, area biopsied, side, date and time.	Formalin fixes the tissue and preserves cellular architecture and composition ready for subsequent examination (Fox et al. 1985, **E**). To ensure that the specimen is assigned to the correct patient. **E**
24	Inspect the puncture site before applying the dressing.	To ensure that the puncture point has sealed and that bleeding has stopped (Rocha et al. 2013, **E**).
25	Steri-Strips should be applied to close the wound.	To aid healing of the wound and minimize the risk of infection (Rocha et al. 2013, **E**).
26	Apply a sterile dressing over the Steri-Strips with pressure to continue compression.	To aid healing of the wound and minimize the risk of infection (Rocha et al. 2013, **E**).
27	Remove gloves and discard waste in the correct containers, for example sharps into a designated receptacle.	To ensure safe disposal and avoid injury to other members of staff or the public (DH 2013, **C**; HSE 2003, **C**).
28	Ensure that the patient is comfortable and arrange to be observed for bleeding through dressing or systematic symptoms such as dizziness or nausea for 30 minutes following injection of local anaesthetic.	To monitor for signs that may indicate adverse reaction to the local anaesthetic such as confusion, respiratory depression and hypersensitivity (Rocha et al. 2013, **E**). To monitor for continued bleeding (Rocha et al. 2013, **E**).

Nipple discharge smear

A nipple discharge smear is undertaken to exclude underlying breast pathology. Nipple discharge can be physiological. Normal cytology results should show a cellular specimen. The presence of ductal epithelial cells is cause for further investigation.

Indications

Λ cytological smear should be sent if one or more of the following criteria are met:

- nipple discharge is:
  - spontaneous
  - bloodstained
  - unilateral and/or uniductal.
- no target lesion palpable or visible on imaging.

Procedure guideline 1.12   Nipple discharge smear

Essential equipment
- Fixative
- Apron
- Non-sterile gloves
- 2 glass slides
- Slide container
- Pencil
- Cytology request form

Pre-procedure

Action	Rationale
1 Inform patient that the intention is to try to elicit nipple discharge for specimen.	To reduce anxieties and manage expectations. **E**
2 Ask patient to remove upper clothes, including bra, behind curtain or screen. Provide a gown for use.	To enable ease of visible inspection and palpation. **E** Provide gown to maintain personal dignity (RCN 2008, **C**).
3 Wash hands with soap and water, dry hands and apply apron and non-sterile gloves.	To minimize risk of infection or cross-contamination (RCN 2017a, **C**).

Procedure

| 4 Gently squeeze the nipple between the thumb and index finger with constant pressure. | In order to elicit discharge, which will come from ducts immediately behind nipple (Derbis and Scott-Connor 2011, **E**). |
| 5 If discharge is seen, make a note of colour and whether it originates from a single duct or multiple. | In order to inform overall clinical impression, assist in diagnosis and assist cytologist in their assessment. **E** |

(continued)

Procedure guideline 1.12   Nipple discharge smear *(continued)*

Action	Rationale
6 Take a clean slide and smear the discharge onto the slide with a single wiping motion.	To transfer discharge cleanly from nipple to slide (Derbis and Scott-Connor 2011, **E**).
7 Apply a second clean slide onto the stained slide and apply gentle and constant downward pressure as you glide the clean slide over the stained one.	To achieve monolayer of cells if cells are present. Clumping of cells will obscure results (Derbis and Scott-Connor 2011, **E**).
Post-procedure	
8 Immediately fix slides with fixative by flooding slide with 95% alcohol solution.	To preserve cell architecture for assessment (Derbis and Scott-Connor 2011, **E**).
9 Give the patient some tissue to wipe the breast.	To help preserve dignity. **E**
10 Label the slides with correct patient demographic information, what the slide is of, and which side discharge is from as well as date.	To ensure results are ascribed to correct patient (Derbis & Scott-Connor 2011, **E**).
11 Remove and dispose of apron and gloves.	To ensure safe disposal and avoid injury to other members of staff or the public (DH 2013, **C**; HSE 2003, **C**).
12 Complete request form.	To ensure results are ascribed to correct patient and to inform cytologist of clinical picture. **E**
13 Ensure patient is aware of plans to get results.	To manage anxiety and expectations. **E**

Post-procedural considerations

Immediate care
Observation of possible complications such as bleeding or infection should be monitored (Rocha et al. 2013).

Education of the patient and relevant others
The patient should be given adequate post-procedural instructions, including care of the biopsy site over the initial 4–48 hours. A contact number should also be provided should any complications arise.

Genetic testing

Definition
Genetic testing assesses the risk of cancer for a specific group of patients and their family. Cancer risk management advice is given to individuals and families who are known to have, or are suspected to have, an increased risk of cancer compared with the general population, due to heritable (germline) mutations in their DNA. Genetic testing is currently available for faults in genes that cause an increased risk of breast, bowel, ovarian, uterine and prostate cancer. Genetic tests are also available for rare faults in genes that may increase the risk of kidney, skin (melanoma), pancreatic and thyroid cancer and retinoblastoma. Initially a blood test is taken followed by assessment, history taking and counselling (Cancer Research UK 2016, Kirk 2005, Kumar and Clark 2016).

Related theory

Important genetic concepts and terminology
In order to provide patients with accurate information and appreciate when a referral to the cancer genetic department would be helpful it is essential to understand the difference between germline and somatic genetic testing.

  Germline testing. This refers to a genetic test that looks for mutations (harmful variants) in genes that people were born with and that may cause an increased risk of cancer. Germline mutations are present in every cell of the person's body, including the reproductive cells of the ova and sperm, meaning that such mutations can be passed down from parent to child (inherited) (Balmain et al. 2003). An example of a germline genetic test is a *BRCA1/2* mutation screen undertaken in a breast cancer patient who has a strong family history of breast cancer.

  Somatic testing. This refers to a genetic test undertaken on the tumour sample of a cancer patient. This type of test looks at the mutations in genes of the tumour cells. These mutations are specific to the tumour cells, would not be found in normal (non-cancerous) cells in the person's body and would not be passed down from parent to child (Stratton et al. 2009). There will be many mutations within the genes of a tumour sample and these mutations are acquired not inherited. Somatic genetic test results can be used to determine treatment options.

Two examples of common somatic gene tests are:

- *HER2* testing in breast cancer. HER2 status is used as a prognostic indicator and to plan treatment, for example HER2-positive patients will benefit from trastuzumab treatment (Wolf et al. 2013).
- *BRAF* testing in metastatic melanoma. A targeted treatment has been developed which is effective specifically for patients with a BRAF mutation in their tumour (Yu et al. 2015).

The genome refers to an organism's complete set of genetic information, including all of the genes. Each genome contains all of the information that organism requires to function. In humans the genome is made up of over 3 billion DNA base pairs and contains over 20,000 genes. Genes make up only approximately 1–5% of the genome. The rest of the DNA is important for regulating the genes and the genome. There is still a lot to learn about how the genome functions (Genomics England 2016).

  In the oncology setting the cancer genome refers to the sequencing of the genes within a tumour sample. The catalogue of mutations within a tumour is specific to that tumour, and the range and types of mutations provide information to cancer researchers and to clinicians treating the patient (Stratton et al. 2009).

Understanding genetic terminology

A cancer predisposition gene is a gene in which germline mutations confer highly or moderately increased risks of cancer (Rahman 2014). For the purposes of this chapter this refers to genes in which rare mutations confer high or moderate risks of cancer (>2-fold relative risks) and at least 5% of individuals with relevant mutations develop cancer (Rahman 2014). A mutation is defined as a permanent change in the DNA sequence (Richards et al. 2015) and this change is also called a variant. Colloquially, 'mutation' is often used to describe a disease-causing (pathogenic) variant in a particular gene (e.g. the patient has a *BRCA1* mutation). However, the genes of any individual will contain many variants and most variants are not harmful (Richards et al. 2015).

Variants can be pathogenic, probably pathogenic, variation of uncertain significance (VUS), likely benign or benign. Pathogenic variants, and probably pathogenic variants are disease-causing changes in the DNA sequence. Information about these variants can be taken into account when assessing genetic risk and making healthcare decisions. Benign and probably benign variants are not harmful and would not be taken into account when assessing genetic risk. Variants of uncertain significance are changes in the DNA code that may or may not be harmful, but there is insufficient evidence to understand how the change in the DNA sequence may alter the function of the gene. The presence of a VUS should not change the management of the patient (Richards et al. 2015).

What proportion of cancer is inherited?

All cancer is caused by the accumulation of pathogenic mutations in the DNA within a cell. Genetic mutations may be acquired (occurring during someone's lifetime) or inherited (also called germline mutations). Most cancer occurs as a result of acquired DNA damage, for example in response to environmental factors such as smoking and radiation. These cancers are called 'sporadic' cancers. Only 2–3% of cancers are linked to inherited pathogenic mutations – they are a very rare cause of cancer, overall (Cancer Research UK 2016, Kluijt et al. 2012). There are specific types of cancer where a small proportion of cases are due to an inherited mutation (Table 1.7).

Most patients with cancer will not require genetic input or testing as most cancers are sporadic. However, it is important to be able to recognize patients who may benefit from a genetics referral, to know how make a referral and to be able to communicate with patients about what to expect at their genetics appointment.

It is also useful to be able to know where to access reliable information about cancer genetics (Kirk 2005).

Rationale

Most germline genetic testing is arranged through a clinical cancer genetics service. The patient's personal history of cancer and their family history of cancer are assessed to determine the likelihood of identifying a germline mutation. If the chance of finding a mutation in a specific cancer predisposition gene or group of genes is significant (usually if there is at least a 10% chance), genetic testing is offered (Jacobs et al. 2014). This information is important for the person undergoing testing as it may inform current or future cancer treatments, preventative options and screening recommendations.

It is also important for the wider family as testing can be carried out in blood relatives to identify who else is at risk and to advise on risk management options. Wherever possible, genetic testing is offered to the patient affected by the cancer, rather than their unaffected relative, in the first instance. If a germline mutation in a cancer predisposition gene is identified, so-called 'predictive' genetic testing can then be offered to the unaffected relatives of the patient (Jacobs et al. 2014) to provide them with genetic information about their risk. It is important that genetic counselling is provided to people considering genetic testing so that a person is informed about all possible outcomes of the genetic test.

Indications

It is important to identify a person who might benefit from genetic services and information. Genetic testing would be undertaken in a person with a strong personal or family history of cancer where the chance of finding a mutation is significant. This is usually if there is at least a 10% chance. Specific clinical features and patterns of cancers in the family that indicate that a genetic referral is warranted are as follows (ACOG 2015, ICR 2016).

In the cancer patient

- Earlier than average age of onset of cancer (e.g. prostate cancer in a man under 50).
- Multiple primary cancers in an individual (e.g. breast and ovarian cancer or bowel and endometrial cancer).
- Bilateral or multifocal disease (e.g. bilateral kidney cancer).
- Specific types of cancer:
  - medullary thyroid cancer
  - triple negative breast cancer

Table 1.7 Proportion of cancer that is inherited

Type of cancer	Population lifetime risk (men)	Population lifetime risk (women)	Proportion of cases estimated to be due to rare inherited mutations
Breast	Rare	1 in 8	5–10% (for women)
Bowel	1 in 14	1 in 19	5–10%
Lung	1 in 13	1 in 17	Not known
Endometrial	n/a	1 in 41	5–10%
Cervical	n/a	1 in 135 (invasive)	Not known
Ovarian	n/a	1 in 52	10%
Prostate	1 in 8	n/a	5–10%
Thyroid	1 in 480	1 in 180	
Medullary thyroid	5–10 in 100 of thyroid cancers		25%
Pancreas	1 in 71		10%
Retinoblastoma	Rare		33%
Melanoma	1 in 54		5–10%

Source: Adapted from Cancer Research UK (2016), Eeles et al. (2014), Leachman et al. (2009); Lu et al. (2007).
n/a, not applicable.

– ovarian, fallopian tube or primary peritoneal cancers
– colorectal cancer with mismatch repair deficiency
– endometrial cancer with mismatch repair deficiency
– retinoblastoma
– adrenocortical cancer
– male breast cancer.

In the cancer patient's family

- Several close relatives from the same side of the family (i.e. related by blood, not marriage) who have been diagnosed with similar cancer or with related cancers (e.g. breast and ovarian or bowel and endometrial cancer).
- One or more close relatives diagnosed at an unusually young age.
- A pattern or more than one case of a less common or rare cancer (e.g. medullary thyroid).
- Pattern of childhood cancers in siblings (Cancer Research UK 2016, Kirk 2005, Kumar and Clark 2016).

Contraindications

- Genetic testing would not be undertaken where the chance of finding a mutation is very low.
- Where a person is uncertain whether they wish to undergo testing.

Legal and professional issues

Genetic tests for cancer predisposition genes should only be requested by health professionals with adequate training in genetic counselling and in interpreting genetic test results. Genetic testing is usually only carried out by clinical geneticists, genetic counsellors and genetic nurses. In some settings genetic tests are ordered by oncologists as part of a patient's diagnostic and treatment pathway, working in close collaboration with a cancer genetics unit.

Genetic competency standards for nurses

The Department of Health commissioned educational guidelines for nurses in 2003 (Kirk et al.), which were revised and updated in 2011 (Kirk et al. 2011a) to establish the skills and knowledge nurses need to have about genetics to be able to benefit their patients. Seven competency standards were agreed as a part of this work (Box 1.3). It is important that nurses identify those who are at risk for or susceptible to genetic–genomic conditions as well as genomic technologies used in the diagnosis and management of diseases such as cancer (Kirk et al. 2011b).

Box 1.3 Genetic testing skills for nurses, midwives and health visitors at registration

1. Identify clients who might benefit from genetic services and information (Gaff 2005).
2. Appreciate the importance of sensitivity in tailoring genetic information and services to clients' culture, knowledge and language level (Middleton et al. 2005).
3. Uphold the rights of all clients to informed decision making and voluntary action (Haydon 2005).
4. Demonstrate a knowledge and understanding of the role of genetic and other factors in maintaining health and in the manifestation, modification and prevention of disease expression, to underpin effective practice (Kirk 2005).
5. Demonstrate a knowledge and understanding of the utility and limitations of genetic testing and information (Bradley 2005).
6. Recognize the limitations of one's own genetics expertise (Benjamin and Gamet 2005).
7. Obtain and communicate credible, current information about genetics, for self, clients and colleagues (Skirton and Barnes 2005).

Consent and confidentiality

Clinical information regarding genetic test results and family histories of cancer is relevant to both the cancer patient and their unaffected relatives. There are nationally agreed guidelines for obtaining correct consent for verifying family histories of cancer and sharing genetic test results and for protecting the confidential information of the patient whilst allowing all at-risk relatives to benefit from genetic risk assessments and test results (Royal College of Physicians, Royal College of Pathologists and British Society for Human Genetics 2011). Patients may express concerns about confidentiality. It is important to inform patients that genetic notes are kept separate from the main hospital notes so confidential genetic information about themselves and their relatives is only available to the genetics team (Skirton and Barnes 2005).

Pre-procedural considerations

Assessment and recording tools

A family history can be recorded using a family history questionnaire or by drawing a 'family tree' or 'pedigree' (Figure 1.17). This can either be done on paper or using specialist computer programs designed to collect family history information (Bennett et al. 1995). The patient's family history is an important tool in determining the likelihood of an inherited cancer predisposition in the patient and their family. Where an inherited cancer predisposition is suspected a referral to a genetics unit would be indicated.

Patients are given a family history questionnaire to complete by the genetics team, ideally ahead of their genetics appointments. Information from this questionnaire is recorded on a pedigree and further details about the family history are recorded on the pedigree at the genetics appointment. The patient is asked to provide information about their relatives' names, dates of birth, dates of death and cancer or other significant medical history, and this information is recorded on the pedigree. The genetics team may also ask the patient to provide copies of death certificates or ask relatives to provide written consent to access their medical records (Bennett et al. 1995).

Non-pharmacological support

Patients seen in the cancer genetic clinic are offered information about their cancer risks and presented with options for genetic testing and/or risk management strategies, if appropriate. The genetics team works with the patient to help them make autonomous choices and to adjust to their genetic risk. This communication process may take place over several appointments over several months or consist of one or two appointments. It is important to tailor information to a specific client's personal situation by listening to and acknowledging an individual's prior experience, recognizing that ethnicity, culture, religion and ethical perspectives may influence their ability to utilize information and services. Communication strategies need to be adapted in relation to the individual's level of understanding of genetic issues (Middleton et al. 2005).

Potential benefits of a genetic risk assessment

When speaking to a patient about a cancer genetic referral, explain the reason for the referral and outline what can be expected at the appointment. Patients may be unaware of the benefits of a referral or that a genetic assessment may have significant implications for their relatives. Before a patient is offered genetic testing they will be provided with information about the condition, the chance of a positive result and the implications of a positive result both for themselves and for their family.

For the cancer patient

- Genetic risk assessment provides an assessment of the genetic basis for their cancer diagnosis.
- Assesses genetic risk to advise on long-term cancer surveillance after treatment.

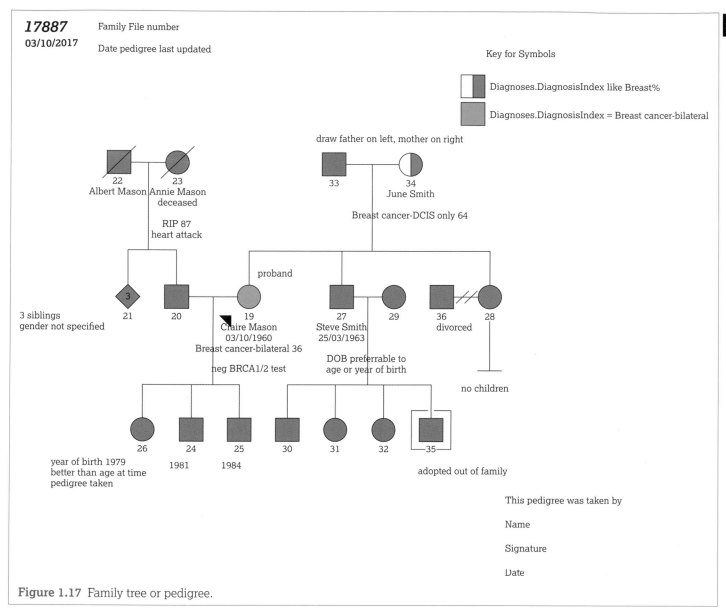

Figure 1.17 Family tree or pedigree.

- May offer genetic testing for germline mutations.
- Assists targeted treatment of cancer based on presence/absence of a germline mutation.
- Provides risk management options that may include the option of risk-reducing surgery.
- Clarifies cancer risk for offspring, siblings, parents and extended family.

For at-risk relatives
- Genetic risk assessment provides an understanding of how their family history of cancer alters their personal risk of cancer.
- Genetic testing for familial germline mutations may clarify their personal risk of cancer.
- Risk management options may include risk-reducing surgery and/or long-term cancer surveillance.
- Knowledge of a germline mutation may influence treatment planning if an at-risk relative develops cancer in the future.
- Cancer risk for offspring, siblings, parents and extended family is assessed (British Society of Genetic Medicine 2016).

Genetic referrals
It is imperative that any referral is discussed with the patient and they agree to the referral. The genetic testing, which is obtained via a blood test, may be offered as part of the risk assessment undertaken at the appointment. However it is not always indicated. The results may take several weeks to process depending on the type of genetic test. Genetics centres will usually accept a referral from any healthcare professional. It does not have to be from the GP or consultant. However, it is good practice to discuss the referral with the treating team, and document it in the patient notes. When making a referral the following information should be supplied:

- name and date of birth of patient
- details of cancer diagnosis including age at diagnosis, pathology details, treatment and surgical summary; include a copy of the histopathology report, if possible
- details on medical history including previous diagnoses of cancer or significant illnesses
- brief description of the family history of cancer including the age of initial diagnosis.

Contact details of the regional genetic services in the UK are available on the British Society for Genetic Medicine website. Each centre's website has referral criteria details and contact details for queries prior to referral (British Society of Genetic Medicine 2016).

Genetic testing for inherited cancer syndromes – future practice

It is likely that more germline genetic testing will be offered directly through oncology clinics as well as genetics clinics. Genetic testing is more likely to be offered at the time of a cancer diagnosis as information about a germline mutation in a cancer predisposition gene can be useful in planning cancer treatment including surgery and chemotherapy (George et al. 2016).

The genetic tests offered are likely to change in the future. Patients are currently offered testing for specific 'high-risk' genes only. Genetic technology has improved significantly and it is now faster and easier to screen patients for mutations in many genes at once, rather than one gene at a time. These multigene tests are often called 'panel tests'. Panel tests may include numerous high- and moderate-risk genes that may contribute to cancer risks (Hall et al. 2014, Selkirk et al. 2014).

Although it is now possible to generate a lot of genetic data using these approaches, it is important that the *clinical utility* (whether the gene test provides useful information about diagnosis, treatment, management or prevention of a disease) and *clinical validity* (whether the genetic variant is clearly linked to the presence, absence or risk of a specific disease) of such tests are determined (Easton et al. 2015). For example, the clinical validity and utility of all the genes included in a panel test need to be clearly defined so that the results of the panel test can be accurately interpreted (Hall et al. 2014, Selkirk et al. 2014). Germline and tumour genetic information will become a key feature in the management of oncology patients in the future as new tests and treatments are developed.

Websites

labtestonline
www.labtestonline.org.uk

NHS Livewell: NHS cancer screening
www.nhs.uk/Livewell/preventing-cancer/Pages/cancer-screening.aspx

Ionising Radiation Regulations 1999 (SI 3232)
www.legislation.hmso.gov.uk/si/si1999/19993232.htm

Ionising Radiation (Medical Exposure) Regulations 2000 (SI 1059)
www.legislation.hmso.gov.uk/si/si2000/20001059.htm

References

Aaronson, D., Walsh, T., Smith, J., Davies, B., Hsieh, M. & Konety, B. (2009) Meta-analysis: does lidocaine gel before flexible cystoscopy provide pain relief? *British Journal of Urology International*, 104(4), 506–510.

Aebi, S., Davidson, T., Gruber, G., & Cardoso, F. (2011) Primary breast cancer: ESMO Clinical Practice Guidelines for diagnosis, treatment and follow-up. *Annals of Oncology*, 22 (Supplement 6), vi12–vi24.

American Congress of Obstetricians and Gynecologists (ACOG) (2015) Hereditary Cancer Syndromes and Risk Assessment, Committee Opinion 634. Available at: http://www.acog.org/Resources-And-Publications/Committee-Opinions/Committee-on-Genetics/Hereditary-Cancer-Syndromes-and-Risk-Assessment (Accessed: 9/5/2018)

Aron, M., Rajeev, T.P. & Gupta, N.P. (2000) Antibiotic prophylaxis for transrectal needle biopsy of the prostate: a randomized controlled study. *British Journal of Urology International*, 85(6), 682–685.

Association for Clinical Biochemistry and Laboratory Medicine (ACB) (2013) *Recommendations as a Result of the ACB National Audit on Tumour Marker Service Provision*. London: ACB.

Association of Breast Surgery (ABS) (2010) *Best practice diagnostic guidelines for patients presenting with breast symptoms*. Available at: https://associationofbreastsurgery.org.uk/media/1416/best-practice-diagnostic-guidelines-for-patients-presenting-with-breast-symptoms.pdf (Accessed: 9/5/2018)

Aydin, M., Salukhe, T., Wilke, I. & Williams, S. (2010) Management and therapy of vasovagal syncope: a review. *World Journal of Cardiology*, 2(10), 308–315.

Balmain, A., Gray, J. & Ponder, B. (2003) The genetics and genomics of cancer. *Nature Genetics*, 33 Supp l, 238–244.

Batura, D. & Gopal Rao, G. (2013) The national burden of infections after prostate biopsy in England and Wales: a wake-up call for better prevention. *Journal of Antimicrobial Chemotherapy*, 68(2), 247–249.

Benjamin, C.M. & Gamet, K. (2005) Recognising the limitations of your genetics expertise. *Nursing Standard*, 20 (6), 49–54.

Bennett, R.L., Steinhaus, K.A., Uhrich, S.B., et al. (1995) Recommendations for standardized human pedigree nomenclature. Pedigree Standardization Task Force of the National Society of Genetic Counselors. *American Journal of Human Genetics*, 56(3), 745–752.

Bootsma, A.M., Laguna Pes, M.P., Geerlings, S.E. & Goossens, A. (2008) Antibiotic prophylaxis in urologic procedures: a systematic review. *European Urology*, 54(6), 1270–1286.

Bozlu, M., Ulusoy, E., Doruk, E., et al. (2003) Voiding impairment after prostate biopsy: does tamsulosin treatment before biopsy decrease this morbidity? *Urology*, 62, 1050–1053.

Bradley, A.N. (2005) Utility and limitations of genetic testing and information. *Nursing Standard*, 20 (5), 52–55.

Brierley, J.D., Gospodaroxicz, M.K. & Whittekind, C. (2017) *UICC TNM Classification of Malignant Tumours*, 8th edn. Oxford: Wiley Blackwell.

British Association of Urological Surgeons (BAUS) and British Association of Urological Nurses (BAUN) (2012a) *Flexible cystoscopy: training and assessment guideline*. Available at: www.baus.org.uk/_userfiles/pages/files/Publications/FlexiGuidelines.pdf (Accessed: 9/5/2018)

British Association of Urological Surgeons (BAUS) and British Association of Urological Nurses (BAUN) (2012b) *Flexible cystoscopy: performance criteria, training and logbook*. Available at: www.baus.org.uk/_userfiles/pages/files/Publications/FlexiLogbook.pdf (Accessed: 9/5/2018)

British Association of Urological Surgeons (BAUS) (2013) *Multidisciplinary Team (MDT) Guidance for Managing Bladder Cancer*, 2nd edn. London: BAUS.

British Association of Urological Surgeons (BAUS) (2017) Transrectal ultrasound-guided biopsies of the prostate gland: Information about your procedure from the British Association of Urological Surgeons (BAUS) May 2017 Leaflet 17/108. Available at: www.baus.org.uk/_userfiles/pages/files/Patients/Leaflets/TRUSP%20biopsies.pdf (Accessed: 9/5/2018)

British Society of Breast Radiology (BSBR) (2012) *Protocol for breast biopsy in patients taking anticoagulant and antiplatelet therapy*. Available at: www.bsbrsociety.org/files/8313/9895/6729/biopsy_guidelines_jul_2012.pdf (Accessed: 9/5/2018)

British Society of Genetic Medicine (2016) *Genetics centres*. Available at: www.bsgm.org.uk/information-education/genetics-centres/ (Accessed: 9/5/2018)

Cancer Research UK (2014) *Breast Cancer Statistics: Breast Cancer Incidence (Invasive)* Available at: www.cancerresearchuk.org/health-professional/cancer-statistics/statistics-by-cancer-type/breast-cancer#heading-Zero (Accessed: 9/5/2018)

Cancer Research UK (2016) *Genetic Testing for Cancer Risk*. Available at: www.cancerresearchuk.org/about-cancer/causes-of-cancer/inherited-cancer-genes-and-increased-cancer-risk/genetic-testing-for-cancer-risk (Accessed: 9/5/2018)

Carey, J.M. & Korman, H.J. (2001) Transrectal ultrasound guided biopsy of the prostate. Do enemas decrease clinically significant complications? *Journal of Urology*, 166(1), 82–85.

Challacombe, B., Dasgupta, P., Patel, U., Amoroso, P. & Kirby, R. (2011) Recognizing and managing the complications of prostate biopsy. *British Journal of Urology International*, 108(8), 1233–1234.

Chernecky, C.C. & Berger, B.J. (2013) *Laboratory Tests and Diagnostic Procedures*, 6th edn. St Louis: Elsevier.

Cherry, S.R., Sorenson, J.A. & Phelps, M.E. (2003) *Physics in Nuclear Medicine*, 3rd edn. Oxford: Saunders.

Chetlen, A.L., Kasales, C., Mack, J., Schetter, S. & Zhu, J. (2013) Hematoma formation during needle core biopsy in women taking antithrombotic therapy. *American Journal of Roentgenology, Diagnostic Imaging and Related Sciences*, 201(1), 215–222.

Chou, C.B. & Corder, A.P (2003) Core biopsy versus fine needle aspiration cytology in symptomatic breast clinic. *European Journal of Surgical Oncology*, 29(4), 374–378.

Cox, C. (2010) Legal responsibility and accountability. *Nursing Management*, 17(3), 18–20.

Derbis, F.M. & Scott-Conner, C.E.H. (2011) *Breast Surgical Techniques and Interdisciplinary Management*. Stanford: Springer.

DH (2000) *Ionising Radiation (Medical Exposure) Regulations No. 1059*. HMSO: London.

DH (2005) *Saving Lives: A Delivery Programme to Reduce Healthcare Associated Infection Including MRSA*. London: Department of Health.

DH (2009) *Reference Guide for Consent to Examination or Treatment*, 2nd edn. Available at: www.gov.uk/government/uploads/system/uploads/attachment_data/file/138296/dh_103653__1_pdf (Accessed: 9/5/2018)

DH (2013) *Environment and sustainability: Health Technical Memorandum 07-01: Safe management of healthcare waste*. London: Department of Health.

DH (2016) *Medical Radiation: Uses, Dose Measurements and Safety Advice*. London: Department of Health. Available at: www.gov.uk/government/collections/medical-radiation-uses-dose-measurements-and-safety-advice (Accessed: 9/5/2018)

Dougherty, L. & Lister, S. (2011) *The Royal Marsden Hospital Manual of Clinical Nursing Procedures*, 8th edn. Oxford: Wiley Blackwell.

Dougherty, L. & Lister, S. (2015) *The Royal Marsden Manual of Clinical Nursing Procedures*, 9th edn. Oxford: Wiley Blackwell.

Duffy, M.J. (2013) Tumour markers in clinical practice: a review focusing on common solid cancers. *Medical Principles and Practice*, 22, 4–11.

Easton, D.F., Pharoah, P.D., Antoniou, A.C., et al. (2015) Gene-panel sequencing and the prediction of breast-cancer risk. *New England Journal of Medicine*, 372(23), 2243–2257.

Eble, J., Sauter, G., Epstein, J. & Sesterhenn, I. (2004) *Pathology and Genetics of Tumours of the Urinary System and Male Genital Organs (IARC WHO Classification of Tumours)*, 1st edn. Geneva: WHO.

Eeles, R., Goh, C., Castro, E., et al. (2014) The genetic epidemiology of prostate cancer and its clinical implications. *Nature Reviews Urology*, 11(1), 18–31.

Ellis, B.W., Fawcett, D.P., Fowler, C.G., Gidlow, A. & Sounes, P. (2000) Nurse cystoscopy. Report of a working party of the British Association of Urological Surgeons, March 2000. London: BAUS.

Ellis, H. & Mahadevan, V. (2013) Anatomy and physiology of the breast. *Surgery*, 31(1), 11–14.

European Association of Urology (EAU) (2015) *Guidelines on Non-muscle-invasive Bladder Cancer (Ta, T1 and CIS)*. Available at: https://uroweb.org/wp-content/uploads/EAU-Guidelines-Non-muscle-invasive-Bladder-Cancer-2015-v1.pdf (Accessed: 9/5/2018)

European Group on Tumour Markers (EGTM) (2018) *Information about Tumour Markers by Professionals*. Available at: https://www.egtm.eu/ (Accessed: 9/5/2018)

Feliciano, J., Teper, E., Ferrandino, M., et al. (2008) The incidence of fluoroquinolone resistant infections after prostate biopsy – are fluoroquinolones still effective prophylaxis? *Journal of Urology*, 179(3), 952–925, discussion 955.

Fornage, B.D., Dogan, B.E., Sneige, N. & Staerkel, G.A. (2014) Ultrasound-guided fine-needle aspiration biopsy of internal mammary nodes: technique and preliminary results in breast cancer patients. *Vascular and Interventional Radiology Clinical Perspective*, 203(2), 213–220.

Fox, C.H., Johnson, F.B., Whiting, J. & Roller, P.P. (1985) Formaldehyde fixation. *Journal of Histochemistry and Cytochemistry*, 33(8), 845–853.

Fraise, A.P. & Bradley, T. (2009) *Ayliffe's Control of Healthcare-associated Infection: A Practical Handbook*, 5th edn. London: Hodder Arnold.

Gaff, C.L. (2005) Identifying clients who might benefit from genetic services and information. *Nursing Standard*, 20(1), 49–53.

Genomics England (2016) *Cancer Genomics*. Available at: www.genomicsengland.co.uk/the-100000-genomes-project/understanding-genomics/cancer-genomics/ (Accessed: 9/5/2018)

George, A., Riddell, D., Seal, S. et al. (2016) Implementing rapid, robust, cost-effective, patient-centred, routine genetic testing in ovarian cancer patients. *Scientific Report*, 13(6), 29506.

Giannarini, G., Mogorovich, A., Valent, F., et al. (2007) Continuing or discontinuing low-dose aspirin before transrectal prostate biopsy: results of a prospective randomized trial. *Urology*, 70(3), 501–505.

Goodson III, W.H., Hunt, T.K., Plotnik, J.N. & Moore II, D.H. (2010) Optimization of clinical breast examination. *The American Journal of Medicine*, 123(4), 329–334.

Gould, D. (2012) Skin flora: implications for nursing. *Nursing Standard*, 26(33), 48–56.

Gould, D. & Brooker, C. (2008) *Infection Prevention and Control: Applied Microbiology for Healthcare*, 2nd edn. Basingstoke: Palgrave Macmillan.

Greene, D., Ali, A., Kinsella, N. & Turner, B. (2015) *Transrectal Ultrasound and Prostatic Biopsy: Guidelines & Recommendations for Training*. BAUS & BAUN. Available at: www.baus.org.uk/_userfiles/pages/files/Publications/Transrectal%20Ultrasound%20%20Prostatic%20Biopsy%20FINAL.pdf (Accessed: 9/5/2018)

Guray, M. & Sahin, A.A. (2006) Benign breast diseases: classification, diagnosis and management. *The Oncologist*, 11, 435–449.

Hall, M.J., Forman, A.D., Pilarski, R., Wiesner, G. & Giri, V.N. (2014) Gene panel testing for inherited cancer risk. *Journal of the National Comprehensive Cancer Network*, 12(9), 1339–1346.

Haydon, J. (2005) Genetics: uphold the rights of all clients to informed decision-making and voluntary action. *Nursing Standard*, 20(3), 48–51.

Health Protection Agency (HPA) (2016) *Notes for Guidance on the Clinical Administration of Radiopharmaceuticals and Use of Sealed Radioactive Sources: Administration of Radioactive Substances Advisory Committee*. London: Public Health England.

Heidenreich, A., Bastian, P.J., Bellmunt, J., et al. (2014) EAU guidelines on prostate cancer. Part 1: screening, diagnosis, and local treatment with curative intent-update 2013. *European Urology*, 65(1), 124–137.

Henkin, R.E. (2006) *Nuclear Medicine*, 2nd edn. St Louis: Mosby.

Higgins, C. (2013) *Understanding Laboratory Investigations for Nurses and Health Professionals*, 3rd edn. Oxford: Blackwell Publishing.

Ho, H.S., Ng, L.G., Tan, Y.H., Yeo, M. & Cheng, C.W. (2009) Intramuscular gentamicin improves the efficacy of ciprofloxacin as an antibiotic prophylaxis for transrectal prostate biopsy. *Annals of Academic Medicine of Singapore*, 38(3), 212–216.

Hori, S., Sengupta, A., Joannides, A., Balogun-Ojuri, B., Tilley, R. & McLoughlin, J. (2010) Changing antibiotic prophylaxis for transrectal ultrasound-guided prostate biopsies: are we putting our patients at risk? *British Journal of Urology International*, 106(9), 1298–1302, discussion 1302.

HSE (2003) *Safe Working and the Prevention of Infection in Clinical Laboratories and Similar Facilities*, 2nd edn. Sudbury: HSE Books.

HSE (2005) *Biological Agents: Managing the Risks in Laboratories and Healthcare Premises*. Sudbury: HSE Books.

HSE (2006) *Information to Accompany Patients Undergoing Nuclear Medicine Procedures*. Available at: www.hse.gov.uk/research/rrpdf/rr416.pdf (Accessed: 9/5/2018)

HSE (2014) *Risk Assessment: A Brief Guide to Controlling Risks in the Workplace*. Available at: www.hse.gov.uk/pubns/indg163.pdf (Accessed: 9/5/2018)

Hughes, L.E. (1991) Classification of benign breast disorders: The ANDI classification based on physiological processes within the normal breast. *British Medical Bulletin*, 47(2), 251–297.

Insinga, R.P., Glass, A.G. & Rush, B.B. (2004) Diagnoses and outcomes in cervical cancer screening: a population based study. *American Journal of Obstetrics and Gynecology*, 191, 105–113.

Institute of Cancer Research (ICR) (2016) *Cancer Genetic Clinical Protocols*. Available at: www.icr.ac.uk/our-research/research-divisions/division-of-genetics-and-epidemiology/genetic-susceptibility/research-projects/cancer-genetic-clinical-protocols (Accessed: 9/5/2018)

Ionising Radiation Regulations (1999) SI 1999/3232. London: Stationery Office. Available at: www.opsi.gov.uk/si/si1999/19993232.htm (Accessed: 9/5/2018)

Ionising Radiation (Medical Exposure) Regulations (IRMER) (2000) SI 2000/1059. London: Stationery Office. Available at: www.opsi.gov.uk/si/si2000/20001059.htm (Accessed: 9/5/2018)

Jacobs, C., Robinson, L. & Webb, P. (2014) *Genetics for Health Professionals in Cancer Care: From Principles to Practice*. Oxford: Oxford University Press.

Kapoor, D.A., Klimberg, I.W., Malek, G.H., et al. (1998) Single-dose oral ciprofloxacin versus placebo for prophylaxis during transrectal prostate biopsy. *Urology*, 52(4), 552–558.

Kierszenbaum, A.L. & Tres, L.L. (2016) *Histology and Cell Biology: An Introduction to Pathology*, 4th edn. Philadelphia: Elsevier.

Kirk, M. (2005) The role of genetic factors in maintaining health. *Nursing Standard*, 20(4), 50–54.

Kirk, M., McDonald, K., Anstey, S. & Longley, M. (2003) *Fit for Practice in the Genetics Era. A Competence Based Education Framework for Nurses, Midwives and Health Visitors.* Pontypridd: University of Glamorgan.

Kirk, M., Tonkin, E. & Skirton, H. (2011a) *Fit for Practice in the Genetics/Genomics Era: A Revised Competence Based Framework with Learning Outcomes and Practice Indicators. A Guide for Nurse Education and Training.* Birmingham: NHS National Genetics Education and Training Centre.

Kirk, M., Calzone, K., Arimori, N., Tonkin, E. & Skirton, H. (2011b) Genetics-Genomics Competencies and Nursing Regulation. *Journal of Nursing Scholarship*, 43(2), 107–116.

Kluijt, I., Sijmons, R.H., Hoogerbrugge, N., et al. (2012) Familial gastric cancer: guidelines for diagnosis, treatment and periodic surveillance. *Familial Cancer*, 11, 363.

Korenstein, D., Falk, R., Howell, E.A., Bishop, T. & Keyhani, S. (2012) Overuse of health care services in the United States: an understudied problem. *Archives of Internal Medicine*, 172(2), 171–178.

Kumar, P.J. & Clark, M.L. (2016) *Kumar & Clark's Clinical Medicine*, 9th edn. Edinburgh: Saunders/Elsevier.

Lange, D., Zappavigna, C., Hamidizadeh, R., Goldenberg, S.L., Paterson, R.F. & Chew, B.H. (2009) Bacterial sepsis after prostate biopsy – a new perspective. *Urology*, 74(6), 1200–1205.

Larkin, A., Millan, E., Wagner, S. & Blum, M. (2011) Radioactivity of blood samples taken from thyroidectomised thyroid carcinoma patients after therapy with (131)I. *Thyroid*, 21(9), 1009–1012.

Leachman, S.A., Carucci, J., Kohlmann, W., et al. (2009) Selection criteria for genetic assessment of patients with familial melanoma. *Journal of the American Academy of Dermatology*, 61(4), 677.e1–677.e14.

Lee, C. & Woo, H.H. (2014), Current methods of analgesia for transrectal ultrasonography (TRUS)-guided prostate biopsy – a systematic review. *British Journal of Urology International*, 113 Suppl 2, 48–56.

Liss, M.A., Johnson, J.R., Porter, S.B., et al. (2015) Clinical and microbiological determinants of infection after transrectal prostate biopsy. *Clinical Infectious Diseases*, 60(7), 979–987.

Loeb, S., Vellekoop, A., Ahmed, A.H., et al. (2013) Systematic review of complications of prostate biopsy. *European Urology*, 64(6), 876–892.

Loveday, H.P., Wilson, J.A., Pratt, R.J., et al. (2014) Epic3: National Evidence-based guidelines for preventing healthcare-associated infections in NHS hospitals in England. *Journal of Hospital Infections*, 86(S1), S1–S7.

Lu, K.H., Schorge, J.O., Rodabaugh, K.J., et al. (2007) Prospective determination of prevalence of Lynch syndrome in young women with endometrial cancer. *Journal of Clinical Oncology*, 25, 5158–5164.

Luini, A., Galimberti, V., Gatti, G., et al. (2005) The sentinel node biopsy after previous breast surgery: preliminary results on 543 patients treated at the European Institute of Oncology. *Breast Cancer Research and Treatment*, 89(2), 159–163.

Marieb, E.N. & Hoehn, K. (2015) *Human Anatomy and Physiology*, 10th edn. San Francisco: Pearson.

Mescher, A.L. (2016) *Basic Histology: Text and Atlas*, 14th edn. London: McGraw-Hill Medical.

Middleton, A., Ahmed, M., & Levene, S. (2005). Tailoring genetic information and services to clients' culture, knowledge and language level. *Nursing Standard*, 20(2), 52–56.

Miller, J., Perumalla, C., & Heap, G. (2005) Complications of transrectal versus transperineal prostate biopsy. *ANZ Journal of Surgery*, 75(1-2), 1445–2197.

Nam, R.K., Saskin, R., Lee, Y., et al. (2013) Increasing hospital admission rates for urological complications after transrectal ultrasound guided prostate biopsy. *Journal of Urology*, 189(1 Suppl), S12–17; discussion S17–18.

NHS Pathology (2014) *Samples and Request Forms.* Surrey: NHS Pathology. Available at: www.nhspathology.fph.nhs.uk/Core-Service/Test-Directory/General_Information_Samples_and_Request_Forms.aspx (Accessed: 9/5/2018)

NHSCSP (2004) *Guidelines on Failsafe Actions for the Follow-Up of Cervical Cytology Reports.* Sheffield: NHS Cancer Screening Programmes. Available at: www.cancerscreening.nhs.uk/cervical/publications/nhscsp21.pdf (Accessed: 9/5/2018)

NHSCSP (2013) *Achievable Standards, Benchmarks for Reporting, and Criteria for Evaluating Cervical Cytopathology*, 3rd edn. Sheffield: NHS Cancer Screening Programmes.

NHSCSP (2015) NHS Cervical Screening (CSP) Programme. London: Public Health England. Available at: www.gov.uk/topic/population-screening-programmes/cervical (Accessed: 9/5/2018)

NHSCSP (2017) *Cervical Sample Taker e-Learning Course.* Available at: https://portal.e-lfh.org.uk/Component/Details/502328. (Accessed 25/06/2018)

NICE (2002) *Improving Outcomes in Breast Cancer.* Available at: www.nice.org.uk/guidance/csg1/resources/improving-outcomes-in-breast-cancer-update-773371117 (Accessed: 9/5/2018)

NICE (2003) *Guidance on the Use of Liquid-Based Cytology for Cervical Screening. Technology Appraisal Guidance 69.* London: NICE.

NICE (2010) *Metastatic Malignant Disease of Unknown Primary Origin in Adults: Diagnosis and Management (CG104).* London: NICE. Available at: www.nice.org.uk/guidance/cg104/chapter/1-guidance (Accessed: 9/5/2018)

NICE (2013) *Familial Breast Cancer: Classification, Care and Managing Breast Cancer and Related Risks in People with A Family History of Breast Cancer* (CG164). Available at: www.nice.org.uk/guidance/CG164 (Accessed: 9/5/2018)

NICE (2014) *Prostate Cancer: Diagnosis and Management (CG175).* London: NICE. Available at: www.nice.org.uk/guidance/cg175?unlid=54952719620161242039 (Accessed: 9/5/2018)

NICE (2015a) *Bladder Cancer: Diagnosis and Management (NG2).* London: NICE. Available at: www.nice.org.uk/guidance/ng2 (Accessed: 9/5/2018)

NICE (2015b) *Suspected Cancer: Recognition and Referral* (NG12). London: NICE. Available at: www.nice.org.uk/guidance/ng12 (Accessed: 9/5/2018)

NICE (2016) *Breast Cancer* (QS12). Available at: www.nice.org.uk/guidance/qs12 (Accessed: 9/5/2018)

NMC (2010a) *Record Keeping Guidance.* London: Nursing and Midwifery Council. Available at: www.nmc.org.uk/standards/code/record-keeping/ (Accessed: 9/5/2018)

NMC (2010b) *Standards for Medicines Management.* London: Nursing and Midwifery Council. Available at: www.nmc.org.uk/globalassets/sitedocuments/standards/nmc-standards-for-medicines-management.pdf (Accessed: 9/5/2018)

NMC (2015) *The Code: Professional Standards of Practice and Behaviour for Nurses and Midwives.* London: Nursing and Midwifery Council. Available at: www.nmc.org.uk/globalassets/sitedocuments/nmc-publications/nmc-code.pdf (Accessed: 9/5/2018)

O'Dwyer, H.M., Lyon, S., Fotheringham, T. & Lee, M. (2003) Informed consent for interventional radiology procedures: a survey detailing current European practice. *Cardiovascular and Interventional Radiology*, 26(5), 428–433.

Osborne, S. (2007) Nurse-led flexible cystoscopy: the UK experience informs a New Zealand nurse specialist's training. *International Journal of Urological Nursing*, 1(2) 58–63.

Pandya, S. & Moore, R.G. (2011) Breast development and anatomy. *Clinical Obstetrics and Gynaecology*, 54(1), 91–95.

Patel, U., Dasgupta, P., Amoroso, P., Challacombe, B., Pilcher, J. & Kirby, R. (2012) Infection after transrectal ultrasonography-guided prostate biopsy: increased relative risks after recent international travel or antibiotic use. *British Journal of Urology International*, 109(12) 1781–1785.

Peter, J.E. & Gambhir, S. (2004) *Nuclear Medicine in Clinical Diagnosis and Treatment*, 3rd edn. Edinburgh: Churchill Livingstone.

Peyronnet, B., Drouin S.J., Gomez, F.D., et al. (2016) Local analgesia during flexible cystoscopy in male patients: a non-inferiority study comparing Xylocaine® gel to Instillagel® Lido. *Progres en Urologie* 26(11-1), 651–655.

Qaseem, A., Alguire, P., Dallas, P., et al. (2012) Appropriate use of screening and diagnostic tests to foster high-value, cost-conscious care. *Annals of Internal Medicine*, 156(2), 147–149.

Raber, M., Scattoni, V., Roscigno, M., et al. (2008) Topical prilocaine-lidocaine cream combined with peripheral nerve block improves pain control in prostatic biopsy: results from a prospective randomized trial. *European Urology*, 53(5), 967–973.

Radhakrishnan, S., Dorkin, T.J., Johnson, P., Menezes, P. & Greene, D. (2006) Nurse-led flexible cystoscopy: experience from one UK centre. *British Journal of Urology International*, 98(2), 256–258.

Rahman, N. (2014) Realizing the promise of cancer predisposition genes. *Nature*, 505(7483), 302–308.

RCN (2008) *Defending dignity: Challenges and opportunities for nursing.* Available at: www.rcn.org.uk/professional-development/publications/pub-003257 (Accessed: 9/5/2018)

RCN (2012) *Advanced nurse practitioners, An RCN guide to advanced nursing practice, advanced nurse practitioners and programme accreditation.* Available at: https://www.rcn.org.uk/professional-development/publications/pub-003207 (Accessed: 9/5/2018)

RCN (2013) *Cervical Screening: RCN Guidance for Good Practice.* London: Royal College of Nursing. Available at: https://www.rcn.org.uk/professional-development/publications/pub-003105 (Accessed: 9/5/2018)

RCN (2016a) *Consent: Advice Guides.* London: Royal College of Nursing. Available at: www.rcn.org.uk/get-help/rcn-advice/consent (Accessed: 9/5/2018)

RCN (2016b) *Chaperoning: The Role of the Nurse and the Rights of Patients.* London: Royal College of Nursing. Available at: https://www.rcn.org.uk/professional-development/publications/pub-001446 (Accessed: 9/5/2018)

RCN (2017a) *Essential Practice for Infection Prevention and Control: Guidance for Nursing Staff.* London: Royal College of Nursing. Available at: https://www.rcn.org.uk/professional-development/publications/pub-005940 (Accessed: 9/5/2018)

RCN (2017b) *Principles of Consent: Guidance for Nursing Staff.* London: Royal College of Nursing. Available at: https://www.rcn.org.uk/professional-development/publications/pub-006047 (Accessed: 9/5/2018)

RCR (2008) *Guidance on Screening and Symptomatic Imaging*, 3rd edn. London: Royal College of Radiologists. Available at: www.rcr.ac.uk/system/files/publication/field_publication_files/BFCR(13)5_breast.pdf (Accessed: 9/5/2018)

Resuscitation Council (2015) *Resuscitation Guidelines.* London: Resuscitation Council. Available at: www.resus.org.uk/resuscitation-guidelines (Accessed: 9/5/2018)

Reynard, J., Brewster, S. & Biers, S. (2013) *Oxford Handbook of Urology*, 3rd edn. Oxford: Oxford University Press.

Reynard, J., Mark, S., Turner, K., Armenakas, N., Fenely, M. & Sullivan, M. (2008) *Oxford Handbook of Urological Surgery.* Oxford: Oxford University Press.

Richards, S., Aziz, N., Bale, S., et al.; ACMG Laboratory Quality Assurance Committee (2015) Standards and guidelines for the interpretation of sequence variants: a joint consensus recommendation of the American College of Medical Genetics and Genomics and the Association for Molecular Pathology. *Genetic Medicine*, 17(5), 405–424.

Rocha, R.D., Pinto, R.R., Tavares, D.P.B. & Goncalves, C. (2013) Step-by-step of ultrasound-guided core-needle biopsy of the breast: review and technique. *Radiologia Brasileira*, 46(4), 234–241.

Rodriguez, L.V. & Terris, M.K. (1998) Risks and complications of transrectal ultrasound guided prostate needle biopsy: a prospective study and review of the literature. *Journal of Urology*, 160(6), 2115–2120.

Royal College of Physicians, Royal College of Pathologists and British Society for Human Genetics (2011) *Consent and Confidentiality in Clinical Genetic Practice: Guidance on Genetic Testing and Sharing Genetic Information*, 2nd edn. Report of the Joint Committee on Medical Genetics. London: RCP, Royal College of Pathologists. Available at: www.bsgm.org.uk/media/678746/consent_and_confidentiality_2011.pdf (Accessed: 9/5/2018)

Russell, C. (1998) Measurement and interpretation of renal transit times. In: Murray, I.P.C. and Ell, P.J. (eds) *Nuclear Medicine in Clinical Diagnosis and Treatment*, 2nd edn. Edinburgh: Churchill Livingstone, pp. 257–262.

Scales, K. (2009) Correct use of chlorhexidine in intravenous practice. *Nursing Standard*, 24(8), 41–46.

Schrenk, P., Woelfl, S., Bogner, S., et al. (2005) The use of sentinel node biopsy in breast cancer patients undergoing skin sparing mastectomy and immediate autologous reconstruction. *Plastic and Reconstructive Surgery*, 116(5), 1278–1286.

Schuiling, K.D. & Likis, F.E. (2013) *Women's Gynecological Health*, 2nd edn. Rochester: Jones & Bartlett Learning.

Selkirk, C.G., Vogel, K.J., Newlin, A.C., et al. (2014) Cancer genetic testing panels for inherited cancer susceptibility: the clinical experience of a large adult genetics practice. *Familial Cancer*, 13(4), 527–536.

Sharp, C., Shrimpton, J.A. & Bury, R.F. (1998) *Diagnostic Medical Exposures: Advice on Exposure to Ionising Radiation during Pregnancy.* Didcot: National Radiological Protection Board.

Siddiqui, M.M., Rais-Bahrami, S., Turkbey, B., et al. (2015) Comparison of MR/ultrasound fusion-guided biopsy with ultrasound-guided biopsy for the diagnosis of prostate cancer. *Journal of the American Medical Association*, 313(4), 390–397.

Sieber, P., Rommel, F., Agusta, V., Breslin, J., Huffnagle, H. & Harpster, L. (1997) Antibiotic prophylaxis in ultrasound guided transrectal prostate biopsy. *The Journal of Urology*, (157)6, 2199–2200.

Singh, S., van Herwijnen, I. & Phillips, C. (2013) The management of lower urogenital changes in the menopause. *Menopause International*, 19(2), 77–81.

Skills for Health (2010a) *CYST1 Undertake Diagnostic and Surveillance Cystoscopy Using a Flexible Cystoscope.* Version 1. Available at: https://tools.skillsforhealth.org.uk/competence/show/html/code/CYST1/ (Accessed: 9/5/2018)

Skills for Health (2010b) *CYST2 Undertake Biopsy Using a Flexible Cystoscope.* Version 1. Available at: http://tools.skillsforhealth.org.uk/competence/show/html/code/CYST2/ (Accessed: 9/5/2018)

Skills for Health (2010c) *CYST3 Remove Ureteric Stent Using a Flexible Cystoscope.* Version 1. Available at: https://tools.skillsforhealth.org.uk/competence/show/html/code/CYST3/ (Accessed: 9/5/2018)

Skills for Health (2010d) *CYST4 Use Cystodiathermy Via Flexible Cystoscope.* Version 1. Available at: https://tools.skillsforhealth.org.uk/competence/show/html/code/CYST4/ (Accessed: 9/5/2018)

Skirton, H. & Barnes, C. (2005) Obtaining and communicating information about genetics. *Nursing Standard*, 20(7), 50–53.

Smith, A., Badlani, G., Preminger, G. & Kavoussi, L. (2012) *Smith's Textbook of Endourology*, 3rd edn. Oxford: Wiley-Blackwell.

Smith, T., Streeter, E., Choi, W., et al. (2015) Are specialist nurse-led check flexible cystoscopy services as effective as doctor-led sessions? *International Journal of Urological Nursing*, 10(2), 65–67.

Society of Nuclear Medicine and Molecular Imaging (SNMMI) (2016) *Resource Center.* Available at: http://interactive.snm.org/index.cfm?PageID=6309 (Accessed: 9/5/2018)

Stratton, M.R., Campbell, P.J. & Futreal, P.A. (2009) The cancer genome. *Nature*, 458(7239), 719–724.

Taylor, A.K., Zembower, T.R., Nadler, R.B., et al. (2012) Targeted antimicrobial prophylaxis using rectal swab cultures in men undergoing transrectal ultrasound guided prostate biopsy is associated with reduced incidence of postoperative infectious complications and cost of care. *Journal of Urology*, 187(4), 1275–1279.

Taylor, J., Pearce, I. & O'Flynn, K. (2002) Nurse led cystoscopy: the next step. *British Journal of Urology International*, 90(1), 45–46.

Tortora, G.J. & Derrickson, B.H. (2014) *Principles of Anatomy and Physiology*, 14th edn. London: Wiley.

Turner, B. & Pati, J. (2010) Nurse practitioner led prostate biopsy: an audit to determine effectiveness and safety for patients. *International Journal of Urological Nursing*, 4(2), 87–92.

Turner, B., Aslet, Ph., Drudge-Coates, L., et al. (2011) *Evidence-based Guidelines for Best Practice in Health Care: Transrectal Ultrasound Guided Biopsy of the Prostate.* European Association of Urology Nurses. Available at: http://nurses.uroweb.org/wp-content/uploads/EAUN_TRUS_Guidelines_EN_2011_LR.pdf (Accessed: 9/5/2018)

Vassalos, A. & Rooney K. (2013) Surviving sepsis guidelines 2012. *Critical Care Medicine*, 41(12), e485–486.

Vialard-Miguel, J., Mazere, J., Mora, S., et al. (2005) I131 in blood samples: management in the laboratory. *Annales de Biologie Clinique (Paris)*, 63(5), 561–565.

Wallis, M., Tarvidon, A., Helbich, T. & Schreer, I. (2006) Guidelines from the European Society of Breast Imaging for diagnostic interventional breast procedures. *European Radiology*, 17(2), 581–588.

Wegerhoff, F. (2006) It's a bug's life – specimen collection, transport, and viability. *Microbe*, 1, 180–184.

Weston, D. (2008) *Infection Prevention and Control: Theory and Clinical Practice for Healthcare Professionals*. Oxford: John Wiley & Sons.

WHO (2014) *Comprehensive Cervical Cancer Control: A Guide to Essential Practice*. Geneva: World Health Organization.

WHO (2015) *Guidance on Regulations for the Transport of Infectious Substances 2015–2016*. Geneva: World Health Organization.

Williamson, D.A., Barrett, L.K., Rogers, B.A., Freeman, J.T., Hadway, P., & Paterson, D.L. (2013) Infectious complications following transrectal ultrasound-guided prostate biopsy: new challenges in the era of multidrug-resistant Escherichia coli. *Clinical Infectious Diseases*, 57(2), 267–274.

Wolf, A.C., Hammond, E.H., Hicks, D.G., et al (2013) Recommendations for Human Epidermal Growth Factor Receptor 2 Testing in Breast Cancer: American Society of Clinical Oncology/College of American Pathologists Clinical Practice Guideline Update. *Journal of Clinical Oncology*, 31, 3997–4013.

Wright, C.A. (2012) Fine-needle aspiration biopsy of lymph nodes. *Continuing Medical Education*, 30(2), 56–60.

Xu, S., Markson, C., Costello, K.L., Xing, C.Y., Demissie, K. & Llanos, A.A. (2016) Leveraging Social Media to Promote Public Health Knowledge: Example of Cancer Awareness via Twitter. *JMIR Public Health and Surveillance*, 2(1), e17.

Yu, B., O'Toole, S.A. & Trent, R.J. (2015) Somatic DNA mutation analysis in targeted therapy of solid tumours. *Translational Pediatrics*, 4(2), 125–138.

Yun, T.J., Lee, H.J., Kim, S.H., Lee, S.E., Cho, J.Y. & Seong, C.K. (2007) Does the intrarectal instillation of lidocaine gel before periprostatic neurovascular bundle block during transrectal ultrasound guided prostate biopsies improve analgesic efficacy? A prospective, randomized trial. *Journal Urology*, 178(1), 103–106.

Zani, E.L., Clark, O.A. & Rodrigues Netto, N. Jr. (2011) Antibiotic prophylaxis for transrectal prostate biopsy. *Cochrane Database of Systematic Reviews* 11(5), CD006576.

Ziessman, H.A., O'Malley, J.P. & Thrall, J.H. (2006) *Nuclear Medicine*, 3rd edn. St Louis, MO: Mosby.

Zuber, T.J. (2002) Punch biopsy of the skin. *American Family Physician*, 65(6), 1161–1162.

Chapter 2

Haematological procedures

Procedure guidelines

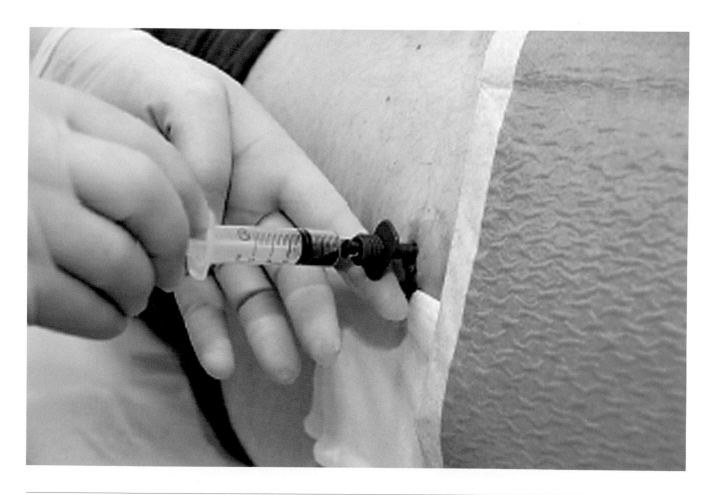

The Royal Marsden Manual of Cancer Nursing Procedures. Edited by Sara Lister and Lisa Dougherty, with Assistant Editor Louise McNamara.
© 2019 The Royal Marsden NHS Foundation Trust. Published 2019 by John Wiley & Sons, Ltd.

Overview

This chapter provides a review of and guide to procedures commonly undertaken by haematology nurses. Haematological procedures include:

- bone marrow procedures
- apheresis procedures
- ribavirin administration
- pentamidine administration.

Definitions

- *Bone marrow procedures* involve the removal of haematopoietic tissue from the medullary cavity of bone. Tissue is removed by either aspiration or biopsy (Al-Ibraheemi et al. 2013, Hoffbrand and Moss 2015, Odejide et al. 2013). Specific procedures include the following.
  - *Aspiration and trephine biopsy.* Biopsy of the bone marrow is an indispensable tool for the study of diseases of the blood and may be the only way in which a correct diagnosis can be made. Marrow is usually obtained by needle aspiration and percutaneous trephine biopsy. If performed correctly, bone marrow aspiration is simple and safe; it can be repeated many times and performed on outpatients (Hoffbrand and Moss 2015, Lewis et al. 2011, Moore et al. 2016). Trephine biopsy is a little less simple, but is invaluable in the diagnosis of conditions which yield a 'dry tap' on bone marrow aspiration (e.g. myelofibrosis, infiltrations) or when disrupted architecture of the marrow is an important diagnostic feature (e.g. Hodgkin's disease, lymphoma). It is also performed on outpatients (Lewis et al. 2011).
  - *Bone marrow harvest.* Traditionally bone marrow harvest was the primary method of collecting stem cells in order to perform a haematopoietic stem cell transplant (Richardson and Atkinson 2006). The process is similar to that of bone marrow aspiration but multiple aspirations are needed from each posterior iliac crest in order to obtain the necessary volume of stem cells (Yarbro et al. 2016). The procedure is performed in the operating room with the donor anaesthetized and this is usually an inpatient procedure (Yarbro et al. 2016).
- *Apheresis* is the generic term applied to blood cell separator procedures, which may be used for donor or therapeutic purposes. Cell separators remove whole blood from a patient or donor and separate this into component parts to allow a desired element to be collected, while returning the remainder to the patient or donor (Corbin et al. 2010). Separation of the blood components can be accomplished by filtration, centrifugation or a combination of both. Filtration takes advantage of differences in particle size to separate blood plasma from the cellular elements. Centrifugation uses differences in specific gravity to separate and isolate blood components (Burgstaler 2010). The specific procedures are described according to the blood element being removed (Kaushansky et al. 2016):
  - leukapheresis (white cell depletion)
  - thrombocytopheresis (platelet depletion)
  - erythrocytapheresis (red cell exchange)
  - therapeutic plasmapheresis (plasma exchange).
- *Ribavirin* is a drug that inhibits a wide range of DNA and RNA viruses by disrupting viral protein synthesis (Joint Formulary Committee 2018). It is generally given by inhalation for the treatment of severe bronchiolitis caused by the respiratory syncytial virus (RSV) and parainfluenza (Dignan et al. 2016, Molinos-Quintana et al. 2013, Raboni et al. 2003). It may occasionally be given intravenously for infection in sites other than the lungs.
- *Pentamidine isetionate* is a synthetic amidine derivative, and is an antiprotozoal and antifungal agent that interferes with DNA replication and function. It is effective in the treatment of some fungal infections, specifically *Pneumocystis jirovecii* (previously *carinii*) pneumonia. It is also useful in treating trypanosomiasis and leishmaniasis (Sun and Zhang 2008).

Bone marrow procedures

Anatomy and physiology

Bone marrow

The maturation of blood cells is termed haematopoiesis (Davē and Koury 2016) and takes place in the bone marrow. At 5–9 months of fetal life, the bone marrow, liver and spleen produce the cellular components of blood. At birth, the marrow of all bones is involved in haematopoiesis. During childhood, there is some replacement of the haematopoietic tissue (red marrow) with fatty tissue (yellow marrow). In adults, the only sites of haematopoiesis are bones such as the pelvis and sternum (Yarbro et al. 2016). Yellow marrow has the ability to revert to haematopoietic tissue in certain circumstances such as haemolytic anaemia (Davē and Koury 2016).

Stem cells

All mature blood cells originate from one precursor cell called a stem cell. The stem cell has the ability for unlimited self-renewal (can produce more stem cells) and differentiation (can develop into any of the mature blood cell types) (Figure 2.1).

The self-renewal and differentiation of stem cells are regulated by acidic glycoprotein molecules called haematopoietic growth factors (Traynor 2006). Some growth factors are found naturally in the plasma but others are only detectable following an inflammatory event or other stimulus (Hoffbrand and Moss 2015). Growth factors include granulocyte-colony stimulating factor (G-CSF), erythropoietin and thrombopoietin (Traynor 2006).

The first step in the differentiation process is a division of the stem cell into two main cell lineages: myeloid and lymphoid. The myeloid progenitor cell divides into red blood cells, platelets, granulocytes (neutrophils, eosinophils and basophils) and monocytes (macrophages). The lymphoid progenitor cell matures into lymphocytes (T and B). Lymphocytes, granulocytes and monocytes are all white cells (Bondurant et al. 2012). The main functions of the blood cells and the haematological values for normal adults are listed in Table 2.1.

Plasma

Plasma gives blood its liquid property to allow it to flow through the vascular system. If the cellular components of whole blood were allowed to sediment in a test tube, around 54% of the volume would be the straw-coloured plasma (Traynor 2006). Plasma consists of water, plasma proteins (e.g. fibrinogen, albumin, globulins), electrolytes (e.g. sodium, potassium, chloride) and metabolites (e.g. urea, creatinine, cholesterol). The functions of these elements include clotting, maintaining blood pressure, controlling plasma viscosity, antibody formation and regulating intra/extracellular pressure.

Aspiration and trephine biopsy

Related theory

Examination of the bone marrow usually involves two separate but inter-related specimens. The first is a cytological preparation of bone marrow cells obtained by aspiration of the marrow and a smear of the cells (Hoffbrand and Moss 2015, Odejide et al. 2013). The aspiration specimen is used to assess cell morphology (Longo 2016). The second specimen is a trephine biopsy of the bone and associated marrow, to assess overall marrow architecture, bone marrow cellularity, fibrosis, infections or infiltrative diseases (Longo 2016). Diagnosis and management of many haematological diseases depend on

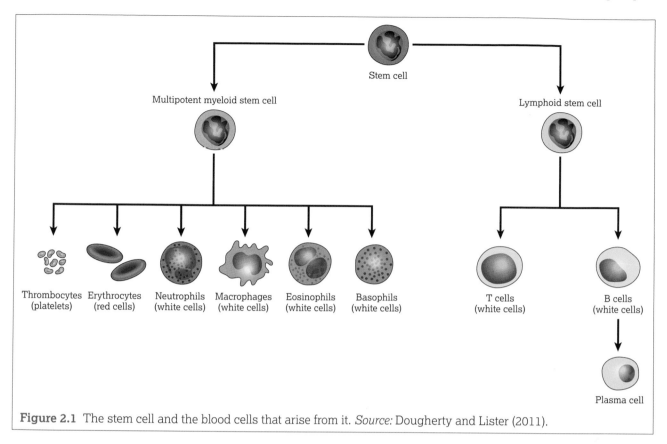

Figure 2.1 The stem cell and the blood cells that arise from it. *Source:* Dougherty and Lister (2011).

Table 2.1 The main function of blood cells and the haematological values for normal adults

Blood cell type and function	Haematological value	Illustration
Red blood cells (erythrocytes) Transport oxygen from the lungs to the tissues and return carbon dioxide from the tissues to be expelled by the lungs	Men: 15±2 g/dL Women: 14±2 g/dL	
Platelets (thrombocytes) Form mechanical plugs during the normal haemostatic response to vascular injury	130–400×10⁹/L	
White blood cells (leucocytes) A group of diverse cells that work together to protect the body from disease and to provide immunity	7.0±3.0×10⁹/L	
White blood cell differential *Neutrophil:* Attracted to sites of infection (chemotaxis); ingests micro-organisms (phagocytosis) and destroys them	2.0–7.0×10⁹/L	
Eosinophil: Same function as the neutrophil; in addition, helps control parasitic infections; has a role in allergic responses	0.04–0.4×10⁹/L	

(continued)

Table 2.1 The main function of blood cells and the haematological values for normal adults *(continued)*

Blood cell type and function	Haematological value	Illustration
Basophil: Has a role in immediate hypersensitivity reactions, allergic and inflammatory responses and in the control of parasitic infections	$0.02–0.1\times10^9$/L	
T lymphocyte: Attacks cells bearing foreign antigens and antibody-coated cells; can help or suppress B cells (part of cell-mediated immunity) *B lymphocyte:* Matures into a plasma cell, which secretes antibodies (humoral immunity) *Natural killer (NK) lymphocyte:* Attacks foreign cells and tumour cells (part of cell-mediated immunity)	$1.0–3.0\times10^9$/L	
Monocyte (differentiates to macrophage in tissues): Has a role in chemotaxis, phagocytosis, killing of some micro-organisms (fungi and mycobacteria), release of IL-1 and TNF which stimulate bone marrow stromal cells to produce GM-CSF, G-CSF, M-CSF and IL-6	$0.2–1.0\times10^9$/L	

Sources: Adapted from Bain (2004), Hoffbrand and Moss (2015), Hughes-Jones et al. (2013), Provan et al. (2015), Turgeon (2014).
G-CSF, granulocyte-colony stimulating factor; GM-CSF, granulocyte-macrophage colony stimulating factor; IL, interleukin; M-CSF macrophage colony stimulating factor; TNF, tumour necrosis factor.

examination of the bone marrow (Hoffbrand and Moss 2015, Odejide et al. 2013).

Evidence-based approaches

Rationale
Before a bone marrow examination is carried out, clear diagnostic goals about the information to be obtained from the procedure should be defined. It should be decided whether any special studies are needed so that all the necessary specimens may be collected and handled correctly (Hoffbrand and Moss 2015). Table 2.2 outlines this in more detail.

Several sites may be used for bone marrow aspiration and biopsy (Figure 2.2). Normally, only aspirations and not biopsies are done on the sternum because of its small size and proximity to vital organs. The site selected may reflect the normal distribution of bone marrow in relation to the age of the patient. Younger children may have marrow taken from the anterior medial tibial area, whereas adult marrow is best sampled from the sternum at the second inter-costal space or from either the anterior or posterior iliac crest area (Hoffbrand and Moss 2015, Koeppen et al. 2011). Sternal marrows do not allow a trephine biopsy to be performed, and several possible complications, including haemorrhage and pericardial tamponade, may occur if the inner table of the sternum is penetrated by the

Table 2.2 Comparison of bone marrow aspiration and trephine biopsy

	Aspiration	Trephine
Site	Posterior/anterior iliac crest or sternum (anterior medial tibial area in children)	Posterior/anterior iliac crest
Result available	1–2 hours	1–7 days (according to decalcification method)
Main indications	Hypoproliferative or unexplained anaemia, leucopenia or thrombocytopenia, suspected leukaemia or myeloma or marrow defect, evaluation of iron stores, work-up of some cases of fever of unknown origin	Performed in addition to aspiration for pancytopenia (aplastic anaemia), metastatic tumour, granulomatous infection (e.g. mycobacteria, brucellosis, histoplasmosis), myelofibrosis, lipid storage disease (e.g. Gaucher's, Niemann–Pick), any case with 'dry tap' on aspiration; evaluation of marrow cellularity
Special tests	Histochemical staining (leukaemias), cytogenetic studies (leukaemias, lymphomas), microbiology (bacterial, mycobacterial, fungal cultures), Prussian blue (iron) stain (assess iron stores, diagnosis of sideroblastic anaemias)	Histochemical staining (e.g. acid phosphatase for metastatic prostate carcinoma), immunoperoxidase staining (e.g. immunoglobulin or cell surface marker detection in multiple myeloma, leukaemia or lymphoma; lysozyme detection in monocytic leukaemia), reticulin staining (increased in myelofibrosis), microbiological staining (e.g. acid-fast staining for mycobacteria)

Sources: Adapted from Hoffbrand and Moss (2015), Longo (2016).

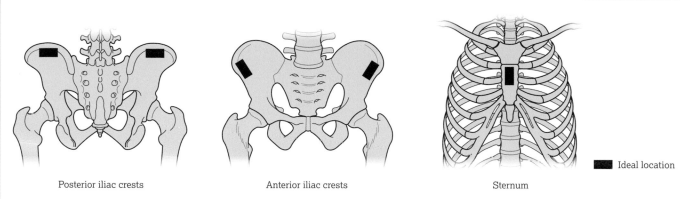

Posterior iliac crests   Anterior iliac crests   Sternum

■ Ideal location

Figure 2.2 Common sites for bone marrow examination, arranged in order of preference. Normally, only aspirations and not biopsies are done on the sternum because of its small size and proximity to vital organs. *Source:* Dougherty and Lister (2011).

needle at areas other than the second intercostal space (Hoffbrand and Moss 2015, Koeppen et al. 2011). In contrast, little morbidity is associated with iliac crest aspiration and biopsy, and the posterior iliac crest is the most common site for bone marrow examinations (Figure 2.3). The anterior iliac crest may be used if previous radiation, surgery or patient discomfort does not allow a posterior approach (Hoffbrand and Moss 2015, Koeppen et al. 2011).

Indications

There are a number of indications for performing a bone marrow examination. These include (Hoffbrand and Moss 2015, Koeppen et al. 2011):

- further work-up of haematological abnormalities observed in the peripheral blood smear
- evaluation of primary bone marrow tumours
- staging for bone marrow involvement by metastatic tumours
- assessment of infectious disease processes, including fever of unknown origin
- evaluation of metabolic storage diseases.

Contraindications

- The only absolute reason to avoid performing a bone marrow examination is the presence of coagulation disorders such as

haemophilia (unless correctable), which may lead to serious bleeding after the procedure.
- If there is a skin or soft tissue infection over the hip, a different site should be chosen (Goldberg et al. 2007).

Principles of care

The procedure should be performed in an aseptic manner with meticulous handwashing to reduce any risk of infection. Any equipment that may cause a needlestick injury must be safely disposed of. Local anaesthetic/general anaesthetic and fasting procedure policies should be followed.

Methods of aspiration and trephine biopsy

- *Aspiration.* An aspirate needle is inserted through the skin into the bone marrow. Once the needle is in the marrow cavity, a syringe is attached and used to aspirate liquid bone marrow (Figure 2.4). This is then spread onto slides (Hoffbrand and Moss 2015) (Figure 2.5).
- *Trephine.* A trephine needle is inserted and anchored in the bony cortex. The needle is then advanced with a twisting motion and rotated to obtain a solid piece of bone marrow. This piece is then removed along with the needle. A trephine biopsy provides a solid core of bone including marrow and is examined as a histological specimen after fixation in formalin, decalcification and sectioning (Hoffbrand and Moss 2015) (Figure 2.6).

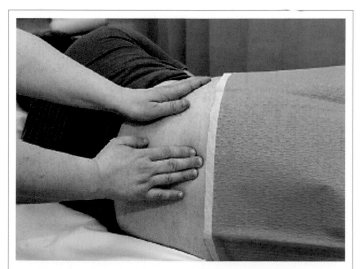

Figure 2.3 Patient lying in the left lateral position, with the head to the left, exposing the lower back and gluteal region with the right posterior iliac crest palpated. *Source:* Dougherty and Lister (2011).

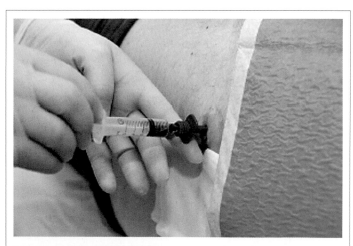

Figure 2.4 Aspiration of bone marrow from the marrow cavity. *Source:* Dougherty and Lister (2011).

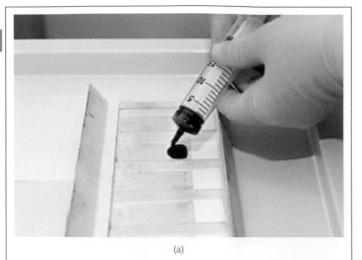

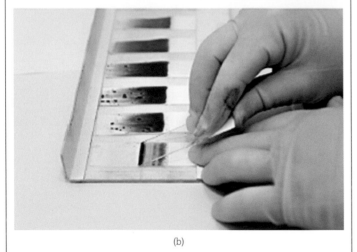

Figure 2.5 (a) Preparation of aspiration smears. (b) Completed aspiration smear. *Source:* Dougherty and Lister (2011).

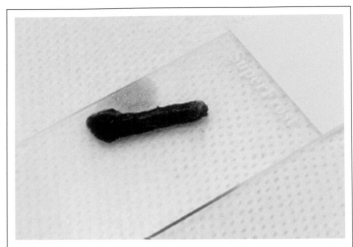

Figure 2.6 Trephine biopsy sample. *Source:* Dougherty and Lister (2011).

Legal and professional issues

Bone marrow biopsies were traditionally performed by physicians but, more recently, a significant number are being performed by specially trained nurses (Lewis et al. 2016, Ruegg et al. 2009). It has long been recognized that, with motivated staff and a structured training programme, it is possible for nurse practitioners to perform the techniques of bone marrow biopsy and obtain specimens of satisfactory quality (Lawson et al. 1999). It has also been suggested that this improves the efficiency of a haematology unit and increases the quality of patient care (Lawson et al. 1999, McNamara 2011).

It is common for bone marrow samples to be required for research purposes. These should be collected according to good clinical practice guidelines (MHRA 2012). Other regulations that set standards include the Human Tissue Authority (2017c) *Code E: Research*.

The administration of local anaesthetic should be in accordance with a Patient Group Direction or a written prescription.

Competencies

A suitable training package should be available for new practitioners. All practitioners should be assessed by a competent practice facilitator prior to performing procedures on their own. Nurses must always operate within their scope of practice as set out by their profession (NMC 2015). Learning tools may include competency-based workbooks.

Consent

The practitioner performing the procedure is responsible for providing information prior to the biopsy and obtaining written consent. In the case of paediatric patients, parental consent is required unless the child is over the age of 16 years (NMC 2015).

Pre-procedural considerations

Equipment

Needles with a range of gauges may be used. Most have a removable introducer (which prevents plugging of the needle before aspiration) and a stylet that may be used to express the bone marrow biopsy sample. Some models, primarily used for sternal bone marrow aspiration procedures, have adjustable guards that limit the extent of needle penetration; there are currently no safety devices available for this procedure (Smock & Perkins 2014). Figure 2.7 shows the more specialist equipment needed to perform a bone marrow biopsy. Procedure guideline 2.1 provides a full list of essential equipment.

Pharmacological support

In most adult cases, bone marrow biopsies may be carried out with little risk of patient discomfort, provided adequate local anaesthesia is administered. Lidocaine 2% (maximum dose 200 mg) is frequently used (Joint Formulary Committee 2018). Patients may describe a 'dragging sensation' during the actual aspiration procedure, even when the site is numb. The duration of the local anaesthetic action is about 90 minutes (Joint Formulary Committee 2018).

Apprehensive patients may be given an oral sedative, Entonox® or intravenous conscious sedation before the procedure, but this is usually not necessary (Hjortholm et al. 2013, McGrath 2013). When intravenous sedation is used, a second practitioner should be present to administer the conscious sedation and to monitor the patient. A local standard operating practice should be in place to support practitioners in practice, for example ensuring that cardiac monitoring, pulse oximetry, oxygen administration, the reversal agent and resuscitation equipment are available in order to adhere to guidance from the Academy of Royal Medical Colleges (Academy of Royal Medical Colleges 2013, Provan et al. 2015).

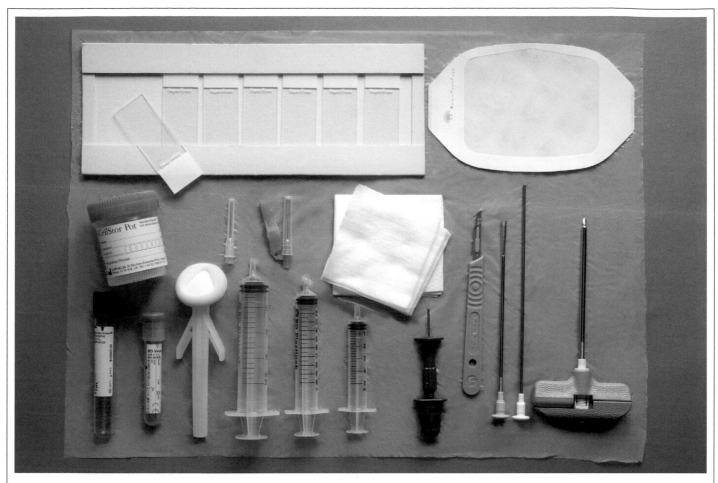

Figure 2.7 Bone marrow biopsy equipment including antiseptic skin cleaning agent with sponge applicator, selection of syringes for bone marrow sampling and administration of local anaesthetic, selection of needles for the administration of local anaesthetic, marrow aspiration needle and guard, trephine biopsy needle, cytology slides and coverslips, specimen bottles, sterile dressing and size 11 scalpel.

Bone marrow biopsy may be more upsetting for paediatric patients and measures to reduce distress include:

- The use of a general anaesthetic.
- The application of a thick layer of topical lidocaine 2.5%/prilocaine 2.5% cream under an occlusive dressing to the site selected for cannulation 1–5 hours before the procedure. *Note*: contraindicated in a child less than 37 weeks' corrected gestational age (Paediatric Formulary Committee 2018).
- The local infiltration of lidocaine to the bone marrow biopsy site for post-operative pain control. The recommended dose for neonates and children less than 12 years is up to 3 mg/kg (0.3 mL/kg of 1% solution) (Paediatric Formulary Committee 2018). If in any doubt, expert advice should be sought.

Non-pharmacological support

Special consideration may also be needed for those who are extremely anxious. Measures include ensuring that the patient has a family member or friend present and complementary therapies such as relaxation, massage and music (Bufalini 2009).

Specific patient preparations

Thrombocytopenia is not a contraindication and bone marrow examination seems to be safe even when thrombocytopenic purpura is present (Lewis et al. 2011). However, the nurse must take a history to assess for risk of bleeding (BCSH 2008). This should include details of family history, previous excessive post-traumatic or post-surgical bleeding, liver disease and the use of antithrombotic drugs. If the bleeding history is negative, no further coagulation testing is indicated. If the bleeding history is positive or there is a clear clinical indication (e.g. liver disease), a haematologist should be consulted as to what screening tests are needed and what actions should be taken. Some of these are outlined in the pharmacological support section. If haemorrhage occurs post bone marrow biopsy, the main reasons (in order of frequency) are (Bain 2005):

- a myeloproliferative disorder
- aspirin treatment
- other platelet dysfunction.

Questions to determine if the patient's posterior iliac crests have undergone previous radiation or surgery or are affected by soft tissue damage or infection will aid appropriate site selection.

Further assessment should determine if the patient has an allergy to any of the medication, cleaning agents, dressings or equipment to be used.

The need to stop taking antithrombotic drugs prior to the procedure should be discussed with the referring medical team. It is usual practice to stop warfarin 3 days and low molecular weight heparin 24 hours before the procedure. If a patient is on warfarin, a blood test to check the international normalized ratio (INR) should be requested. The result of this should be within the range stipulated by local policy prior to performing the procedure, for example ≤ 1.5.

Some patients, such as those with multiple myeloma, will require careful positioning due to the infiltration of disease in their bones. These patients may also find bone marrow biopsies more uncomfortable as maintaining the correct position may be difficult. An environment that facilitates the patient's need for privacy and dignity is essential for bone marrow biopsy procedures (NMC 2015).

Education

The patient's co-operation is essential to ensure the procedure is undertaken safely. All patients should be given access to information and support in a manner that they understand (DH 2005a, NMC 2015). Written information should be available and patients often access information via the internet at sites such as www.macmillan.org.uk. Consideration must be given to those patients with learning disabilities, language barriers or sensory deficit (DH 2009).

Procedure guideline 2.1   Bone marrow aspiration and trephine biopsy

Essential equipment
- Antiseptic skin cleaning agent (e.g. chlorhexidine gluconate 2% in alcohol 70%)
- Sterile dressing pack
- Sterile gloves
- Plastic apron
- Eye protection
- Selection of syringes for bone marrow sampling and administration of local anaesthetic (2, 5 and 10 mL)

Medicinal products
- Local anaesthetic, for example lidocaine 2%
- Selection of needles for administration of local anaesthetic (25, 23 and 21 G)
- Marrow aspiration needle and guard
- Trephine biopsy needle
- Cytology slides and coverslips
- Specimen bottles (e.g. plain, formalin, EDTA and heparin)
- Sterile dressing
- Size 11 scalpel

Pre-procedure

Action	Rationale
1 Explain and provide written information about the bone marrow examination.	To ensure the patient is properly informed about the procedure (DH 2005a, **C**; NMC 2015, **C**).
2 Obtain written informed consent.	To enable patients to actively participate in and comply with their treatment (NMC 2015, **C**).
3 Check that blood parameters are within safe limits.	To decrease the risk of haemorrhage, which has been identified as the most common and serious adverse event associated with bone marrow examination (Bain 2006, **E**).
4 Consider oral (e.g. lorazepam), Entonox or intravenous (e.g. midazolam) sedation for very anxious patients (Giannoutsos et al. 2004).	To ensure that the procedure is performed safely and with minimal distress to the patient. **E**
5 Prepare the procedure trolley and ensure that all the necessary equipment and specimen containers are readily available.	To ensure the procedure is performed efficiently and that all the necessary specimens are collected and handled correctly (Smock and Perkins 2014, **E**).
6 Ensure patient privacy by drawing the curtains and making use of a sheet or blanket.	An environment that facilitates the patient's need for privacy and dignity is essential for bone marrow biopsy procedures (NMC 2015, **C**).
7 Assist the patient into the correct position, which is usually the left or right lateral position with the knees drawn up to the chest.	To access the posterior iliac crest, the most common biopsy site in adults. **E**

Procedure

Action	Rationale
8 Open pack and then open all the equipment onto sterile field.	To maintain asepsis throughout the procedure to minimize the risk of infection (Fraise and Bradley 2009, **E**).
9 Wash hands and apply sterile gloves.	To maintain asepsis throughout the procedure to minimize the risk of infection (Fraise and Bradley 2009, **E**).
10 Reassure and observe the patient throughout the procedure.	To allay anxiety and facilitate the patient's maximum co-operation. **P**
11 Clean the skin thoroughly at the biopsy site with an antiseptic solution (Perkins 2003), for example chlorhexidine 0.5%, and alcohol solution and allow to dry.	To maintain asepsis throughout the procedure to minimize the risk of infection (Fraise and Bradley 2009, **E**).
12 Administer local anaesthetic (e.g. lidocaine 2%) intradermally and subcutaneously at the site of the biopsy. Warn the patient that the drug can result in a 'stinging' sensation during administration.	To minimize pain during the procedure (Ruegg et al. 2009, **R1**).

13	Make a small cut in the skin overlying the biopsy site with a scalpel.	To allow for better insertion of the biopsy needle through the skin and to avoid a skin 'plug'. **E**
14	Insert the aspiration needle through the skin and subcutaneous tissues. Penetrate the marrow cortex 3–10 mm, with a slight rotating motion (Provan et al. 2015). Entry of the needle into the bone marrow cavity may be sensed as a slight give.	To access the bone marrow for aspiration. **E**
15	Remove the introducer, attach a 5 mL syringe to the needle and aspirate a volume of 0.2–2 mL marrow (bloody fluid) (Smock et al. 2014). Aspiration may cause a very brief, sharp, dragging sensation.	To aspirate liquid bone marrow in order to prepare specimens for further investigation (Hoffbrand and Moss 2015, **C**).
16	Disconnect the syringe and smear the marrow quickly onto the cytology slides.	To avoid clotting. **E**
17	Perform additional aspirations if necessary.	To provide material for flow cytometry, cytogenetics, culture or other special studies as required (Provan et al. 2015, **C**).
18	Perform the trephine biopsy using the same skin incision if the aspirate has been performed in the iliac crest area. Use a separate biopsy needle, slightly larger than the aspirate needle (Smock et al. 2014).	In order to minimize the number of skin entry sites. **E**
19	Advance the trephine needle to penetrate the bone cortex (Provan et al. 2015). The biopsy needle may require more pressure to enter the bone because of the larger bore size.	To access the bone for biopsy. **E**
20	Position the trephine needle away from the area where the aspiration was performed.	To avoid collection of a specimen with extensive artefact induced by the aspiration procedure (Smock et al. 2014, **E**).
21	Remove the introducer and use firm hand pressure to advance the needle another 2 cm	To provide a solid core of bone (Provan et al. 2015, **E**).
22	Insert a stylet into the back of the needle.	To give an approximation of the size of the bone core within the needle (Smock et al. 2014, **E**).
23	Ensure the length of the trephine specimen is in the range of 1.6–2 cm (Bain 2001, Bishop et al. 1992, Campbell et al. 2003).	The analysis of the relation between length of trephine and the rate of positivity for neoplasia yielded a minimum adequate length of 1.6 cm before processing (Bishop et al. 1992, **C**).
24	Remove the needle from the bone and use the stylet to express the specimen into the appropriate container (Smock et al. 2014).	To collect the solid core of bone and marrow to examine as a histological specimen after fixation in formalin, decalcification and sectioning (Hoffbrand and Moss 2015, **C**).
25	Apply manual pressure to the site for several minutes until the bleeding stops.	To achieve haemostasis (Smock et al. 2014, **E**).
26	Apply a sterile pressure dressing.	To achieve haemostasis and decrease the risk of infection at the biopsy site (Provan et al. 2015, **E**).

Post-procedure

27	Apply pressure bandages and check the site for prolonged bleeding if a patient is thrombocytopenic (Smock et al. 2014).	To minimize bruising, prevent haematoma and decrease the risk of haemorrhage (Bain 2006, **C**).
28	Dispose of sharps as per local policy.	To ensure the safe handling and disposal of needles and other sharp instruments and to protect staff, patients and visitors from exposure to bloodborne pathogens (Loveday et al. 2016, **C**).
29	Label specimens as per trust policy and send them to the appropriate laboratory department.	To prevent incorrect diagnosis and disease management through incorrectly labelled specimens (BCSH 2012, **C**).
30	Record the necessary information in the appropriate documents as per local policy.	To maintain accurate records (NMC 2015, **C**).
31	Ensure the patient has returned to pre-procedure functional status before discharge.	To ensure the safe management and recovery of patients receiving sedation. **E**
32	Give the patient appropriate aftercare instructions (see 'Education of patient and relevant others').	To ensure the safe management of patients and to enable them to actively participate in and comply with their treatment (NMC 2015, **C**).

Problem-solving table 2.1 Prevention and resolution (Procedure guideline 2.1)

Problem	Cause	Prevention	Action
Anxiety	Fear of pain or anticipatory anxiety due to a previous adverse experience (Lidén et al. 2009) Pre-existing pain (Lidén et al. 2009) Anxiety about the diagnostic outcome (Lidén et al. 2009)	Provide reassurance and support	Answer all questions and consider non-pharmacological support, for example relaxation therapy Consider anxiolytics, for example oral or intravenous benzodiazepines (Smock et al. 2014)
Difficulty locating posterior iliac crest	An inexperienced practitioner Difficulty in palpating the posterior iliac crest, for example in bariatric patients Altered anatomy, for example multiple myeloma patients who have experienced collapsed vertebrae and loss in height or patients who have had back surgery Patients who are unable to maintain the correct position due to, for example, pre-existing pain	Competency-based learning Guidance and support from an experienced practitioner Elective radiological guided procedure Adequate pain control	Recheck surface landmarks Ask for the assistance of a more experienced practitioner Consider a radiological guided procedure, especially in the case of bariatric patients
Uncontrollable pain	Inadequate administration of local anaesthetic Anticipatory anxiety associated with a previous experience which may augment the experience of pain (Lidén et al. 2009) Pre-existing pain related to disease process or co-morbidity	Administer sufficient local anaesthetic and wait for this to take effect Ensure adequate reassurance and support as anxiety may enhance the perception of pain Ensure correct positioning and direct approach Review pain control and consider referral to colleagues in the pain control team for advice	Reassess positioning. It is unusual for the procedure to be unbearably painful if the approach is correct and sufficient local anaesthesia has been used The procedure should be aborted if the pain continues and assistance should be sought Consider sedation for future procedures
No dragging sensation noted by the patient and no marrow obtained	Faulty technique, fibrosis, hyper- or hypocellularity (Humphries 2006)	Ensure correct positioning Ensure guidance and support for new practitioners	Rotate the needle and apply suction again. If no marrow is obtained, another sampling site may be required (Smock et al. 2014)
No marrow can be aspirated (dry tap)	Faulty technique, fibrosis, hyper- or hypocellularity (Humphries 2006)	Ensure correct positioning Ensure guidance and support for new practitioners	Make touch preparations from the biopsy (trephine roll) (Smock et al. 2014)

Post-procedural considerations

Immediate care
The patient should be advised to lie on their back, exerting pressure downwards on the biopsy site to assist in achieving haemostasis (Bain 2006). The biopsy site should be checked before the patient leaves the department to ensure that there is no bleeding. The patient should not experience any discomfort at the biopsy site immediately after the procedure due to the ongoing action of the local anaesthetic (Joint Formulary Committee 2018). The patient should return to pre-procedure functional status immediately after the procedure if no sedation has been used. A medical review should be requested if the patient has any unexpected pain or loss of mobility.

Ongoing care
This comprises wound care, pain control and monitoring for signs of infection. This is discussed further in 'Education of patient and

relevant others', as a bone marrow examination is usually an outpatient procedure (Lewis et al. 2011).

Documentation
The operator is responsible for documenting the procedure details to ensure accurate records are kept (NMC 2015). These should include:

- the site used and number of puncture sites
- volume and percentage of local anaesthetic
- information about any other medication used
- a list of samples obtained
- any unexpected incidents or adverse events
- dressings and wound care
- follow-up advice and information provided.

Education of patient and relevant others
The patient should be encouraged to contact the hospital if there are any concerns about post-procedural care. Contact

telephone numbers and the following advice should be given to patients.

- *Wound care.* The patient should be instructed to check the site frequently and to reapply pressure if the biopsy site does start to ooze. Intermittent application of an ice pack may also help to achieve haemostasis. It is routine practice to advise the patient to keep the dressing dry for 24 hours. The patient may then remove the dressing and wash as normal. Patients are also advised to monitor the biopsy site for any signs of infection such as redness, pain, swelling, failure to heal or exudate (Radhakrishnan 2017).
- *Pain.* Once the local anaesthetic has worn off, mild discomfort lasting 12–24 hours is common after a bone marrow examination (Radhakrishnan 2017). The patient should be advised that this may be dealt with by simple analgesia such as paracetamol (Provan et al. 2015).

Complications
Although adverse events after trephine biopsies and bone marrow aspirates are rare, they can have considerable impact on individual patients (Bain 2005).

- *Cardiac tamponade.* The actual risks associated with a sternal puncture are extremely small but penetration of the bone and damage to underlying structures are possible as the sternum is only approximately 1 cm thick in adults (Smock et al. 2014). The use of a guarded needle helps in preventing too deep an insertion. Tamponade is managed with an emergency call to the cardiac arrest team for immediate intervention.
- *Bone fractures.* These may occur particularly in small children owing to the pressure exerted. They are managed with analgesia, radiological investigation and referral to the orthopaedic team if indicated.

Bone marrow harvest

Related theory
Collecting haematopoietic stem cells by means of a bone marrow harvest or apheresis is well established in the transplant setting. More recently, transplants have also been facilitated through stem cells obtained from umbilical cords. Cord blood transplantation remains a specialized procedure more relevant for some areas of transplantation than others (Richardson and Atkinson 2006). The protocol for harvesting this alternative source of stem cells is beyond the scope of this chapter.

Evidence-based approaches

Rationale
Every year in the United Kingdom about 38,760 people are diagnosed with a haematological malignancy such as leukaemia, lymphoma or myeloma (Haematological Malignancy Research Network 2016). A stem cell transplant is one possible treatment option for these diseases (Atkinson 2005). A stem cell transplant aims to replace a patient's own diseased bone marrow with healthy stem cells. Before the patient receives the stem cells, they receive a combination of chemotherapy and radiation to destroy their own bone marrow. The healthy stem cells are collected from a patient when in remission (autologous) or from a donor (allogeneic) (Richardson and Atkinson 2006). The stem cells are then introduced into the patient's bloodstream much in the same manner as a blood transfusion. If the donated stem cells 'engraft', they begin producing normal blood cells (Atkinson 2005). The principles and process of collecting bone marrow apply to both allogeneic and autologous donors.

Indications
Although the use of stem cells collected by apheresis has superseded bone marrow in both the autologous and allogeneic setting in many transplant centres (Richardson and Atkinson 2006), indications for bone marrow harvest include:

- allogeneic donors under the age of 16 years
- allogeneic donors providing cells for a recipient with a nonmalignant disorder, for example aplastic anaemia
- donor preference.

Contraindications
Contraindications to donating stem cells by means of bone marrow include:

- a history of back problems
- donors who are unable to undergo a general anaesthetic.

Principles of care
The care of bone marrow donors is guided by a duty of care, encompassing the physical, emotional, psychological, social and spiritual dimensions of well-being (Be the Match Registry 2010). Ethical considerations should be incorporated into local policy and guidelines are available that outline the expected standards of care for unrelated (Hurley and Raffoux 2004, World Marrow Donor Association 2017) and related (van Walraven et al. 2010) donors. The procedure should be performed as a sterile procedure under general anaesthetic and all perioperative principles apply. Bone marrow harvests are performed under general anaesthesia because:

- The procedure may last for approximately 1 hour compared with 15–30 minutes for an aspiration and biopsy.
- Multiple puncture sites are used.
- The procedure may be painful.

Methods for bone marrow harvest
The procedure is undertaken by:

- two trained practitioners to perform the harvest (either two doctors, or a doctor and a nurse)
- one theatre nurse to oversee the equipment, sterile trolley and infusion of bone marrow into the sterile kit
- theatre staff
- an anaesthetist.

Bone marrow is aspirated directly from the marrow with a bone marrow harvest needle and syringe. A volume of 800–1000 mL is aspirated from the posterior iliac crest (in order to acquire sufficient cells per kilogram of the recipient's body weight) (Outhwaite 2008). The marrow is either frozen and stored or given fresh to the recipient (Richardson and Atkinson 2006).

Anticipated patient/donor outcomes
The anticipated outcome from the procedure is to collect a sufficient dose of stem cells in order to carry out a haematopoietic stem cell transplant. The anticipated outcome for the donor is to:

- remain infection free
- have no nerve, tissue or bone damage
- return to pre-donation levels of activity within 1 month of the harvest
- adequately manage any pain or discomfort experienced due to the bone marrow harvest.

Legal and professional issues
Standards that regulate bone marrow donation include the Human Tissue Authority (2017b) *Code G: Donation of Allogeneic Bone Marrow and Peripheral Blood Stem Cells for Transplantation* and FACT-JACIE's (2015) *International Standards for Cellular Therapy Product Collection, Processing and Administration.*

Competencies

It is a requirement that practitioners performing this procedure have experience and training in bone marrow harvesting (FACT-JACIE 2015). Competence must be demonstrated and documented.

Consent

Before consent is taken, donors should be carefully informed about the risks and benefits of the donation procedure in a manner that they understand. Although transplant centres usually have a preference for the source of stem cells, donors should be given a choice whether to donate bone marrow or stem cells by means of apheresis. Consent is an ongoing process and donors have the right to refuse to proceed (FACT-JACIE 2015). They should, however, be warned what the consequences of this would be for the recipient, if they do so after the conditioning regimen for transplant has been commenced.

Children acting as donors require further consideration. Laws and regulations governing minors who act as a donor for a sick sibling differ from country to country. Rarely, adult donors with severe developmental or psychological problems rendering them mentally incapable of informed consent are considered as stem cell donors for a relative. These can be either donors who have always been mentally challenged (e.g. Down's syndrome) or those who are suffering from a psychiatric illness. It is advised to first establish whether the aspirant donor would be able to endure the donation procedure (both physically and mentally) before performing tissue type testing (van Walraven et al. 2010).

In the United Kingdom, evidence must be documented that the Human Tissue Authority (2017a) *Code A: Guiding Principles and the Fundamental Principle of Consent* has been applied. All information should be managed within a strict framework of confidentiality (FACT-JACIE 2015).

Pre-procedural considerations

Equipment

Bone marrow harvest needles are usually 11 G with a removable introducer. Harvested bone marrow must be filtered to remove particulate matter prior to final processing and packaging for distribution or transplantation (FACT-JACIE 2015). This process must be performed under sterile conditions in the operating room at the time of harvest or in an appropriate sterile setting in the processing laboratory (FACT-JACIE 2015). Sterile in-line filters are available commercially in a collection set. The filter size may range from coarse (500 μm) to medium (300 μm) to fine (200 μm). All harvested marrow should ultimately pass through a fine filter, while other sizes may only be necessary if the marrow has a large amount of particulate matter (FACT-JACIE 2015).

Pharmacological support

The bone marrow harvest is performed under general anaesthesia and local policy with regard to perioperative care should be followed. Local anaesthetic, for example lidocaine 2%, is usually instilled into the harvest sites for postsurgery pain relief. Postoperative pain should be monitored and is usually managed with non-opioids and mild opioids. Iron supplements may be prescribed to facilitate haemoglobin recovery post harvest.

Specific patient/donor preparation

There should be donor evaluation procedures in place to protect the safety of the donor and recipient. All stem cell donors (autologous or allogeneic) should be given a medical examination to confirm they are physically and emotionally fit to undergo anaesthesia and the marrow harvest (Be the Match Registry 2010). The donor's medical history, physical examination and laboratory test results should be performed and documented according to the *International Standards for Cellular Therapy Product Collection, Processing and Administration* (FACT-JACIE 2015). Both the potential for disease transmission from the donor to the recipient and the risks to the donor from the collection procedure should be assessed (FACT-JACIE 2015). The allogeneic donor's suitability must be documented before the recipient's high-dose therapy has begun.

The psychosocial needs of the donor should be assessed (Scott and Sandmaier 2016). Key areas for support are: childcare arrangements, transportation, past and present drug and alcohol usage, unique cultural, religious, literacy and language needs and employment issues (Scott and Sandmaier 2016). An appropriately trained healthcare professional should be available to offer donors counselling, reassurance and support.

Education

It is widely agreed that donors require good-quality information to reduce their anxiety, to enable them to give informed consent and to enable them to actively participate with the donation process (Chapman and Rush 2003, NMC 2015). An increasing number of people are obtaining information from the internet and may be quite informed (or misinformed) based on the quality of the information they acquire. Transplant facilities and donor registries should develop their own centre-specific information which can be posted on their website or mailed to donors in advance of their first clinic visit to meet some of the education needs (Scott and Sandmaier 2016).

Procedure guideline 2.2 Bone marrow harvest

Essential equipment

- Skin cleaning agent, for example 2% chlorhexidine solution
- A sterile collection set with transfer packs and in-line filters (e.g. 500 and 200 μm) containing specified anticoagulant, for example anticoagulant citrate dextrose (ACDA) solution
- 250 mL 0.9% sodium chloride with 50 mL of heparin (1000 units per mL preservative free)
- Two 11 G bone marrow harvest needles flushed with heparinized saline
- 20 mL syringes containing 1 mL of heparinized saline × 6
- Selection of syringes and needles for administration of local anaesthetic
- Dressings
- Sterile gauze
- Sterile drapes

- Two receivers
- Facemasks
- Sterile gowns
- Sterile gloves
- Sterile pack containing jug, gallipot, gauze swabs, forceps, towel clips
- Documentation as per accreditation and local policy requirements

Medicinal products

- General anaesthesia (as per local policy)
- Lidocaine 2%

Pre-procedure

Action	Rationale
1 Explain and provide written information about the bone marrow harvest.	To ensure the donor is properly informed about the procedure (DH 2009, **C**; NMC 2015, **C**).

2 Obtain written informed consent.	To enable donors to actively participate in and comply with their treatment (FACT-JACIE 2015, **C**; Human Tissue Authority 2017a, **C**; NMC 2015, **C**).
3 Ensure that two units of cross-matched, allogeneic packed red cells are available on the day of harvest. These should only be used in exceptional circumstances, for example massive haemorrhage.	To reduce the risks associated with allogeneic blood transfusion (Confer et al. 2016, **E**).
4 Prepare the sterile procedure trolley and ensure that all the necessary equipment is available.	To ensure the procedure is performed efficiently and that the cells are collected and handled correctly. **E**
5 Bring the donor into the operating room when anaesthetized and position correctly on the operating table. In adults, this is usually the prone position with hands placed above the head.	To allow marrow to be collected simultaneously from both the left and right posterior iliac crest by two practitioners (Confer et al. 2016, **E**).
6 Ensure the harvest is performed as a sterile procedure. (a) Don facemasks. (b) Scrub hands meticulously. (c) Don sterile gowns. (d) Don sterile gloves.	To maintain asepsis throughout the procedure to minimize the risk of infection (Fraise and Bradley 2009, **E**).

Procedure

7 Clean the skin over the posterior iliac crests thoroughly with an antiseptic solution and allow to dry.	To maintain asepsis throughout the procedure to minimize the risk of infection (Fraise and Bradley 2009, **E**).
8 Place four sterile drapes over the patient to maintain a sterile field. (a) One drape placed above the posterior iliac crests and spread towards the donor's head. (b) One drape placed below the posterior iliac crests and spread towards the donor's feet. (c) Two drapes spread left and right of the harvest site respectively.	To create a sterile field around the harvest site and to maintain asepsis throughout the procedure to minimize the risk of infection (Fraise and Bradley 2009, **E**).
9 Place two receivers on the sterile towels. (a) One should contain two 11 G harvest needles (flushed with heparinized saline). (b) One should contain six 20 mL syringes (flushed with heparinized saline and drawn up to 1 mL with heparinized saline).	To ensure the harvest equipment is easily accessible. The heparinized saline prevents the marrow from clotting in the syringe. **E**
10 Locate the posterior iliac spine through palpation (Confer et al. 2016).	To ensure the preferred site for harvest is located. **E**
11 Insert the harvest needle through the skin and subcutaneous tissues, and penetrate the marrow cortex 3–10 mm, with a slight rotating motion. Entry of the needle into the bone marrow cavity may be sensed as a slight give.	To access the marrow within the bony cortex (Confer et al. 2016, **E**).
12 Remove the introducer and attach the harvest needle to a 20 mL syringe. Aspirate a volume of 10–20 mL of marrow (bloody fluid) by applying vigorous suction.	To aspirate marrow from the donor. Short, vigorous aspirations are generally thought to produce a higher concentration of marrow cells relative to peripheral blood (Confer et al. 2016, **E**).
13 Place filled syringes in the receiver.	To allow the nurse responsible for transferring the marrow into the sterile collection set to access them. **E**
14 If using ACDA, the nurse should add 70 mL of ACDA to the main collection bag prior to each harvest of 420 mL.	To prevent any clotting. **E**
15 Remove the filled syringe from the receiver and dispel any air from the syringe.	To ensure that the correct amount of marrow is aspirated. **E**
16 Ensure the marrow volume is recorded by a member of the theatre staff.	To keep a running total to ensure that the correct amount of marrow is aspirated. **E**
17 The nurse should gently add the marrow to the collection bag and gently agitate the collection bag to mix the marrow with the anticoagulant.	To prevent any clotting. **E**
18 Flush the syringe with heparinized saline (leaving 1 mL in the syringe).	To prevent any clotting. **E**
19 Return it to the receiver ready for subsequent aspirations.	To ensure the practitioners performing the harvest have a supply of appropriately prepared syringes to perform the aspirations. **E**

(continued)

Procedure guideline 2.2   Bone marrow harvest (continued)

Action	Rationale
20 Advance the harvest needle several millimetres and repeat the process.	To allow for several aspirations from a single bone puncture as the needle is repeatedly advanced (Confer et al. 2016, **E**).
21 After a number of aspirations from the same site, replace the introducer and move the position of the harvest needle to another place in the bone approximately 2 cm from the first entry site.	To allow the bone to be entered multiple times through a single skin entry site. A typical collection may involve 70 marrow aspirations obtained through only a few skin punctures. **E**
22 (a) Once a total of 420 mL of marrow has been collected, open the clips to allow the marrow to pass through the in-line filters (the 500 µm filter and then the 200 µm filter) from the collection bag to the first transfer pack. Then close the two clips prior to adding a second volume of 70 mL of ACDA to the collection bag and beginning bone marrow aspirations for a second transfer pack.	To ensure that transfer packs are not overfilled and that the correct amount of anticoagulant is added to prevent clotting (**E**) and to remove particulate matter (FACT-JACIE 2015, **C**).
(b) The total volume in each bag should approximate 420 mL of marrow and 70 mL of ACDA. If less than 420 mL of marrow is required for subsequent bags, the ACDA should be reduced accordingly to maintain a ratio of 1:7 ACDA:marrow.	To prevent any clotting. **E**
23 Aspirate a small sample from the first transfer pack when this has been filled.	To allow the adequacy of the collection to be determined by a nucleated cell count (Confer et al. 2016, **E**).
24 Place the sample in an EDTA specimen container.	This is the preferred medium for nucleated cell count analysis (Confer et al. 2016, **E**).
25 Label specimen container.	To ensure safe and correct processing of sample (BCSH 2012, **C**).
26 Send sample to the laboratory for a white cell count.	To allow the adequacy of the collection to be determined by a nucleated cell count (Confer et al. 2016, **E**).
27 This process should be repeated for each transfer pack filled.	To allow the adequacy of the entire collection to be determined by a nucleated cell count (Confer et al. 2016, **E**).
28 Document in the hospital notes the number of puncture holes made.	To facilitate post-operative wound care and to maintain accurate records (NMC 2015, **C**).
29 The nurse should seal the transfer packs as per local policy, using an approved heat sealer.	To maintain asepsis, minimize the risk of infection and facilitate the safe transport of the cells (Fraise and Bradley 2009, **E**).
30 The nurse should record the respective volume of bone marrow on the outside of the transfer pack in millilitres, using FACT-JACIE approved labels.	To establish total amount of bone marrow in each bag. **E**
31 Withdraw the harvest needles from the posterior iliac crest, pack sterile gauze over the left and right harvest sites respectively and maintain digital pressure until the bleeding has stopped.	To achieve haemostasis, minimize leakage and prevent the formation of a haematoma. **E**
32 Instil lidocaine 2% intradermally into the harvest sites up to the maximum recommended dose.	To help with pain control immediately post-operatively. **E**

Post-procedure

Action	Rationale
33 Dispose of sharps as per local policy.	To ensure the safe handling and disposal of needles and other sharp instruments and to protect staff, patients and visitors from exposure to bloodborne pathogens (DH 2005b, **C**; Loveday et al. 2016, **C**).
34 Inspect the puncture sites for bleeding. Mepore and a pressure dressing may be applied over the sterile gauze.	To achieve haemostasis and decrease the risk of infection at the harvest sites. **E**
35 Take the donor to the recovery room.	To ensure appropriate post-operative care. **E**
36 Label each transfer pack as per local policy with FACT-JACIE compliant labels.	To ensure correct management of the product (FACT-JACIE 2015, **C**).

37	Place the transfer packs in a secondary container (e.g. a zip-type resealable bag) prior to transfer to the appropriate processing facility.	To prevent the loss of a portion of the collection, to minimize the potential of post-collection contamination of the component and to prevent potential spillage of biohazard material in areas where it may pose a risk to employees, visitors or patients (FACT-JACIE 2015, **C**).
38	Transport the marrow to the appropriate processing facility with the necessary forms and in a FACT-JACIE compliant container.	To allow for cell measurement, storage and/or issue of the marrow. **E**
39	Record the necessary information in the appropriate documents as per local policy.	To maintain accurate records (NMC 2015, **C**).
40	Ensure post-donation care is appropriately managed (see 'Post-procedural considerations').	To ensure the safe management of patients and to enable them to actively participate in and comply with their treatment (NMC 2015, **C**).

Problem-solving table 2.2 Prevention and resolution (Procedure guideline 2.2)

Problem	Cause	Prevention	Action
Reactions to the anaesthetic agents and associated morbidity (Rosenmayr et al. 2003)	Allergic reactions, hypersensitivity reactions or idiosyncratic reactions (Confer et al. 2016)	Careful preassessment	Instigate urgent treatment and mechanical ventilation as necessary (Confer et al. 2016)
Haemorrhage, which can result in life-threatening blood loss and can also create severe pain from the compression of soft tissues (Confer et al. 2016)	Poor technique Antiplatelet drugs Anticoagulant drugs Coagulopathies	Careful preassessment Experienced practitioners	Pressure dressing Platelet transfusion Correction of clotting derangement Analgesia
Target cell dose not achieved through aspiration from the posterior iliac crests	This may occur if the marrow space of the crest has been compromised by, for example, trauma or radiation (Confer et al. 2016). This is particularly applicable to autologous donors	Careful preassessment Experienced practitioners	Marrow may then also be collected from the anterior iliac crests or the sternum (Confer et al. 2016)

Post-procedural considerations

Immediate care
Immediate post-donation care includes:

- all usual post-operative nursing care measures
- post-operative full blood count
- adequate analgesia and antiemetic cover
- wound and dressing check before discharge.

Documentation
Bone marrow harvests should be strictly regulated within a quality management system with clear standard operating procedures and documentation. Archived documentation should be maintained according to governmental, regulatory or institutional policy, whichever is longer (FACT-JACIE 2015). Due to the strict regulatory nature of bone marrow harvests, a record-keeping system must be in place to ensure the authenticity, integrity and confidentiality of all documents (FACT-JACIE 2015). All nursing records must be clearly maintained to ensure accurate data (NMC 2015).

Education of patient and relevant others
All donors should be informed that it is normal to experience some pain, bruising and stiffness, feel more tired than usual and run a low-grade fever during the first week after donation. Soreness at the collection site usually eases off in around a week with pain relief (Be the Match Registry 2010). Further guidelines to be given to donors post procedure are detailed in Box 2.1.

Box 2.1 Guidelines to be given to bone marrow harvest donors post procedure

- The discomfort at the harvest site should resolve in about 1 week.
- Analgesia should be taken as directed.
- Aspirin should be avoided during the first week after the donation unless instructed by the medical team.
- The harvest site should be checked daily for bleeding or increasing erythema.
- The harvest site should be kept dry the night after the procedure.
- Bandages should be removed 24 hours after surgery, and replaced with an adhesive dressing.
- Some wound drainage is expected.
- Showers rather than baths should be taken for the first 2–3 days to decrease the risk of infection.
- The adhesive dressings should be changed daily after a shower until the wounds have healed.
- If bleeding occurs, firm pressure should be applied for 5 minutes, followed by an ice pack. The patient should be advised, if the bleeding does not stop after 10 minutes of constant direct pressure, to contact the hospital.
- It is common to experience 'hard lumps' at the harvest sites where the needles were inserted. These may take a few weeks to resolve.

Source: Adapted from Be the Match Registry (2010).

Box 2.2 Reported bone marrow harvest transfusion practice

- Units of autologous blood may be collected from donors a few weeks prior to the harvest for transfusion after the procedure. This practice is becoming less common.
- Autologous red cells may be recovered from the collected bone marrow. This process has been successfully applied in child donors without compromising the quality of the marrow donation.
- Administration of erythropoietin (EPO) may also diminish the likelihood of allogeneic blood transfusion. A theoretical concern about pretreatment of donors with EPO is diminished quality of the collected marrow.

Source: Adapted from Confer et al. (2016).

Furthermore, all donors should receive written instructions to contact the hospital if they experience any of the following symptoms (Be the Match Registry 2010):

- temperature of 38°C or higher
- increased redness, bleeding, swelling, drainage or pain at the collection area
- muscle weakness or severe headache within 2 weeks of donation
- pain more than 14 days after the donation.

Complications

The complications of bone marrow harvest are rare but it remains a significant procedure and not without physical risk or psychological consequences (Scott and Sandmaier 2016). There is potential for bone, nerve or other tissue damage at the aspiration sites (Rosenmayr et al. 2003). Sciatic pain, lasting up to 18 months, has been reported in a related donor (Confer et al. 2016). Other complications include:

- A potential for *infection* at the aspiration sites (Rosenmayr et al. 2003). This may occur due to poor practitioner technique or inadequate wound care. Hand decontamination, infection control and wound care policies should be followed as essential preventive measures (Fraise and Bradley 2009). Antibiotics should be used to treat infections if indicated (Confer et al. 2016).
- *Anaemia*, due to the large amount of bone marrow aspirated (Rosenmayr et al. 2003). Resultant allogeneic transfusions may cause transfusion reactions or transmit viral infections and, rarely, bacterial infections (Confer et al. 2016). Transfusion practice for bone marrow donation varies depending on the collection physician (see Box 2.2). Discharge medication should include ferrous sulfate.
- *Fatigue* related to procedure-induced anaemia. The severity of anaemia is determined entirely by the donor's pre-operative haemoglobin level and the net blood loss. Treatment with transfusion has already been described. Other measures include:
  - a gradual return to work (usually after 1 week)
  - ensuring rest between periods of work
  - avoiding strenuous activity for 3–4 weeks
  - a 1-month follow-up appointment for check-up and repeat full blood count.

In the event of complications, donors should be referred to the medical team, physiotherapist and the wider multidisciplinary team as necessary.

Apheresis

Related theory

Apheresis was introduced in the late 1960s and was innovative as it served to remove the major blood cell constituents or plasma rapidly, while efficiently processing large volumes of blood (Kaushansky et al. 2016). The earliest procedures were performed on patients with chronic myeloid leukaemia. In these instances, the procedure served to lower the patient's white cell count (Kaushansky et al. 2016).

With scientific advances, apheresis is no longer only used on patients in order to remove blood components or exchange them for therapeutic purposes; it is now possible to harvest blood components such as stem cells to be used for donation. Stem cells can be 'mobilized' into the peripheral blood following treatment with cytotoxic chemotherapy and/or the administration of the haematopoietic growth factor G-CSF, with or without plerixafor (an immunostimulant). The use of stem cells collected by means of apheresis has superseded bone marrow in many transplant centres (Richardson and Atkinson 2006). Exact protocols vary according to underlying disease, treatment regimens, local practice and the type of stem cell donor; for example, cytotoxic chemotherapy and plerixafor are not used to mobilize stem cells from healthy donors.

Another, newer application of apheresis in the haematooncology setting is extracorporeal photopheresis (ECP) (Knobler et al. 2014). This involves a specialized cell separator machine that additionally incorporates a light box that exposes the patient's collected lymphocyte product to ultraviolet light following the administration of a photo-sensitizing drug. Indications for use are cutaneous T cell lymphoma, and chronic graft-versus-host disease post allogeneic stem cell transplant (Howell et al. 2015).

Evidence-based approaches

Rationale

Apheresis is used for a number of donor and therapeutic purposes. A therapeutic procedure is when a blood component is removed from a patient to decrease the number of defective cells or deplete a disease mediator (Schwartz et al. 2013). A donor procedure is when a blood component (e.g. stem cells, lymphocytes, platelets) is removed to be used for therapeutic purposes (e.g. peripheral blood stem cell transplant, donor lymphocyte infusion, platelet transfusion).

Indications

The American Society for Apheresis (ASFA) Applications Committee reviews and categorizes the indications for therapeutic apheresis every 7 years. It aims to provide uniformity, is as evidence-based as possible and provides comprehensive information which could be shared with patients and clinical services requesting the use of therapeutic apheresis (Schwartz et al. 2013). Some apheresis applications and indications are outlined in Table 2.3.

Contraindications

Contraindications will depend on the reason for undertaking the procedure, that is, donor or therapeutic.

- *Donors*. There are strict processes in place that regulate whether an individual may donate a blood component for therapeutic use. These include FACT-JACIE's (2015) *International Standards for Cellular Therapy Product Collection, Processing and Administration* for stem cell and lymphocyte donors and the regulations that national blood services put forward for platelet and granulocyte donors. Contraindications should be stated in the cell separator facility's standard operating procedure manual. An example of a contraindication for allogeneic donors is a diagnosis of human immunodeficiency virus (HIV).
- *Patients*. It is a medical decision as to whether a patient is fit to proceed with a cell separator procedure for therapeutic reasons. It may be appropriate to undertake a cell separator procedure in a very unwell patient if it is considered to be a life-saving intervention. For example, some patients with acute myeloid leukaemia present with a high white cell count and are at risk of leucostasis and are therefore referred for white cell depletion. All decisions must be documented in the patient's medical notes.

Table 2.3 Apheresis applications and indications

Applications	Indications
Therapeutic apheresis	
Plasma exchange:	
Removal of a patient's own plasma and replacement with appropriate fluids, for example albumin, FFP. This is in order to remove disease mediators including: • alloantibodies • autoimmune antibodies • antigen–antibody complexes • abnormal or increased amounts of plasma protein • very high cholesterol levels • high levels of plasma metabolic waste products • plasma-bound poisons or drugs	• Thrombotic thrombocytopenia purpura (TTP) • Guillain–Barré syndrome • Myasthenia gravis
Red blood cell exchange:	
Removal of large volumes of patient red blood cells and replacement with normal donor red blood cells	• Sickle cell disease • Malaria • Babesiosis
Cellular depletion:	
Rapid removal of greatly elevated numbers of cells from the intravascular space. Decreases the risk associated with vascular stasis, for example: • White blood cell depletion • Platelet depletion	• Symptomatic leucocytosis in, for example, a patient newly diagnosed with acute myeloid leukaemia • Symptomatic thrombocytosis in a patient with thrombophilia
Photopheresis:	
Use of apheresis technology, light-activated drugs and ultraviolet light to modulate lymphocyte activity	• Cutaneous T cell lymphoma • Pemphigus vulgaris • Chronic graft-versus-host disease • Acute and chronic graft rejection
Immunoadsorption:	
Removal of a disease mediator from the patient's plasma and the subsequent return of the treated plasma to the patient	• Immune thrombocytopenic purpura (ITP) • Rheumatoid arthritis • Platelet refractoriness • Haemolytic uraemic syndrome
Dendritic cell collection:	
Removal of dendritic cells in order to manipulate them *in vitro* by providing them with tumour antigen so that they are capable of activating T lymphocytes to fight malignancy	• Prostate cancer • Melanoma • Multiple myeloma • Small cell lung cancer • Renal cell carcinoma • Breast cancer
LDL apheresis:	
Selective removal of LDL cholesterol from a patient's plasma through secondary processing	• Familial hypercholesterolaemia unresponsive to drug therapy
Donor apheresis	
Peripheral blood stem cell collection:	
White cell procedure to collect haematopoietic stem cells. The collected stem cells may be used fresh or cryopreserved for both malignant and non-malignant conditions	• Autologous stem cell collection (patient's own stem cells) • Allogeneic stem cell collection (collected from an HLA-matched related or unrelated donor) • Syngeneic stem cell collection (collected from the patient's identical twin) • Haploidentical stem cell collection (collected from either the mother or father of the patient)
Granulocyte collection:	
White cell procedure to collect granulocytes (neutrophils) from suitable donors	• Transfuse to neutropenic patients in order to provide adequate numbers of functional neutrophils to fight bacterial, fungal or yeast infections
Lymphocyte collection:	
White cell procedure to collect lymphocytes from a related or unrelated donor for a patient following an allogeneic stem cell transplant (the donor of the graft cells is also the donor of the lymphocytes)	• Post allogeneic stem cell transplantation in the event of malignancy relapse • Non-myeloablative allogeneic stem cell transplant • Production of targeted cytotoxic T lymphocytes
Platelet collection:	
Collection of platelets from healthy donors. Primarily the role of the blood transfusion service	• For patients who, for a multitude of reasons, require a platelet transfusion

Source: Adapted from Choi and Foss (2010), Schwartz et al. (2013), Strauss (2010).
FFP, fresh frozen plasma; LDL, low density lipoprotein.

74

Principles of care

There has been an increase in the clinical use of cell separators for the treatment of a greater variety of clinical conditions and to collect a greater range of therapeutic products. It is therefore important that careful consideration is given to the likely clinical conditions to be treated, blood products to be collected, the most suitable type of equipment to use and the appropriate training of staff when setting up a cell separator service (Howell et al. 2015).

The decision to use a cell separator for donor or therapeutic purposes is the responsibility of a medical consultant. In view of the known risks and complications associated with the use of cell separators, appropriately trained medical and nursing staff must be in attendance (Howell et al. 2015).

Methods for apheresis

The procedure for performing apheresis is complex and differs depending on the system and application. The basic steps in apheresis are:

- removal of whole blood from a patient or donor into a cell separator
- addition of an anticoagulant to the blood to prevent clotting in the extracorporeal circuit
- centrifugation and/or filtration to achieve separation of the blood components
- removal/collection of the desired blood component
- return of the rest of the blood to the patient with or without replacement products.

The ability of various techniques and equipment to carry out these basic steps determines collection efficiency and product purity (Burgstaler 2010). Further information can be gained from the respective apheresis operators' manuals.

Anticipated patient/donor outcomes

Anticipated patient/donor outcomes are dependent on the indication for carrying out the procedure. It is anticipated that cell separator procedures do no harm to patients or donors. Local standard operating procedures should be followed to ensure that desired end-points are reached and the efficacy of the procedure is within an expected range, irrespective of the operator.

Legal and professional issues

Other regulations that require compliance for apheresis procedures, if being used in the field of stem cell transplantation, include the Human Tissue Authority (2013) *Code of Practice 6: Donation of Allogeneic Bone Marrow and Peripheral Blood Stem Cells for Transplantation* and FACT-JACIE's (2015) *International Standards for Cellular Therapy Product Collection, Processing and Administration.*

Cell separator procedures should only be performed after a written and signed order from the medical team. The administration of any drugs and fluids used should be in accordance with a Patient Group Direction or a written prescription.

Competencies

Apheresis should only be performed by specially trained operators who are deemed competent to work at an advanced level. Nurses must always operate within their scope of practice (NMC 2015). Training packages should address the theoretical base and clinical skills needed to work as an apheresis nurse and should be carried out in accordance with local standard operating procedures. It is usual for the manufacturers of cell separator machines to offer training days and supply training materials, for example workbooks. This is often supported by work-based learning with a mentor or practice facilitator. Academic modules at university level are offered in some countries. Training should cover the assessment and management of patients and donors (including paediatrics if appropriate) undergoing apheresis, as well as the technology used to carry out the applications. Other training needs, dependent on particular centres, may include:

- principles of basic haematology, coagulation and immunology
- stem cell mobilization procedures and principles of stem cell transplant
- knowledge of the diseases for which apheresis is required
- collection of specific blood components by apheresis
- recognition and treatment of common complications
- validation of procedures and processes within a quality management system
- regulatory, legal and professional issues.

A suitable assessment, designed to determine the level of competence, must be performed and documentation of knowledge and technical ability must be maintained (FACT-JACIE 2015, Howell et al. 2015). Apheresis nurses must also ensure that their cardiopulmonary resuscitation training is up to date (FACT-JACIE 2015).

Consent

The routine of obtaining consent from patients and donors undergoing apheresis represents good clinical practice (MHRA 2012). Clearly written explanatory literature or other forms of information should be available to assist in obtaining informed consent. This should include any drugs or replacement fluids that may be used (Howell et al. 2015).

If the apheresis procedure is being undertaken as part of a stem cell transplantation procedure, all regulations and principles pertaining to consent apply, as discussed in the Bone marrow harvest section.

Pre-procedural considerations

Equipment

Numerous types of cell separator machines are now available, but all operate on either a continuous or intermittent flow principle, allowing for the rapid return of anticoagulated blood (Figure 2.8). These systems consist of a device that will carry out whole-blood separation, normally using a sterile, functionally closed-system, single-use disposable apheresis kit (Howell et al. 2015) with a citrate or heparin anticoagulant solution. All equipment must conform to relevant safety requirements. Regular servicing should be undertaken according to manufacturers' guidelines with service records kept (Howell et al. 2015). It is recommended that a service contract exists to ensure that an engineer can be contacted to repair the machine within a stipulated timeframe. Cell separator machines must be regularly cleaned with a suitable decontaminating agent and a standard procedure for dealing with blood spillage must be used (Howell et al. 2015). It is recommended that cell separator facilities undertake a risk assessment and prepare a business continuity plan to manage untoward incidents (FACT-JACIE 2015).

Vascular access

High blood flow rates are required for apheresis, so particular care must be taken over the peripheral venous assessment and vein selection of patients and donors. A rigid 16/17 G needle, cannula or equivalent is placed in the antecubital fossa for access (Figure 2.9) and a 20 G cannula or equivalent is sited in a peripheral vein for return. Peripheral access and return are usually sited in opposing arms. Side-effects from needle insertion may include pain, bleeding and haematoma. In addition, patients and donors may suffer from needle phobia, resulting in anxiety and vasovagal reactions (Association of Anaesthetists of Great Britain and Ireland 2016, Dougherty and Lister 2015).

When there is poor venous access, a central venous catheter needs to be placed to undertake the procedure (NHS Blood and Transplant 2010). This has been identified as the greatest risk that patients and donors face (Stroncek et al. 2000). Standard alternatives to peripheral access include rigid percutaneous polyurethane or tunnelled silicone catheters (Pertine et al. 2002).

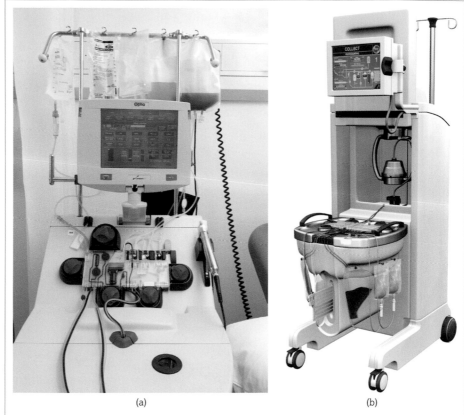

Figure 2.8 (a) Optia™ cell separator machine during stem cell collection procedure. (b) Therakos Celex™ photophoresis machine.

An estimated 1% of central catheter placements are associated with haemorrhage, pneumothorax or infection (Stroncek et al. 2000). These risks are reduced by experienced personnel inserting the catheters with the assistance of ultrasound. In addition, placing the catheters in the femoral vein eliminates the risk of pneumothorax and these types of catheters are well tolerated for a short time (Stroncek et al. 2000). Further information about the general management of venous access devices can be found in Dougherty and Lister (2015) *The Royal Marsden Manual of Clinical Nursing Procedures, Ninth Edition*: Chapter 14 Vascular Access Devices: Insertion and Management.

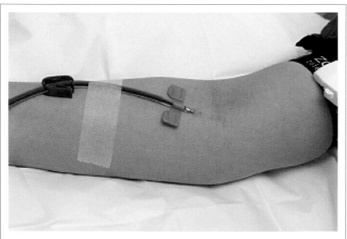

Figure 2.9 Peripheral venous access for cell separator procedures. *Source:* Dougherty and Lister (2011).

Assessment and recording tools

It is standard practice to make use of a pre-prepared apheresis worksheet, and this should form part of a wider quality management and document control system. Information detailed usually contains at least the information included in Box 2.3.

Box 2.3 Information included on an apheresis worksheet

- The date, patient/donor details, indication for apheresis and application requested.
- Confirmation that consent has been obtained and re-confirmed pre procedure.
- Confirmation that the cell separator has been cleaned as per standard operating procedure before initiating the procedure.
- Blood tests requested and pertinent results (before and after procedure).
- The patient/donor's blood pressure, pulse, temperature and oxygen saturation dependent on condition and indication for procedure (initial and subsequent).
- A log of what machine, reagents, replacement fluids and kit were used with details of the lot numbers and expiry dates to ensure traceability.
- The patient/donor's height, weight and gender to calculate the total blood volume.
- Target values and expected outcomes for the procedure.
- A record of venous access devices used and where they were sited.
- Medication administered, complications experienced and actions taken.
- The final run results and the patient/donor's fluid balance.
- The operator's signature with the date and time.

Pharmacological support

It is good practice to apply a local anaesthetic cream to peripheral venous access sites to minimize pain and discomfort during cannulation. Apprehensive patients may be given an oral sedative to relieve anxiety.

Anticoagulants used to prevent blood clotting in the extracorporeal circuit are usually citrate based; however, heparin is used for some procedures. If a citrate-based anticoagulant is used, it is important that nurses are aware that electrolyte supplements may be needed during the procedure if the patient/donor experiences any signs of citrate toxicity. One example is tetany related to hypocalcaemia. An algorithm of drug management for citrate toxicity should be used to guide staff.

Replacement fluids that may be used during exchange procedures include sodium chloride 0.9%, human albumin solutions, fresh frozen plasma (FFP), cryo-poor FFP, solvent/detergent plasma and human red cell concentrates.

Predosage of donors with corticosteroids and G-CSF to enhance the yield of granulocyte collections is sometimes undertaken. Records of cumulative doses for each donor must be kept (Howell et al. 2015).

G-CSF is routinely used for patients and donors to stimulate haematopoietic stem cell release and improve collection efficiency during stem cell collections by means of apheresis. Plerixafor is a more recent drug intervention that can be utilized to enhance the mobilization of stem cells for collection and subsequent autologous transplantation in patients with lymphoma and multiple myeloma who have failed to mobilize adequately with first-line mobilization therapy, that is, chemotherapy with G-CSF or G-CSF alone (Chen et al. 2012). Plerixafor is an antagonist that blocks stromal cell-derived factor (SDF)-1-alpha to the cellular receptor CXCR4, resulting in stem cell release from bone marrow (National Cancer Institute 2010). An additional application of plerixafor to a standard G-CSF mobilization regimen may lead to a significant increase in stem cell release (Chen et al. 2012). Both G-CSF and plerixafor should be used in accordance with the manufacturer's recommendations and local guidelines.

Nurses working in cell separator facilities with responsibility for patient/donor care must have knowledge of the side-effects of any fluids and drugs used and also any drugs patients may already be taking that may affect the apheresis procedure, for example angiotensin-converting enzyme (ACE) inhibitors (Howell et al. 2015).

Non-pharmacological support

An apprehensive patient will experience a sympathetic nervous system response and consequently vasoconstriction. This will diminish blood flow to the cell separator and result in a less efficient procedure. All measures should be taken to reassure and calm patients and provide them with support.

Specific patient/donor preparations

Cell separator procedures can take up to 5 hours and it is important to ensure that patients and donors are as comfortable as possible. Some considerations include the following.

- The positioning of the donor/patient on a bed or apheresis chair. Pillows should be used for support as necessary.
- The need to encourage patients and donors to eat and drink as normal; however, care must be taken if there is a need to use the toilet, as it is not usually possible to interrupt the cell separator procedure. This is due to the need to maintain a functionally closed system for sterility purposes.
- Distractions such as access to a television, DVDs, radio, music and reading material.
- The use of a heated blanket at the venous access or return sites to ease any discomfort that may occur due to vasoconstriction.
- Asking if patients and donors would like a friend or family member to accompany them during the procedure. Space constraints usually limit additional visitors.

There should be sufficient space in the cell separator facility to allow staff to operate all equipment without danger to themselves, donors/patients or visitors. The area should also be adequate to allow a cardiac arrest team to operate, and resuscitation equipment must be available (FACT-JACIE 2015).

Education

All patients and donors should be given access to information and support in a manner that they understand (DH 2005a, NMC 2015). Consideration must be given to those patients with learning disabilities, language barriers or sensory deficit.

Procedure guideline 2.3   Apheresis

This is a general guide as it is beyond the scope of this chapter to detail each procedure.

Essential equipment
- Cell separator machine
- Disposable tubing set compatible with cell separator machine and application needed, for example stem cell, white blood cell, therapeutic plasma exchange, red blood cell exchange kit or ECP kit
- Sterile gloves
- For peripheral venous access: a rigid 16/17 G needle, cannula or equipment for insertion (see *The Royal Marsden Manual of Clinical Nursing Procedures, Ninth Edition*: Chapter 14 Vascular Access Devices: Insertion and Management)
- For peripheral venous return: 20 G device, for example cannula and equipment for insertion (see *The Royal Marsden Manual of Clinical Nursing Procedures, Ninth Edition*: Chapter 14 Vascular Access Devices: Insertion and Management)
- For central venous access and return: equipment to access (see *The Royal Marsden Manual of Clinical Nursing Procedures, Ninth Edition*: Chapter 14 Vascular Access Devices: Insertion and Management)

- Documentation as per local policy and dependent on procedure type
- Apheresis system operator's manual
- Access to patient/donor medical notes/prescription chart

Medicinal products
- Anticoagulant, for example 500 mL ACDA anticoagulant (number of bags needed is usually stipulated by length of procedure)
- 1000 mL 0.9% sodium chloride
- Local anaesthetic cream for venous access if indicated
- Replacement fluids as indicated dependent on the type of procedure, for example sodium chloride 0.9%, human albumin solutions, FFP, cryo-poor FFP, solvent/detergent plasma, and human red cell concentrates
- Methoxypsoralen and heparin if performing ECP
- Electrolyte supplements, for example calcium, as per the local policy for the management of citrate toxicity

Pre-procedure

Action	Rationale
1 Explain and provide written information about the apheresis procedure.	To ensure the patient or donor is properly informed about the procedure (DH 2005a, **C**; NMC 2015, **C**).
2 Check that written informed consent has been taken and re-confirmed and that the patient has a good understanding of the procedure.	To enable patients or donors to actively participate in and comply with their treatment (FACT-JACIE 2015, **C**; Human Tissue Authority 2017a, **C**; NMC 2015, **C**).
3 Check that all documentation, which may vary according to local policy and also procedure type, is complete.	To maintain accurate records and comply with regulatory policy (FACT-JACIE 2015, **C**; Human Tissue Authority 2017a, **C**; NMC 2015, **C**).
4 Ensure the patient or donor is wearing a wristband correctly labelled with their name, hospital number and date of birth.	To prevent patient safety incidents and near misses relating to missing or incorrect wristbands (FACT-JACIE 2015, **C**).
5 Check that pertinent serological tests have been carried out within the timeframes stipulated by local and/or regulatory policy.	To prevent cross-infection with bloodborne infections (FACT-JACIE 2015, **C**; Human Tissue Authority 2017a, **C**).
6 Consider oral sedation (e.g. lorazepam) for very anxious patients.	To ensure that the procedure is performed safely and with minimal distress to the patient. **E**
7 Document which apheresis machine is being used.	To ensure traceability of procedures and assist in the audit of collection efficiency (FACT-JACIE 2015, **C**).
8 Obtain and record the patient or donor's biological parameters, for example height, weight and gender, to calculate total blood volume.	To ensure accurate data input and machine settings. **E**
9 Obtain and record the patient or donor's baseline observations, for example temperature, pulse rate, blood pressure.	Subsequent observations can be compared against the baseline to assist in accurately informing the need for intervention if the patient or donor's condition appears to deteriorate during the procedure. **E**
10 Check and record pertinent blood results (e.g. haemoglobin, haematocrit, platelet count, white cell differential, blood group, electrolytes, plasma viscosity, haemoglobin S, peripheral CD34-positive count and clotting). The blood tests required will differ depending on procedure type. Local policy should be followed.	To ensure accurate data input, machine settings, disease monitoring and patient/donor safety (Human Tissue Authority 2017a, **C**; JACIE 2015, **C**).
11 Ensure solutions and drugs needed for the procedure have been prescribed.	To ensure good medicines management (NMC 2010, **C**).
12 If a central venous catheter has been placed with the tip in the superior vena cava, check the documentation of the catheter tip position prior to use. This should be documented in the medical records after a chest X-ray.	High flow rates are required for apheresis so good venous access is essential (FACT-JACIE 2015, **C**).
13 Check that the apheresis machine has been cleaned and maintained as per local policy. This must be documented.	Environmental conditions must be controlled for surface contaminants to minimize the risk of contamination or cross-contamination (FACT-JACIE 2015, **C**).
14 Prepare the procedure trolley and ensure that all the necessary equipment and specimen containers are readily available.	To ensure the procedure is performed efficiently and that all the necessary specimens are collected and handled correctly (Smock and Perkins 2014, **E**).
15 Visually examine all reagents used for damage or evidence of contamination prior to use. Note the lot numbers and expiry dates of all reagents. Ensure local incident reporting systems are used if any reagents are not suitable for use.	To ensure an effective quality management plan is established and maintained and to minimize the risk of contamination or cross-contamination (FACT-JACIE 2015, **C**).
16 Select and load the disposable set and reagents. The set will differ depending on what procedure is undertaken and which type of cell separator is used.	To prepare the apheresis machine prior to connecting the patient and to ensure that it is in good working order (Choi and Foss 2010, **E**; Strauss 2010, **E**; Terumo BCT 2011, **C**)
17 Prime the disposable tubing set with 0.9% sodium chloride and anticoagulant.	To expel air from the disposable tubing set. **E**
18 Perform alarm tests and checks.	To prepare the apheresis machine prior to connecting the patient and to ensure that it is in good working order (Choi and Foss 2010, **E**; Strauss 2010, **E**; Terumo BCT 2011, **C**).
19 If the apheresis machine alarm sounds during the procedure, refer to the troubleshooting section of the operator's manual and follow the relevant instructions.	To prepare the apheresis machine prior to connecting the patient and to ensure that it is in good working order (Choi and Foss 2010, **E**; Strauss 2010, **E**; Terumo BCT 2011, **C**).

(continued)

Procedure guideline 2.3   Apheresis *(continued)*

Action	Rationale
20 Enter the patient or donor's biological parameters and pertinent blood results into the apheresis machine as prompted. Amend settings as required by local policy.	To customize and optimize the procedure (Choi and Foss 2010, **E**; Strauss 2010, **E**; Terumo BCT 2011, **C**).
21 Document target run results and pertinent information as required by local policy.	To maintain accurate records (NMC 2015, **C**).
22 Ensure patient privacy by drawing the curtains as per patient preference. A blanket or sheet may be needed if vascular access is via a femoral, percutaneous or tunnelled central venous catheter.	An environment that facilitates the patient's need for privacy and dignity is essential (NMC 2015, **C**).
23 Assist the patient into the correct position, which is usually the supine position with arms comfortably rested at their sides. The back of the bed or apheresis chair is usually slightly elevated, but this is guided by patient preference.	To maintain patient comfort and access either peripheral or central venous access devices. **E**
24 Wash hands and apply gloves. Non-sterile gloves must be used when handling biological specimens (JACIE 2015).	To protect the nurse from any contamination (European Commission 2011, **C**).

Procedure

Action	Rationale
25 Place the sterile field under the patient's venous access and clean the end of the needlefree connector attached to the vascular access device.	To maintain asepsis throughout the procedure to minimize the risk of infection (Fraise and Bradley 2009, **E**).
26 Connect the patient or donor to the apheresis machine via the preselected venous access devices. There must be one lumen for access and one for return of blood. Check that all venous access devices are patent by withdrawing blood and flushing with 10 mL 0.9% sodium chloride. No resistance should be felt.	High flow rates are required for apheresis so good venous access is essential (NHS Blood and Transplant 2010, **C**).
27 Proceed with the run as per the operator's manual depending on procedure type.	To achieve therapeutic or donation targets (Kaushansky et al. 2016, **E**).
28 Monitor the condition of the patient or donor and also the progress of the procedure and intervene as required (see Problem-solving table 2.3 for troubleshooting).	To ensure the procedure runs smoothly and the patient or donor is safely managed. **E**
29 Dependent on the procedure type, perform a rinseback when the procedure targets have been met. A rinseback is when the cell separator is flushed through with sodium chloride 0.9% to ensure that any blood remaining in the machine is returned to the patient (Burgstaler 2010).	To ensure accurate fluid balance and haemodynamic stability (Howell et al. 2015, **C**). For this reason, it is unusual to perform a rinseback in, for example, paediatric cases (where a blood prime has been used) or after red cell exchanges for patients with sickle cell disease (Burgstaler 2010, **E**).

Post-procedure

Action	Rationale
30 If undertaking a donation procedure, permanently seal the product bags, preferably by using a heat sealer. As a contingency, three sealing clips closed by clamp may be used.	To ensure safe handling and protect product from exposure to pathogens (DH 2005b, **C**; Loveday et al. 2016, **C**).
31 Take any post-collection blood sampling, for example full blood count, from the access device prior to removal.	To monitor cellular loss as a result of the apheresis procedure (Crookston and Novak 2010, **E**) and to make corrections or give advice as necessary.
32 Disconnect the donor/patient from the machine before unloading the pumps and removing the disposable set from the apheresis machine.	To ensure the safety of the patient/donor. **E**
33 Dispose of sharps and waste products as per local policy.	To ensure the safe handling and disposal of needles and other sharp instruments and to protect staff, patients and visitors from exposure to bloodborne pathogens (DH 2005b, **C**; HSE 2013, **C**; Loveday et al. 2016, **C**; European Commission 2011, **C**).
34 Inspect the cannulation sites for bleeding. A pressure dressing may be applied over sterile gauze.	To achieve haemostasis and decrease the risk of infection. **E**
35 For donation products, label collection bags and complete documentation for release of products from the collection facility. JACIE (2015) compliant labels and paperwork must be used.	To ensure correct management of the product (JACIE 2015, **C**).
36 Place the collection bags in a secondary container (e.g. a zip-type resealable bag) prior to transfer to the appropriate processing facility (for donation procedures).	To prevent the loss of a portion of the collection, to minimize the potential for post-collection contamination of the component and to prevent potential spillage of biohazard material in areas where it may pose a risk to employees, visitors or patients (JACIE 2015, **C**).

37	For donation procedures, transport the collection bags to the appropriate processing facility with the necessary forms and in a JACIE 2015 compliant container.	To allow for cell measurement, storage and/or issue of the donated product. **E**
38	Record the necessary information in the appropriate documents as per local policy.	To maintain accurate records (NMC 2015, **C**).
39	Ensure post-donation care is appropriately managed (see 'Post-procedural considerations').	To ensure the safe management of patients and to enable them to actively participate in and comply with their treatment (NMC 2015, **C**).
40	Remove the disposable tubing set from the apheresis machine as per the operator's manual and dispose of it in a hazardous waste container.	To ensure the safe handling and disposal of clinical waste to protect staff, patients and visitors from exposure to bloodborne pathogens (DH 2005b, **C**; Loveday et al. 2016, **C**).
41	Clean the apheresis machine with a suitable decontaminating agent as per local policy (Howell et al. 2015)	To protect staff, patients and visitors from exposure to bloodborne pathogens (JACIE 2015, **C**).

Problem-solving table 2.3 Prevention and resolution (Procedure guideline 2.3)

Problem	Cause	Prevention	Action
Vascular access, for example high return pressure or low access pressure	Haematoma Kinking in tubing Valves in closed position Vascular inadequacy Needle phobia Vasovagal episode	Careful venous pre-assessment Central venous catheter insertion Experienced practitioners	Reassurance Check tubing for kinks Check position of valves Reduce inlet flow Adjust or resite access or return devices Central venous catheter insertion
Citrate toxicity	Electrolyte imbalance if citrate formulation is used as anticoagulant	Consider administration of electrolyte supplements (IV or oral), for example calcium Ensure correct anticoagulant rate settings	Decrease flow rate Consider administration of calcium supplements (IV or oral) Pause/stop procedure
Under-anticoagulation which may manifest as clotting or unstable interface	Incorrect biometric measurement Incorrect data input Incorrect settings with a lower AC:inlet ratio than needed	Ensure correct anticoagulant rate settings	Check tubing for kinks Increase AC:inlet ratio Stop procedure
Fluid overload	Cardiac impairment Renal impairment Paediatric patient	Careful pre-assessment Do not perform a rinseback in the paediatric setting if a blood prime has been performed Careful data input	Operate at negative fluid balance Request medical review Stop procedure
Hypotension	Hypovolaemia Paediatric patient Vasovagal episode	Blood prime Careful pre-assessment Careful data input Reassurance	Operate at positive fluid balance Increase colloid:crystalloid ratio
Chilling	Cold environment Cold replacement fluids	Use blood warmer Ensure adequate climate control	Increase room temperature Provide additional blankets Use blood warmer
Adverse reaction	Allergic reaction to replacement fluids or anticoagulant Incompatible transfusion Septicaemia Anaphylaxis	Careful preassessment Careful monitoring Adherence to blood product administration protocols	Request urgent medical review Instigate treatment as indicated, for example administer antimicrobials, antihistamine, hydrocortisone and emergency treatment Stop procedure

Sources: Dougherty and Lister (2015), Freshwater and Maslin-Prothero (2005), Howell et al. (2015), Stroncek et al. (2000).

Post-procedural considerations

Immediate care

During the procedure, blood is prevented from clotting in the extracorporeal circuit by a citrate-based anticoagulant. This functions by binding the calcium in the blood and removing it from the clotting cascade. Donors may experience symptoms of hypocalcaemia, such as muscular irritability, tetany, numbness and 'pins and needles' in extremities, light-headedness, nausea and vomiting (Freshwater and Maslin-Prothero 2005). This side-effect is known as citrate toxicity and is controlled by giving the donor calcium supplements or reducing the dose of citrate administered by decreasing the blood flow rate (Stroncek et al. 2000).

Different procedures may produce varying haemodynamic effects. Fluid overload may be a problem for patients with cardiac or renal impairment, whereas hypovolaemia may be of concern in the paediatric setting (Crookston and Novak 2010). Blood pressure in particular should be monitored, as hypotension may occur.

With red cell and plasma exchanges, patients may experience transfusion reactions, for example fever, chills and allergic reactions (see *The Royal Marsden Manual of Clinical Nursing Procedures, Ninth Edition*: Chapter 7 Nutrition, Fluid Balance and Blood Transfusion).

There is a potential for cellular loss, particularly platelets, as large volumes of donor or patient blood circulate through the apheresis machine and blood cells are intentionally or incidentally removed. Studies show that individual apheresis procedures produce only modest decreases in circulating blood cell counts, which are not associated with immediate toxicity (Crookston and Novak 2010). Patients with underlying instabilities or those undergoing repeated procedures may need to be supported by blood component transfusion. These are monitored closely by the apheresis nurse who is providing one-to-one care with the patient. Repeated monitoring of blood counts throughout the procedure is necessary.

Any adverse reaction must be dealt with promptly and must be documented. The patient/donor must have recovered as fully as possible before being allowed to leave the facility (Howell et al. 2015).

Ongoing care

Patients and donors should be encouraged to rest and take refreshment before leaving the cell separator facility. A full blood count should be taken at the end of the procedure and advice given depending on the result. For instance, there is a potential for platelet loss during stem cell collections by means of apheresis and patients and donors should be advised to moderate alcohol consumption and avoid strenuous exercise and activities that may put them at risk of bleeding or bruising. The platelet count usually recovers within a few days (Crookston and Novak 2010).

Documentation

Apheresis should be strictly regulated within a quality management system with clear standard operating procedures and documentation. Archived documentation should be maintained according to governmental, regulatory or institutional policy, whichever is longer (FACT-JACIE 2015). Due to the strict regulatory nature of apheresis, a record-keeping system must be in place to ensure the authenticity, integrity and confidentiality of all documents (MHRA 2009). All nursing records must be clearly maintained to ensure accurate data (NMC 2015).

Education of patient/donor and relevant others

If the donor or patient is likely to feel fatigued, it is sensible that someone accompanies them home. Advice needs to be customized to the particular procedure undertaken.

Complications

Overall rates of adverse reactions have decreased significantly over the past two decades. Greater understanding of the physiology of apheresis has guided continued improvements in technology and the potential for untoward effects has been minimized so that most procedures are performed without adverse events. This is especially true of donation procedures, which have become very routine (Crookston and Novak 2010). Caution is in order if cell or plasma removal exceeds current guidelines or if patients have underlying instabilities that predispose them to untoward events (Crookston and Novak 2010).

The use of central venous catheters can be associated with well-described complications and these complications lead to the majority of fatalities associated with apheresis (Stroncek et al. 2000). Subclavian and superior vena caval catheters can be associated with perforation, haemothorax, pneumothorax, infection and thrombosis. The use of femoral catheters can be associated with the occurrence of haemorrhage, thrombosis and infection (Howell et al. 2015). These risks are reduced by experienced personnel inserting the catheters with the assistance of ultrasound (Stroncek et al. 2000).

Ribavirin administration

Related theory

Respiratory syncytial virus (RSV) is known to be a frequent cause of lower respiratory tract infection, which can be severe and fatal in haemato-oncology patients (Dignan et al. 2016). Mortality may be as high as 80% depending upon other haematopoietic progenitor cell transplant complications, the timing of the transplant and degree of immunosuppression. There is a poor prognosis if these infections go untreated, and it is important to diagnose them early and treat promptly (Dignan et al. 2016; see also Chapter 1).

RSV should be suspected and routinely tested for in any coryzal patient undergoing high-dose chemotherapy treatment. RSV and other influenza pathogens are best detected by a nasopharyngeal aspirate (NPA) sample (Dignan et al. 2016). An NPA should be done at the earliest opportunity following the presentation of respiratory symptoms (see *The Royal Marsden Manual of Clinical Nursing Procedures, Ninth Edition*: Chapter 10 Interpreting Diagnostic Tests). The detection of viral antigen is performed using indirect immunofluorescence, with specific monoclonal antibodies for RSV, adenovirus, influenza A and B and the parainfluenza group (type 1, 2 and 3). This method is highly sensitive, specific, rapid and low cost (Blaschke et al. 2011, Raboni et al. 2003, Tunsjo et al. 2015).

Ribavirin is classed as a substance hazardous to health under the statutory requirements of the Control of Substance Hazardous to Health Regulations (COSHH 2002) and the accompanying Approved Code of Practice for Carcinogens. Under the regulations, the risk of exposure to ribavirin must be reduced 'to as low a level as is reasonably practicable' where use cannot be eliminated.

Evidence-based approaches

Rationale

It is recommended by Dignan et al. (2016) that aerosolized ribavirin is administered to allogeneic transplant patients with lower respiratory tract infection with RSV.

Indications

- Allogeneic transplant patients with lower respiratory tract infection with RSV (Shah et al. 2013).
- Allogeneic transplant patients with upper respiratory tract infection with RSV and multiple risk factors for progression to lower respiratory tract infection (Dignan et al. 2016).
- Furthermore:
  - Oral ribavirin may be an alternative in allogeneic transplant patients with lower respiratory tract infection with RSV if aerosolized ribavirin is not available.

– It is also recommended that intravenous immunoglobulin is administered to allogeneic transplant patients with RSV infection (DH 2011).

Contraindications

- Patients who are pregnant, breastfeeding or undergoing fertility treatment should not be administered ribavirin.
- Treatment with ribavirin is not recommended for patients with upper respiratory tract infection with parainfluenza or metapneumovirus.
- Patients with uncontrolled diarrhoea, vomiting or haemorrhagic cystitis (Donovan et al. 2012).
- Patients dependent on high flow or high percentages of oxygen.

Risks and safe handling

Pregnancy

Pregnancy is a contraindication for the administration of ribavirin as animal reproduction studies involving small animals such as rabbits and rodents have shown that it induced embryo death and teratogenicity (Kilham and Ferm 1977). Other small studies involving larger animals and humans did not demonstrate adverse effects, but due to the limited experience with ribavirin administration during pregnancy, concerns about potential effects on humans and in particular the developing fetus have been raised (Gladu and Ecobichon 1989, Harrison et al. 1988, Linn et al. 1995, MHRA 2014, Munzenberger and Walker 1994).

As previously noted, due to the potential teratogenic effects of exposure to ribavirin, healthcare workers who suspect or know that they are pregnant, who are breastfeeding or who are undergoing fertility treatment should not reconstitute or administer ribavirin or care for patients receiving it via nebulization. In addition, they should not enter the patient's room during administration of ribavirin by nebulization.

All staff involved in the direct care of patients receiving ribavirin therapy must have their names recorded on an administration record sheet (see Figure 2.10 for the record sheet used at the Royal Marsden) and this record must be kept and returned to occupational health within the Trust.

Protective eyewear

There has been one anecdotal report of ribavirin leaving deposits on contact lenses. Some staff may wish to wear glasses instead if they are reconstituting ribavirin.

Asthma

People suffering from asthma are advised not to enter the room while ribavirin is being administered and for 15 minutes following the procedure (Donovan et al. 2012).

In order to ensure compliance with COSHH (2002) and provide a written record of the control measures applied during the use of ribavirin, an administration record sheet should be completed for each patient receiving treatment (example in Figure 2.10). It is the responsibility of the ward manager and the nurse on duty to ensure that the administration record sheet (example in Figure 2.10) is completed each time a new patient receives ribavirin. All staff should record when they administer ribavirin to a patient (see Figure 2.10) in order to keep a record of exposure. This is because ribavirin should be regarded as a substance hazardous to health, and the risk of exposure should be reduced to as low a level as is reasonably practicable where use is indicated. Records of exposure are retained in occupational health (COSHH 2002).

Legal and professional issues

Competencies

A suitable training package should be available for new nurses. Nurses should be assessed by a competent practice facilitator

This form should be completed for each administration of ribavirin (Virazole®). At the end of the treatment period, it is expected that a copy of the form should be sent the Hospital's Occupational Health Department.

The completion of this form will constitute a written assessment of the risks to the health and safety of healthcare workers, patients and visitors for the administration of ribavirin (Virazole®) and the identification of the control measures to reduce those risks.

It is recognized that the decision to use ribavirin (Virazole®) will require a clinical judgement of the patient's needs and an awarenes of the associated health and safety risks to healthcare workers. For example, a clinician may need to decide if treatment should proceed if a single room is not immediately available. It is ultimately the responsibility of the clinician to determine whether the treatment should proceed given the circumstances of use. If there is any doubt, advice should be sought from the most senior nurse manager on duty.

Part A – Treatment details

Name of patient	
Hospital number	
Ward	

Part B – A list of staff involved in the administration of ribavirin (Virazole®) to the above patient.

Date of treatment	List of staff attending to patient
Day 1:	
Day 2:	
Day 3:	
Day 4:	
Day 5:	

Figure 2.10 The safe use of ribavirin (Virazole®) – administration record sheet.

prior to setting up the equipment, to develop their competence in the procedure. Nurses must always operate within their scope of practice as set out by their profession (NMC 2015).

Pre-procedural considerations

Only negative-pressure rooms or positive-pressure lobbied rooms (which all have sufficient extraction) are to be used where ribavirin is administered via a nebulizer. During nebulized administration of the drug, entry to the room should be limited as far as is practically possible. A warning sign 'Respiratory Isolation: Do Not Enter: Ribavirin Administration In Progress' must be placed on the patient's door during the time that the Aiolos nebulizer is in operation to ensure that staff and visitors do not unknowingly enter the room. Signs should be available from the infection control team. If an appropriate room is not available, consideration should be given to delaying the use of nebulized ribavirin, and intravenous or oral administration may be considered.

Equipment

Ribavirin is administered via an aerosol generator such as the ICN small particle aerosol generator (SPAG) model. It is important to read the operator's manual for instructions prior to use (Valeant 2014).

The aerosol can be delivered to an infant oxygen hood from the aerosol generator. Administration by facemask or oxygen tent may be necessary if a hood cannot be employed. However, the volume of distribution and condensation area are larger in a tent and efficacy of this method of administering the drug has been evaluated in only a small number of patients. Ribavirin should not be administered with any other aerosol generating device or from the same reservoir as other aerosolized medications (Valeant 2014).

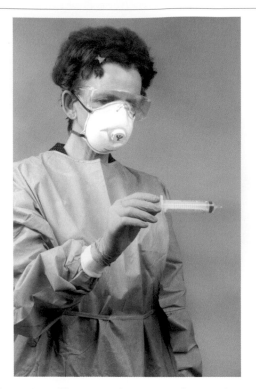

Figure 2.11 Nurse wearing personal protective equipment (PPE) for the administration of ribavirin.

It is important to use the recommended drug concentration as recommended by the manufacturer of the aerosol generator.

Personal protective equipment is necessary to administer ribavirin. A filtering facepiece 2 (FFP2) mask, a disposable apron, gloves and fitting goggles are required (Figure 2.11).

Assessment and recording tools

It is vital that patients are assessed for their suitability to be treated with ribavirin and that they have a good performance status. This is to ensure that they can safely be left alone for the 2-hour administration of the drug.

Pharmacological support

It is recommended that pharmacy reconstitute ribavirin in a controlled environment with extraction facilities (COSHH 2002), however the drug can be drawn up with PPE in the patient's room if required out of hours.

Non-pharmacological support

Thought should be given to the patient and their relatives as isolation is required during administration. Relatives should be advised not to enter the room during administration. This can often leave the patient feeling isolated and vulnerable; equally relatives should be kept regularly informed about when it is safe to enter the room so they can offer support to the patient (Ghosh et al. 2000).

Procedure guideline 2.4 Ribavirin administration

Essential equipment

- Aerosol generator
- Aerosol generator equipment may vary dependent on the make and model. Additional equipment may be required and nurses should check the manufacturer's instructions
- Compressed air/oxygen source. Use air or oxygen that meets specifications for medical breathing use. (Choice dependent upon patient's condition)
- Facemasks (FFP2 or FFP3)
- Gloves, non-sterile
- Eye protection – protective goggles

- Clean plastic apron
- Sterile disposable gown
- Extra bed sheets
- Pharmaceutical/chemotherapy disposal sharps bin
- Red bag/alginate bag

Medicinal products

- Ribavirin (Virazole®)

Pre-procedure

Action	Rationale
1 Explain and provide written information about the nebulization procedure.	To ensure the patient is properly informed about the procedure (DH 2005a, **C**; NMC 2015, **C**).
2 Ensure the patient is in a negative-pressure room.	To comply with COSHH guidance (2002, **C**).
3 Ensure the prescription chart is available and the ribavirin has been correctly prescribed and it has been indicated whether oxygen or pressurized air is required for nebulization.	To comply with medicines management regulations (NMC 2010, **C**).
4 Apply the safety equipment (facemasks, gloves, eye protection and clean apron) as per local Trust guidance and reconstitute the ribavirin inside the room when a course of treatment is required.	Ribavirin is usually reconstituted in a pharmacy, but due to its short shelf-life it may need to be made up by nurses. To comply with COSHH guidance (2002, **C**).
5 Prepare the equipment as per the manufacturer's instructions.	To comply with the manufacturer's instructions for use. **C**
6 Ask all visitors to leave the room during administration to reduce risk of unnecessary secondary exposure.	To minimize unnecessary exposure (COSHH 2002, **C**).

7	Ensure the patient can be observed during treatment and has easy access to call for assistance in case of emergency.	To react quickly to any deterioration in the patient (NPSA 2007, **C**).
8	Instruct and ensure patient understanding in administration procedure of the nebulizer.	To ensure patient understanding and safety of staff (COSHH 2002, **C**).

Procedure

9	Apply the safety equipment (facemasks, gloves, eye protection and clean apron) as per local Trust guidance.	To comply with COSHH guidance (2002, **C**).
10	Prepare the ribavirin.	To comply with the manufacturer's instructions for use. **C**
11	Ensure facemask is fully fitted to patient and cover patient with extra bed sheet, to lessen spread of ribavirin particles to the environment. If using a hood or tent, ensure this is correctly set up.	To comply with COSHH guidance (2002, **C**). To comply with manufacturer's instructions for use. **C**
12	Commence ribavirin administration in accordance with the manufacturer's instructions.	To comply with the manufacturer's instructions for use. **C**
13	Check the system components as per manufacturer's guidelines as the medicine solution may form crystal deposits on the inner surfaces of the equipment and these can affect the flow.	To comply with the manufacturer's instructions for use. **C**

Post-procedure

14	At the end of the treatment, staff should enter the room to check if the machine was switched off. Staff should immediately leave the room and wait 5–10 minutes before re-entering to minimize exposure to the medicine's dust particles, which remain in the air following administration.	To ensure patient and staff safety (NPSA, 2007, **C**).
15	Discard the ribavirin disposables in a pharmaceutical cytotoxic bin.	To comply with safe management of healthcare waste (DH 2013, **C**).
16	Place the equipment to one side ready for cleaning in the room.	To prevent bacterial contamination and cross-contamination (NHS Professionals 2013, **C**)
17	Apply gloves and clean the equipment as recommended by the manufacturer.	To prevent bacterial contamination and cross-contamination (NHS Professionals 2013, **C**)
18	Dispose of any remaining ribavirin in accordance with local policy. Manage any spillage/leakage in accordance with the local spillage policy.	To comply with safe management of healthcare waste (DH 2013, **C**).
19	Dispose of extra linen. The top pillow case must be disposed of in a red linen bag.	To comply with safe management of healthcare waste (DH 2013, **C**).
20	Clean all surfaces. Bed sides must be cleaned with soap and water after each dose.	To prevent bacterial contamination and cross-contamination (NHS Professionals 2013, **C**).
21	Continue to wear full PPE while the room is being damp dusted. Respiratory precautions will continue as this patient will have a confirmed respiratory virus; goggles may be omitted or removed if not required at this point.	To prevent bacterial contamination and cross-contamination (NHS Professionals 2013, **C**).
22	Ensure that cleaning staff wait 2 hours before entering the room to clean the floor with soap and water.	To comply with safe management of healthcare waste (DH 2013, **C**).
23	Dispose of cleaning material according to local waste management rules.	To comply with safe management of healthcare waste (DH 2013, **C**).
24	Document administration is completed in nursing notes. Sign for administration of the medicine on the prescription chart and the administration record sheet.	To comply with medicines management regulations (NMC 2010, **C**).

Problem-solving table 2.4 Prevention and resolution (Procedure guideline 2.4)

Problem	Cause	Prevention	Action
Medication crystal formation	Ribavirin crystals	Make sure equipment is cleaned between doses and correctly assembled according to manufacturer's instructions	If the crystal deposit exceeds 1 mm, rinse using sterile water or fit new tubing
There is little or no aerosol	The equipment is not correctly assembled	Check equipment before use	Reassemble equipment
	The flow meter is turned off, or is not fully adjusted	Maintenance of equipment as recommended by the manufacturer	Adjust the flow meter to administer the correct flow
	The equipment is dirty or clogged		Replace faulty components
	The equipment is broken		

Post-procedural considerations

Immediate care

Care of the patient and their relatives is important as the patient is isolated for a number of hours per day during treatment. This can be particularly traumatic for some patients and it is vital that psychological issues are taken into account when proceeding with treatment.

Care must be taken to minimize the exposure to healthcare workers to comply with COSHH guidance (2002).

Ongoing care

It is recommended by Dignan et al. (2016) that patients with respiratory viruses are monitored for signs of respiratory failure and that the critical care team is involved where required. They also advise that oral ribavirin can be used in patients who do not tolerate aerosolized ribavirin. Dignan et al. (2016) advocate that intravenous immunoglobulin is administered to allogeneic transplant patients with RSV infections.

Education of patient and relevant others

Patients should be given a patient information sheet to advise them of the risks and benefits of treatment and should be advised to minimize contact with others during the treatment period.

Complications

Toxicities associated with the administration of aerosolized ribavirin include bronchospasm, cough, claustrophobia, nausea, rash, reduced pulmonary function, mucus plugging and conjunctival irritation (Shah and Chemaly 2011).

There is a potential risk that ribavirin is teratogenic and mutagenic so patients and staff should be made aware of the risks (Donovan et al. 2012).

Intravenous ribavirin has been associated with haemolysis, leucopenia and hyperbilirubinaemia, and oral ribavirin has been associated with anaemia and nausea (Shah and Chemaly 2011).

Pentamidine isetionate administration

Related theory

Pneumocystis jirovecii pneumonia is a fungal infection of the lungs. The disease has also been referred to as *Pneumocystis carinii* or PCP pneumonia (Anevlavis et al. 2012). The fungus is common within the environment and rarely causes illness in healthy people. However, in patients with a weakened immune system and those undergoing stem cell transplantation it can lead to a lung infection that can be fatal (Anevlavis et al. 2012).

Prophylaxis against *Pneumocystis jirovecii* pneumonia is indicated in all haematopoietic stem cell transplant and severely immunocompromised patients (Joint Formulary Committee 2018). Co-trimoxazole by mouth is the first-line drug recommended for prophylaxis against pneumocystis pneumonia (Joint Formulary Committee 2018). Where this is contraindicated, or a patient is unable to tolerate co-trimoxazole, nebulized pentamidine isetionate is indicated (Brown and Cutler 2012, Joint Formulary Committee 2018). Pentamidine isetionate is given by inhalation of a nebulized solution at 300 mg every 4 weeks (Joint Formulary Committee 2018).

Pentamidine isetionate is classed as a substance hazardous to health. In accordance with COSHH Regulations (2002), exposure to pentamidine isetionate must be reduced to 'as low a level as is reasonably practicable', where its use cannot be eliminated.

Evidence-based approaches

Rationale

Indications

More commonly in the haemato-oncology setting:

- pneumonia caused by *Pneumocystis jirovecii*
- prophylaxis against *Pneumocystis jirovecii* pneumonia for severely immunocompromised patients.

Other:

- prevention of *Pneumocystis jirovecii* pneumonia in patients infected by HIV who have experienced a previous episode of PCP (EMC 2015, Joint Formulary Committee 2018).
- cutaneous leishmaniasis
- early phase African sleeping sickness caused by *Trypanosoma brucei gambiense*.

Contraindications

- Patients who are pregnant, breastfeeding or undergoing fertility treatment should not be administered pentamidine isetionate. Although there is no evidence of the safety of pentamidine isetionate use in human pregnancy, one miscarriage within the first trimester of pregnancy has been reported following aerosolized prophylactic administration (EMC 2015).
- Caution should be taken for patients with hypotension or hepatic impairment, and dose reductions are indicated for patients with renal impairment (Joint Formulary Committee 2018).

Legal and professional issues

Competencies

Pentamidine isetionate should be administered by trained healthcare professionals, operating within their scope of practice (NMC 2015). A suitable training package and assessment should be undertaken to determine the competence of the administrator. Nurses should be assessed by a competent practice facilitator prior to setting up the equipment, to develop their competence in the procedure.

Pre-procedural considerations

Patients should be counselled by a trained healthcare professional on the side-effects and procedure prior to the administration of the drug. The patient should be counselled by the healthcare professional to self-administer the nebulizer. The healthcare professional should remain outside the room for the duration of the nebulized treatment unless a severe reaction necessitates intervention. The healthcare professional should ensure that exposure is kept to the minimum level possible.

Pentamidine isetionate should be delivered in a negative-pressure room to reduce the exposure, and no-one should enter the room during administration unless a medical emergency is indicated.

Equipment

Personal protective equipment (FFP3 facemasks, goggles, gloves and aprons) must be worn by health professionals administering the drug (European Commission 2011).

The equipment required to perform the procedure is a standard nebulizer consisting of a chamber and mask to deliver salbutamol to the patient prior to the pentamidine inhalation. A pentamidine nebulizer kit, which consists of a Filta-Guard™ with a purple chamber and mouthpiece, is used to administer the pentamidine.

Assessment and recording tools

It is vital that patients are assessed for their suitability to be treated with pentamidine isetionate and that they have a good performance status. This is to ensure that they can be left safely and are able to self-administer the pentamidine isetionate nebulizer for the 1-hour administration of the drug in accordance with COSHH guidelines (2002).

Pentamidine isetionate is known to cause hypotension in some patients (Joint Formulary Committee 2018). A full set of observations should be taken prior to administration and post administration; these should be documented within the nursing notes.

Pharmacological support

It is recommended that pharmacy make up pentamidine isetionate in a controlled environment with extraction facilities (COSHH 2002).

Bronchospasm has been reported to occur following the use of nebulized pentamidine isetionate, particularly in patients who have a history of smoking or asthma. This should be controlled by prior use of bronchodilators (Joint Formulary Committee 2018).

Non-pharmacological support

An apprehensive patient may experience anxiety during the procedure. Counselling prior to administration should be undertaken by a trained professional to calm patients and provide them with information. The patient should be given the call bell so that they can attract nursing staff attention should they require it. Relatives should be advised not to enter the room during administration. Due to possible complications of administration it is advisable that the patient is accompanied to the hospital and that someone accompanies them home.

Procedure guideline 2.5   Pentamidine isetionate administration

Essential equipment

- Salbutamol nebulizer kit (SideStream with blue chamber and mask)
- Pentamidine nebulizer kit (Filta-Guard with purple chamber and mouthpiece)
- Non-sterile gloves, goggles (sealed if wearing contact lenses) and disposable apron
- Facemask FFP3 (particulate filter respirator and surgical mask)
- Upright chair designed for patient comfort
- Completed prescription chart

- Pharmaceutical/chemotherapy disposal bin
- Red bag/alginate bag

Medicinal products

- Pentamidine solution 300 mg (pre-prepared into syringe in pharmacy)
- Salbutamol solution 2.5 mg
- Compressed medical air or oxygen outlet with flow meter. Use air or oxygen that meets specifications for medical breathing use. (Choice dependent upon patient's condition)

Pre-procedure

Action	Rationale
1 Ensure pentamidine isetionate is prescribed on prescription chart.	To comply with medicines management regulations and Trust policy (NMC 2010, **C**).
2 Explain and discuss the procedure with the patient. This must include: – details of the drugs and equipment – why the procedure is necessary – the possible side-effects.	To ensure that the patient understands the procedure and gives their valid consent (DH 2009, **C**; NMC 2015, **E**). The routine of obtaining verbal consent from patients undergoing pentamidine administration represents good clinical practice (MHRA 2009, **C**).
3 Gain consent and assess patient's current condition.	To ensure the patient has no underlying medical problems and is suitable to undergo the procedure. **E**
4 Ensure the patient is wearing a wristband correctly labelled with their name, hospital number and date of birth.	To identify correct patient and prevent patient safety incidents and near misses relating to missing or incorrect wristbands (NPSA 2005, **C**).
5 Obtain a baseline blood pressure and record on the observation chart.	To monitor the effect of pentamidine administration on blood pressure as it is known to cause hypotension in some patients (Joint Formulary Committee 2018, **C**).
6 Consult the patient's prescription chart to ascertain the following: – drug – dose – date and time of administration – route and method of administration – diluent as appropriate – validity of prescription – signature of doctor.	To ensure that the patient is given the correct drug in the prescribed dose using the appropriate diluent and by the correct route (NMC 2010, **C**).

Procedure

7 Take the prepared dose to the patient and check the patient's identity by asking them to verbally identify themselves (where possible) and check against the patient's identification wristband. Also ask about and check allergy status.	To prevent error and confirm patient's identity (NMC 2015, **C**; NPSA 2005, **C**; 2007, **C**).
8 Assess the patient to ensure they are capable and competent to switch from the salbutamol to pentamidine.	To ensure patient understanding and safety of staff (COSHH 2002, **C**).

(continued)

Procedure guideline 2.5 Pentamidine isetionate administration *(continued)*

Action	Rationale
9 Treat all patients receiving pentamidine in a negative-pressure room designated only for the administration of pentamidine.	As pentamidine is classed as a substance hazardous to health, exposure needs to be reduced to as low a level as is reasonably practicable (COSHH 2002, **C**).
10 The door must be kept closed at all times with a visible DO NOT ENTER: PENTAMIDINE ADMINISTRATION IN PROGRESS sign on the door.	To minimize unnecessary exposure (COSHH 2002, **C**).
11 Due to the teratogenic effects of the drug, ask all staff and relatives to leave the room prior to and while pentamidine is being administered unless there is a clinical need.	To minimize unnecessary exposure (COSHH 2002, **C**).
12 Wash hands using a bactericidal handrub.	To minimize the risk of infection (Loveday et al. 2016, **C**).
13 Apply goggles, gloves and a plastic apron to administer the pentamidine.	Pentamidine is classed as a substance hazardous to health. Exposure needs to be reduced to as low a level as is reasonably practicable (COSHH 2002, **C**).
14 Sit the patient in an upright chair in a negative-pressure room where they can be observed from the outside.	To minimize dyspnoea and allow maximum lung expansion in order to ensure medication reaches the bronchioles. This aids gravitational sedimentation (settling), and diffusion (Gardenhire et al. 2013, **E**).
15 Ensure the patient can be observed and a nurse call bell is easily accessible in the event of the patient seeking assistance. Observe the patient intermittently throughout the procedure.	To react quickly to any deterioration in the patient (NPSA 2007, **C**).
16 Wherever possible, the patient should be instructed to switch on the nebulizer themselves.	This allows the nurse to leave the room. To ensure patient understanding and safety of staff (COSHH 2002, **C**).
17 Instruct the patient in the use of the nurse call system and ensure the bell is within easy reach.	To react quickly to any deterioration in the patient (NPSA 2007, **C**).
18 Administer salbutamol first. – Put prescribed salbutamol into the reservoir of the salbutamol nebulizer and secure. – Attach the oxygen tubing to one end and connect the other end to the oxygen/medical air outlet. – Secure the mask safely and securely on the patient's face and adjust straps to fit to ensure there is no leakage.	To dilate the bronchus and minimize the risk of bronchospasm from the pentamidine (Joint Formulary Committee 2018, **C**).
19 Turn on oxygen/medical air to flow at 6 litres per minute. Instruct the patient to breathe normally until all of the solution of salbutamol has been inhaled (this takes approximately 10 minutes).	To ensure at least 65% of the droplets are of a size that enables drug penetration into the distal airways (Downie et al. 2007, **E**).
20 On completion dispose of nebulizer in clinical waste bin.	To comply with safe management of healthcare waste (DH 2013, **C**).
21 To change the salbutamol over to the pentamidine inhalation the nurse should ensure that they put on their PPE (facemask, goggles and gloves).	Pentamidine is classed as a substance hazardous to health. Exposure needs to be reduced to as low a level as is reasonably practicable (COSHH 2002, **C**).
22 Place the syringe of prescribed pentamidine solution into the reservoir and secure.	To ensure correct administration (manufacturer's instructions, **C**).
23 Attach the reservoir with mouthpiece to the Filta-Guard breathing filter at the clear plastic end.	To ensure correct administration (manufacturer's instructions, **C**).
24 Attach one end of the tubing to the reservoir and the other end to the oxygen/medical air outlet.	As pentamidine is classed as a substance hazardous to health, exposure needs to be reduced to as low a level as is reasonably practicable (COSHH 2002, **C**). To ensure correct administration (manufacturer's instructions, **C**).
25 Instruct patient to place lips firmly on the mouthpiece.	To ensure correct administration (manufacturer's instructions, **C**).
26 Turn oxygen/medical air on to 10 litres per minute.	To ensure correct administration (manufacturer's instructions, **C**).
27 Instruct patient to breathe in slowly. After inspiration, the patient should pause briefly before exhaling.	To promote greater disposition of medication in the airways (Perry 2016, **E**).
28 Leave the room and dispose of aprons and gloves into orange clinical waste bin.	To ensure safety of staff (COSHH 2002, **C**).

29	This should continue until the nebulized medication is completely administered (this takes approximately 10 minutes).	To ensure correct administration (manufacturer's instructions, **C**).
30	Instruct the patient to remain in the room for 30 minutes after the procedure has completed.	This allows for adequate ventilation, thereby minimizing the risk of pentamidine inhalation by staff/relatives before the room is used again (COSHH 2002, **C**).

Post-procedure

31	Ensure all equipment is disposed of in the cytotoxic/cytostatic (purple-topped) waste bins.	To comply with the safe management of healthcare waste (DH 2013, **C**).
32	Check and record blood pressure once the patient has completed the 30 minutes post procedure.	To monitor the effect of pentamidine administration on blood pressure as it is known to cause hypotension in some patients (Joint Formulary Committee 2018, **C**).
33	Document and sign administration has been completed on prescription chart and in relevant nursing notes.	To comply with medicines management regulations (NMC 2010, **C**). There must be a clear, accurate and immediate record of all medicine administered, intentionally withheld or refused by the patient, ensuring the signature is clear and legible (NMC 2010, **C**).

Post-procedural considerations

All pentamidine and salbutamol nebulizer masks are single use only and must be discarded appropriately after each use, according to COSHH (2002) guidance. Staff should refrain from entering rooms in which pentamidine has been administered for a further 30 minutes to allow for the drug to settle or be extracted via the ventilation system.

All linen from these rooms should be dealt with as infected and placed in a water-soluble bag within a red plastic bag.

Rooms should be damp dusted, including all furniture around the nebulizer or patient's chair. The wipes should then be discarded into the purple-lidded cytotoxic/cytostatic waste stream.

Immediate care

During the procedure, the patient may experience severe reactions, sometimes fatal, due to hypotension. They may also experience nausea and vomiting, dizziness, syncope, flushing, hyperglycaemia, rash, taste disturbances, bronchoconstriction, cough and shortness of breath (Joint Formulary Committee 2018). The patient should be advised prior to administration to alert a healthcare professional, using the call bell, if any reaction is experienced. The healthcare professional will need to stop the nebulizer and monitor and stabilize the patient, who will require a medical review. Any adverse reaction must be documented in accordance with the NMC (2015). The patient must have recovered as fully as possible before being allowed to leave the facility.

Ongoing care

In the longer term, pentamidine isetionate is known to cause hypoglycaemia, pancreatitis, arrhythmias, leucopenia, thrombocytopenia, acute renal failure and hypocalcaemia in some patients. The patient's full blood count and urea and electrolytes should be monitored regularly to detect any early signs of deterioration following the administration of pentamidine in the longer term.

Complications

If bronchospasm occurs during or after pentamidine therapy, make sure that a bronchodilator is prescribed and call for assistance from the medical team or critical care outreach team.

The patient may complain of a burning sensation in the back of the throat, usually occurring in the latter part of therapy. This is usually resolved by temporarily discontinuing therapy and allowing the patient to have a drink of some liquid. Other rare complications include chest pain, palpitations, syncope, confusion, seizure, or marked desaturation (Joint Formulary Committee 2018). If any of these occurs, immediate attention from the medical and critical care outreach team will be required (NPSA 2007).

Websites

Bloodwise
https://bloodwise.org.uk/all-blood-cancers/understanding-blood-cancers

British Society for Haematology
www.b-s-h.org.uk

European Society for Blood and Marrow Transplantation
www.ebmt.org

US Food and Drug Administration: Drugs
www.fda.gov/Drugs

Health and Safety Executive: Control of Substances Hazardous to Health
www.hse.gov.uk/coshh

Medicines and Healthcare products Regulatory Agency
www.mhra.gov.uk

UK Government
https://www.gov.uk/

U.S. National Library of Medicine: MedlinePlus®
www.nlm.nih.gov/medlineplus

Sanofi: Pentacarinat (pentamidine isetionate) 300mg
https://www.medicines.org.uk/emc/medicine/948

References

Academy of Royal Medical Colleges (2013) *Safe Sedation Practice for Healthcare Procedures, Standards and Guidance.* London: Academy of Royal Medical Colleges. Available at: https://www.rcoa.ac.uk/system/files/PUB-SafeSedPrac2013.pdf (Accessed: 18/4/2018)

Al-Ibraheemi, A., Pham, T., Chen, L., et al. (2013) Comparison between 1-needle technique versus 2-needle technique for bone marrow aspiration and biopsy procedures. *Archive of Pathology and Laboratory Medicine*, 137, 974–978.

Anevlavis, S., Kaltsas, K. & Bouros, D. (2012) Prophylaxis for Pneumocystis pneumonia (PCP) in non-HIV infected patients. *Pneumon*, 4(25), 348–350.

Association of Anaesthetists of Great Britain and Ireland (2016) Safe vascular access. *Anaesthesia*, 71(5), 573–585. Available at: http://onlinelibrary.wiley.com/doi/10.1111/anae.13360/full (Accessed: 18/4/2018)

Atkinson, M. (2005) Communicating news of patients' deaths to unrelated stem cell donors. *Nursing Standard*, 19(32), 41–47.

Bain, B. (2001) Bone marrow trephine biopsy. *Journal of Clinical Pathology*, 54, 737–742.

Bain, B. (2004) *A Beginner's Guide to Blood Cells*, 2nd edn. Boston, MA: Blackwell Publishing.

Bain, B. (2005) Bone marrow biopsy morbidity: review of 2003. *Journal of Clinical Pathology*, 58(4), 406–408.

Bain, B. (2006) Morbidity associated with bone marrow aspiration and trephine biopsy – a review of 2004. *Haematologica*, 91, 1293–1294.

BCSH (2008) Guidelines on the assessment of bleeding risk prior to surgery or invasive procedures. Available at: https://onlinelibrary.wiley.com/doi/epdf/10.1111/j.1365-2141.2007.06968.x (Accessed: 18/4/2018)

BCSH (2012) Guidelines for pre-transfusion compatibility procedures in blood transfusion laboratories. *Transfusion Medicine*, 23, 1. Available at: http://onlinelibrary.wiley.com/doi/10.1111/j.1365-3148.2012.01199.x/pdf (Accessed: 18/4/2018)

Be the Match Registry (2010) Understanding your commitment. Available at: https://bethematch.org/support-the-cause/donate-bone-marrow/join-the-marrow-registry/before-you-join/ (Accessed: 18/4/2018)

Bishop, B., McNally, K. & Harris, M. (1992) Audit of bone marrow trephines. *Journal of Clinical Pathology*, 45, 1105–1108.

Blaschke, A.J., Allison, M.A., Meyers, L., et al. (2011) Non-invasive sample collection for respiratory virus testing by multiplex PCR. *Journal of Clinical Virology*, 52, 210–214.

Bondurant, M., Mahmud, N. & Rhodes, N. (2012) Origin and development of blood cells. In: Greer, J. et al. (eds) *Wintrobe's Clinical Hematology*, 13th edn. Philadelphia: Lippincott, Williams and Wilkins, pp. 79–89.

Brown, M. & Cutler, T. (2012) *Haematology Nursing*. Oxford: Wiley-Blackwell.

Bufalini, A. (2009) Role of interactive music in oncological pediatric patients undergoing painful procedures. *Minerva Pediatric*, 61(4), 379–389.

Burgstaler, E. (2010) Current instrumentation for apheresis. In: McLeod, B., Szczepiorkowski, Z.M., Weinstein, R. & Winters, J.L. (eds) *Apheresis: Principles and Practice*, 3rd edn. Bethesda, MD: AABB Press, pp. 71–110.

Campbell, J., Matthews, J. & Seymour, M. (2003) Optimum trephine length in the assessment of bone marrow involvement in patients with diffuse large cell lymphoma. *Annals of Oncology*, 14, 273–276.

Chapman, K. & Rush, K. (2003) Patient and family satisfaction with cancer-related information: a review of the literature. *Canadian Oncology Nursing Journal*, 13(2), 107–116.

Chen, A., Bains, T., Murray, S., et al. (2012) Clinical experience with a simple algorithm for plerixafor utilization in autologous stem cell mobilization. *Bone Marrow Transplantation*, 47,1526–1529.

Choi, J. & Foss, F.M. (2010) Photopheresis. In: McLeod, B., Szczepiorkowski, Z.M., Weinstein, R. & Winters, J.L. (eds) *Apheresis: Principles and Practice*, 3rd edn. Bethesda, MD: AABB Press, pp. 615–634.

Confer, D.L., Miller, J.P. & Chell, J.W. (2016) Bone marrow and peripheral blood cell donors and donor registries. In: Forman, S.J., Negrin, R.S., Antin, J.H. & Appelbaum, F.R. (eds) *Thomas' Hematopoietic Cell Transplantation*, 5th edn. Boston, MA: Blackwell Publishing, pp. 423–432.

Control of Substances Hazardous to Health (COSHH) (2002) Available at: www.hse.gov.uk/coshh/index.htm (Accessed: 18/4/2018)

Corbin, F., Cullis, H.M., Freireich, E.J., et al. (2010) Development of apheresis instrumentation. In: McLeod, B., Szczepiorkowski, Z.M., Weinstein, R. & Winters, J.L. (eds) *Apheresis: Principles and Practice*, 3rd edn. Bethesda, MD: AABB Press, pp. 1–26.

Crookston, K.P. & Novak, D.J. (2010) Physiology of apheresis. In: McLeod, B., Szczepiorkowski, Z.M., Weinstein, R. & Winters, J.L. (eds) *Apheresis: Principles and Practice*, 3rd edn. Bethesda, MD: AABB Press, pp. 45–70.

Davē, U.P. & Koury, M.J. (2016) Structure of the marrow and the hematopoietic microenvironment. In: Kaushansky, K. et al. (eds) *Williams Hematology*, 9th edn. London: McGraw-Hill, pp. 53–84.

DH (2005a) *Creating a Patient-Led NHS – Delivering the NHS Improvement Plan*. London: Department of Health.

DH (2005b) *Hazardous Waste (England) Regulations*. London: Department of Health.

DH (2009) *Reference Guide to Consent for Examination or Treatment*, 2nd edn. London: Department of Health.

DH (2011) *Clinical Guidelines for Immunoglobulin Use: Update to Second Edition*. London: Department of Health. Available at: https://assets.publishing.service.gov.uk/government/uploads/system/uploads/attachment_data/file/216671/dh_131107.pdf (Accessed: 18/4/2018)

DH (2013) *Environment and Sustainability. Health Technical Memorandum 07-01: Safe Management of Healthcare Waste*. London: Department of Health. Available at: https://www.gov.uk/government/uploads/system/uploads/attachment_data/file/167976/HTM_07-01_Final.pdf (Accessed: 18/4/2018)

Dignan, F.L., Clark, A., Aitken, C., et al.; Haemato-oncology Task Force of the British Committee for Standards in Haematology; British Society for Blood and Marrow Transplantation and the UK Clinical Virology Network (2016) BCSH/BSBMT/UK clinical virology network guideline: diagnosis and management of common respiratory viral infections in patients undergoing treatment for haematological malignancies or stem cell transplantation. *British Journal of Haematology*, 173(3), 380–393. Available at: https://onlinelibrary.wiley.com/doi/full/10.1111/bjh.14027 (Accessed: 18/4/2018)

Donovan, L., Fairest, M., Graves, L., et al. (2012) *Ribavirin Nebulisation Guidance Document. Guidance for the preparation, administration and safety considerations of nebulised ribavirin using the Aiolos nebuliser.* EBMT-NAP Group UK. Available at: http://ebmt.co.uk/wp-content/uploads/2012/03/Revised-Guidance-Document-September-2012.pdf (Accessed: 18/4/2018)

Dougherty, L. & Lister, S. (eds) (2011) *The Royal Marsden Manual of Clinical Nursing Procedures: Professional Edition*, 8th edn. Oxford: Wiley-Blackwell.

Dougherty, L. & Lister, S. (eds) (2015) *The Royal Marsden Manual of Clinical Nursing Procedures: Professional Edition*, 9th edn. Oxford: Wiley-Blackwell.

Downie, G., MacKenzie, J. & Williams, A. (2007) Medicine management. In: Downie, G., Mackenzie, J. & Williams, A. (eds) *Pharmacology and Medicines Management for Nurses*, 3rd edn. London: Churchill Livingstone, pp. 44–91.

EMC (2015) Summary of Product Characteristics, Pentacarinat 300 mg. www.medicines.org.uk/emc/medicine/948

European Commission (2011) *Occupational Health and Safety Risks in the Healthcare Sector*, Luxembourg: Publications Office of the European Union. Available at: http://ec.europa.eu/social/BlobServlet?docId=7167&langId=en (Accessed: 18/4/2018)

FACT-JACIE (2015) *International Standards for Cellular Therapy Product Collection, Processing and Administration*. Available at: www.jacie.org/standards/6th-edition-2015 (Accessed: 18/4/2018)

Fraise, A.P. & Bradley, T. (eds) (2009) *Ayliffe's Control of Healthcare-associated Infection: A Practical Handbook*, 5th edn. London: Hodder Arnold.

Freshwater, D. & Maslin-Prothero, S. (eds) (2005) *Blackwell's Nursing Dictionary*. Oxford: Blackwell Publishing.

Gardenhire, D., Ari, A., Hess, D. & Myers, T.R. (2013) *A Guide to Aerosol Delivery Devices for Respiratory Therapists*, 3rd edn. American Association for Respiratory Care. Available at: http://www.irccouncil.org/newsite/members/aerosol_guide_rt.pdf (Accessed: 18/4/2018)

Ghosh, S., Champlin, R.E., Englund, J., et al. (2000) Respiratory syncytial virus upper respiratory tract illnesses in adult blood and marrow transplant recipients: combination therapy with aerosolized ribavirin and intravenous immunoglobulin. *Bone Marrow Transplantation*, 25(7), 751–755.

Giannoutsos, I., Grech, H., Maboreke, T. & Morgenstern, G. (2004) Performing bone marrow biopsies with or without sedation: a comparison. *Clinical and Laboratory Haematology*, 26(3), 201–204.

Gladu, J-M. & Ecobichon, D.J. (1989) Evaluation of exposure of health care personnel to Ribavirin. *Journal of Toxicology and Environmental Health*, 28, 1–12.

Goldberg, C., Vergidis, D. & Sacher, R. (2007) *Bone Aspiration and Biopsy*. Medscape, New York. emedicine.medscape.com/article/207575-overview#section-author_information.

Haematological Malignancy Research Network (2016) Quickstats. Available at: www.hmrn.org/Statistics/quick (Accessed: 18/4/2018)

Harrison, R., Bellows, J. & Rempel, D. (1988) Accessing exposures of health-care personnel to aerosols of Ribavirin. *Morbidity and Mortality Weekly Report*, 37(36), 560–563.

Hjortholm, N., Jannidi, E., Halaburda, K., et al. (2013) Strategies of pain reduction during the bone marrow biopsy. *Annals of Hematology*, 92(2), 145–149.

Hoffbrand, A.V. & Moss, P.A.H. (2015) *Hoffbrand's Essential Haematology*, 7th edn. Oxford: Wiley-Blackwell.

Howell, C., Douglas, K., Cho, G., et al. (2015) Guideline on the clinical use of apheresis procedures for the treatment of patients and collection of cellular therapy products. British Committee for Standards in Haematology. *Transfusion Medicine*, 25, 57–78. [This document replaces the BCSH Joint Working Party of the Transfusion and Clinical Haematology Task Forces (1998) Guidelines for the clinical use of blood cell separators. *Clinical and Laboratory Haematology*, 20, 265–278.]

HSE (2013) Health and Safety (Sharp Instruments in Healthcare) Regulations 2013. Guidance for employers and employees. Available at: www.hse.gov.uk/pubns/hsis7.pdf (Accessed: 18/4/2018)

Hughes-Jones, N., Wickramasinghe, S. & Hatton, C. (2013) *Lecture Notes on Haematology*, 9th edn. Oxford: Blackwell Publishing.

Human Tissue Authority (2013) *Code of Practice G: Donation of Allogeneic Bone Marrow and Peripheral Blood Stem Cells for Transplantation*. Available at: https://www.hta.gov.uk/sites/default/files/Code%20G%20-%20Bone%20Marrow%20Final.pdf (Accessed 8/7/2018)

Human Tissue Authority (2017a) *Code A: Guiding Principles and the Fundamental Principle of Consent*. Available at: www.hta.gov.uk (Accessed: 18/4/2018)

Human Tissue Authority (2017b) *Code G: Donation of Allogeneic Bone Marrow and Peripheral Blood Stem Cells for Transplantation*. Available at: www.hta.gov.uk (Accessed: 18/4/2018)

Human Tissue Authority (2017c) *Code E: Research*. Available at: www.hta.gov.uk (Accessed: 18/4/2018)

Humphries, J. (2006) Dry tap bone marrow aspiration: clinical significance. *American Journal of Hematology*, 35(4), 247–250.

Hurley, C. & Raffoux, C. (2004) Special report: World Marrow Donor Association: International Standards for unrelated hematopoietic stem cell registries. *Bone Marrow Transplantation*, 34, 97–101.

JACIE (2015) *JACIE Standards*, 6th edn. Available at: www.jacie.org/document-centre (Accessed: 18/4/2018)

Joint Formulary Committee (2018) *British National Formulary*. London: BMJ Group, Pharmaceutical Press and RCPCH Publications. Available at: http://www.medicinescomplete.com (Accessed: 18/4/2018)

Kaushansky, K., Lichtman, M., Prchal, J.T., et al. (2016) *Williams' Hematology*, 9th edn. London: McGraw-Hill.

Kilham, L. & Ferm, V.H. (1977) Congenital anomalies induced in hamster embryos with Ribavirin. *Science*, 195, 413–414.

Knobler, R., Berlin, G., Calzavara-Pinton, P., et al. (2014) Guidelines on the use of extracorporeal photopheresis. *Journal of the European Academy of Dermatology and Venereology*, 28(1), 1–37.

Koeppen H, Bueso-Ramos, C. & Konoplev, S.N. (2011) Traditional diagnostic approaches. In: Faderl, S. & Kantarjian, H. (eds) *Leukaemias, Principles and Practices of Therapy*. Oxford: Wiley-Blackwell.

Lawson, S., Aston, S., Baker, L. et al. (1999) Trained nurses can obtain satisfactory bone marrow aspirates and trephine biopsies. *Journal of Clinical Pathology*, 52(2), 154–156.

Lewis, S.L., Bucher, L., Heitkemper, M.M., Harding, M.M., Kwong, J. & Roberts, D. (2016) *Medical-Surgical Nursing: Assessment and Management of Clinical Problems*, 10th edn. St Louis, MO: Mosby.

Lewis, S.M., Bain, B.J. & Bates, I. (2011) *Dacie and Lewis Practical Haematology*, 11th edn. London: Churchill Livingstone.

Lidén, Y., Landgren, O., Arnér, S., et al. (2009) Procedure related pain among adult patients with hematologic malignancies. *Acta Anaesthesiologica Scandinavica*, 53(3), 354–363.

Linn, W.S., Gong, H., Anderson, K.R., Clark, K.W. & Shamoo, D.A. (1995) Exposure of health care workers to Ribavirin aerosol; a pharmacokinetic study. *Archives of Environmental Health*, 50(6), 445–451.

Longo, D. (2016) Examination of blood smears and bone marrow. In: Kasper, D., Braunwald, E. & Fauci, A. (eds) *Harrison's Manual of Medicine*, 19th edn. New York: McGraw-Hill, pp. 265–267.

Loveday, H.P., Wilson, J.A., Prieto, J. & Wilcox, M.H. (2016) epic3: revised recommendation for intravenous catheter and catheter site care. *Journal of Hospital Infection* 92(4), 346–348.

McGrath, P. (2013) Procedural care for adult bone marrow aspiration and biopsy: qualitative research findings from Australia. *Cancer Nursing*, 36(4), 309–316.

McNamara, L. (2011) Bone marrow biopsy training for nurses. *Cancer Nursing Practice*, 10, 9, 14–19.

MHRA (2009) Drug Safety Update: Volume 2, Issue 9. London: Medicines and Healthcare products Regulatory Agency.

MHRA (2012) *Good Clinical Practice Guide*. London: Medicines and Healthcare products Regulatory Agency.

MHRA (2014) *Summary of product characteristics, Virazole (Ribavirin) Aerosol*. London: Medicines and Healthcare products Regulatory Agency. Available at: http://www.mhra.gov.uk/home/groups/spcpil/documents/spcpil/con1493963375390.pdf (Accessed: 18/4/2018)

Molinos-Quintana, A., Pérez-de Soto, C., Gómez-Rosa, M., Pérez-Simón, J.A. & Pérez-Hurtado, J.M. (2013) Intravenous ribavirin for respiratory syncytial viral infections in pediatric hematopoietic SCT recipients. *Bone Marrow Transplantation*, 48, 265–268.

Moore, G., Knight, G. & Blann, A. (2016) *Haematology*, 2nd edn. Oxford: Oxford University Press.

Munzenberger, P.J. & Walker, P.C. (1994) Protecting hospital employees and visitors from aerolised Ribavirin. *American Journal of Hospital Pharmacy*, 51, 823–826.

National Cancer Institute (2010) NCI drug dictionary. Bethesda, MD: National Cancer Institute. Available at: https://www.cancer.gov/publications/dictionaries/cancer-drug (Accessed: 18/4/2018)

NHS Blood and Transplant (2010) Haematopoietic stem cell transplant services. Available at: https://www.nhsbt.nhs.uk/what-we-do/transplantation-services/stem-cells/ (Accessed: 18/4/2018)

NHS Professionals (2013) *Standard Infection Prevention and Control Guidelines Clinical Governance Version 4*. NHS Professionals, UK. Available at: https://www.nhsprofessionals.nhs.uk/en/members/elibrary/publications/cg1%20stanard%20infection%20prevention%20and%20control%20guidelines (Accessed: 18/4/2018)

NMC (2010) *Standards for Medicine Management*. London: Nursing & Midwifery Council.

NMC (2015) *The Code: Professional Standards of Practice and Behaviour for Nurses and Midwives*. London: Nursing & Midwifery Council.

NPSA (2005) *Safer Patient Identification*. London: National Patient Safety Agency. Available at: www.nrls.npsa.nhs.uk/resources/patient-safety-topics/patient-admission-transfer-discharge/?entryid45=59799 (Accessed: 18/4/2018)

NPSA (2007) Recognising and responding appropriately to early signs of deterioration in hospitalised patients. London: National Patient Safety Agency. Available at: www.npsa.nhs.uk/EasySiteWeb/GatewayLink.aspx?alId=6240 (Accessed: 18/4/2018)

Odejide, O., Cronin, A. & DeAngelo, D. (2013) Improving the quality of bone marrow assessment: Impact of operator techniques and use of a specimen preparation checklist. *Cancer*, 119(19), 3472–3478.

Outhwaite, H. (2008) Blood and marrow transplantation. In: Grundy M. (ed.) *Nursing in Haematological Oncology*, 2nd edn. Edinburgh: Baillière Tindall, pp. 140–155.

Paediatric Formulary Committee (2018) *BNF for Children*. London: BMJ Group, Pharmaceutical Press and RCPCH Publications. Available at: http://www.medicinescomplete.com (Accessed: 18/4/2018)

Perkins, S. (2003) Bone marrow examination. In: Greer, J. et al. (eds) *Wintrobe's Clinical Hematology*, 11th edn. Lippincott, Williams and Wilkins, Philadelphia, pp. 3–22.

Perry, A.G. (2016) Administration of nonparenteral medications. In: Perry, A.G., Potter, P. A. & Ostendorf, W.R. (eds) *Nursing Interventions and Clinical Skills*, 6th edn. St Louis, MO: Elsevier, pp.555–596.

Pertine, B., Razvi, S. & Weinstein, R. (2002) Prospective investigation of a subcutaneous, implantable central venous access device for therapeutic plasma exchange in adults with neurological disorders. *Journal of Clinical Apheresis*, 17(1), 1–6.

Provan, D., Baglin, T., Dokal, I. & de Vos, J. (2015) *Oxford Handbook of Clinical Haematology*, 4th edn. Oxford: Oxford University Press.

Raboni, S.M., Nogueira, M.B., Tsuchiya, L.R., et al. (2003) Respiratory tract viral infections in bone marrow transplant patients. *Transplantation*, 76, 142–146.

Radhakrishnan, N. (2017) Bone Marrow Aspiration and Biopsy. Available at: http://emedicine.medscape.com/article/207575-overview (Accessed: 18/4/2018)

Richardson, C. & Atkinson, J. (2006) Blood and marrow transplantation. In: Grundy M. (ed.) *Nursing in Haematological Oncology*. Edinburgh: Baillière Tindall, pp. 265–291.

Rosenmayr, A., Hartwell, L. & Egeland, T. (2003) Informed consent – suggested procedures for informed consent for unrelated haematopoietic stem cell donors at various stages of recruitment, donor evaluation, and donor workup. *Bone Marrow Transplantation*, 31, 539–545.

Ruegg, T., Curran, C. & Lamb, T. (2009) Use of buffered lidocaine in bone marrow biopsies: a randomized, controlled trial. *Oncology Nursing Forum*, 36(1), 52–60.

Schwartz, J., Winters, J.L., Padmanabhan, A., et al. (2013) Guidelines on the use of therapeutic apheresis in clinical practice – evidence based approach from the writing committee of the American Society for Apheresis: the sixth special issue. *Journal of Clinical Apheresis*, 28, 145–284.

Scott, B.L. & Sandmaier, B.M. (2016) The evaluation and counseling of candidates for hematopoietic cell transplantation. In: Forman, S.J., Negrin, R.S., Antin, J.H. & Appelbaum, F.R. (eds) *Thomas' Hematopoietic Cell Transplantation*, 5th edn. Boston, MA: Blackwell Publishing, pp. 349–365.

Shah, D.P., Ghantoji, S.S., Shah, J.N., et al. (2013) Impact of aerosolized ribavirin on mortality in 280 allogeneic haematopoietic stem cell transplant recipients with respiratory syncytial virus infections. *Journal of Antimicrobial Chemotherapy*, 68, 1872–1880.

Shah, J.N. & Chemaly, R.F. (2011) Management of RSV infections in adult recipients of hematopoietic stem cell transplantation. *Blood*, 117, 2755–2763.

Smock, K.J. & Perkins, S.L. (2014) Examination of the blood and bone marrow. In: Greer, J., Arber, D.A., Glader, B.E., et al. (eds) *Wintrobe's Clinical Hematology*, 13th edn. Philadelphia: Lippincott, Williams and Wilkins, pp. 3–22.

Strauss, R. (2010) Granulocyte (neutrophil) transfusion. In: McLeod, B., Szczepiorkowski, Z.M., Weinstein, R. & Winters, J.L. (eds) *Apheresis: Principles and Practice*, 3rd edn. Bethesda, MD: AABB Press, pp. 215–228.

Stroncek, D., Confer, D. & Leitman, S. (2000) Peripheral blood progenitor cells for HPC transplants involving unrelated donors. *Transfusion*, 40, 731–741.

Sun, T. & Zhang, Y. (2008) Pentamidine binds to tRNA through non-specific hydrophobic interactions and inhibits aminoacylation and translation. *Nucleic Acids Research*, 36(5), 1654–1664.

Terumo BCT (2011) Operational manual for Optia™: Mononuclear cell collection, Plasma Exchange, and White blood cell collection. Available at: www.terumobct.com (Accessed: 18/4/2018)

Traynor, B. (2006) Haematopoiesis. In: Grundy M. (ed.) *Nursing in Haematological Oncology*, 2nd edn. Edinburgh: Elsevier, pp. 3–20.

Tunsjo, H.S., Berg, A.S., Inchley, C.S., Roberg, I.K. & Leegaard, T.M. (2015) Comparison of nasopharyngeal aspirate with flocked swab for PCR-detection of respiratory viruses in children. *APMIS*, 123(6), 473–477.

Turgeon, M.L. (2014) *Clinical Haematology, Theory and Procedures*, 5th edn. Philadelphia: Lippincott, Williams and Wilkins.

Valeant Canada LP (2014) *Product monograph.* Pr*VIRAZOLE® (Ribavirin for Inhalation Solution, USP)*. Quebec: Valeant.

Van Walraven, A., Nicoloso-de Faveri, G., Axdorph-Nygell, U., et al. for the WMDA Ethics and Working Groups (2010) Family donor care management: principles and recommendations. *Bone Marrow Transplantation*, 45(8), 1269–1273.

World Marrow Donor Association (2017) *International Standards for Unrelated Hematopoietic Progenitor Cell Donor Registries.* Available at: www.wmda.info/wp-content/uploads/2018/02/20170101-STDC-WMDA-standards-cleared-version.pdf (Accessed: 18/4/2018)

Yarbro, C.H., Wujcik, D.L. & Gobel, B.H. (2016) *Cancer Nursing: Principles and Practice*, 8th edn. Sudbury, MA: Jones and Bartlett.

Chapter 3

Cancer pain assessment and management

Procedure guidelines

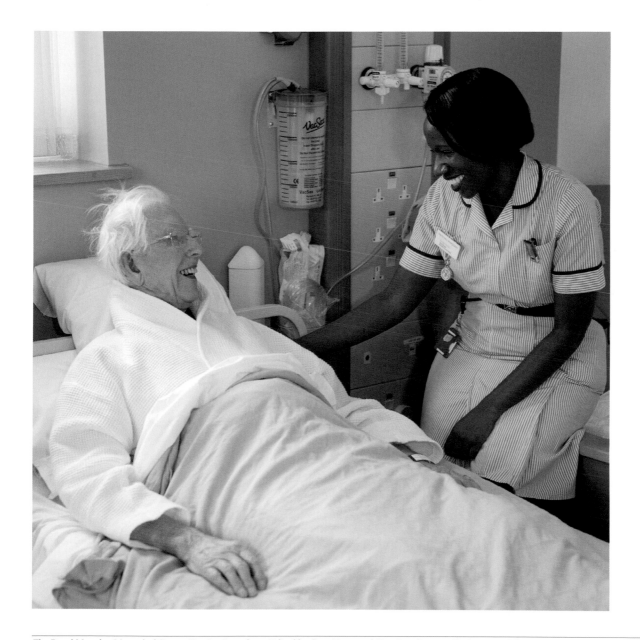

The Royal Marsden Manual of Cancer Nursing Procedures. Edited by Sara Lister and Lisa Dougherty, with Assistant Editor Louise McNamara.
© 2019 The Royal Marsden NHS Foundation Trust. Published 2019 by John Wiley & Sons, Ltd.

Overview

The aim of this chapter is to present an overview of cancer pain, pain assessment and pain management.

Cancer pain is arguably one of the most common symptoms reported by cancer patients (Lang and Patt 2004). The prevalence of cancer pain has been estimated at 39.3% after curative treatment, 55.0% during anticancer treatment and 66.4% in advanced, metastatic or terminal disease (van den Beuken et al. 2016). Despite this high incidence of pain and advances in moderate treatment methods, up to 50% of patients continue to be undertreated (Deandrea et al. 2008) with 67% of patients reporting their experience of pain as distressing (Breivik et al. 2009). This high incidence of untreated pain results in a reduction in patient quality of life and can impact on the regular activities of daily living (Portenoy 2011).

Definition

Pain is a complex phenomenon that has physiological, psychological and social factors that influence the individual patient experience. It is subjective so the patient's perspective is important to understand. It has both a physical and an affective (emotional) component. To reflect this, the International Association for the Study of Pain (IASP 1994) published the following definition of pain: 'An unpleasant sensory and emotional experience associated with actual or potential tissue damage, or described in terms of such damage'. As pain is subjective, another favoured definition for use in clinical practice, proposed originally by McCaffrey (1968) and cited in McCaffrey (2000, p. 2), is: 'Pain is whatever the experiencing person says it is, existing whenever the experiencing person says it does'.

Pain in patients with cancer is often not a purely physical experience but involves many other factors. Pain may have psychological, physical, social and spiritual components.

Anatomy and physiology

Pain mechanisms (anatomy and physiology) are usually described in terms of nociceptive pain or neuropathic pain. As with acute and chronic pain, it is common for pain to be both nociceptive and neuropathic in origin rather than purely one or the other; it is often then referred to as mixed nociceptive and neuropathic pain.

Nociceptive pain

Nociceptive pain is the 'normal' pain pathway that occurs in response to tissue injury or damage (Figure 3.1). It consists of four components: transduction, transmission, perception and modulation. Nociceptors are free nerve endings found at the end of pain neurones. They occur in skin and subcutaneous tissue, muscle, visceral organs, tendons, fascia, joint capsules and arterial walls (Godfrey 2005). Nociceptors respond to noxious thermal stimuli (heat and cold) and mechanical stimuli (stretching, compression, infiltration) and to the chemical mediators released as part of the inflammatory response to tissue injury. These chemical mediators include prostaglandins, bradykinin, substance P, serotonin and adenosine. As a result of this stimulation process, an action potential is generated in the nerve (*transduction*).

The pain signal is then transmitted along the peripheral nervous system (A delta and C fibres) to the central nervous system, arriving at the dorsal horn of the spinal cord. Neurotransmitters are released to allow the pain signal to be transmitted from the endings of the peripheral nerves to the nociceptors in the dorsal horn. The message is then transmitted to the brain where perception of the pain occurs (*transmission*). *Perception* is the end-result of the neuronal activity of pain transmission. The perception of pain includes behavioural, psychological and emotional components as well as physiological processes.

Modulation occurs when the transmission of pain impulses in the spinal cord is changed or inhibited. Modulatory influences on pain perception are complex, involving a gating system which is linked to a descending modulatory pathway. Modulation can occur as a result of a natural release of inhibitory neurotransmitter

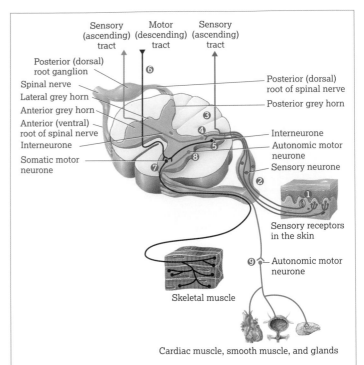

Figure 3.1 Processing of sensory input and motor output by the spinal cord. *Source:* Tortora and Derrickson (2011). Reproduced with permission from John Wiley & Sons.

chemicals that inhibit transmission of pain impulses and therefore produce analgesia. Other interventions, including distraction, relaxation, sense of well-being, heat/cold therapy, massage and transcutaneous electrical nerve stimulation (TENS), can also help to modulate pain perception. Analgesic medications work by inhibiting some of the chemicals involved in pain transduction and transmission and thus modulating pain perception (Figure 3.2). Pain signals can also be increased by certain factors such as anxiety, fear and low mood/depression.

Neuropathic pain

Neuropathic pain is not pain that originates as part of 'normal' pain pathways. It has been described as pain related to abnormal processing within the nervous system (Mann 2008). Nerve injury or dysfunction can be caused by a range of conditions such as infection, trauma, metabolic disorder, chemotherapy, surgery, radiation, neurotoxins, nerve compression, joint degeneration, tumour infiltration and malnutrition (Mann 2008).

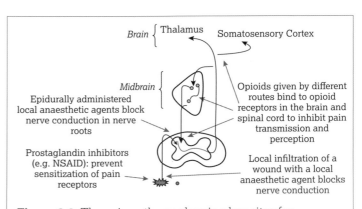

Figure 3.2 The pain pathway showing key sites for particular analgesic interventions. NSAID, non-steroidal anti-inflammatory drug. *Source:* Dougherty and Lister (2015).

The following are currently thought to contribute to the mechanisms by which neuropathic pain is generated and maintained (Baron et al. 2010, Mann 2008, Nickel et al. 2012).

- Damage or abnormalities in the nerves change the way in which nerves communicate with each other.
- Pain receptors require less stimulation to initiate pain signals both in peripheral nerves and the central nervous system, where it is often referred to as central sensitization.
- Pain transmission is altered from its normal sequence.
- There may be an increase in the release of chemical neurotransmitters.
- There can be increased and chaotic firing of nerves.
- Damaged nerves spontaneously generate impulses in the absence of any stimulation.
- The descending inhibitory systems may also be reduced or lost.

The nervous system changes its structure and function in response to the input it receives throughout an individual's life course and this is termed **neuroplasticity**, also known as **brain plasticity** or **neural plasticity**. Neuroplasticity is evident at all levels from the nociceptor to the brain (cortex). Individuals who suffer from persistent pain experience prolonged pain at sites that may have been previously injured, yet are otherwise currently healthy. This phenomenon is related to neuroplasticity due to a maladaptive reorganization of the nervous system, both peripherally and centrally. These mechanisms result in increased activity or transmission of pain signals despite less input from the peripheral nervous system, and even become responsive to innocuous stimuli. Pain can be spontaneous, may be triggered by non-painful stimuli such as touch (allodynia) or may be an exaggerated pain response (hyperalgesia); patients may also experience non-painful sensations such as pins and needles and tingling (paraesthesias).

Related theory

Many factors influence the expression of pain and may be associated with the patient, the nurse or the clinical environment (organizational aspects) (Briggs 2010, Carr and Mann 2000). Pain can have many dimensions including physical, psychological, spiritual and sociocultural.

Pain in cancer patients can be categorized into three main types:

- acute pain
- persistent or chronic pain
- breakthrough pain.

There are several ways to categorize the types of pain that occur, for example nociceptive (somatic or visceral) or neuropathic. It is increasingly recognized that acute and chronic pain may represent a continuum rather than being distinct entities (Macintyre et al. 2010) and may combine different pain mechanisms and vary in duration.

Acute pain

The IASP has defined acute pain as: 'Pain of recent onset and probable limited duration. It usually has an identifiable temporal and causal relationship to injury or disease' (Ready and Edwards 1992, p.1). Acute pain is produced by a wide range of physiological processes, and includes inflammatory, neuropathic, sympathetically maintained, visceral and cancer pain (Walker et al. 2006). Acute pain serves a purpose by alerting the individual to a problem and acting as a warning of actual or potential tissue damage. Pain may be the presenting symptom that causes patients to seek healthcare review leading to their subsequent cancer diagnosis. If left untreated, acute pain may result in severe consequences; for example, not seeking help for acute abdominal pain may result in an emergency such as bowel obstruction. Acute pain occurs in response to any type of injury to the body and resolves when the injury heals.

Common causes of acute pain in patients with cancer include:

- diagnostic interventions (e.g. biopsy, lumbar puncture, repeated venepuncture, wound care, endoscopy)
- therapeutic interventions (e.g. surgery, tumour embolization, catheterization)
- anticancer treatments (e.g. chemotherapy, radiotherapy, surgery)
- infection and/or vascular events (e.g. venous thromboembolism, cellulitis)
- acute tumour-related pain (e.g. pathological fractures, vertebral collapse, ureteric obstruction, bowel obstruction).

Persistent or chronic pain

Chronic pain is usually prolonged. It is defined as pain that exists for more than 3 months, lasting beyond the usual course of the acute disease or expected time of healing (IASP 1996). It is often associated with major changes in personality, lifestyle and functional ability (Orenius et al. 2013). Chronic pain in patients with cancer may also worsen or intensify with time depending on the status of the underlying disease. Chronic or persistent cancer pain syndromes can be associated with direct tumour invasion or cancer therapy (Chapman 2012).

Types of chronic cancer- or cancer-treatment-related pain include the following:

- tumour-related pain – direct infiltration, compression, distension or stretching, e.g. pancreatic cancer or liver capsule pain
- bone metastases or skeletal muscle tumours
- neuropathic pain from infiltration of the tumour into peripheral nerves, nerve plexuses and spinal cord
- chemotherapy-induced peripheral neuropathy
- chronic pain after surgery syndromes (e.g. thoracotomy pain, post-mastectomy pain syndrome, phantom limb pain)
- pain in cancer survivors.

Breakthrough cancer pain

Breakthrough cancer pain (BTCP) has been recognized as a burdensome, psychologically distressing symptom that is inadequately treated and often unresolved in many cancer patients. The scope guidelines developed by the European Oncology Nursing Society (EONS) describe and explain BTCP as an independent phenomenon with distinct clinical symptoms, and provide guidance on the assessment, identification and management of BTCP (EONS 2013). Although several definitions of BTCP exist, as yet there is no universally accepted definition, or agreed upon term, to describe BTCP. An expert group in palliative care defined BTCP as 'A transient exacerbation of pain that occurs either spontaneously, or in relation to a specific predictable or unpredictable trigger, despite relatively stable and adequately controlled background pain''' (Davies et al. 2009). BTCP is differentiated from background pain by being transient or episodic and breaking through the stable, controlled chronic background pain. Consequently, the treatment of BTCP demands a different management strategy. The term 'breakthrough cancer pain' is used in practice; however, other ways to describe this include 'episodic', 'transient' or 'flare up' pain.

Characteristics of BTCP

The two widely identified and accepted categories of BTCP are spontaneous pain and incident pain and these can be described as follows.

- Spontaneous pain ('idiopathic pain' – Davies et al. 2009). These episodes are not related to an identifiable trigger and so are more unpredictable.
- Incident pain ('precipitated pain'). These episodes are related to an identifiable precipitant, and can be generally predictable in

nature. Incident pain is usually sub-classified into one of three categories:
- volitional incident pain which can be brought on by situations such as walking
- non-volitional incident pain precipitated by an involuntary act such as coughing
- procedural pain related to an intervention such as changing of a wound dressing.

One of the key factors in the management of BTCP is that BTCP must not be confused with episodes of pain that occur in situations where the patient does not have controlled background pain. One example of such a situation is where episodes of pain occur during initiation or titration of opioid analgesics for the treatment of background pain – such episodes should be termed either a 'background pain flare', or simply an 'exacerbation of background pain'. Another example is where episodes of pain occur before the administration of opioid analgesics in end-of-dose failure. It should be noted, however, that end-of-dose failure is regarded as a subtype of breakthrough pain by some experts in the field (Davies et al. 2009).

Examples of difficult to manage pain syndromes

Cancer-related bone pain
Many common cancers such as breast, lung, prostate and kidney are frequently associated with bone metastases. Bone metastases are associated with pain, hypercalcaemia, increased susceptibility to skeletal fractures, compression of the spinal cord, spinal instability and decreased mobility.

Cancer-related bone pain is caused by:

- local bone destruction
- causation of pathological fractures
- infiltration of surrounding tissues
- secondary muscle spasm
- compression of neurological structures.

Related theory
Cancer-related bone pain has overlapping but distinct features of both inflammatory and neuropathic pain. The most important changes are in bone homeostasis. These changes correspond with events in the peripheral and central nervous system.

In healthy bone osteoclasts and osteoblasts are highly regulated to maintain balanced reabsorption and formation of bone respectively (Kane and Bennett 2015). In the presence of bone metastases this relationship is disrupted leading to increased osteoclast activity and bone destruction.

Cancer cells also stimulate local inflammatory mediators, creating a highly acidic environment. This sensitizes the peripheral nerve endings within the bone marrow and bone matrix (Mantyh 2014). Combined with the destruction of nerve endings through cancer invasion, the resulting pain is a mixture of ongoing inflammatory and neuropathic processes, leading to central sensitization in the spinal cord (Mantyh 2014).

For patients, cancer bone pain is constant, with high sensitivity for movement. Bone pain remains one of the most difficult to control, as metastases are often not limited to one site. This can be extremely debilitating in patients who may already have limited life expectancy.

Management of bone pain
Management of bone pain includes a thorough assessment to diagnose this as the cause of the pain.

Once diagnosed, the treatment of bone pain may include the following:

- radiotherapy – to directly treat the cancer
- surgery – to stabilize pathological fractures (e.g. long bones, joints and spinal vertebrae)
- analgesia
- bisphosphonates, which inhibit osteoclast-mediated bone reabsorption, alleviate pain and hypercalcaemia and reduce skeletal events
- interventional pain management techniques (e.g. nerve blocks, epidurals).

Abdominopelvic pain
Abdominal and pelvic pain in cancer can be visceral pain or can be mixed pain and also have a neuropathic component. Tumours of the stomach, pancreas and liver can all cause visceral pain due to compression or stretching within the organ or obstruction of ducts or vessels.

Pain can also be very severe if the coeliac plexus is invaded by tumours of the pancreas or stomach. Patients describe pain in the upper abdomen which can also radiate through to the back between the scapulae, spreading to the left and right (Bennett 2014).

Pelvic pain can be caused by tumours of the rectum or colon, or gynaecological or urological cancers. These tumours can cause pain by compression of the organ, infiltration into surrounding nerve and muscle structures or bowel obstruction.

Patients can also develop pain and tenesmus following surgical resection of the colon or rectum that may be so severe that they are unable to sit (Peat and Hester 2012).

Management options for abdominal pain
These include oncological treatment of the primary tumour, analgesia, surgery or interventional radiology procedures to relieve obstructed ducts, vessels or organs. After careful assessment of the position of the tumour to assess suitability, a coeliac plexus block may be considered.

Management options for pelvic pain
These include oncological treatment of the primary tumour, analgesia, surgery or interventional radiology procedures to relieve obstructed ducts, vessels or organs or interventional analgesia procedures (sacral nerve blocks, saddle blocks, epidural or intrathecal analgesia).

Thoracic pain
Thoracic pain in cancer patients can be caused by lung cancers and mesothelioma. Pain is often poorly localized and patients often describe a generalized area of pain in the chest wall. Severe intractable pain, particularly in mesothelioma, is caused by the tumour compressing the remaining lung, pleural effusion, and infiltration of tumour into the chest wall and nerve structures (Sharma and Gupta 2014).

Cancer survivors who have had surgery for thoracic cancer may also develop persistent thoracic postsurgical pain.

Management of thoracic pain
Treatment options for thoracic pain caused by tumour include:

- oncological management of the primary tumour
- analgesia
- intercostal and paravertebral nerve blocks
- epidural or intrathecal analgesia
- cervical cordotomy.

Nerve plexus invasion
Tumour invasion can occur in a number of different types of nerve plexus, causing severe pain. The pain is typically neuropathic in nature and referred within the distribution of the nerves affected (Peat and Hester 2012).

Examples include:

- invasion of the lumbar plexus from pelvic tumours such as advanced cervical or prostate cancer, or any tumour that spreads into the psoas compartment or paravertebral space at L2, 3, 4 (Peat and Hester 2012)

- invasion of the brachial plexus from advanced breast cancer or lung 'Pancoast' cancer (Peat and Hester 2012).

Treatment options include analgesic drug therapy, oncological therapy and interventional techniques. Analgesia is often more successful with a combination of opioids and adjuvant drugs such as gabapentin, amitriptyline and steroids (Raphael et al. 2010).

Chemotherapy-induced peripheral neuropathy

Background
Chemotherapy-induced peripheral neuropathy (CIPN) can be argued to be the most common and debilitating symptom following cancer treatment (Majithia et al. 2016). It is becoming a major issue in cancer survivorship as chemotherapy agents are increasingly being used as first-line treatment (Majithia et al. 2016).

The exact incidence of CIPN is difficult to determine due to the variety of cancer treatments being used and under-reporting from patients. Under-reporting is often due to the fear of having treatment doses reduced or stopped in consequence. It is most commonly associated with platinum- and taxane-based treatments (Brewer et al. 2016, Kuroi and Shimozuma 2004). Hershman et al. (2014) estimated the incidence of CIPN in patients receiving multiple agent treatment at 38% and Brown et al. (2014) estimated its prevalence at 30%.

Ventzel et al. (2016) found that out of 174 patients 63.6% reported CIPN 1 year after completion of treatment. Majithia et al. (2016) found that patients were reporting symptoms lasting years after completion of treatment. In patients who report symptoms lasting longer than 6 months the condition becomes virtually irreversible. It is estimated that around 60% of patients fall into this group (Beijers et al. 2014).

Pathophysiology
The exact pathophysiology of CIPN is complex and not fully understood as it is highly dependent on the chemotherapy agent being administered (Brown et al. 2014).

Different theories have been suggested as to the cause of CIPN. Causes include: changes to the structure of mitochondria in cells (Flatters and Bennett 2006); alteration in pain mediators in peripheries and the central nervous system (Cavaletti et al. 2002); and abnormal transmission of pain impulses via A delta, A beta and C fibres in vincristine, paclitaxel and oxaliplatin treatment (Xiao and Bennett 2008). The alteration in pain mediators can also include a reduction in nerve growth factor that results in nerve damage (Cavaletti et al. 2002).

The side-effect profiles of chemotherapy agents are well known and documented. However their neurotoxic effects can vary depending on the individual and this can make predicting CIPN challenging (Tzatha and DeAngelis 2016). There are associated risk factors and other co-morbidities that can predispose the nervous system to injury. These include (Tzatha and DeAngelis 2016):

- previous treatment with neurotoxic agents
- diabetes
- vitamin deficiencies
- thyroid dysfunction
- HIV
- reduced creatinine clearance.

Symptoms
The initial presenting symptoms for CIPN normally include abnormal and/or loss of sensation, which usually starts in fingertips and toes and can spread to upper and lower extremities depending on severity (Tofthagen et al. 2013). Brown et al. (2014) and Kuroi and Shimozuma (2004) reported that the most common presenting symptoms included:

- paraesthesia
- numbness

- temperature changes
- loss of proprioception
- dysaesthesia
- neuropathic pain
- loss of balance.

Impaired fine motor function
CIPN can have a negative impact on the patient's quality of life with many reporting difficulty with or inability to perform daily tasks such as buttoning clothes, holding objects, opening jars/bottles, loss of balance and pain on standing/walking/climbing stairs (Beijers et al. 2014, Driessen et al. 2012).

A 2014 study (Beijers et al. 2014) surveyed 43 patients, of whom 48% reported a direct decrease in quality of life indicators as a result of CIPN symptoms. It also found that CIPN had a profound impact on emotional well-being and patients became more dependent on others to assist with daily tasks.

Assessment of CIPN
Despite the wide use of treatments that cause CIPN and the severity of the side-effects there is no clinical agreement on how best to assess severity and monitor changes in symptoms (Cavaletti et al. 2002). Tofthagen et al. (2013) suggest that simple direct questioning of the patient at every visit (asking if they have any new altered sensation, i.e. numbness, pins and needles, etc.) would be the simplest way of identifying patients with CIPN. However, patients are often reluctant to report symptoms of CIPN for fear of having their treatment stopped or simply not wanting to disturb healthcare staff (Tofthagen 2010). As CIPN is not always painful, patients may not report this when asked about their pain, and because it falls out of the normal pain characteristics the patient may not make the association between CIPN and pain (Tofthagen et al. 2013).

Ellen et al. (2014) surveyed 408 oncology nurses regarding their knowledge and assessment of patients with CIPN. They found that 86% were collecting data on patient-reported sensory symptoms but only 41% were performing physical examination and the use of assessment tools was infrequent.

A wide variety of assessment tools can be used to aid CIPN diagnosis. However these rely heavily on subjective questions (Brown et al. 2014). The tools most commonly used are the World Health Organization (WHO) CIPN grading scale, the Eastern Cooperative Oncology Group (ECOG) neuropathy scale and the National Cancer Institute Common Toxicity Criteria (NCI-CTC) neuropathy score (Cavaletti et al. 2010).

Given the subjective nature of the symptoms, the most accurate assessment tool is one that relies on the patient's report of their symptoms (Postma et al. 2005). The European Organisation for Research and Treatment of Cancer (EORTC) performed literature reviews and a survey of healthcare professionals on CIPN issues that led to the development of a 20-item questionnaire to identify symptoms of CIPN. Called the EORTC CIPN20 (Postma et al. 2005), it has been shown to be a valid and accurate tool to score the severity of symptoms and impact on the patient's quality of life. The authors of this study went on to develop the Rasch-built overall disability scale (R-ODS) based on the limitations from CIPN20. They recommend the use of this scale in future research to ascertain validity (Binda et al. 2013).

Cancer pain assessment and management

Pain assessment

Evidence-based approaches
Pain is a common symptom in patients with cancer (Chapman 2012). Causes of cancer pain can be multifactorial and are related to either the effects of cancer treatment such as surgery,

radiotherapy or chemotherapy, or pain can be caused by the cancer itself such as in patients with bone metastases or where the cancer has caused injury to nerves. Cancer pain can be both acute and chronic and requires careful assessment and attention to detail, including a detailed history of previously tried medications and responses to these pharmacological interventions. Assessment, treatment plan and review are key to the management of cancer pain.

Methods of pain assessment

Cancer pain is multidimensional and complex and therefore a comprehensive and holistic assessment is essential in formulating an effective management plan (Burton et al. 2014). Cancer pain may change depending on disease progression and response to treatment; it is complex and as stated previously can be a mix of acute treatment-related episodes alongside chronic disease-related pathways. Pain assessment is not a one-off episode, pain is dynamic and changes, and therefore pain assessment should be dynamic in order to ensure the appropriate management strategy is in place.

Total pain

The term 'total pain' was first used by Dame Cicely Saunders (1978) with the aim of identifying the impact that pain has on the individual as a whole. Dame Cicely suggested that pain is influenced by psychological, social, emotional and spiritual factors that contribute to the individual's overall pain experience. The physical aspects of the pain could be a result of treatment side-effects or caused by the cancer itself; psychological factors that will heighten perception of pain are anxiety, depression and previous episodes of poorly controlled pain; social aspects can be loss of income due to ill health and financial concerns; and spiritual factors can be loss of faith, fear of the unknown and loss of meaning/purpose (IASP 2009). It is for this reason that pain assessment must be multidimensional and holistic in order to address the needs of the patient.

Assessment tools

A variety of assessment tools have been validated for use in clinical practice.

- One-dimensional tools are effective in monitoring pain intensity (Hjermstad et al. 2011). These are most commonly used in acute pain as they are a quick and convenient method of assessing pain at the bedside and allow us to quantify baseline pain scores that can be used to assess response to treatment (Chapman 2012).
- Multidimensional tools are used to measure the patient's overall pain experience. Given that cancer pain is complex and multidimensional, these tools can be more effective in performing a comprehensive pain assessment.

One-dimensional tools

The simplest techniques for pain measurement involve the use of a verbal rating scale, numerical rating scale or visual analogue scale. Patients are asked to match pain intensity to the scale. Three principles apply to the use of these scales:

1 The patient must be involved in scoring his or her own pain intensity. It provides the patient with an opportunity to express their pain intensity and also what it means to them and the effect it has on their lives. This is important because healthcare professionals frequently underestimate the intensity of a patient's pain and effectiveness of pain relief (Alemdar and Aktas 2014, Drayer et al. 1999, Idvall et al. 2002, Loveman and Gale 2000).
2 Pain intensity assessment should incorporate different components of pain. It should include assessment of static (rest) pain and dynamic pain (on sitting, coughing or moving the affected part). For example, in a post-operative patient this is important to prevent complications of delayed recovery such as chest infections and emboli (deep vein thrombosis, pulmonary embolism) and to determine if analgesia is adequate for return of normal function (Hobbs and Hodgkinson 2003, Macintyre and Schug 2015).
3 It is important to remember that a complete picture of a patient's pain cannot be derived solely from the use of a pain scale (Burton et al. 2014). Ongoing communication with the patient is required to uncover and manage any psychosocial factors that may be affecting the patient's pain experience.

Lim et al. (2015) surveyed 551 patients on their satisfaction with pain assessment scales and found that 79% were in favour of using the scales and that they were beneficial in managing their pain symptoms.

Multidimensional tools

A variety of multidimensional assessment tools can be used to assess other aspects of cancer pain.

1 The McGill Pain Questionnaire Short Form (1987) lists 15 descriptors of pain that the patient can then score as none, mild, moderate or severe. The terms used include throbbing, shooting, sharp, cramping. The multidimensional nature of this scale takes the form of four final descriptors of tiring – exhausting, sickening, fearful and punishing-cruel – to assess the impact the pain experience is having on the patient as a whole. This is a quick and easy tool that can be utilized in a clinic setting (Ngamkham et al. 2012).
2 The Brief Pain Inventory (BPI) (Cleeland and Ryan 1994) consists of three main sections:
   a. A front and back body diagram that allows the patient to mark the area of pain.
   b. Pain severity. Patients are asked to score pain using a 0–10 scale where 0 is no pain and 10 is most severe.
   c. Pain impact on daily function. Patients are asked to score the level of interference they are experiencing from pain where 0 is no interference and 10 is complete interference.
   The brief pain inventory is a widely used and validated method of pain assessment in both cancer patients and in a chronic pain population (Furler 2013).
3 The MD Anderson Symptom Inventory (MDASI) (Cleeland et al. 2000) is based on the BPI and has been expanded on to include a variety of symptoms other than pain that impact the cancer population. The MDASI tool has been used to identify symptoms of pain, fatigue, nausea, disturbed sleep, emotional distress, shortness of breath, lack of appetite, drowsiness, dry mouth, sadness, vomiting, memory difficulties and numbness and tingling (Burton et al. 2014). On the same principles as the BPI, patients are asked to score the level of their symptoms based on a 0–10 scale with 0 being not present and 10 being the worst level imaginable. This comprehensive assessment tool allows the clinician to assess fully the impact of the patient's condition at the time and allow a review of multiple factors, not just pain.

Given the variety of assessment tools available it is important to find one that both the patient and the clinician understand and are able to use and engage with. It is important to understand that the patient's self-reporting and classification of symptoms is more accurate than the clinician's perception of the patient's pain (Brunelli et al. 2014).

Pain assessment can be difficult to achieve. For example, the tendency suggested by both research and clinical practice is for the patient not to report any pain or to do so inadequately or inaccurately, minimizing the pain experience (Bell and Duffy 2009, McCaffery and Beebe 1989). Nurses are influenced by a number of variables when assessing the amount of pain a patient is suffering (Kitson 1994). Pargeon and Hailey (1999) demonstrated that healthcare providers usually over- or underestimate a patient's pain. McCaffery and Ferrell (1997) found that nurses were more likely to accept a patient's report of pain if they were showing signs of visible distress than if they did not. It has also been suggested that nurses do not possess sufficient knowledge to care for patients in pain (Drayer et al. 1999, McCaffery and Ferrell 1997). A survey of over 3000 nurses (McCaffery and Robinson 2002) demonstrated that nurse education has improved confidence in the pain assessment process but that further education continues to be required in the pharmacology of pain medications and addressing nurses' fears of opioid addiction and respiratory depression, which continue to contribute to the undertreatment of pain.

A variety of pain assessment tools exist to assist nurses to assess pain and plan nursing care. They enable pain to be successfully assessed and monitored (McCaffery and Beebe 1989, Twycross et al. 1996, Walker et al. 1987) and improve communication between staff and patients (Raiman 1986). Higginson (1998, p. 150) notes that: 'Taking assessments directly from the patient is the most valid way of collecting information on their quality of life'. Encouraging patients to take an active role in their pain assessment by using pain tools helps to increase their confidence and makes them feel part of the pain management process. It is important to remember that pain is whatever the patient reports it is at that time. However McCaffery and Ferrell (1997) found that less than half of nurses surveyed agreed that patients' self-reporting of pain was reliable.

Some degree of caution, however, must be exercised with the use of pain assessment tools. The nurse must be careful to select the tool that is most appropriate for a particular type of pain experience: for example, it would not be appropriate to use a pain assessment tool designed for use with patients with chronic pain to assess post-operative pain. Furthermore, pain tools should not be used indiscriminately. Walker et al. (1987) found that pain tools appeared to have little value in cases of unresolved or intractable pain.

Accurate pain assessment and reassessment are crucial to develop an understanding and baseline measure of the pain. The role of the nurse is crucial in the assessment and management of the patient's pain as they spend the most time with the patient. The key is to ask appropriate questions, which should seek to cover the following areas. The SOCRATES pain assessment framework is a mnemonic commonly used by healthcare professionals.

S – *severity:* none, mild, moderate, severe
O – *onset:* when and how did it start?
C – *characteristic:* is it shooting, burning, aching – ask the patient to describe it
R – *radiation:* does it radiate anywhere else?
A – *additional factors:* what makes it better?
T – *time:* is it there all the time, is there a time of day when it is worse?
E – *exacerbating factors:* what makes it worse?
S – *site:* where is the pain?

In addition to this, questions relating to the following psychosocial elements should also be addressed (Mackintosh and Elson 2008).

- The effect of pain on mood.
- Are relationships affected by the pain?
- Physical limitations caused by the pain.
- Social effects: has the pain resulted in a loss of work or loss of role?
- Other types of pain affecting the patient.
- Previous treatments for pain and their effects.
- Other co-morbidities.
- Allergies.

Neuropathic pain may require a specific assessment tool. Patients may describe spontaneous pain (arising without detectable stimulation) and evoked pain (abnormal responses to stimuli) (Bennett 2001). The Leeds Assessment of Neuropathic Symptoms and Signs (LANSS) pain scale (Bennett 2001) was developed to more accurately assess this type of pain.

New UK National Guidelines to help healthcare professionals recognise and assess pain in older people have been published in 2018. The guidelines were developed by the British Geriatric Society, British Pain Society and Royal College of Nursing in collaboration with researchers. In adults with no or mild to moderate cognitive impairment, both numerical rating scales (0–10) and verbal descriptor rating scales (no pain, mild, moderate or severe pain) are reliable and valid for patients' self-report of pain intensity. The new UK guidelines include recognising that patient self-reporting is the most reliable and accurate measure. Assessment may need to include the use of related terms such as 'soreness, aching, or discomfort' and also recommends that re-wording questions to elicit the presence of pain such as 'Do you hurt anywhere?' can help to identify the presence or absence of pain (Schofield 2018). For older or vulnerable adults with moderate-to-severe cognitive/communication impairment Pain in Advanced Dementia (PAINAD) and Doloplus2 are recommended (Schofield 2018). Doloplus2 and PAINAD scales continue to show positive results in terms of reliability and validity. There has been no recent evaluation of the Abbey pain scale (Abbey et al. 2004) but it remains widely used throughout the UK due to its ease of use (Schofield 2018). Similarly, for patients who have a learning disability who cannot communicate their pain verbally, the use of pictorial or non-verbal assessment tools may be appropriate and questioning those around the patient who know them well can be a great asset in assessing the pain needs of the person with a learning disability.

Fixed times for reviewing the pain have been omitted intentionally to allow for flexibility. It is suggested that, initially, the nurse review the patient's pain every 4 hours. When a patient's level of pain has stabilized, recordings may be made less frequently, for example 12-hourly or daily. The chart should be discontinued if a patient's pain becomes totally controlled.

Pain management

Evidence-based approaches

Pain management uses a multidisciplinary team approach that matches therapy to the individual patient. In some instances, simple analgesia can be sufficient to control pain. Simple or non-opioid analgesics include paracetamol and non-steroidal anti-inflammatory drugs (NSAIDs) used either individually or in combination.

Multimodal analgesia

Multimodal or balanced analgesia involves the use of more than one analgesic compound or method of pain control to achieve additive (or synergistic) pain relief while minimizing adverse effects (Schug and Chong 2009). This allows for lower doses of individual drugs. It combines different analgesics that act by different mechanisms and at different sites in the nervous system. The aim is to achieve greater analgesia than each of the individual drugs could provide alone.

Opioids, non-opioids (such as paracetamol, NSAIDs, cyclo-oxygenase-2-selective inhibitors [COX-2]), local anaesthetics and anticonvulsants are all examples of drugs that may be used as part of a multimodal analgesic approach. An example of multimodal analgesia to manage acute post-operative pain would be a continuous epidural infusion of a combined opioid and local anaesthetic solution in combination with paracetamol and an NSAID (if not contraindicated). Another example would be a continuous peripheral nerve block with paracetamol and an NSAID. Both of these approaches combine different analgesic compounds and analgesic approaches (oral route, epidural route and peripheral nerve block).

A multimodal approach may also include non-pharmacological approaches such as relaxation therapy, imagery, TENS and heat therapy.

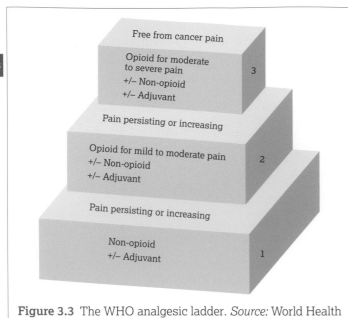

Figure 3.3 The WHO analgesic ladder. *Source:* World Health Organization (1996). Reproduced with permission of WHO.

Table 3.1 The use of adjuvant drugs (co-analgesics)

Type	Use	Examples
Non-steroidal anti-inflammatory drugs	Bone pain Muscular pain Inflammation Visceral pain	Diclofenac Naproxen Ibuprofen Nabumetone
Steroids	Pressure Bone pain Inflammation Raised intracranial pressure	Dexamethasone Prednisolone
Tricyclic antidepressants	Neuropathic pain	Amitriptyline Nortriptyline
Anticonvulsants		Sodium valproate Carbamazepine Gabapentin Pregabalin
Antibiotics	Infection	Flucloxacillin Trimethoprim
Benzodiazepines	Anxiety	Diazepam Clonazepam
Antispasmodics	Spasms	Baclofen
Bisphosphonates	Bone pain	Zoledronic acid

Management of persistent chronic and cancer pain

The control of pain is directed by the 'analgesic ladder', which was presented by the World Health Organization (WHO) in 1996 as a guide to the management of persistent cancer pain (Figure 3.3). It is also often used to guide the management of chronic persistent pain. It involves a stepwise approach to the use of analgesics, including non-opioids (step 1), opioids for mild-to-moderate pain (step 2) and opioids for moderate-to-severe pain (step 3). Adjuvant drugs are those that contribute to pain relief but are not primarily indicated for pain management. They can be used at all steps of the ladder. Examples include antidepressant and anticonvulsant drugs, corticosteroids, benzodiazepines, antispasmodics and bisphosphonates.

The WHO treatment guide recommends the following five points for the correct use of analgesics.

- Administered orally if appropriate.
- Given at regular intervals.
- Prescribed according to assessment of pain intensity evaluated using a pain intensity scale.
- The dose of the analgesic should be adapted to the individual. There is no standard dose to treat certain types of pain.
- Analgesia should be prescribed with ongoing review, monitoring for effectiveness and side-effects (WHO 1996).

Therefore, some patients who present with severe pain will need to start on step 3 of the ladder; it would not be appropriate to progress through each step in this circumstance. Treatment of chronic/cancer pain does not necessarily begin with step 1, progress to step 2 and follow with step 3 (Eisenberg et al. 2005).

It is important to remember that the patient will experience different types of pain due to different aetiological and physiological changes. Each pain needs to be assessed individually, since the pain may need to be managed in a different manner and one analgesic intervention or route will rarely be sufficient. Often the best practice is to combine different types of analgesia in order to achieve maximum pain control (Table 3.1). It is also important to utilize non-pharmacological interventions at all stages of the treatment plan. Whilst the pain ladder has been questioned as to further iterations of its current format which might include patients being moved from step 1 to step 3, thus excluding step 2 (Reid and Davies 2004), it remains one of the most used tools in the management of pain in cancer.

Accurate ongoing assessment is imperative for efficient and effective pain control.

Methods of pain management

Using the WHO analgesic ladder
The analgesic ladder was designed as a framework for the management of cancer pain (see Figure 3.3). There are several drugs available to manage cancer pain and the analgesic ladder allows the flexibility to choose from the range according to the patient's requirements and tolerance (Hanks et al. 2004). For acute pain management, the WHO ladder can be used as a guide in reverse, starting at step 3 for immediate post-operative pain and moving down through step 2 and then step 1 as post-operative pain improves.

Step 1: non-opioid drugs
Examples of non-opioid drugs include paracetamol, aspirin and NSAIDs that are effective for mild-to-moderate pain. These drugs are especially effective for musculoskeletal and visceral pain (Twycross et al. 2014).

Step 2: opioids for mild-to-moderate pain
Examples of opioids for mild-to-moderate pain include codeine, dihydrocodeine, tramadol and low-dose oxycodone (steps 2 and 3). These drugs are used when adequate pain management is not achieved with non-opioids and are usually used in combination formulations. It is not recommended to administer another analgesic from the same group if the drug being used is not controlling the pain. Uncontrolled pain needs to be assessed and managed with the titration of an opioid by moving up the ladder. The exception to this would be if the patient was experiencing intolerable side-effects on the weak opioid and an alternative drug might be beneficial.

Step 3: opioids for moderate-to-severe pain
Examples of opioids for moderate-to-severe pain include morphine, oxycodone, fentanyl, diamorphine, methadone, buprenorphine, hydromorphone and alfentanil.

Methods of drug delivery

Oral analgesia
The oral route is invariably the chosen method of drug delivery. This is based mainly on the ease of use for the patient. This

obviously is dependent on the patient being able to tolerate oral medications and absorb them. This route can be limited by a number of factors, mainly nausea and/or vomiting.

Subcutaneous analgesia

Opioids are often given subcutaneously to manage chronic cancer pain. This is usually influenced by the patient's ability to take medication by the oral route and if there are issues such as bowel obstruction that may impact on drug absorption. Consent from the patient for this method of delivery is key in achieving concordance with drug administration.

Intramuscular analgesia

Until the early 1990s, regular 3–4-hourly intramuscular injections of opioids such as pethidine and morphine were routinely used for the management of post-operative pain. Because alternative techniques such as patient-controlled analgesia (PCA) and epidural analgesia are now available, intramuscular analgesia is used less frequently. Some useful algorithms have been developed to give guidance on titrating intramuscular analgesia (Harmer and Davies 1998, Macintyre and Schug 2015. Absorption via this route may be impaired in conditions of poor perfusion (e.g. in hypovolaemia, shock, hypothermia or immobility). This may lead to inadequate early analgesia (the drug cannot be absorbed properly and reach the systemic circulation and so forms a drug depot) and late absorption of the drug depot (where the drug has remained in the muscular tissue and is absorbed only once perfusion is restored) (Macintyre et al. 2010).

Transdermal analgesia

Transdermal analgesia is a simple method of giving analgesia. It is convenient, and often very acceptable to patients, particularly those who dislike tablets or have many to take. A number of patch formulations have been developed to allow the delivery of drugs across the skin (such as fentanyl, buprenorphine or local anaesthetics). Disadvantages of giving strong opioids such as fentanyl by this route include inflexibility (the patient usually has to be on a stable dose of an opioid and it takes a long time for a dose increase to take effect) and breakthrough doses must be given by another route (oral, buccal or sublingual).

Buccal or sublingual analgesia

Buccal means that the analgesia is placed between the upper lip and the lining of the upper gum. A sublingual drug is placed under the tongue. Drugs given by this route pass directly into the systemic circulation and bypass first-pass metabolism. Their speed of onset is often rapid (Stannard and Booth 2004).

Intranasal administration

Intranasal administration is a non-invasive method of drug delivery because drugs can be absorbed into the systemic circulation through the nasal mucosa. It is suggested that it offers advantages such as ease of administration, rapid onset of action and avoidance of first-pass metabolism, which consequently offers for example an alternative to subcutaneous, oral transmucosal, oral or rectal administration in the management of pain with opioids. Fentanyl-containing formulations have been approved and marketed for the treatment of breakthrough cancer pain (Grassin-Delyle et al. 2012).

Pre-procedural considerations

Pharmacological support

Non-opioid analgesics

Paracetamol and paracetamol combinations

The use of non-opioid analgesics such as paracetamol or paracetamol combined with a weak opioid such as codeine is recommended for managing pain following minor surgical procedures or when the pain following major surgery begins to subside (McQuay et al. 1997). It is also used in cancer patients with pain related to the cancer itself, procedure or treatment-related pain. Paracetamol can also be given rectally if the oral route is contraindicated. An intravenous preparation of paracetamol is now available and can provide effective analgesia after surgical procedures (Romsing et al. 2002). It is more effective and of faster onset than the same dose given enterally. The use of the intravenous form should be limited to patients in whom the enteral route cannot be used. With regard to dosing schedules for parenteral administration of paracetamol, the dose should be reduced for those who weigh 50 kg or under. For example, patients who weigh 33–50 kg should not exceed a maximum daily dose of 60 mg/kg, not exceeding 3 g. For patients over 50 kg with an additional risk factor for hepatotoxicity, the maximum daily dose should be 3 g in 24 hours, and for those patients over 50 kg with no risk factor then the maximum daily dose can be up to 4 g (Bristol-Myers Squibb 2012).

Paracetamol taken in the correct dose of not more than 4 g per day is relatively free of side-effects. When used in combination with codeine preparations, the most frequent side-effect is constipation.

Non-steroidal anti-inflammatory drugs

Non-steroidal anti-inflammatory drugs (NSAIDs) have been shown to provide better pain relief than paracetamol combinations for acute pain (McQuay et al. 1997). These drugs can be used alone or in combination with both opioid and non-opioid analgesics. Two commonly used NSAIDs are diclofenac, which can be administered by the oral, parenteral, enteral or rectal route, and ibuprofen, which is available only as an oral or enteral preparation. The disadvantage of both of these is that often side-effects such as coagulation problems, renal impairment and gastrointestinal disturbances limit their use. Newer COX-2-specific NSAIDs have the advantage that they have similar analgesic and anti-inflammatory effects (Reicin et al. 2001) but have no effect on platelets or the gastric mucosa (Rowbotham 2000). As a result, coagulation problems and gastrointestinal irritation are likely to be significantly reduced. However, several of these drugs have been withdrawn from the market due to long-term cardiovascular side-effects and it will take time for newer products with an improved safety profile to re-establish themselves in practice (Macintyre et al. 2010).

A meta-analysis has suggested that there is little evidence to suggest that any of these drugs are safe in cardiovascular terms. Compared with placebo, rofecoxib was associated with the highest risk of myocardial infarction and ibuprofen with the highest risk of stroke followed by diclofenac. Diclofenac and lumiracoxib were associated with the highest risk of cardiovascular death. Naproxen is viewed as being least harmful for cardiovascular safety but this advantage should be weighed against gastrointestinal toxicity (Trelle et al. 2011). The decision to prescribe an NSAID should be based on an assessment of a person's individual risk factors, including any history of cardiovascular and gastrointestinal illness (NICE 2015). Naproxen (1000 mg a day or less) and low-dose ibuprofen (1200 mg a day or less) are considered to have the most favourable thrombotic cardiovascular safety profiles of all NSAIDs. The lowest effective dose should be used for the shortest duration necessary to control symptoms. A person's need for symptomatic relief and response to treatment should be re-evaluated periodically.

Opioids for mild-to-moderate pain

Tramadol

In studies, tramadol has been recognized as being efficacious in the management of chronic cancer pain of moderate severity (Davis et al. 2005).

It is uncertain whether tramadol is more effective than other opioids for mild-to-moderate neuropathic pain; one report suggests a reduction in allodynia (pain from stimuli which are not normally painful) (Sindrup and Jensen 1999, Twycross and Wilcock 2001). It is uncertain whether tramadol is more effective in neuropathic pain than other opioids for mild to moderate pain (Dühmke et al. 2004). Tramadol has been associated with seizures, notably when the total daily dose exceeds 400 mg or when tramadol has been prescribed alongside other medications that may lower the seizure threshold, for example tricyclic antidepressants and selective serotonin reuptake inhibitors (SSRIs) (Twycross et al. 2014). It is available in immediate- and modified-release preparations. A warning about tramadol from the US Food and Drug Administration (FDA) suggested an increased risk of suicide in those patients who were emotionally unstable and in particular those already taking anti-depressants and tranquillizers.

Codeine phosphate
Codeine is metabolized by the hepatic cytochrome CYP2D6 to morphine. Approximately 7% of Caucasians and 1–3% of the Asian population are poor CYP2D6 metabolizers and therefore do not experience effective analgesia with codeine.

Codeine is available in tablet and syrup formulations. Doses of 30–60 mg po qds are generally prescribed to a maximum of 240 mg/24 h. It is also available in combination preparations with a non-opioid. The combination preparations are available in varying strengths of codeine and paracetamol, including co-codamol 8 mg/500 mg, 15 mg/500 mg and 30 mg/500 mg.

Morphine
A large amount of information and research is available concerning morphine and therefore it tends to be the first-line opioid (of choice). It is available in oral, rectal, parenteral and intraspinal preparations.

All strong opioids require careful titration from an expert practitioner. Where possible, modified-release preparations should be used at regular intervals in the management of persistent pain (British Pain Society [BPS] 2010). For patients who are requiring in excess of 120–180 mg of morphine or equivalent, advice from a pain specialist should be sought. Patients should be informed of potential side-effects such as constipation, nausea and increased sleepiness, in order to allay any fear. The patient should also be told that nausea and drowsiness are transitory and normally improve within 48 hours, but that constipation can be an ongoing problem and it is recommended that a laxative should be prescribed when the opioid is started.

Patients often have many concerns about commencing strong drugs such as morphine. Fears frequently centre around addiction and abuse (Cherny et al. 2003). Time should be taken to reassure patients and their families and verbal and written information provided (NICE 2016).

Although morphine is still considered to be the opioid drug of choice for moderate-to-severe pain (Hanks et al. 2004), alternative opioids allow the practitioner to carefully assess the patient on an individual basis and select the most appropriate one to use. From a palliative care perspective, guidance available from NICE supports safe prescribing of opioids (NICE 2016).

Durogesic (fentanyl)
Fentanyl is a strong opioid, available in a patch, which is recommended in patients who have stable pain requirements. Transdermal patches are available in doses of 12, 25, 50, 75 or 100 μg per hour. It is reported to have an improved side-effect profile in comparison to morphine in relation to constipation (Urban et al. 2010), although some patients experience nausea and mild drowsiness. Use of the patch has increased because it frees the patient from taking tablets.

Changing of the patch is recommended every 3 days but in some circumstances patients may require a dosing interval of 2 days (Urban et al. 2010). The patch should be applied to skin that is free from excess hair and any form of irritation and should not be applied to irradiated areas. It is advisable to change the loca-

Table 3.2 Recommended conversion rate guide from oral morphine to 72-hour fentanyl patch

Morphine dose in 24 hours (mg)	Fentanyl TTS (μg/h)
30	12
60	25
120	50
180	75
240	100

TTS, transdermal therapeutic system.

tion on the body to avoid an adverse skin reaction. Occasionally difficulties arise relating to the titration of the patch as each patch is equivalent to a range of morphine (Table 3.2).

Methadone
Methadone is a synthetic opioid developed more than 40 years ago (Riley 2006). It is available in oral, rectal and parenteral preparations. There has been some reluctance amongst professionals to use methadone, which arose from the difficulties experienced in titrating the drug due to its long half-life (15 hours) that caused accumulation to occur, especially in the elderly (Gannon 1997). There are different methods of achieving effective titration (Gannon 1997); for example, one regimen is to calculate one-tenth of the total daily dose of morphine (maximum starting dose must not exceed 30 mg). Administer the methadone to the patient on an as-required basis but not within 3 hours of the last fixed dose. The total dose required over a 24-hour period is calculated after 5–6 days, divided and given as a two or three times daily regimen and this avoids the build-up of methadone within the body (Morley and Makin 1998). Titration is recommended in a hospital setting to ensure accurate administration. This can be difficult for patients because they have to experience pain before they are administered a dose of methadone in the titration period.

Methadone can be a cheap, effective alternative to morphine if titration is supervised by the specialist pain or palliative care team (Gardner-Nix 1996).

It is particularly useful in patients with renal failure. Morphine is excreted via the kidneys and, if renal failure occurs, this may lead to the patient experiencing severe drowsiness as a result of accumulation of morphine metabolites (Gannon 1997). Methadone is lipid soluble and is metabolized mainly in the liver. About half of the drug and its metabolites are excreted by the intestines and half by the kidneys. Methadone should be used with the advice of a pain/palliative care specialist.

Oxycodone
Oxycodone is available as an immediate- or modified-release preparation and titration should occur in the same way as morphine. Oxycodone is a useful alternative to morphine (Riley 2006). It has similar properties and can be administered orally, rectally and parenterally. Oxycodone has similar side-effects and is usually given 4–6 hourly. It has an analgesic potency 1.5–2.0 times higher than morphine. It has similar side-effects to morphine, although oxycodone has been found to cause less nausea (Heiskanen and Kalso 1997) and significantly less itchiness (Mucci-LoRusso et al. 1998).

A study by Riley (2012) identified that on a population level there is no difference between morphine and oxycodone in terms of analgesia efficacy and tolerability.

Targinact
This drug is a combination of modified-release oxycodone and naloxone. The aim of this combination is to prevent the potential negative effects of opioids on bowel function. It is suggested that

approximately 97% of the naloxone is eliminated by first-pass metabolism (the drug is absorbed into the gastrointestinal tract through the portal vein into the liver which means only a proportion of the drug reaches the circulation) in the healthy liver, preventing it from significantly affecting analgesic effects (Vondrackova et al. 2008).

Tapentadol
Tapentadol is a centrally acting opioid analgesic supported by evidence for the management of acute and severe chronic pain (Schwartz et al. 2011, Wild et al. 2010). It is available in oral preparations in immediate- and modified-release forms. The conversion factor for tapentadol from oral morphine is 2.5:1. Therefore 10 mg oral morphine is equivalent to 25 mg of tapentadol. Side-effects associated with tapentadol are similar to other opioids, including dizziness, headaches, somnolence, nausea and constipation.

Diamorphine
Diamorphine is used parenterally in a syringe pump for the control of moderate-to-severe pain when patients are unable to take the oral form of morphine. It is calculated by dividing the total daily dose of oral morphine by three. Breakthrough doses are calculated by dividing the 24-hour dose of diamorphine by six and administering on an as-required basis (Fallon et al. 2010).

Buprenorphine
Buprenorphine is an alternative strong opioid available in patch form. The patch has similar advantages to fentanyl but does not contain a reservoir of the drug. Instead, it is contained in a matrix form with effective levels of the drug being reached within 24 hours. Titration is recommended with an alternative opioid initially and then transfer to the patch when stable requirements have been reached. A lower dose patch (Butrans) is available in strengths of 5, 10 and 20 μg/h that should be worn continuously by the patient for 7 days. The higher dose patch (Transtec) of 35, 52.5 and 70 μg/h is licensed to be used up to 96 hours or twice weekly for patient convenience. Conversion is based on the chart supplied by the pharmaceutical company which demonstrates equivalent doses. Buprenorphine is also available as a sublingual tablet, which is titrated from 200 to 800 μg 6 hourly. Conversion is based on multiplying the total daily dose of buprenorphine by 100 to give the total daily dose of morphine (i.e. 200 μg buprenorphine/8-hourly = 600 μg buprenorphine/24 hours = 60 mg morphine/24 hours) (Budd 2002).

Transmucosal opioids such as fentanyl citrate (Actiq), Abstral, Effentora and intranasal preparations such as PecFent are licensed to be used for the treatment of cancer breakthrough pain. There are some circumstances when these agents are used off licence but they should always be used under the guidance of a specialist.

Oral transmucosal fentanyl citrate (Actiq)
Licensed for the management of breakthrough pain in patients who are already on an established maintenance dose of opioid for cancer pain, oral transmucosal fentanyl citrate (OTFC) is a lozenge which is rubbed against the oral mucosa on the side of the cheek, leading to the lozenge being dissolved by the saliva. The advantage of OTFC is its fast onset via the buccal mucosa (5–15 minutes) and its short duration (up to 2 hours). It is available in a range of doses (200–1600 μg) but there is no direct relation between the baseline analgesia and the breakthrough dose. Titration can be difficult and lengthy as the recommended starting dose is 200 μg with titration upwards (Portenoy et al. 1999). It is recommended that the lozenge be removed from the mouth if the pain subsides before it has completely dissolved. The lozenge should not be reused but should be dissolved under running hot water.

Fentanyl buccal tablet
Fentanyl buccal tablets are licensed medications for breakthrough pain in adults with cancer who are already receiving a maintenance opioid for chronic cancer. The brand names for these medications are Effentora and Abstral. Patients receiving maintenance opioid therapy are those who are taking at least 60 mg of oral morphine daily, at least 25 μg of transdermal fentanyl per hour, at least 30 mg of oxycodone daily, at least 8 mg of oral hydromorphone daily or an equi-analgesic dose of another opioid for a week or longer.

Effentora buccal tablet is available in 100, 200, 400, 600 and 800 μg. It is placed on the oral mucosa above the third upper molar which leads to the tablet being dissolved by the saliva. It usually takes 15–25 minutes for the tablet to dissolve. It is recommended that if the tablet has not completely dissolved within 30 minutes then the remainder of the tablet should be swallowed with water as it is thought that the tablet will then only be likely to consist of inactive substances rather than active fentanyl (Darwish et al. 2007).

Abstral is an oral transmucosal delivery formulation of fentanyl citrate, indicated for the management of breakthrough pain in patients using opioid therapy for chronic cancer pain (Rauch et al. 2009). The tablet is administered sublingually and it rapidly disintegrates, ensuring the fentanyl dissolves quickly. Abstral is available in six dosing strengths: 100, 200, 300, 400, 600 and 800 μg fentanyl citrate.

Adjuvant drugs (co-analgesics)
Most chronic pain contains elements of neuropathic pain. Patients with nociceptive pain are likely to gain some benefit from conventional medications such as NSAIDs but these drugs come with a strong side-effect profile. Individuals with neuropathic pain are likely to gain some relief from co-analgesics such as tricyclic antidepressants (e.g. amitriptyline and nortriptyline) and anticonvulsant drugs (e.g. gabapentin and pregabalin) (Mackintosh and Elson 2008).

The WHO analgesic ladder recommends the use of these drugs in combination with non-opioids, opioids for mild-to-moderate pain and opioids for moderate-to-severe pain (see Figure 3.3).

Cannabis
Studies are currently examining the potential benefits of using cannabis for the management of chronic conditions, for example multiple sclerosis and cancer. There is some evidence for relief of spasticity and neuropathic pain and for improvement in sleep (Lynch and Campbell 2011). For those patients who may present wishing to use medications such as cannabis oil, local policies should be consulted.

Education of patient

Opioids and driving
In the UK, patients who are prescribed opioids are permitted to drive. The BPS has suggested that under certain circumstances patients who are taking opioids should not drive. These circumstances include:

- The condition for which they are being treated has physical consequences that might impair their driving ability.
- They feel unfit to drive.
- They have just started opioid treatment.
- The dose of opioid has been recently adjusted upwards or downwards (as withdrawal of opioids can also have an impact on driving).
- They have consumed alcohol or drugs that can produce an additive effect.

The Driving and Vehicle Licensing Agency (DVLA) is the only legal body that can advise a patient about their right to hold a driving licence. Patients starting opioids should be advised to inform the DVLA that they are now taking opioids, and prescribers should document that this advice has been given (BPS 2010). More recent guidance has been published for professionals to guide practice and support patients (Department of Transport 2014).

Complications

The use of opioids in renal failure

Renal failure can cause significant and dangerous side-effects due to the accumulation of the drug. A systematic review in patients with cancer pain has concluded that fentanyl, alfentanil and methadone, with caveats, are the medications likely to cause least harm in patients with renal impairment when used appropriately (King et al. 2011). Basic guidelines for pain management in renal failure include the following:

- Reduce analgesia dose and/or dose frequency (6-hourly instead of 4-hourly).
- Select a more appropriate drug (not renally excreted).
- Avoid modified-release preparations.
- Seek advice from a specialist pain/palliative care team and/or pharmacist (Farrell and Rich 2000).

The use of opioids in liver failure

As the liver is the main site for the metabolism of most drugs, hepatic impairment may lead to changes in the pharmacokinetics which can include:

- accumulation of the drug or its metabolites
- prolonged half-life
- increased bioavailability.

The severity will depend on the degree of damage to the liver (Twycross et al. 2014). The recommendation would be to avoid hepatotoxic drugs or use with care and specialist support.

Management of breakthrough cancer pain (BTCP)

The management of cancer-related breakthrough pain involves several modalities of care. These include lifestyle changes, non-pharmacology interventions, pharmacology, optimizing round the clock medication, rescue medication and where necessary interventional techniques (EONS 2013). Rapid-onset opioids have been developed specifically for the treatment of BTCP. Fentanyl has been the opioid of choice for the development of BTCP medications that use the oral transmucosal and intranasal routes of administration. Transmucosal administration of lipophilic substances has gained popularity in recent years due to the rapid, clinically observable effect occurring 10–15 minutes after drug administration. The oral and nasal mucosae are easily accessible and convenient sites for drug delivery because they allow for a non-invasive, less threatening approach to patients than other routes of administration, such as intravenous or intramuscular (Zepettella 2011). There are many rapid-onset fentanyl products for the treatment of BTCP on the market, each with diverse features. The most commonly used are listed in Box 3.1. Further information can be sourced from Breakthrough Cancer Pain Guidelines (EONS 2013).

Management of chemotherapy-induced peripheral neuropathy (CIPN)

There is little evidence to support the use of pharmacological agents in the treatment of CIPN (BPS 2010). Given the lack of

Box 3.1 Examples of rapid-onset fentanyl preparations

- Oral transmucosal fentanyl citrate
- Fentanyl buccal tablet
- Fentanyl sublingual tablet
- Fentanyl buccal soluble film
- Intranasal fentanyl spray
- Fentanyl pectin nasal spray

pharmacological treatments available to patients, non-pharmacological treatments should also be considered in a multimodal treatment plan (Taverner 2015).

Pharmacology

NICE (2017) neuropathic pain guidelines suggest first-line treatment with amitriptyline, duloxetine, gabapentin or pregabalin. However this is specific not to CIPN but to all neuropathic pain. Chu et al. (2014) performed a systematic review into the use of drugs affecting the central nervous system and found limited evidence to support the use of these drugs in the management of CIPN.

One randomized controlled trial (RCT) found that the use of duloxetine had a positive impact in reducing pain score and improving quality of life when compared with a placebo (Ellen et al. 2013). Use of oxycodone has also been shown to have benefits in a small trial of patients undergoing treatment with oxaliplatin. Patients receiving oxycodone were more likely to complete the full course of treatment compared with those who were not (Nagashima et al. 2014).

Rao et al. (2007) performed a double-blind RCT into the effectiveness of gabapentin versus placebo effect. Given the use of gabapentin in management of other neuropathic pains, its role in treating CIPN could have a positive outcome for patients. Rao et al. (2007) found that pain scores improved by 20–30% over the course of the 6-week trial regardless of the treatment method. They found there was no difference between the placebo and gabapentin group.

Topical treatments

Topical treatments are also used to treat CIPN, often off licence. Capsaicin 0.025% cream, capsaicin 8% patches and lidocaine plasters/patches have all been shown to have benefit in other neuropathic pain states although there is minimal evidence for their use in CIPN, and menthol cream has some demonstrated efficacy in CIPN (Farquhar-Smith and Brown 2016).

The use of topical capsaicin has shown some benefit in two separate Cochrane reviews (Derry et al. 2009, 2013) into the reduction of pain related to CIPN and is also recommended by NICE (2017). Capsaicin is derived from chilli peppers and has action in the depletion and prevention of substance P in the peripheries. Substance P is responsible for the transmission of pain impulses from peripheries to the CNS (Tofthagen et al. 2013). The most common side-effect from application is local erythema and skin irritation, however long-term side-effects are as yet unknown (Dworkin et al. 2010).

The use of topical lidocaine can be very beneficial in reducing pain as a result of CIPN (Fallon 2013). This works by using a localized anaesthetic effect to prevent the conduction of normal nerve impulses in the chosen area of application. The patches are applied for 12-hour periods (Tofthagen et al. 2013). These patches can have a cooling and soothing effect on the area which can be very beneficial to patients reporting classic neuropathic symptoms of burning pain. The most common side-effect from this treatment is local skin irritation (Dworkin et al. 2010).

Proudfoot et al. (2006) found that activation of TRPM8 found in the sensory nerve through cooling resulted in analgesic effect in neuropathic and chronic pain pathways. The method by which they achieved this cooling effect was with topical menthol cream.

Fallon et al. (2015) trialled the use of 1% menthol cream on 51 patients complaining of CIPN over a course of 4–6 weeks and found 82% showed a marked reduction in pain scores when assessed with brief pain inventory. They also showed improved fine motor skills and improvements in walking ability and mood.

Non-pharmacological

Taverner (2015) recommends the use of occupational therapy and psychological support in order to empower patients to manage their pain via alternative methods. The use of occupational and physical therapies can improve overall function and fine motor skills that can be affected as a result of CIPN symptoms (Brewer et al. 2016).

Wong and Sagar (2006) reported in a case review of five patients a decrease in pain scores and increase in quality of life following a course of acupuncture. Schroeder et al. (2012) showed that patients receiving acupuncture treatment for CIPN had a reduction in pain scores and increase in nerve conduction studies. The mechanism of action for acupuncture is thought to be a release of nerve growth factor (NGF), gamma-aminobutyric acid (GABA) and adenosine (Filshie et al. 2016).

Non-pharmacological methods of managing pain

Optimal pain control is more likely to be achieved by combining non-pharmacological with pharmacological techniques. Despite the lack of research evidence to support the effectiveness of many non-pharmacological techniques, their benefits to patients and families should not be underestimated.

Psychological interventions

Psychological interventions can help patients to cope with pain by reducing stress and muscle tension (Chapman 2012). Encouraging activities such as reading, listening to music and, where possible, interacting with family and friends can all improve the patient's perception of the pain.

A number of simple psychological interventions can improve a patient's pain control by:

- reducing anxiety, stress and muscle tension
- distraction (distraction plays a role in pain management by pushing awareness of pain out of central cognition)
- increasing control and pain-coping mechanisms
- improving general well-being.

Some simple interventions include the following:

Creating trusting therapeutic relationships

By creating trusting relationships with patients, nurses are instrumental in reducing anxiety and helping patients to cope with pain. Nurses may underestimate the benefits and comfort they bring by staying with a patient who is experiencing pain (Mann and Carr 2006). Nurses can help to create a trusting relationship by:

- listening to the patient
- believing the patient's pain experience
- acting as a patient advocate
- providing patients with appropriate physical and emotional support.

Information/education

Patient information/education can make all the difference between effective and ineffective pain relief. Information/education helps to reduce anxiety (Chapman 2012) and enables patients to make informed decisions about their care. Patients should be given specific information about why pain control is important, what to expect in terms of pain relief, how they can participate in their management and what to do if pain is not controlled. Some caution is required, however, because not all patients respond positively to the same level of information. Patients with high levels of anxiety may find that detailed information can increase their anxiety and influence their pain control. NICE guidance on the safe prescribing of opioids suggests that all patients who start on opioids should be offered written information to support them (NICE 2016).

Relaxation/guided imagery

This can be used to help patients manage pain and anxiety. It helps by engaging the patient in a more pleasant activity and provides distraction from the pain or may change the perception of a painful experience such as venepuncture/cannulation (Chapman 2012). Relaxation techniques are further discussed in the section on 'Cancer-related fatigue (CRF) and sleep' in Chapter 8.

Music

The use of music in the healthcare setting can also provide relaxation and distraction from pain (Heiser et al. 1997). Setting up a library of music (e.g. easy listening, classical) and having personal listening devices available for patient use is a simple way to provide patients with relaxing music. Vaajoki et al. (2012) reported significantly lower pain intensity and pain distress in bedrest on the second post-operative day in a music group compared with a control group after elective abdominal surgery.

Art

A literature review highlighted that art therapy could be used to alleviate physical symptoms in some patients. Therapeutic art-making was shown to be beneficial in improving the quality of life for patients. Art therapy allows patients emotional safety and assists them to resolve the personal struggles that contribute to their pain (Angheluta and Lee 2011).

Physical interventions

In addition to psychological interventions, a number of physical interventions can be helpful in reducing pain.

Comfort measures

Simple comfort measures such as positioning pillows and bed-linen (e.g. to support a painful limb) (Mann and Carr 2006) can help the patient feel more relaxed and improve patient comfort and pain control. Other comfort measures include ensuring that interruptions and noise are minimized to promote rest and ensuring the ambient temperature is comfortable.

Exercise

Physiotherapy and occupational therapy can help to reduce pain and to improve function and quality of life for patients (BPS 2010). A variety of measures can be used for this including therapeutic exercise, pacing of daily activity and lifestyle adjustment (BPS 2010).

Transcutaneous electrical nerve stimulation

Transcutaneous electrical nerve stimulation (TENS) (Figure 3.4) is thought to work by sending a weak electrical current through the skin to stimulate the sensory nerve endings. Depending on the stimulation parameters used, TENS is thought to modulate pain impulses by closing the gate to pain transmission within the spinal cord by stimulating the release of natural pain-relieving chemicals in the brain and spinal cord (King 1999).

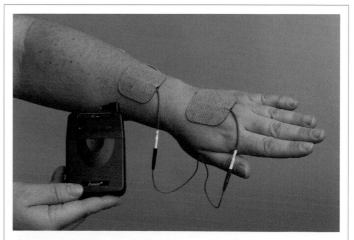

Figure 3.4 TENS machine. *Source:* Dougherty and Lister (2015).

Evidence for the use of TENS is variable. Johnson and Martinson (2007) reported significant decreases in pain at rest and on movement in a meta-analysis of 38 studies on TENS and peripheral nerve stimulation for chronic musculoskeletal pain. The evidence for TENS for post-operative pain is often negative, but this may be due to how the studies are conducted.

Heat therapies

For decades, superficial heat therapy has been used to relieve a variety of muscular and joint pains, including arthritis, back pain and period pain. There is much anecdotal and some scientific evidence to support the usefulness of heat as an adjunct to other pain treatments (French et al. 2006).

Heat works by:

- stimulating thermoreceptors in the skin and deeper tissues, thereby reducing the sensitivity to pain by closing the gating system in the spinal cord
- reducing muscle spasm
- reducing the viscosity of synovial fluid which alleviates painful stiffness during movement and increases joint range (Carr and Mann 2000).

In the home environment, people use a variety of different methods for applying heat therapies, such as warm baths, hot water bottles, wheat-based heat packs and electrical heating pads. In the hospital setting, caution is required with this equipment as it does not reach health and safety standards (no even and regular temperature distribution) and there have been incidences of serious burns (Barillo et al. 2000). Carr and Mann (2000) note that heat therapy should not be used immediately following tissue damage as it will increase swelling. The Medicines and Healthcare products Regulatory Agency (MHRA 2005) has documented evidence of burns caused by using heat patches or packs and therefore urges caution in their use and also recommends regular checking of skin throughout therapy.

Cold therapies

Cold therapies can also be used to stimulate nerves and modulate pain (Carr and Mann 2000). Cold may be particularly valuable following an acute bruising injury where it can help to reduce inflammation and limit further damage. Cold can be applied in the form of crushed ice or gel-filled cold packs which should be wrapped in a towel to protect the skin from an ice burn.

Acupuncture

Background and definition

Acupuncture is a therapeutic technique that involves the insertion of fine needles into the skin and underlying tissues at specific points for therapeutic or preventive purposes (White et al. 2008). The use of acupuncture has been growing in popularity and it is now commonly used alongside conventional treatments for pain and symptom control in the cancer and palliative care setting (Filshie and Thompson 2009). Leng (2013) carried out a survey into the use of acupuncture in the hospice and palliative care setting across the UK and found that 59% of centres were actively using acupuncture for symptom control.

The management of pain and nausea has improved significantly with the use of conventional medical treatments. However, there is a lack of management for other common symptoms of fatigue, anxiety and depression. As cancer patients will normally present with numerous symptoms it is ideal to address as many of these symptoms at once to ensure a positive outcome for the patient. Sagar and Capsulet (2005) discussed that the use of complementary therapies to manage the wide spectrum of cancer patients' symptoms can be beneficial. Lim et al. (2011) compared the use of acupuncture with supportive care from a specialist nurse in managing patients' symptoms. Out of the 42 patients surveyed they found a reduction in symptoms of 22% following acupuncture treatment compared with 14% following support care appointment. Hu et al. (2015) performed a systematic review of 20 articles and found that acupuncture in combination with conventional analgesic treatment results in longer episodes of no pain, increased response time in pain relief, increase in length of analgesic duration, improved quality of life and reduction of analgesic side-effects due to decrease in use.

Anatomy and physiology

Acupuncture has been used in China for over 2000 years; the history of Western medical acupuncture started in the 1970s when a medically qualified doctor took a rational, scientific approach to exploring acupuncture and its benefits (White et al. 2008). We still do not know exactly how acupuncture works but due to numerous scientific studies there is evidence to show that acupuncture works on the nervous system and the muscles.

Five mechanisms have been identified and these can overlap (White et al. 2008).

Local effects

The acupuncture needles activate action potentials in nerve fibres in the skin and muscle. Various substances are released as a result and this causes an increase in local blood flow. This can often be seen as a red mark around the acupuncture needle during treatment. The local effect can also cause an increase in the blood supply in the deeper tissue that can aid wound healing. It can also be used near an underactive salivary gland in the treatment of xerostomia (White et al. 2008) which can be a common side-effect following radiotherapy.

Segmental effects

The action potentials activated by the local effects continue to travel up the nerve to the spinal cord and reduce the painful stimuli by reducing activity at the dorsal horn. This is the main mechanism by which acupuncture relieves pain.

Extrasegmental effects

This is a response in which the effect of acupuncture is not restricted to a single area. The action potentials continue to the brainstem; this then affects every segment of the spinal cord (White et al. 2008). This allows for the treatment of multiple symptoms, which is extremely useful for cancer patients as they often report a variety of different symptoms (Sagar and Capsulet 2005).

Central effects

Acupuncture affects other structures in the brain such as the hypothalamus and limbic system. In these areas acupuncture can have a regulatory effect; this can be used to treat nausea, hormone imbalances and drug addiction. These effects have been shown on MRI scans. This can be very effective in managing hot flushes following hormone treatment; it has been shown to reduce incidence of hot flushes by 50% (Hervik and Mjaland 2009).

Myofascial trigger point effect

People can experience pain due to 'tight bands' or 'pressure/trigger points' in their muscles. Acupuncture is effective in treating this pain; the needles are inserted directly into the painful area and often the patient experiences instant pain relief. It is thought that acupuncture was originally developed for this type of pain. There is limited evidence on the incidence of myofascial trigger points in cancer patients, however careful examination and palpation of the site of pain should be performed to identify the possibility (Hasuo et al. 2016).

Evidence-based approaches

Acupuncture is now being used widely in the management of multiple symptoms in the cancer and supportive care setting. It has been shown to improve quality of life of patients through the improvement of one or multiple symptoms related to their cancer or treatment (Dean-Clower et al. 2010). Towler et al. (2013) looked at 17 systematic reviews into the effectiveness of acupuncture for symptom management in cancer patients. They found benefit was shown in the management of multiple symptoms and recommended its use in the control of symptoms when other treatments have failed.

Indications

Filshie et al. (2016) list the following indications for the use of acupuncture in symptom management:

- pain acute and chronic (e.g. persistent pain following breast surgery)
- radiotherapy complications/side-effects
- chemotherapy-induced peripheral neuropathy
- joint pains secondary to aromatase inhibitors
- breathlessness
- nausea and vomiting
- hot flushes
- xerostomia
- anxiety
- fatigue.

Figure 3.5, Figure 3.6 and Figure 3.7 show some common acupuncture points used in practice.

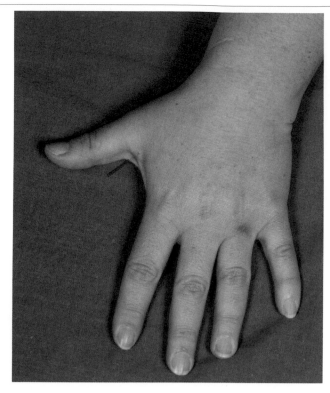

Figure 3.6 A point used for pain relief. *Source:* Dougherty and Lister (2015).

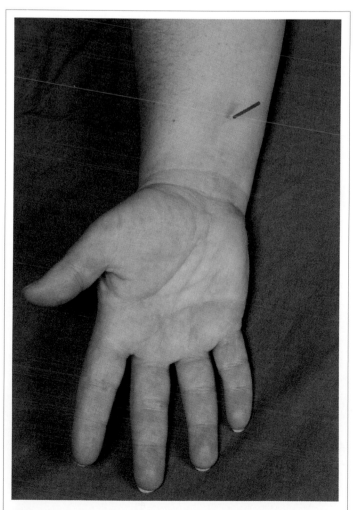

Figure 3.5 A point used for acupuncture. *Source:* Dougherty and Lister (2015).

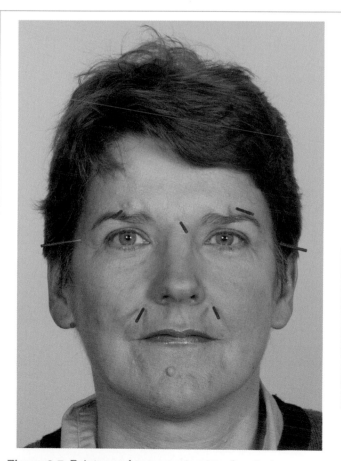

Figure 3.7 Points used to treat migraines/headaches. *Source:* Dougherty and Lister (2015).

Date at first presentation	Ref.	Age	Sex	Diagnosis or presenting complaint (PC)	Duration of PC (months)	No. of Rx	Response

(BMAS 2013)

Figure 3.8 Acupuncture treatment record chart. *Source:* Adapted from BMAS (2013).

Contraindications

Acupuncture is contraindicated in patients who:

- refuse, e.g. in cases of extreme needle phobia
- have pain originating from an unknown cause
- are unable to give informed consent or co-operate with treatment
- have severe clotting dysfunction or who bruise spontaneously.

In addition needling should be avoided:

- directly onto a tumour nodule or into an area of ulceration
- in lymphoedematous limbs or limbs prone to lymphoedema
- in the ipsilateral arm in patients who have undergone axillary dissection (risk of development of swelling and lymphoedema after insertion of any needle)
- in areas of spinal instability due to potential risk of cord compression (due to acupuncture's muscle-relaxing properties)
- into a prosthesis (could cause leakage of saline/silicone)
- over intracranial deficits following neurosurgery.

Caution should be taken with:

- patients who are underweight (not to needle too deeply over the chest wall)
- patients who are confused
- patients who are agitated
- patients with a metal allergy
- patients receiving anticoagulation therapy
- patients who are immunocompromised
- patients with peripheral vascular disease
- patients with bloodborne infections, e.g. HIV
- patients who are pregnant
- patients who are prone to keloid scar formation
- all cancer patients as they may be very sensitive to acupuncture, so close supervision is advised, especially during the first treatment.

Legal and professional issues

All acupuncture practitioners must have completed a recognized, validated, formal training course within their scope of professional practice (for example, the Foundation Course in Acupuncture provided by the British Medical Acupuncture Society [BMAS]). Any nurse who practises acupuncture should check with their union to ensure they have appropriate indemnity cover.

Pre-procedural considerations

Equipment

Acupuncture needles consist of a shaft and a handle. The handle is made of either plastic or metal. The needles are single use, disposable and covered by a safety guide tube.

There are different dimensions of needles available:

- 0.25 or 0.30 mm diameter needles are standard
- 25 or 40 mm length needles are standard.

Assessment and recording tools

Record the patient's treatment in the hospital notes/hospital computer system (e.g. condition, acupuncture points used, outcome) (Figure 3.8).

Patient preparation

Patients should be treated in a comfortable well-supported position on a couch, either lying down or sitting, with the facility to lie down quickly in case they feel faint during or after the procedure. A healthcare professional should remain with the patient throughout their first treatment as their reaction to acupuncture is unknown.

Consent

All patients must sign a consent form to agree to treatment. An example of a consent form to use can be found on the BMAS website (www.medical-acupuncture.co.uk).

Procedure guideline 3.1   Acupuncture: preparation and administration

Essential equipment
- Hand-washing facilities
- Couch and pillows to support the patient
- Cotton wool swabs
- Sharps bin
- Tray to hold needles
- Needles
- Facilities for record keeping

Procedure

Action	Rationale
1 Take a full medical history from the patient.	To ensure acupuncture is not contraindicated and to ascertain which treatment points need to be used.
2 Explain the procedure to the patient and give the patient an information sheet.	
3 Take patient's consent.	Patient needs to agree to treatment (NMC 2015).
4 Ask the patient to lie down.	To reduce the risk of the patient fainting (White et al. 2008, **E**).
5 Wash hands.	To minimize the risk of infection (Preston 2005, **C**).
6 Give treatment.	
7 Count the needles used (use the empty introducers on the tray as a reminder).	To ensure no needles are lost/miscounted (White et al. 2008, **E**).
8 Leave needles *in situ* for 20 minutes; remove if the patient cannot tolerate them. Stay with the patient throughout.	To ensure safe treatment.
9 Remove the needles and count them as they are removed. Dispose of needles in a designated sharps container.	To ensure no needles are lost/miscounted (White et al. 2008, **E**). To minimize risk of infection and needlestick injury.
10 Ensure the patient feels OK; let the patient rest on the couch if they feel dizzy, etc.	To reduce the risk of the patient fainting (White et al. 2008, **E**).
11 Document needling points used on patient record.	To ensure that the treatment can be replicated/adjusted at the next appointment according to response (White et al. 2008, **E**).

Post-procedural considerations

If patients are having treatment in an outpatient setting, they can travel home immediately after treatment. If the patient feels dizzy/faint, they should rest and drink fluids until the feeling passes.

Complications

Acupuncture, when performed by a competent practitioner, is a very safe treatment. Macpherson et al. (2001) found that in a study of 34,407 treatments there were 43 reports of mild adverse effects as a result of acupuncture and no serious event occurred. Complications can be categorized into three groups: mild, significant and serious (White et al. 2008).

Mild events
- Bleeding (more than a small drop) 3%.
- Exacerbation of symptoms 1–2%.
- Pain on insertion of needle 1%.
- Drowsiness 1%.
- Fainting less than 0.5%.

Significant events

These events are extremely rare and can include skin infections at insertion sites, peripheral nerve injury, exacerbation of asthma and seizures (commonly occur when the patient is treated sitting upright and then faints).

Serious events
- Pneumothorax: 54 cases reported caused by a practitioner with poor anatomical knowledge (Park et al. 2010).
- Cardiac tamponade: 9 cases reported.
- Damage to blood vessels, i.e. pseudoaneurysm: 10 reported cases.
- Brain/spinal cord injury: 12 reported cases.
- Infection: HIV (4 reported cases), hepatitis B (148 reported cases) caused by reuse of needles.

Interventional techniques for managing complex cancer-related pain

Effective management of pain can be achieved in approximately 90% of patients using pharmacological analgesia such as opioids, non-opioids and adjuvants (Jain 2014). However, for some patients, despite thorough assessment and treatment, it is difficult to attain and maintain adequate pain control and these patients may benefit from interventional techniques (FONS 2013).

Examples of complex pain where interventional techniques may be considered include (Bennett 2014, Peat and Hester 2012):

- nerve plexus invasion (brachial plexopathy or lumbosacral plexopathy)
- visceral upper abdominal pain (liver, pancreas or stomach cancers)
- fractures (rib, pelvic, spinal or limb fractures)
- chest wall pain (infiltration of chest wall and mesothelioma)
- rectal pain (tumour or persistent following surgery)
- perioperative management of patients dependent on high-dose opioids
- opioid toxicity preventing titration of analgesia.

Effective control can be achieved by a variety of different types of blocks which can reduce intractable cancer pain caused by tumour invasion of soft tissues, nerves or organs. The interventions aim to interrupt the neural pathways of pain transmission. They can be given as:

- single nerve blocks and injections (such as trigger point and joint injections)
- regional peripheral and plexus blocks that target individual nerves, plexuses or ganglia (such as intercostal blocks, lumbar plexus blocks)
- neuraxial (spinal) blocks (such as epidural and intrathecal).

These interventions can be useful but careful consideration and assessment must take place to ensure that any potential side-effects are discussed with the patient (interventional techniques may severely limit the patient's activities) and that future planning is addressed with the patient and family as some interventions may limit discharge options for the patient who is dying.

Simpson (2011) describes the following general principles to follow when considering a nerve block:

- Pain must be carefully assessed and investigated.
- Careful explanation and informed consent.
- Patients and carers must be given time to consider interventions.
- Those involved in the patient's care must understand the procedure, what it can achieve, aftercare, and beneficial and adverse effects.
- Nerve blocks must not cause functional defects.
- Neuro-destructive procedures must be selective of sensory or autonomic nerves and leave motor paths and sphincters intact.
- Nerve blocks should not be regarded as a treatment in isolation but must form part of a strategy for analgesia.
- Nerve blocks must not be left as a last resort when the patient may be too ill to tolerate the technique or to come to a hospital for complex procedures.

Single nerve blocks and injections

Single peripheral nerve blocks and injections such as trigger point and joint injections can provide excellent symptomatic relief. They can be used when pain occurs in the field of one or more peripheral nerves (Ripamonti et al. 2012). Examples include intercostal nerve blocks for pathological rib fractures and trigger point injections in areas of severe muscle spasm or spasticity. These are performed as 'single shot' injections and can be repeated every 3–6 months. They are usually combined with other pain treatments as it is rare that these techniques alone will provide sufficient pain relief.

Regional peripheral and plexus nerve blocks and infusions

Definition

The term 'regional anaesthesia' refers to the loss of sensation in a region of the body produced by application of an anaesthetic agent to all the nerves supplying that region. Regional analgesia includes peripheral nerve blocks to the arm, leg or head.

Regional analgesia can be used for patients with cancer-related pain when the oral route is failing or cannot be escalated further due to severe side-effects. It can either be a single injection ('single shot') or a continuous infusion such as a continuous peripheral nerve block (CPNB). CPNB can also be delivered as an ambulatory service where patients are discharged home with the infusion.

Anatomy and physiology and related theory

Regional analgesia blocks transmission of pain impulses through a nerve or a nerve plexus by depositing an analgesic drug (usually local anaesthetic with or without an opioid) close to the nerve, cutting off sensory innervation to the region it supplies. Pain impulses are inhibited but some sensation of touch and muscle functions are intact. Regional analgesia gives relief of pain on movement.

Specific regional analgesia nerve blocks

Specific types of regional analgesia nerve blocks can be used for different types of cancer pain. Table 3.3 lists examples of different regional nerve blocks and the procedures they can be used for.

Table 3.3 Examples of regional analgesia blocks

Type of block	Remarks
Brachial plexus block	The brachial plexus is the major nerve bundle going to the shoulder and arm. This block can be used to manage intractable cancer pain from tumours invading the brachial plexus such as those involving the breast and chest wall
Coeliac plexus block	For severe pain due to pancreatic cancers. This is a neurolytic block using an injection of alcohol or phenol into the coeliac plexus – this destroys the neural pathways that cause pain. It can be performed by two approaches: percutaneous and endoscopic
Hypogastric plexus block	For visceral pain from advanced cervical, bladder, rectal and prostate cancer
Saddle block	For uncontrolled pain of the perineum, scrotum, penis or anus

Evidence-based approaches

Rationale

Regional analgesia approaches can be used for several reasons. The ability to provide selective analgesia with minimal adverse effects can be beneficial, particularly in older patients who may have co-existing conditions (Macintyre and Schug 2015, Parizkova and George 2009a, b). By using a nerve block or a continuous infusion of local anaesthetic, pain relief can be superior to the use of opioids alone, and the use of opioids can be minimized in the post-operative setting, resulting in fewer adverse effects such as nausea, vomiting, sedation and pruritus (D'Arcy 2011, Le Wendling and Enneking 2008, Richman et al. 2006). Pain relief and functionality may also be improved.

Contraindications for regional analgesia nerve blocks

There are few contraindications for the use of regional nerve blocks but consideration must be given to the risk of bleeding and infection, particularly if the patient is on anticoagulant therapy. The risk of haematoma and developing an infection should be carefully explained along with any other risks associated with the procedure. In patients with cancer these techniques may be more technically challenging due to the loss of traditional 'landmarks' to guide correct placement of the needle or catheter. These landmarks can be difficult to find due to oedema (palpation of pulses and bony prominences can be difficult or impossible) and neuro-anatomy can be distorted by tumour or scarring near the nerves to be blocked (Peat et al. 2012).

Classes of drugs used in regional analgesia and mechanism of action

In peripheral nerve blocks the most common drug used is a local anaesthetic.

Commonly used local anaesthetic agents include bupivacaine, levobupivacaine and ropivacaine. Local anaesthetics bind directly within the intracellular portion of voltage-gated sodium channels. The degree of block produced by local anaesthetics is dependent upon how the nerve has been stimulated and on its resting membrane potential. Local anaesthetics are only able to bind to sodium channels in their charged form and when the sodium channels are open. They will cause numbness and loss of sensation and there may also be some loss of muscle function depending on the purpose of the block.

The dose of a local anaesthetic agent will also determine which nerves are blocked. Low concentrations of bupivacaine (e.g. 0.100–0.125%) preferentially block nerve impulses in the smallest diameter nerve fibres, which include the pain and temperature sensory fibres. As the larger diameter motor fibres are less likely to be blocked with concentrations of 0.100–0.125% bupivacaine, the incidence of motor weakness is reduced and the patient is able to mobilize.

In certain blocks a steroid may be combined with the local anaesthetic to reduce inflammation and pain; an example of a steroid used is methylprednisolone.

Legal and professional issues
There should be formal induction courses and regular updates for doctors, nurses, theatre and recovery staff who will be responsible for supervising patients receiving CPNBs.

Staff competency
Nursing competencies for the nurse who monitors the patient with a CPNB should include knowledge of:

- anatomy and physiology of the spinal cord and column and neurological system
- purpose of the regional nerve block for pain management
- untoward reactions to medication and management of complications.

Nursing care responsibilities include:

- observation
- any necessary procedures (e.g. reinforcing dressing)
- documentation of care.

Pre-procedural considerations
Prior to a CPNB procedure the following areas need to be considered:

- Does the patient have capacity to make an informed choice?
- Can the patient physically sustain a suitable position while the intervention is performed?
- Does the patient have an uncorrectable coagulopathy?
- Are there any considerations for aftercare?

Post-procedural considerations

Immediate and ongoing care

Monitoring the patient
When caring for a patient receiving regional analgesia, it is important to monitor the patient for the following:

- drug-related side-effects
- pain intensity
- signs of complications due to the regional analgesia procedure.

Complications
Complications can:

- be drug related
- arise from the insertion of the needle or catheter
- arise from the indwelling catheter.

Neuraxial (spinal) blocks: epidural and intrathecal analgesia

Definition
The term 'spinal analgesia' refers to both the epidural and intrathecal route (Day 2001, Sloan 2004). The spinal cord rests in a medium of cerebrospinal fluid (CSF), which is contained by the protective membrane of the dura mater. Analgesics applied outside the dura mater are termed 'epidural analgesia', and medications given into the CSF are termed 'intrathecal analgesia' (Sloan 2004).

Anatomy and physiology
The spinal cord (Figure 3.9 and Figure 3.10) is covered by the meninges; the *pia mater* is closely applied to the cord and the *arachnoid mater* lies closely with the outer, tough covering of the *dura mater* (Behar et al. 2007). The epidural space lies outside all three membranes, encasing the spinal cord between the spinal dura and ligamentum flavum. The contents of the epidural space include a rich venous plexus, spinal arterioles, lymphatics and extradural fat.

The intrathecal space (also termed the subarachnoid space) lies between the arachnoid mater and pia mater and contains the CSF (Chapman and Day 2001).

There are 31 pairs of spinal nerves of varying size which pass out through the intervertebral foramina between each vertebra (Chapman and Day 2001). There are two main groups of nerve fibres.

- *Myelinated:* myelin is a thin, fatty sheath that protects and insulates the nerve fibres and prevents impulses from being transmitted to adjacent fibres.
- *Unmyelinated:* delicate fibres, more susceptible to hypoxia and toxins than myelinated fibres.

The spinal nerves are composed of a posterior and anterior root, which join to form the nerve.

- *Posterior root:* transmits ascending sensory impulses from the periphery to the spinal cord.
- *Anterior root:* transmits descending motor impulses from the spinal cord to the periphery by means of its corresponding spinal nerve (Chapman and Day 2001, Day 2001, Gelinas and Arbour 2014).

Specific skin surface areas are supplied/innervated by each of the spinal nerves. These skin areas are known as dermatomes (Figure 3.11).

Evidence-based approaches
Epidural analgesia is the administration of analgesics (local anaesthetics and opioids with or without adjuvants such as corticosteroids and clonidine) into the epidural space via an indwelling catheter (Macintyre et al. 2010). This technique enables analgesics to be injected close to the spinal cord and spinal nerves where they exert a powerful analgesic effect. It is one of the most effective techniques available for the management of acute pain (Macintyre and Schug 2015, Wheatley et al. 2001).

Intrathecal (spinal) analgesia is the administration of analgesic drugs directly into the CSF in the intrathecal space (Gelinas and Arbour 2014). The intrathecal space is also referred to as the subarachnoid space. Analgesic drugs given via this route are 10 times as potent as those given into the epidural space so doses given are much smaller.

Spinal blocks are forms of anaesthesia that temporarily interrupt sensation from the chest, abdomen and legs by injection of local anaesthetic medication into the vertebral canal, which contains the spinal cord, spinal nerves and CSF. They are typically given as a single injection which will last for 2–6 hours depending on the type and volume of local anaesthetic given. If an opioid is given, such as morphine, this can produce analgesia lasting 12 hours (Macintyre et al. 2010).

In chronic pain, this method (intrathecal drug delivery – ITDD) can be utilized for the delivery of continuous infusions of analgesia in patients with:

- chronic non-cancer pain unresponsive to other analgesics or when analgesia leads to intolerable side-effects

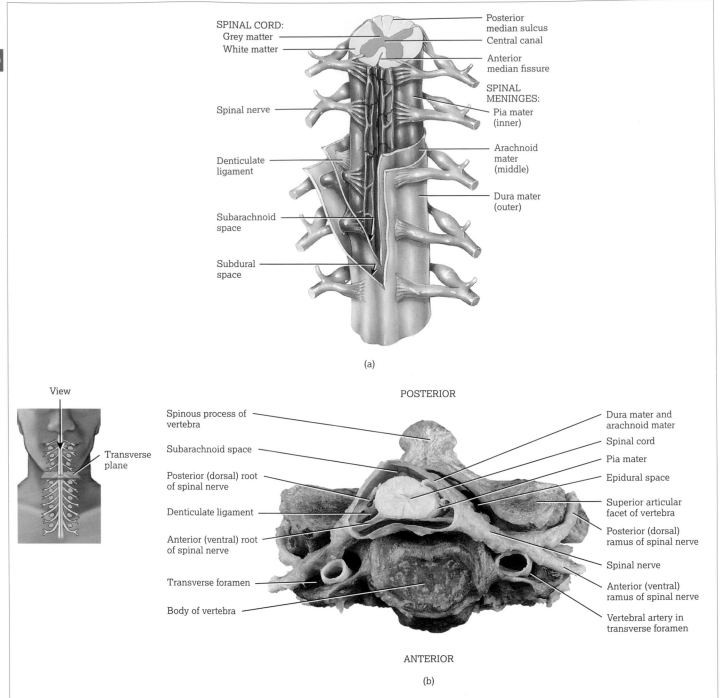

Figure 3.9 Gross anatomy of the spinal cord. (a) Posterior view and transverse section through spinal cord. (b) Transverse section of the spinal cord within a cervical vertebra. *Source:* Tortora and Derrickson (2011). Reproduced with permission from John Wiley & Sons.

- cancer pain that is uncontrolled with appropriate systemic opioids or when analgesia leads to intolerable side-effects
- spasticity.

Several different types of drug delivery systems are available.

- Percutaneous catheters (tunnelled or not) used with an external pump, which are easy to place and may be appropriate if the patient has limited life expectancy.

- Fully implantable ITDD systems with an injection port to enable top-up of the analgesic medication, and a programmable function to allow for adjustments in dose and rate settings from an external device.

Local anaesthetics, opioids and other drugs such as clonidine can be given via this route.

The use of drugs via either the epidural or the intrathecal route can cause both a loss of sensation (anaesthesia) and a loss of pain (analgesia).

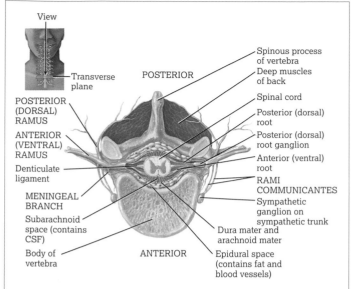

Figure 3.10 Branches of a typical spinal nerve, shown in cross-section through the thoracic portion of the spinal cord: transverse section. *Source:* Tortora and Derrickson (2011). Reproduced with permission from John Wiley & Sons.

Rationale

There are two main advantages to using epidural or intrathecal analgesia.

- It has the potential to provide effective dynamic pain relief for many patients (D'Arcy 2011).
- The combination of local anaesthetic agents with opioids has a synergistic action that allows the concentration of each drug to be reduced. This limits the unwanted side-effects of each drug (Hurley et al. 2010).

Indications
- Provision of post-operative analgesia in patients undergoing palliative surgery for cancer. Epidural analgesia has been used since the late 1940s as a method of controlling post-operative pain (Chapman and Day 2001).
- Provision of analgesia for pain resulting from cancer invasion of local structures such as pathological fractures.
- Management of intractable pain in patients with cancer who experience the following:
  - unacceptable side-effects with systemic opioids
  - unsuccessful treatment with opioids via other routes despite escalating doses
  - severe neuropathic pain due to tumour invasion or compression of nerves (Day 2001, Mercadante 1999, Smitt et al. 1998).
- To relieve muscle spasm and pain resulting from lumbar cord pressure due to disc protrusion or local oedema and inflammation.

For cancer patients who do not obtain pain relief from treatment with opioids administered orally, rectally, by injection or continuous infusion, there is evidence that both epidural and intrathecal analgesia can be effective (Ballantyne and Carwood 2005). Intrathecal analgesia can either be delivered via an external infusion pump or can be part of a fully implantable reservoir system (Dickson 2004).

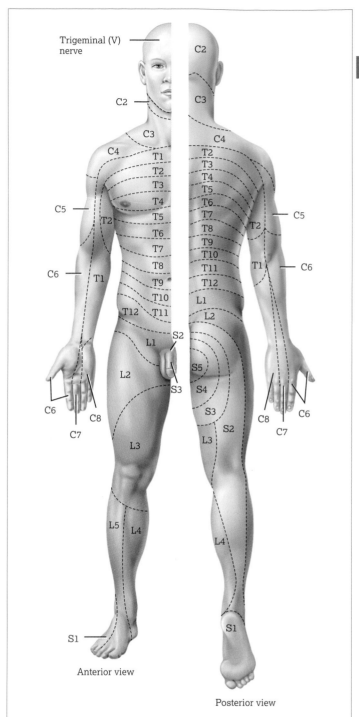

Figure 3.11 Distribution of dermatomes. *Source:* Tortora and Derrickson (2011). Reproduced with permission from John Wiley & Sons.

Contraindications
These may be absolute or relative.

Absolute
- Patients with coagulation defects, which may result in haematoma formation and spinal cord compression, for example iatrogenic (anticoagulated patient) or congenital (haemophiliacs), or thrombocytopenia due to disease or as the result of anticancer treatment (Horlocker et al. 2010).

- Local sepsis at the site of proposed epidural or intrathecal injection; the result might be meningitis or epidural abscess formation.
- Proven allergy to the intended drug.
- Unstable spinal fracture.
- Patient refusal to consent to the procedure.

Relative
- Unstable cardiovascular system.
- Spinal deformity.
- Raised intracranial pressure (risk of herniation if a dural tap occurs).
- Certain neurological conditions, for example multiple sclerosis, where an epidural may result in an exacerbation of the disease (Hall 2000).
- Unavailability of staff trained in the management of epidural or intrathecal analgesia (Macintyre and Schug 2015). Hall (2000) notes that staff managing patients with epidural or intrathecal analgesia should have undertaken a period of formal training to care for patients safely and competently.

Methods of administration

Continuous infusion
Continuous infusions of intrathecal analgesic drugs have been shown to be effective in the management of chronic intractable cancer pain (Ballantyne and Carwood 2005).

Continuous infusions can be given by either a syringe pump or a designated infusion pump system. The effectiveness of this method of administering drugs is dependent on a number of factors including the combination of drugs used, the position of the catheter at a level appropriate to the site of pain (Weetman and Allison 2006) and the volume of the local anaesthetic agent infused (Chapman and Day 2001, Hall 2000).

Patient-controlled epidural analgesia
The use of patient-controlled epidural analgesia (PCEA) has gained popularity in recent years because it enables patients to control their analgesia. For patients with persistent pain, PCEA is used more effectively in combination with a low-dose background infusion (Wheatley et al. 2001). This ensures a baseline level of analgesia that can then be supplemented by the patient when required.

Bolus injections
Bolus injections of local anaesthetic agents and/or opioids are used infrequently but can be given to top up and re-establish analgesia if pain is uncontrolled. This procedure is usually performed by the doctor or bolus doses of low-dose concentrations may be given by nursing staff as part of an advanced practice role, according to local policy. This should follow an agreed period of education and supervised practice, which must be documented.

This is a clean aseptic procedure. Most epidural/intrathecal infusion pumps allow a bolus dose to be programmed and delivered from the pump. This prevents the administration line and bacterial filter being accessed and thus minimizes the risk of introducing infection. Intrathecal bolus doses are usually only given by the doctor.

Classes of epidural and intrathecal drugs and mechanism of action
Three classes of drugs are commonly used to provide epidural or intrathecal analgesia: opioids, local anaesthetic agents and adjuvant drugs such as corticosteroids and clonidine.

Opioids
A number of different opioids have been used for epidural and intrathecal analgesia; two of the most commonly used are diamorphine and fentanyl (Bannon et al. 2001, Cook et al. 1997, Romer and Russell 1998). When either of these opioids is injected into the *epidural* space, part of the opioid dose:

- crosses the dura and arachnoid membrane and enters the CSF. From the CSF, a proportion of the drug is taken up into the spinal cord and reaches the opioid receptors in the spinal cord. Once bound to the opioid receptors, this results in blocking of pain impulses
- enters the systemic circulation and contributes to analgesia
- binds to the epidural fat and does not contribute to analgesia.

When opioids are placed directly into the CSF in the intrathecal space, they attach directly to the opioid spinal cord receptor sites (Urdan et al. 2006).

Fentanyl differs from diamorphine in that it is more lipid soluble. This means that it passes more easily into the CSF, gaining faster access to the opioid receptors and having a more rapid onset of action. Fentanyl also has a shorter duration of action (1–4 hours) compared with diamorphine (6–12 hours) (Macintyre and Schug 2015).

Local anaesthetic drugs
Commonly used local anaesthetic agents include bupivacaine, levobupivacaine and ropivacaine. They inhibit pain transmission by blocking sodium ion channels that are involved in the propagation of electrical impulses along the spinal nerves. In epidural analgesia, these drugs gain access to the nerve roots and the spinal cord by crossing the dura and subarachnoid membranes (Macintyre and Schug 2015).

The dose of a local anaesthetic agent will also determine which nerves are blocked. Low concentrations of bupivacaine (e.g. 0.100–0.125%) preferentially block nerve impulses in the smallest diameter nerve fibres, which include the pain and temperature sensory fibres. As the larger diameter motor fibres are less likely to be blocked with concentrations of 0.100–0.125% bupivacaine, the incidence of leg weakness is reduced and the patient is able to mobilize.

Adjuvant drugs

Corticosteroids
Corticosteroid 'single shot' injections are often used to relieve back pain caused by degenerative disc disease and radicular pain from inflammatory irritation of nerve roots from a 'trapped nerve' or a disc prolapse (Farquhar-Smith 2012).

Clonidine
Adrenergic alpha-2 receptors are found in the spinal cord and are thought to be activated by descending inhibitory pathways and release of endogenous agonists. Clonidine is a mixed adrenergic alpha-2 agonist and is thought to be active at the spinal level (Farquhar-Smith 2012).

Legal and professional issues
There should be formal induction courses and regular updates for doctors, nurses, theatre and recovery staff who will be responsible for supervising patients receiving continuous epidural analgesia (Royal College of Anaesthetists 2010). The acute pain service or a clearly designated consultant anaesthetist from the anaesthesia department will be responsible for the immediate supervision of patients receiving local anaesthetic infusions. The National Patient Safety Agency (NPSA 2007) recommends that in addition to routine training and regular updates, additional training occurs when changes are made to protocols, medicine products or medical devices. Routine training should include a programme to help healthcare staff gain competence and confidence in using infusion devices employed to deliver epidural/intrathecal analgesia, a theoretical understanding of how the drugs work, and the monitoring required to detect both drug- and procedure-related side-effects and complications (Table 3.4).

There have been reported fatal cases where epidural medicines have been administered by the intravenous route and intravenous

Table 3.4 Example of competency role development profile for epidural analgesia for pain. Intended learning outcomes and elements of practitioner competency

Knowledge and understanding	Skills

You are expected to possess knowledge and understanding of the following.
 • The normal anatomy of the spinal cord.
 • The physiology of pain and measures of pain management.
 • Education and information needs of the patient/family/carer with regard to the implications of having an epidural, to ensure valid consent is given.
 • Contraindications for epidural analgesia.
 • Infection control considerations before, during and after insertion of an epidural.
 • Principles of epidural care and management including side-effects and complications of epidural insertion and epidural analgesia.
 • Observations required during the administration of epidural analgesia and the rationale for the frequency of:
   – respiratory rate/sedation levels
   – cardiovascular status
   – temperature
   – epidural site
   – dermatomal blockade
   – pain assessment.
 • The standard prescription for epidural analgesia for acute pain management.
 • Deviations from the standard prescription available and situations in which they may be used.
 • Pharmacology of epidurally administered local anaesthetics and opioids and their side-effects.
 • The optimum infusion rate.
 • When to stop and remove an epidural catheter.
 • Implications of anticoagulant therapy prior to removing the epidural catheter.
 • Considerations for analgesia once epidural analgesia is stopped.
	You are expected to possess the following skills.
	 • Ability to care for the patient before, during and immediately after epidural insertion.
	 • Ability to check the epidural site; frequency of checks and what problems to look for.
	 • How to redress the epidural site and frequency of epidural site dressing changes.
	 • How to assess pain and the frequency of assessment.
	 • How to carry out a dermatomal blockade assessment and where to document it.
	 • Ability to change epidural infusion rate.
	 • Ability to change epidural infusion bag and awareness of the frequency of infusion bag changes.
	 • Ability to change and prime the infusion administration set and awareness of the frequency of change.
	 • Ability to deal with equipment problems:
	   – proximal occlusion alarm
	   – distal occlusion alarm
	   – cassette not fitted
	   – low battery.
	 • Ability to deal with administration problems:
	   – catheter disconnection from bacterial filter
	   – catheter occlusion
	   – catheter leakage
	   – the patient still has pain
	   – side-effects of analgesia
	   – complications of epidural catheter insertion.
	 • Procedure for removing an epidural catheter.
	 • Safe disposal of unused epidural infusion bags after discontinuing therapy.

medicines have been administered by the spinal route. In response to this, the NPSA (2009) issued a Patient Safety Alert recommending that all epidural, spinal (intrathecal) and regional anaesthesia infusions and bolus doses should be given with devices with connectors that *will not* also connect with intravenous equipment – so-called 'safer connectors'. Non-Luer connectors for devices used for epidural, spinal (intrathecal) procedures and regional blocks have now been introduced to avoid the accidental, but potentially fatal, connection of an intravenous infusion or injection. The new international standard (ISO 80369 2010) for these connectors is now available and includes a dedicated connector for these devices known as NRFit™ (ISO 80369-6 2016) that is not compatible with Luer connectors.

Pre-procedural considerations

Equipment
Epidural or intrathecal catheters are inserted using:

- a Tuohy needle (a bevelled curved-tip needle to reduce the risk of accidental dural puncture, with 1 cm length markings, either 16 G or 18 G)
- an epidural/intrathecal catheter (a relatively stiff catheter made of polyamide, length 1000 mm with clear blue markings completely embedded in the catheter material)
- a bacterial filter (filters provide an additional degree of safety and control to prevent bacterial infections. Minimal dead space enables accurate dosing. A high-pressure resistance up to 7 bar enhances safety during manual injection)
- connector (to ensure safe catheter fixation)
- loss of resistance device (to aid clear identification of the epidural space).

The equipment often comes in prepared sterile disposable epidural trays or packs (Parizkova and George 2009a, b).

Dressings
The dressing over the epidural/intrathecal exit site needs to fulfil the following three functions:

- to help secure the epidural/intrathecal catheter
- to minimize the risk of infection
- to allow observation of the site without disturbing the dressing.

A transparent moisture-responsive occlusive dressing fulfils these functions. The dressing needs to be waterproof, adhesive and breathable, so that it allows exchange of oxygen and moisture while protecting the skin from outside contamination. The epidural/intrathecal site should be inspected daily and the dressing changed at least once weekly or more frequently if there is any serous discharge from the site (see Procedure guideline 3.3: Epidural/intrathecal exit site dressing change).

Pharmacological support

Combination of drugs used
Epidural or intrathecal infusions of local anaesthetic and opioid combinations are commonly used in the UK (Baker et al. 2004, Wheatley et al. 2001). The rationale behind their combined use is based on the observation that better analgesia is achieved with lower doses of each drug, therefore minimizing drug-related side-effects produced by higher concentrations (Curatolo et al. 1998, Fotiadis et al. 2004). Although the solutions used will vary with the clinical situation, combinations of fentanyl and a local anaesthetic such as levobupivacaine are often used. The use of

premixed bags is recommended to minimize medication errors involving the epidural/intrathecal route (NPSA 2007).

Specific patient preparation

Patients undergoing epidural/intrathecal analgesia should always have a venous access device *in situ* before the procedure. This is because, although rare, a reaction to the opioid or local anaesthetic solution (e.g. respiratory depression or sympathetic blockade) may require immediate access to the venous system. The procedure should be performed in a clinical area with access to full resuscitation equipment.

Patient information and consent prior to using epidural/intrathecal analgesia for intractable chronic or cancer pain

The following issues should be addressed with the patient, family and primary healthcare team prior to using epidural/intrathecal analgesia for intractable chronic or cancer pain.

- *Drug-related side-effects.* The concentration of analgesics needed to provide sufficient analgesia for patients with chronic cancer pain is often higher than the concentrations used postoperatively. As a result, drug-related side-effects such as motor weakness and urinary retention can occur. Some patients find these side-effects unacceptable and may prefer to avoid epidural/intrathecal analgesia altogether. Therefore, a discussion must take place with the patient and family to ensure that they are aware of these potential side-effects and are willing to continue with epidural/intrathecal analgesia (Wallace 2002).

- *Increased time in hospital.* The patient should also be informed that they will need to spend a period of time in hospital following insertion of the catheter, to allow for dose adjustment and ensure that side-effects are minimized and optimum pain management achieved.

Position of epidural or intrathecal catheter

Local anaesthetic drugs block nerve fibres at spinal segments adjacent to their site of administration. To ensure the local anaesthetic agent spreads to the dermatomes or nerves supplying the area of pain (e.g. the surgical site or the pain location caused by a tumour), the tip of the spinal catheter should be placed within the mid-dermatomal distribution of the pain site (Table 3.5). This achieves optimal analgesia using the least amount of drugs. If the catheter is placed below the dermatomes supplying the pain site then analgesia is likely to be inadequate (Macintyre and Schug 2015).

Table 3.5 Optimal catheter location for different anatomical sites

Anatomical site	Catheter location
Thoracic	T6–T9
Upper abdominal	T7–T10
Lower abdominal	T9–L1
Hip/knee	L1–L4

Procedure guideline 3.2 Epidural/intrathecal sensory blockade: assessment

Essential equipment
- Ice or single-use proprietary cold pack. These can be discarded after each test to reduce cross-infection risk.
- Ethanol spray
- Copy of a dermatome distribution figure or chart (see Figure 3.11)

Pre-procedure

Action	Rationale
1 Explain and discuss the procedure with the patient. Obtain informed verbal consent from the patient.	To ensure that the patient understands the procedure and gives their valid consent and to ensure the patient has time to assess information and ask questions (NMC 2015, **C**).

Procedure

Action	Rationale
2 Ensure patient's privacy and dignity are maintained throughout the procedure by use of curtains or screens.	To maintain privacy and dignity.
3 Explain to the patient that they need to report: • if the temperature of the ice/cold changes or becomes warmer • if they cannot feel the ice/cold sensation at all.	This will indicate the dermatome level at which the epidural/intrathecal analgesia is working.
4 Remove any clothing that may restrict the assessment.	The ice or spray needs to be applied directly to the skin to undertake the assessment. **E**
5 Test the ice/cold pack or spray on an area of the body that should not be affected by the epidural/intrathecal infusion (the face or the back of the hand).	To ensure the patient can feel the cold sensation. **P**
6 Starting at the top of the chest (just above nipple level), place the ice/cold pack/spray above the incision or level of pain and ask the patient if this feels as cold as when placed on the test area. Continue this procedure down the torso and the legs if appropriate for the level of epidural/intrathecal analgesia and on the right and left of the body.	To check sensory block level and assess effectiveness and safety of epidural block.
7 Replace patient's clothing.	To maintain privacy and dignity.

Post-procedure

Action	Rationale
8 Document at what level the patient can detect a change as per the dermatome chart (see Figure 3.11).	To maintain accurate patient record.

Procedure guideline 3.3   Epidural/intrathecal exit site dressing change

Essential equipment

- Sterile dressing pack including gloves
- Disposable apron
- Bactericidal handrub
- Skin-cleaning agent, for example chlorhexidine in 70% alcohol
- Transparent occlusive dressing

Pre-procedure

Action	Rationale
1 Explain and discuss the procedure with the patient.	To ensure that the patient understands the procedure and gives their valid consent (NMC 2015, **C**).
2 Wash hands with soap and water. Clean the trolley or other appropriate surface according to local policy.	To minimize cross-infection (Preston 2005, **C**). To provide a clean working surface (Parker 2004, **E**).
3 Position the patient comfortably on their side or sitting forward so that the site is easily accessible without undue exposure of the patient.	To maintain the patient's dignity and comfort. This is especially important when carers are attending to an area that is not visible to the patient (Chapman and Day 2001, **E**).
4 Prepare trolley or tray with sterile field and cleaning solution.	To minimize risk of infection and ensure equipment is available (Preston 2005, **C**).

Procedure

5 Remove old dressing and place in disposable bag.	To prevent cross-infection (Loveday et al. 2014, **E**).
6 Wash hands with bactericidal handrub. Put on gloves and personal protective apron.	To minimize the risk of microbial contamination (Fraise and Bradley 2009, **E**).
7 Observe site for any signs of infection such as redness, swelling or purulent discharge. If any of these are present contact the hospital anaesthetic/pain team for advice.	To ensure careful monitoring of site to minimize the chance of any infection (Royal College of Anaesthetists 2010, **C**).
8 Clean site with skin-cleaning agent (chlorhexidine in 70% alcohol).	To minimize the risk of infection (Hebl 2006, **R5**; Kinirons et al. 2001, **R1b**; Mimoz et al. 1999, **R1b**).
9 Apply transparent occlusive dressing over the whole area.	To anchor the epidural/intrathecal catheter, minimize the risk of infection and allow observation of the epidural/intrathecal site (Burns et al. 2001, **R1b**; Royse et al. 2006, **E**).
10 Ensure that the patient is comfortable.	

Post-procedure

11 Remove gloves and apron and dispose of all material in the clinical waste bag.	To prevent environmental contamination (Preston 2005, **C**).
12 Wash hands with soap and water.	To reduce the risk of cross-infection (Preston 2005, **C**).

Procedure guideline 3.4   Epidural/intrathecal catheter removal

Essential equipment

- Sterile dressing pack including gloves
- Skin-cleaning agent, for example chlorhexidine 0.5% in 70% alcohol
- Specimen container (if epidural catheter needs to be sent for bacterial culture)
- Occlusive dressing
- Alcohol handrub

Pre-procedure

Action	Rationale
1 Explain and discuss the procedure with the patient.	To ensure the patient understands the procedure and gives their valid consent (NMC 2015, **C**).
2 Wash hands with bactericidal soap and water or bactericidal alcohol handrub. Clean trolley (or plastic tray in the community) with chlorhexidine in 70% alcohol with a paper towel.	To minimize cross-infection (Preston 2005, **C**). To provide a clean working surface (Parker 2004, **E**).
3 Open dressing pack.	

(continued)

Procedure guideline 3.4   Epidural/intrathecal catheter removal *(continued)*

Procedure

4	Wash hands and remove tape and dressing from catheter insertion site.	To minimize risk of cross-infection (Preston 2005, **C**).
5	Wash hands with bactericidal handrub. Put on gloves and personal protective apron.	To minimize the risk of microbial contamination (Loveday et al. 2014, **E**).
	Gently, in one swift movement, remove the catheter.	To ensure the catheter is removed intact with the minimum of discomfort to the patient. **E**
	Check that the catheter is intact. This can be done by observing that the tip of the catheter is marked blue and that the 1 cm marks along the length of the catheter are all intact.	
6	Clean around the catheter exit site using skin-cleaning agent.	To minimize contamination of site by micro-organisms. **E**
7	Apply an occlusive dressing and leave *in situ* for 24 hours.	To prevent inadvertent access of micro-organisms along the tract. **E**

Post-procedure

8	The epidural/intrathecal tip may be sent for culture and sensitivity if infection is suspected, or according to local policy.	
9	Remove gloves and apron and dispose of all material in the clinical waste bag. Wash hands with soap and water.	To prevent environmental contamination (Preston 2005, **C**).
10	Document that the catheter was removed intact in nursing notes.	To maintain accurate patient record.

Problem-solving table 3.1 Prevention and resolution (Procedure guidelines 3.2, 3.3, 3.4)

Problem	Cause	Prevention	Suggested action
Headache.	Dural puncture.	Expertise of practitioner inserting the epidural.	Bedrest: headache will be less severe if patient lies flat. Replacement fluids either intravenously or orally to encourage formation of CSF. Administer analgesics for headache. If headache does not settle, contact the anaesthetic team who may consider an epidural blood patch to seal the puncture (Gaiser 2006).
Sedation and respiratory depression (opioid toxicity). Circumoral tingling and numbness, twitching, convulsions and apnoea (local anaesthetic toxicity).	If catheter migrates into a blood vessel, signs of opioid or local anaesthetic toxicity can occur.	Expertise of practitioner inserting the epidural. Careful monitoring of the patient to detect early symptoms.	Stop epidural infusion. Contact pain/anaesthetic team or summon emergency assistance. Treat the patient for complications of opioid or local anaesthetic overdose (Chapman and Day 2001).
Apnoea, profound hypotension and unconsciousness.	If an epidural catheter migrates from the epidural space into the intrathecal space to the CSF, the analgesic solution may reach as high as the cranial subarachnoid space. If this occurs the respiratory muscles are paralysed together with the cranial nerves, resulting in apnoea, profound hypotension and unconsciousness. This is because intrathecal doses are calculated as one-tenth of the epidural dose and migration from the epidural space to the intrathecal space leads to a drug overdose.	Expertise of practitioner inserting the epidural. Careful monitoring of the patient to detect early symptoms.	Stop epidural infusion. Summon emergency assistance. Prepare emergency equipment to support respiration and ventilate lungs. Prepare emergency drugs and intravenous fluids and administer as directed. Above actions to be discussed with medical team and to be undertaken if symptoms are thought to be acute and due to epidural/ intrathecal infusion rather than deterioration in condition due to underlying disease.

Problem	Cause	Prevention	Suggested action
Back pain and tenderness and nerve root pain with sensory and motor weakness.	Epidural haematoma.	Assessment of coagulation status before insertion and removal of the epidural/intrathecal catheter.	Urgent neurological assessment. Computed tomography (CT) or magnetic resonance imaging (MRI) scan may be performed to diagnose if there is nerve or spinal cord compression. If a haematoma is diagnosed patient may be referred for urgent surgery (Chapman and Day 2001). To avoid haematoma on removal of epidural in patients treated with prophylactic anticoagulants, see guidelines for timing of removal.
Back pain and tenderness. May have redness and purulent discharge from catheter exit site. May also develop nerve root signs with neuropathic pain and sensory/motor weakness.	Epidural abscess.	Maintain aseptic technique when accessing the epidural/intrathecal analgesic system. Monitor temperature regularly and check insertion site for evidence of infection.	Treat with antibiotics. CT or MRI scan may be performed and patient may be referred for urgent neurosurgery to prevent paraplegia dependent on their current prognosis. Discussion with all of team, patient and family on risks/benefits of stopping and removing epidural/intrathecal catheter. Infection does not always require removal of the catheter (O'Neill 2012).
Headaches, fever, neck stiffness, photophobia.	Meningitis.	Maintain aseptic technique when accessing the epidural/intrathecal analgesic system. Monitor temperature regularly.	Assist anaesthetist/doctor to obtain CSF sample for microbiology analysis. Initiate antibiotic therapy as per hospital policy. Non-pharmacological measures for symptom management, for example dim lights. If the infection does not respond to antibiotics it may be necessary to remove the catheter and convert back to systemic analgesia until meningitis has resolved (Mercadante 1999).
Pain, paraesthesia, numbness in lower extremities that may progress to paresis.	Intrathecal catheter granuloma (an inflammatory mass that forms around the catheter tip).	In long-term therapy intrathecal may be preferable to epidural to minimize the development of a granuloma due to the presence of the CSF.	MRI scan to diagnose the problem. Stop infusion (granulomas may resolve on their own once the infusion is stopped) (Du Pen 2005).

Post-procedural considerations

Immediate care

Volume of infusion
The medication 'spread' within the epidural space is determined by the site of the epidural catheter, the patient's age and the volume of the drug being infused (Rockford and DeRuyter 2009). It is therefore important to maintain the hourly infusion rate at a volume that keeps the appropriate nerves blocked.

Effectiveness of blockade
The spinal nerves supply specific areas of skin known as dermatomes (see Figure 3.11). Sensitivity to changes in temperature (such as the cold of ice) along the sensory dermatome can be used to assess the level of epidural/intrathecal block (see Proce-

dure guideline 3.2: Epidural/intrathecal sensory blockade: assessment). This level should be checked to ensure that the epidural/intrathecal block is providing pain relief by covering the area of the site of pain, but is also necessary to maintain safety during the administration of epidural/intrathecal infusions. If the sensory block is too high (above T4) then there is an increased risk of respiratory and cardiac symptoms as a result of the local anaesthetic effects on nerves at this level, and if it is too dense it will cause unnecessary motor blockade.

Ongoing care
When caring for a patient receiving epidural or intrathecal analgesia, it is important to monitor the patient for the following:

- drug-related side-effects
- pain intensity

- signs of complications due to the procedure (see Problem solving table 3.1)
- equipment-related problems, such as the catheter or the infusion pump (see Problem solving table 3.1).

Drug-related side-effects

There are a number of drug-related side-effects associated with epidural/intrathecal opioids and local anaesthetic agents.

Opioids

- *Respiratory depression.* This is due to the action of opioids on the respiratory centre. Potential respiratory depression may occur at two different time intervals.
  - *Early:* usually within 2 hours of the opioid injection. This may occur if high blood levels of the opioid follow absorption from the epidural space into the systemic circulation (Macintyre and Schug 2015).
  - *Late:* this may not be seen for 6–12 hours after an opioid is given. It results from rostral migration of the drug in the CSF to the brainstem and respiratory centre (Macintyre and Schug 2015). This is less likely to occur with lipid-soluble opioids such as fentanyl.
  - Patients referred for epidural/intrathecal infusions for intractable pain are not opioid naïve and have often been taking adjuvant medications that can include sedation.
- *Sedation.* Although there may be many different causes of sedation, epidural/intrathecal opioids can cause sedation owing to their effect on the CNS. Opioid-induced sedation is often an early warning sign of respiratory depression.
- *Nausea and vomiting.* Nausea and vomiting is caused by the action of opioids on the vomiting centre in the brainstem and stimulation of the chemoreceptor trigger zone in the fourth ventricle of the brain.
- *Pruritus.* Although the exact mechanism is unknown, pruritus is presumed to be centrally mediated via an itch centre

in the medulla and as a consequence of disinhibition of itch neurones in the dorsal horn of the spinal cord (Macintyre and Schug 2015).

- *Urinary retention.* This is due to opioid inhibition of the micturition reflex which is evoked by increases in bladder volume.

Local anaesthetic agents

- *Hypotension.* This can be caused by two mechanisms. First, local anaesthetic agents can spread outside the epidural/intrathecal space, blocking the sympathetic nerves. This results in peripheral vasodilation and hypotension. It is most likely to occur if a bolus dose of local anaesthetic agent (e.g. 10 mL of 0.25% bupivacaine) is given to improve pain control (Macintyre and Schug 2015). Second, if the local anaesthetic agent spreads above the T4 dermatome (nipple line), the cardio-accelerator nerves may become blocked, leading to bradycardia and hypotension (Macintyre and Schug 2015).
- *Motor blockade.* This will depend on the concentration and total dose of local anaesthetic agent used and the position of the epidural/intrathecal catheter (Hall 2000). Motor blockade occurs when the local anaesthetic agent blocks the larger diameter motor nerves. Leg weakness will occur if the motor nerves supplying the legs are blocked.
- *Urinary retention.* As with epidural/intrathecal opioids, blockade of the nerves supplying the bladder sphincter can cause urinary retention.

Routine monitoring of the patient for these side-effects must be carried out to facilitate early management. The patient's pulse, blood pressure, respiratory rate and peripheral tissue oxygenation and temperature should be recorded regularly and then according to local policy and as the patient's condition dictates (O'Neill 2012).

For guidance on managing the side-effects associated with epidural/intrathecal opioids and local anaesthetic agents, see Table 3.6.

Table 3.6 Epidural/intrathecal infusions of local anaesthetic agents and opioids: management of side-effects

Problem	Cause	Suggested action
Respiratory depression	Increasing age Elderly patients are more susceptible to the side-effects of opioids due to age-related alterations in the distribution, metabolism and excretion of drugs	If respiratory rate falls to 8 breaths a minute or below: (a) Stop the epidural/intrathecal infusion (b) Summon emergency assistance (c) Commence oxygen via facemask and encourage the patient to take deep breaths (d) Review current analgesic prescription and consider reducing opioid and local anaesthetic doses before resuming the infusion (Macintyre and Schug 2015)
	Concurrent use of systemic opioids or sedatives Patients receiving opioids by epidural/intrathecal infusion should not be given opioids by any other route unless given in the palliative care setting for breakthrough pain	(a) Stop the epidural/intrathecal infusion (b) Stay with the patient and monitor respiratory rate, sedation score and peripheral tissue oxygenation (using a pulse oximeter) continuously (c) Commence oxygen therapy (d) Consider giving naloxone if prescribed by anaesthetist or patient unrousable and naloxone already prescribed (when utilized for acute pain management) (e) Review analgesia: stop any other opioids prescribed and consider changing parameters of epidural/intrathecal infusion (McCaffery and Pasero 1999)
Sedation: *Mild:* patient drowsy but easy to rouse *Severe:* patient difficult to rouse	See Respiratory depression	(a) If patient has mild sedation, consider reducing the rate of the infusion or the dose of opioid or taking the opioid out of the infusion (b) If patient is difficult to rouse and opioid toxicity/overdose is suspected, follow management for respiratory depression

Problem	Cause	Suggested action
Hypotension	Patients with hypovolaemia Patients with a high thoracic epidural in whom the concentration of local anaesthetic agent and volume of infusion cause blockade of the cardio-accelerator nerves	If blood pressure falls suddenly: (a) Stop the epidural/intrathecal infusion (b) Summon emergency assistance (c) Administer oxygen via facemask or nasal cannula (d) Stay with the patient and monitor blood pressure at 5-minute intervals (e) Ensure intravenous replacement therapy is available and use if prescribed by the anaesthetist (f) Vasoconstrictor agents such as ephedrine or metaraminol may need to be given by the anaesthetic team if hypotension does not respond to an intravenous fluid challenge (Macintyre and Schug 2015)
Motor blockade	More likely to occur when higher concentrations of local anaesthetic agents are given by continuous infusion If a high concentration of a local anaesthetic agent is administered via a low lumbar epidural/intrathecal catheter then the lumbar motor nerves are likely to be blocked, causing leg weakness	Do not attempt to mobilize patient if leg weakness is evident Contact pain or anaesthetic team for advice: reducing the concentration of the local anaesthetic agent or the rate of the epidural/intrathecal infusion may help to resolve this problem (Pasero and McCaffrey 2011)
Nausea and vomiting	Previous episodes of nausea and vomiting with opioids Exacerbated by low blood pressure	Regular administration of antiemetics Treat other causes, for example low blood pressure Consider use of non-pharmacological methods (e.g. stimulation of the P6 acupressure point)
Pruritus (usually more marked over the face, chest and abdomen)	Previous pruritus with opioids	Administer an antihistamine such as chlorphenamine (may be contraindicated in patients who are becoming increasingly sedated) or a small dose of naloxone (administer with caution as this can easily reverse analgesia) If pruritus does not resolve, consider switching to another opioid or removing the opioid from the infusion (Macintyre and Schug 2015)
Urinary retention	More likely to occur if opioids and local anaesthetic agents are infused in combination	Catheterize patient

Assessment of pain for patients with epidural analgesia

Pain should be assessed (at rest and on movement) at the same time that the patient's routine observations are carried out. Simple numerical (e.g. 0–10 where 0 is no pain and 10 is the worst pain imaginable) or verbal rating scales (e.g. none, mild, moderate, severe or very severe) can be used.

When used for intractable cancer pain management, the aim of epidural/intrathecal analgesia is to improve the overall quality of life of the patient. Although it is acceptable to use simple pain assessment rating scales, a more in-depth pain assessment scale may also be used such as the BPI (Tan et al. 2004).

Equipment and prescription safety checks

When a patient is receiving a continuous infusion of epidural/intrathecal analgesia, it is advisable to carry out the safety checks given in Table 3.7 at least once per shift.

Removal of epidural/intrathecal catheter

Before an epidural/intrathecal catheter is removed, it is essential to consider the clotting status of the patient's blood. If the patient is fully anticoagulated, a clotting profile must be performed and advice sought from the anaesthetic/pain management/medical staff as to when the catheter can be safely removed. If the patient is receiving a prophylactic anticoagulant, the following guidelines are recommended (Gogarten et al. 2010, Harrop-Griffiths et al. 2013, Horlocker et al. 2010, Horlocker 2011).

Low-dose low molecular weight heparin

If this is given once daily, the epidural/intrathecal catheter should be removed at least 12 hours after the last injection and several

Table 3.7 Epidural/intrathecal analgesia: safety checklist

Checklist	Rationale
Check the prescription and rate of the epidural/intrathecal infusion	To ensure epidural/intrathecal drugs are being administered correctly
Check the epidural/intrathecal infusion/syringe pump extension set is connected to the epidural catheter and not to any other access device	To ensure drugs are administered via the correct route
Check the bacterial filter is securely attached to the epidural/intrathecal catheter	To prevent accidental disconnection of the catheter from the filter
Check that the dressing over the epidural/intrathecal catheter exit site is secure	To prevent catheter dislodgement and minimize the risk of contamination of the catheter site

hours prior to the next dose. The timing will depend on the manufacturer's recommended guidelines but it is recommended that epidural or intrathecal catheters are removed and the next dose should not be given for minimum of 4 hours after removal.

Unfractionated heparin

The epidural/intrathecal catheter should be removed following local guidelines and the advice of the anaesthetic/pain management team.

Discharge planning

If it is anticipated that the patient will go home with a continuous epidural or intrathecal infusion, the patient's general practitioner and community nursing team should be consulted at the outset to determine whether they are willing to be involved and/or trained in the management of epidural/intrathecal analgesia care.

Arrangements should also be made with the primary healthcare team for the provision of a suitable epidural/intrathecal pump and the supply of reconstituted syringes/infusion bags. Primary care teams, patients and their families will need to be trained and supplied with the appropriate equipment, drugs, catheter filters, information about the infusion pump, how to identify a catheter-related or systemic infection and what to do if pain occurs or complications arise. For implanted ITDD devices, the patient must be provided with all information to manage the system at home, when they will need to return for the pump to be refilled and who to contact in an emergency.

Contact numbers must be provided in case specialist advice is needed.

Complications

Pain

If pain is not controlled and the infusion has already been titrated according to hospital guidelines, the pain/anaesthetic team should be contacted for advice after checking the following.

- The catheter is still *in situ.*
- The catheter is still connected to the bacterial filter.
- There are no leaks within the system.
- The height of the epidural/intrathecal block. This will indicate whether the block has fallen below the upper limit of the incision or pain site. To check the height of the block, use a small piece of ice or cold solution (ethyl alcohol). Start at the top of the chest above the patient's incision or pain site. Gently dab the ice (or apply the cold solution) down each side of the patient's body (one side and then the other). Use a dermatome map to assess the upper and lower limits of where the sensation changes (see Figure 3.11).

If the height of the block has fallen below the upper limit of the incision or pain site, the pain/anaesthetic team may undertake the following: give the patient a bolus dose of local anaesthetic agent to re-establish the block, and reposition the epidural catheter. If either of these fails, other methods of analgesia need to be considered.

Haematoma

An epidural haematoma can arise from trauma to an epidural blood vessel during catheter insertion or removal. Although the incidence of a haematoma occurring is extremely low, particular care must be taken in patients receiving thromboprophylaxis. Initial symptoms include back pain and tenderness. As the haematoma expands to compress the nerve roots or the spinal cord, this proceeds to sensorimotor weakness (Chapman and Day 2001).

Abscess formation

Infection can be introduced into the epidural/intrathecal space from an exogenous source such as contaminated equipment or drugs or breaches of aseptic technique during insertion and maintenance of spinal catheters (including management of disconnections) or from an endogenous source during episodes of bacteraemia or migration of bacteria through the insertion site (Macintyre and Schug 2015). Alternatively, the catheter can act as a wick through which the infection tracks down from the entry site on the skin to the epidural/intrathecal space (Wheatley et al. 2001). The risk of infection is increased in patients with a malignancy or diabetes or those who are immunocompromised or intravenous drug users. Symptoms include increasing and persistent back pain and tenderness accompanied by signs of infection (redness and/or discharge from the catheter exit site) (Day 2001, Macintyre and Schug 2015).

Complications specific to epidural analgesia

Dural puncture

This occurs when the dura mater is inadvertently punctured during the placement of the epidural catheter. The main symptom is a headache, which arises from leakage of CSF through the dura.

Catheter migration

Catheter migration is extremely rare, occurring in less than 0.2% of patients (Wheatley et al. 2001). The catheter may migrate into either a blood vessel or the CSF. If it migrates into a blood vessel, opioid or local anaesthetic toxicity will occur. Opioid toxicity results in sedation and respiratory depression. Local anaesthetic toxicity results in circumoral tingling, numbness, twitching, convulsions and apnoea (D'Arcy 2011). If the catheter migrates into the CSF, the epidural opioids and local anaesthetic agents may reach as high as the cranial subarachnoid space. If this occurs the respiratory muscles are paralysed together with the cranial nerves, resulting in apnoea, profound hypotension and unconsciousness (Macintyre and Schug 2015).

Complications specific to intrathecal analgesia

Meningitis

Meningitis is a rare complication of intrathecal analgesia. The epidural route is often considered safer as the intact dura serves as an effective barrier to the spread of infection to the subarachnoid space. In fact, similar infection rates are reported with both intrathecal and epidural administration (Mercadante 1999). The incidence of major infections varies widely but is reported by Ballantyne and Carwood (2005) as zero and as approximately 5% by Sloan (2004) for epidural and intrathecal therapy with external pump systems. If the patient presents with headaches, fever, neck stiffness or photophobia, they must be reviewed as a matter of urgency by the medical/anaesthetic team. If meningitis is suspected, CSF samples can be obtained and sent to microbiology for analysis, and antibiotic therapy initiated promptly (Baker et al. 2004, Day 2001).

Entonox (nitrous oxide) administration

Definition

Entonox (nitrous oxide) is a gaseous mixture of 50% nitrous oxide (N_2O) and 50% oxygen (O_2). It is a patient-controlled, inhaled analgesic which is used for the short-term relief of acute pain (BOC 2000). Nitrous oxide is a colourless, sweet-smelling gas with powerful analgesic properties, supplied in premixed cylinders (Bruce and Franck 2000). The gas is inhaled and self-administered by the patient using a demand valve system attached to a facemask or mouthpiece. The nitrous oxide component of the gas acts as an analgesic, producing similar physiological effects to opioids (Emmanouil and Quock 2007), whilst the oxygen component has an antihypoxic effect (Faddy and Garlick 2005) and ensures good cerebral perfusion and enhanced recovery (Peate and Lancaster 2000).

Related theory

Nitrous oxide has been used in clinical practice for over 150 years. The exact mechanism of action of nitrous oxide has never been fully understood (Emmanouil and Quock 2007). Research suggests that its mode of action is due to a release of endogenous opioid peptide that then activates opioid receptors and the descending GABA and noradrenergic pathways; this then modulates pain response in the spinal cord (Emmanouil and Quock 2007).

N-methyl-D-aspartate (NMDA) receptor currents are inhibited by nitrous oxide and it is known that these receptors are involved with many CNS pathways (Jevtovic-Todorovic et al. 2003). The release of these neurotransmitters is thought to activate descending pain pathways which modulate pain transmission in the spinal cord (Maze and Fujinaga 2000). Pulmonary transfer of nitrous oxide is rapid, with onset of effect in seconds and full analgesic effect within 1–2 minutes. It is also rapidly eliminated from the blood, via the lungs, when inhalation ceases (Trojan et al. 1997).

Evidence-based approaches

Rationale
There are several advantages to using Entonox.

- As the gas is inhaled, it is painless when compared to systemic methods of administering analgesia (such as injections).
- It has a rapid onset of effect.
- The side-effects are few and are self-limiting as the gas is self-administered.
- It does not depress respiratory or cardiovascular function when used as directed.
- Effects wear off rapidly, usually within 5 minutes.
- The patient is in full control which provides reassurance that they have instant self-regulated access to analgesia, which also provides a focus or distraction from the procedure taking place. Both of these can help reduce anxiety. Entonox also has sedative properties which can act as an anxiolytic (BOC 2016).

Because of these properties, Entonox is an ideal agent for short-term pain relief following injury or trauma and during therapeutic and investigative procedures. Although its use is mainly in emergency care (O'Sullivan and Benger 2003), obstetrics (Rosen 2002), paediatrics (Bruce and Franck 2000, Pickup and Pagdin 2000) and endoscopy/biopsy procedures (Forbes and Collins 2000, Manikandan et al. 2003), there is a place for Entonox in the oncology setting. Parlow et al. (2005) performed a case review of the use of Entonox in the management of breakthrough cancer pain. Although the review was small they noted that five of the seven patients achieved pain control when compared with placebo.

Indications
- Wound dressing, wound debridement.
- Changing or removal of packs and drains.
- Removal of sutures from sensitive areas, for example the vulva.
- Invasive procedures such as catheterization and sigmoidoscopy.
- Removal of radioactive intracavity gynaecological applicators.
- Altering the position of a patient who experiences incident pain.
- Manual evacuation of the bowel in severe constipation.
- Physiotherapy procedures, particularly post-operatively.

Contraindications
Entonox should not be used with any of the following conditions.

- Maxillofacial injuries (BOC 2000). This could be as a result of surgery or local disease-altering anatomy. The patient may not be able to hold the mask tightly to the face or use the mouthpiece adequately. There is a risk of causing further injury and there may also be a significant risk of blood inhalation if there are any open wounds or aggravation at the surgical site.
- Heavily sedated patients, as they would be unable to breathe in the Entonox on demand, and to potentiate sedation further may be hazardous.
- Intoxicated patients or those with impaired level of consciousness related either to disease state or concurrent medications. Aspiration would be a hazard in the event of vomiting.

- Any condition in which gas is entrapped within the body and where its expansion may be dangerous, such as:
  - pneumothorax (artificial, traumatic or spontaneous)
  - air embolism
  - severe bullous emphysema
  - abdominal distension or bowel obstruction
  - decompression sickness or following a recent dive
  - following air encephalography
  - during myringoplasty
  - in patients who have received a recent intraocular injection of gas (BOC 2016).
  The nitrous oxide constituent of Entonox passes into any air-filled cavity within the body faster than nitrogen passes out. As the gas expands, this is likely to result in a build-up of tension, which will increase the patient's symptoms.
- Laryngectomy patients, as they will be unable to use the apparatus.
- Temperatures of below –6°C, as the gases separate (BOC 1995). If this occurs the cylinders will initially deliver a high concentration of oxygen but will eventually deliver nearly pure nitrous oxide.

Use during pregnancy and lactation
Although this may be rare in the cancer setting, it is important to consider if your patient is trying to become pregnant that prolonged exposure to high levels of nitrous oxide may affect a woman's ability to become pregnant (Axelsson et al. 1996). However, there is no published material to show that nitrous oxide is toxic to the human fetus, therefore there is no absolute contraindication to its use in the first 16 weeks of pregnancy.

There are no known adverse effects to using Entonox during the breast-feeding period (BOC 2016).

Principles of care

Cautions
Prior to Entonox use, consideration should be given to the following:

- The high level of oxygen (50%) in Entonox may depress respiration in patients who have chronic obstructive pulmonary disease and are carbon dioxide (CO_2) retainers.
- Entonox should not be used as a replacement for intravenous analgesia or general anaesthesia in procedures requiring increased levels of medical intervention.
- If Entonox is used as the sole analgesic/sedative agent, BOC's 2016 data sheet recommends that driving or operating complex machinery is not recommended until:
  - the healthcare professional has judged that the patient has returned to normal mental status (Entonox can cause psychotropic effects)
  - the patient feels they are competent to drive after the relevant procedure is completed
  - at least 30 minutes has elapsed after the administration of Entonox has ceased.
- Additional care is needed when Entonox is administered to a patient who has been given concomitant medication.

Legal and professional issues
Healthcare professionals involved in the assessment, administration and continuing care of patients receiving Entonox should have undergone training to do so. To maintain patient safety, healthcare professionals need to understand the properties, applications and prescribing practices for any medicinal product, which includes all medical gases (BOC 2016). They should be able to demonstrate knowledge of the properties of the gas, precautions to be taken, actions in the event of an emergency and the correct operating procedures for equipment. Training should include:

- physical properties of the medical gas Entonox
- indications for its use

- protocols or policies for safe administration
- known side-effects and contraindications
- any other safety precautions
- methods of safe operation of the gas.

Training can be supplied by BOC Healthcare or a designated trainer and certificated.

Prescribing of Entonox

In a number of healthcare settings, nurses, physiotherapists and radiographers may be able to administer Entonox without a written prescription from a doctor providing there is a local Patient Group Direction to allow this. Where this is the case, Entonox can be used more readily and time is not wasted waiting for a medical prescription. Non-medical prescribers who have completed the relevant training as an independent prescriber may also prescribe Entonox if this is within their area of competence.

Pre-procedural considerations

Equipment

Cylinders

Entonox cylinders are available from the BOC in a variety of sizes. All cylinders have blue and white markings on their shoulder (Figure 3.12). The lightweight smaller cylinders have the following advantages:

- They are easier to carry.
- They have a live contents gauge.
- Changing an empty cylinder is simple because it is not necessary to fit a regulator or use a cylinder key.

Demand apparatus

There are a number of different companies that supply the demand apparatus for self-administered Entonox use. Examples include the Ease demand valve (Sabre Medical) and the Carnet single patient use demand valve (Figure 3.13).

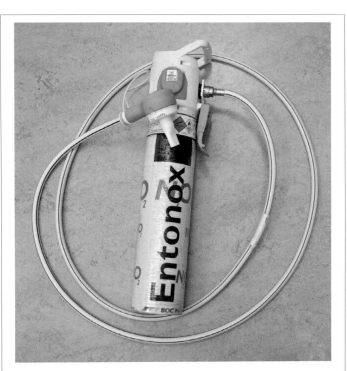

Figure 3.12 Entonox cylinder and hose. *Source:* Dougherty and Lister (2015).

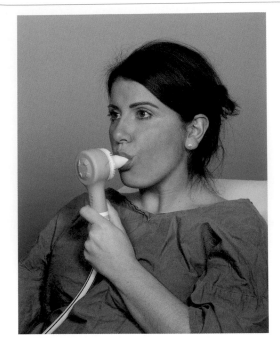

Figure 3.13 Patient using Entonox demand valve. *Source:* The Royal Marsden.

Bacterial filters and mouthpieces/facemasks

Because Entonox equipment is a potential source of cross-infection, bacterial filters (single use only) should be fitted between the facemask or mouthpiece and demand valve if the demand valve is not for single use (Chilvers and Weisz 2000). Facemasks and mouthpieces must also be single use only and disposed of once therapy ceases. Local policies must also be followed for the cleaning/sterilization of non-disposable equipment between patients.

Assessment

The patient's ability to administer Entonox safely and effectively (particularly the very young or old) must be assessed prior to use. Patients should be able to:

- understand the instructions for Entonox use
- hold the demand valve to self-administer the gas
- inhale the gas through the mask or mouthpiece while breathing normally (patients who have impaired lung function may not be able to inhale the gas sufficiently to provide adequate analgesia).

Pharmacological support

Entonox is designed for self-administration by the patient. This method of administration makes use of a demand unit which safeguards the patient from excessive inhalation of Entonox. The demand unit ensures that gas can be obtained only by the patient inhaling from the mouthpiece or mask and producing a negative pressure. The gas flow stops when the patient stops inhaling and removes the mouthpiece or mask from their face. Thus patients are able to self-regulate the dose of Entonox (a method of patient-controlled analgesia). Therefore, the patient must hold the mask firmly over the face or mouthpiece to the lips to produce an airtight fit and breathe in before the gas will flow. Expired gases escape by the expiratory valve on the handpiece. It is essential to adhere to this method of self-administration as it is then impossible for patients to overdose themselves because, if they become drowsy, they will relax their grip on the handset and the gas flow will cease when no negative pressure is applied. However, should inhalation continue, light anaesthesia supervenes and the mask drops away as the patient relaxes. Entonox may be self-regulated, but additionally may be administered by attendant medical personnel trained in its use, for example within obstetric/accident and emergency units, and accident ambulances.

Entonox has an oxygen content 2.5 times that of air and is therefore a good way of giving extra oxygen as well as providing analgesia.

Duration and frequency of administration
The duration and frequency of Entonox administration should always be tailored to individual patient needs. Because prolonged exposure to Entonox causes inactivation of vitamin B_{12}, impaired folate metabolism and pernicious anaemia (BOC 2016), it is recommended that:

- Entonox is used on a short-term rather than a long-term basis.
- It should not be used for more than a total of 24 hours, or more frequently than once every 4 days (BOC 2016).
- If daily use is required for more than 4 days, this should be accompanied by close supervision and haematological monitoring (blood tests) to check for changes in red and white blood cells (BOC 2016). Consideration should also be given to the administration of B_{12} and folate supplements.

Procedure guideline 3.5 Entonox administration

Essential equipment
- Entonox cylinder and head
- Sterile bacterial filter
- Facemask and/or mouthpiece × 2
- Method of documentation

Pre-procedure

Action	Rationale
1 Explain and discuss the procedure with the patient and perform hand-washing technique at bedside.	To ensure that the patient understands the procedure and gives their valid consent (NMC 2015, **C**). To reduce patient anxiety (Royal College of Anaesthetists 2006, **C**). To ensure the patient has no underlying medical problems that contraindicate the use of Entonox (BOC 2016, **C**).

Procedure

Action	Rationale
2 Ensure that the patient is in as comfortable a position as possible.	To promote patient comfort (BOC 2015, **C**).
3 Turn on the Entonox supply from the cylinder.	To ascertain whether there is any Entonox in the cylinder (BOC 2015, **C**).
4 Examine the gauge to determine how much gas is in the cylinder.	To ensure an adequate supply of gas throughout the procedure (BOC 2015, **C**).
5 Demonstrate how to use the apparatus by holding the mask tightly to your face, replacing the mask/mouthpiece that you have used (ensure that the Entonox is turned off at this point). Explain to the patient that when they breathe in and out regularly and deeply, a hissing sound will be heard, indicating that the gas is being inhaled.	To ensure that the patient understands what to do and what to expect before any painful procedure commences (BOC 2015, **C**).
6 Allow the patient to practise using the apparatus.	To enable the patient to adopt the correct technique and for the nurse to observe the analgesic effect of the gas before the procedure commences (BOC 2015, **C**).
7 Encourage the patient to breathe gas in and out for at least 2 minutes before commencing any painful procedure.	To allow sufficient time for an adequate circulatory level of nitrous oxide to provide analgesia. When the patient inhales, gas enters first the lungs then the pulmonary and systemic circulations. It takes 1–2 minutes to build up reasonable concentrations of nitrous oxide in the brain (BOC 2015, **C**).
8 During the procedure, encourage the patient to breathe in and out regularly and deeply.	To maintain adequate circulatory levels, thus providing adequate analgesia (BOC 2015, **C**).
9 Evaluate the effectiveness of Entonox with the patient throughout and following the procedure, by verbal questioning and encouraging the patient to self-assess the analgesic effect.	To establish whether the Entonox has been a useful analgesic for the procedure. This should then be documented to assist any subsequent procedures, for example dressing changes (BOC 2015, **C**).
10 At the end of the procedure observe the patient every 5–10 minutes until the effects of the gas have worn off. Observe the patient for up to 30 minutes.	Some patients may feel a transient drowsiness or giddiness and should be discouraged from getting out of bed until these effects have worn off. It is rare for the patient to experience transient amnesia (BOC 2015, **C**).

(continued)

Procedure guideline 3.5   Entonox administration (continued)

Post-procedure

11 Turn off the Entonox supply from the cylinder.	To avoid potential seepage of gas from the apparatus (BOC 2015, **C**).
12 Depress the diaphragm under the demand valve.	To remove residual gas from tubing (BOC 2015, **C**).
13 Follow local policies/guidelines for the cleaning and sterilization of expiratory valve and tubing, and facemask (or disposal if single use). Filters and mouthpieces should be discarded after use.	To reduce the risk of cross-infection (BOC 2015, **C**).
14 Record the administration on appropriate documentation.	To promote continuity of care, maintain accurate records and provide a point of reference in the event of any queries (BOC 2015, **C**; NMC 2010, **C**).

Problem-solving table 3.2 Prevention and resolution (Procedure guideline 3.5)

Problem	Cause	Prevention	Suggested action
Patient not experiencing adequate analgesic effect.	Entonox cylinder empty. Apparatus not properly connected.	Check before procedure commences.	Change to a full cylinder.
	Patient not inhaling deeply enough (BOC 2000).	Education of patient prior to starting procedure.	Encourage the patient to breathe in until a hissing noise can be heard from the cylinder. Reassess suitability of patient for Entonox use. The patient may not be strong enough to inhale deeply or may have reduced lung capacity.
	Patient inhaling pure oxygen, that is, cylinder has been stored below −6°C and nitrous oxide has liquefied and settled at the bottom of the cylinder.	All cylinders should be stored horizontally at a temperature of 10°C or above for 24 hours before use (BOC 1995).	Initially safe, but later the patient may inhale pure nitrous oxide and be asphyxiated. Discontinue the procedure. Ensure adequate warming of the cylinder and inversion of the cylinder to remix the gases adequately.
	Not enough time has been allowed for nitrous oxide to exert its analgesic effect.	Allow at least 2 minutes of Entonox use before commencing the procedure.	Stop procedure. Allow 2 minutes of Entonox use. Restart procedure.
Patient experiences generalized muscle rigidity.	Hyperventilation during inhalation (BOC 2000).	Education of patient prior to starting procedure.	Discontinue Entonox and allow the patient to recover. Explain the procedure again, stressing deep and regular inspiration. Use a mouthpiece in place of a mask.
Patient unable to tolerate a mask.	Smell of rubber, feeling of claustrophobia.	Assess patient preference to use either mask or mouthpiece before Entonox use.	Use a mouthpiece in place of a mask.
Patient feels nauseated, drowsy or giddy.	Effect of nitrous oxide accumulation (BOC 2000).	None.	Discontinue Entonox administration: the effect will then rapidly disappear. Restart Entonox use; if the same effect occurs, stop using Entonox and use alternative analgesia.
Patient afraid to use Entonox.	Associates gases with previous hospital procedures, for example anaesthesia before surgery (BOC 2000).	Assess suitability of patient for Entonox use. Address fear and anxiety issues before starting Entonox use.	Reassure patient and reiterate instructions for use and short-term effects.

Complications

Effects such as euphoria, disorientation, sedation, nausea, vomiting, dizziness and generalized tingling are commonly described. These are generally minor and rapidly reversible (BOC 2016).

Inappropriate inhalation of Entonox will ultimately result in unconsciousness, passing through stages of increasing light-headedness and intoxication. The treatment is moving to fresh air, mouth-to-mouth resuscitation and, if necessary, the use of an oxygen resuscitator (BOC 1995).

References

Abbey, J., Piller, N., De Bellis, A., et al. (2004) The Abbey pain scale: a 1-minute numerical indicator for people with end-stage dementia. *International Journal of Palliative Nursing*, 10(1), 6–13.

Alemdar, D. & Aktas, Y. (2014) Comparison of nurses and patients assessments of postoperative pain. *International Journal of Caring Sciences*, 7(3), 882–888.

Angheluta, A.M. & Lee, B.K. (2011) Art therapy for chronic pain: applications and future directions. *Canadian Journal of Counselling and Psychotherapy*, 45(2), 112–131.

Axelsson, G., Ahlborg, G. Jr. & Bodin, L. (1996) Shift work, nitrous oxide exposure, and spontaneous abortion among Swedish midwives. *Occupational and Environmental Medicine*, 53(6), 374–378.

Baker, L., Lee, M., Regnard, C., Crack, L. & Callin, S. (2004) Evolving spinal analgesia practice in palliative care. *Palliative Medicine*, 18(6), 507–515.

Ballantyne, J.C. & Carwood, C.M. (2005) Comparative efficacy of epidural, subarachnoid, and intracerebroventricular opioids in patients with pain due to cancer. *Cochrane Database of Systematic Reviews*, 1, CD005178.

Bannon, L., Alexander-Williams, M. & Lutman, D. (2001) A national survey of epidural practice. *Anaesthesia*, 56(10), 1021.

Barillo, D.J., Coffey, E.C., Shirani, K.Z. & Goodwin, C.W. (2000) Burns caused by medical therapy. *Journal of Burn Care & Rehabilitation*, 21(3), 269–273.

Baron, R., Binder, A. & Wasner, G. (2010) Neuropathic pain: diagnosis, pathophysiological mechanisms and treatment. *Lancet Neurology*, 9(8), 807–819.

Behar, J.M., Gogalniceanu, P. & Bromley, L. (2007) Anaesthesia: regional anaesthesia. *Student BMJ*, 15, 186–189.

Beijers, A., Mold, F., Dercksen, W., Driessen, C. & Vreucigdenhil, G. (2014) Chemotherapy induced peripheral neuropathy and impact on quality of life 6 months after treatment with chemotherapy. *Journal of Community and Supportive Oncology*, 12(11), 401–406.

Bell, L. & Duffy, A. (2009) Pain assessment and management in surgical nursing: a literature review. *British Journal of Nursing*, 18(3), 153–156.

Bennett, M. (2001) The LANSS Pain Scale: the Leeds assessment of neuropathic symptoms and signs. *Pain*, 92(1–2), 147–157.

Bennett, M.I. (2014) Chapter 1. Definition and pathophysiology of complex cancer pain. In: Sharma, M., Simpson, K.H., Bennett, M.I. & Gupta, S. (eds) *Practical Management of Complex Cancer Pain*. Oxford: Oxford University Press.

Binda, D., Vanhoutte, E.K. & Cavaletti, G. (2013) Rasch-built Overall Disability Scale for patients with chemotherapy induced peripheral neuropathy (CIPN-R-ODS). *European Journal of Cancer*, 49(13), 2910–2918.

BOC (1995) *BOC Gases Data Sheet: Entonox*. Manchester: BOC Group.

BOC (2000) *Entonox: Controlled Pain Relief Reference Guide*. Manchester: BOC Medical.

BOC (2015) *Entonox: The Essential Guide*. Manchester: BOC Healthcare Ltd.

BOC (2016) *Entonox: Essential safety information. Summary of Product Characteristics*. Manchester: BOC Healthcare Ltd.

Breivik, H., Cherny, N., Collett, B., et al. (2009) Cancer related pain: a pan-European survey of prevalence, treatment and patient attitudes. *Annals of Oncology*, 20, 1420–1433.

Brewer, J.R., Morrison, G., Dolan, M.E. & Fleming, G.F. (2016) Chemotherapy-induced peripheral neuropathy: current status and progress. *Gynecologic Oncology*, 140(1), 176–183.

Briggs, E. (2010) Assessment and expression of pain. *Nursing Standard*, 25(2), 35–38.

Bristol-Myers Squibb (2012) *Perfalgan, Dosing Tool*. Uxbridge: Bristol-Myers Squibb Pharmaceuticals.

British Medical Acupuncture Society (BMAS) (2013) Treatment Record Chart. London: BMAS. Available at: http://www.medical-acupuncture.co.uk/Default.aspx?tabid=64 (Accessed: 17/4/2018)

British Pain Society (BPS) (2010) *Cancer Pain Management*. London: BPS. Available at: https://www.britishpainsociety.org/static/uploads/resources/files/book_cancer_pain.pdf (Accessed: 17/4/2018)

Brown, M., Ramirez, J. & Farquhar-Smith, P. (2014) Pain in cancer survivors. *British Journal of Pain*, 8(4), 139–155.

Bruce, E. & Franck, L. (2000) Self-administered nitrous oxide (ENTONOX) for the management of procedural pain. *Paediatric Nursing*, 12(7), 15–20.

Brunelli, C., Kaasa, S. & Knudsen, A.K. (2014) Comparisons of patients and physician assessment of pain related domains in cancer pain classification: results from a large international multicentre study. *Journal of Pain*, 15, 59–67.

Budd, K. (2002) *Evidence-based Medicine in Practice. Buprenorphine: A Review*. Newmarket: Haywood Medical.

Burns, S.M., Cowa, C.M., Barclay, P.M. & Wilkes, R.G. (2001) Intrapartum epidural catheter migration: a comparative study of three dressing applications. *British Journal of Anaesthesia*, 86(4), 565–567.

Burton A., Chai T. & Smith L. (2014) Cancer Pain Assessment. *Supportive and Palliative Care*, 8(2), 112–116.

Carr, E. & Mann, E.M. (2000) Recognising the barriers to effective pain relief. In: *Pain: Creative Approaches to Effective Management*. Basingstoke: Palgrave Macmillan, pp. 109–129.

Cavaletti, G., Pezzoni, G., Pisano, C., et al. (2002) Cisplatin-induced peripheral neurotoxicity in rats reduces the circulating levels of nerve growth factor. *Neuroscience Letters*, 322, 103–106.

Cavaletti, G., Frigeni, B., Lanzani, F., et al. (2010) Chemotherapy-induced peripheral neurotoxicity assessment: a critical revision of the currently available tools. *European Journal of Cancer*, 46(3), 479–494.

Chapman, S. (2012) Cancer pain part 2: assessment and management. *Nursing Standard*, 26(48), 44–49.

Chapman, S. & Day, R. (2001) Spinal anatomy and the use of epidurals. *Professional Nurse*, 16(6), 1174–1177.

Cherny, N.I., Catane, R. & European Society of Medical Oncology Taskforce on Palliative and Supportive Care (2003) Attitudes of medical oncologists toward palliative care for patients with advanced and incurable cancer: report on a survey by the European Society of Medical Oncology Taskforce on Palliative and Supportive Care. *Cancer*, 98(11), 2502–2510.

Chilvers, R.J. & Weisz, M. (2000) Entonox equipment as a potential source of cross-infection. *Anaesthesia*, 55(2), 176–179.

Chu S.H, Lee Y.J, Lee E.S, Geng, Y., Wang, X.S. & Cleeland, C.S. (2014) Current use of drugs affecting the central nervous system for chemotherapy-induced peripheral neuropathy in cancer patients: a systematic review. *Support Cancer Care*, 25, 513–524.

Cleeland, C.S. & Ryan, K.M. (1994) Pain assessment: global use of the Brief Pain Inventory. *Annual Academic Medicine Singapore*, 23, 129–138.

Cleeland, C.S., Mendoza, T.R. & Wang, X.S. (2000) Assessing symptom distress in cancer patients: the M.D Anderson Symptoms Inventory. *Cancer*, 89, 1634–1646.

Cook, T.M., Eaton, J.M. & Goodwin, A.P. (1997) Epidural analgesia following upper abdominal surgery: United Kingdom practice. *Acta Anaesthesiologica Scandinavica*, 41(1 Pt 1), 18–24.

Curatolo, M., Petersen-Felix, S., Scaramozzino, P. & Zbinden, A.M. (1998) Epidural fentanyl, adrenaline and clonidine as adjuvants to local anaesthetics for surgical analgesia: meta-analyses of analgesia and side-effects. *Acta Anaesthesiologica Scandinavica*, 42(8), 910–920.

D'Arcy, Y. (2011) Regional techniques for postoperative pain relief. In: D'Arcy, Y (ed.) *Acute Pain Management*. New York: Springer Publishing Company.

Darwish, M., Kirby, M. & Giang, J.D. (2007) Effect of buccal dwell time on the pharmacokinetic profile of fentanyl buccal tablet. *Expert Opinion in Pharmacotherapy*, 8, 2011–2016.

Davies, A.N., Dickman, A., Reid, C., Stevens, A.M. & Zeppetella G; Science Committee of the Association for Palliative Medicine of Great

Britain and Ireland (2009) The management of cancer-related breakthrough pain: recommendations of a task group of the Science Committee of the Association for Palliative Medicine of Great Britain and Ireland. *European Journal of Pain*, 2009, 13(4), 331–338.

Davis, M.P., Glare, P. & Hardy, J. (2005) *Opioids in Cancer Pain*. Oxford: Oxford University Press.

Day, R. (2001) The use of epidural and intrathecal analgesia in palliative care. *International Journal of Palliative Care*, 7(8), 369–374.

Dean-Clower, E., Doherty-Gilman, A.M., Keshaviah, A., et al. (2010) Acupuncture as palliative therapy for physical symptoms and quality of life for advanced cancer patients. *Integrated Cancer Therapy*, 9(2), 158–167.

Deandrea, S., Montanari, M., Moja, L. & Apolone, G. (2008) Prevalence of undertreatment in cancer pain. A review of published literature. *Annals of Oncology*, 19(12),1985–1991.

Department of Transport (2014) *Guidance for Healthcare Professionals on Drug Driving*. London: Department of Transport.

Derry, S., Lloyd, R. & Moore, R.A. (2009) Topical capsaicin for chronic neuropathic pain in adults. *Cochrane Database of Systematic Reviews*, 4, CD007393.

Derry, S., Sven-Rice, A., Cole, P., Tan, T., & Moore, R.A. (2013). Topical capsaicin (high concentration) for chronic neuropathic pain in adults. *Cochrane Database of Systematic Reviews*, 2, CD007393.

Dickson, D. (2004) Risks and benefits of long-term intrathecal analgesia. *Anaesthesia*, 59(7), 633–635.

Dougherty, L. & Lister, S. (Eds) (2015) *The Royal Marsden Manual of Clinical Nursing Procedures*, 9th edn. Oxford: Wiley-Blackwell.

Drayer, R.A., Henderson, J. & Reidenberg, M. (1999) Barriers to better pain control in hospitalized patients. *Journal of Pain and Symptom Management*, 17(6), 434–440.

Driessen, C.M.L., de Kleine-Bolt, K.M.E., Vingerhoets, A.J.J.M., Mols, F. & Vreugdenhil, G. (2012). Assessing the impact of chemotherapy-induced peripheral neurotoxicity on the quality of life of cancer patients: the introduction of a new measure. *Supportive Care in Cancer*, 20(4), 877–881.

Dühmke R.M., Cornblath D.D. & Hollingshead J.R.F. (2004) Tramadol for neuropathic pain. *Cochrane Database of Systematic Reviews*, 2, CD003726.

Du Pen, A. (2005) Care and management of intrathecal and epidural catheters. *Journal of Infusion Nursing*, 28(6), 377–381.

Dworkin, R.H., O'Connor, A.B, Audette, J., et al. (2010) Recommendations for the pharmacological management of neuropathic pain: an overview and literature update. *Mayo Clinic Proceedings*, 85(3 suppl), S3–14.

Eisenberg, E., Marinangeli, F., Birkhahn, J., Paladini, A. & Varrassi, G. (2005) Time to modify the WHO analgesic ladder? *Pain Clinical Updates*, 13, 1–4.

Ellen, M., Smith, L., Pang, H., et al. (2013) Effect of duloxetine on pain, function, and quality of life among patients with chemotherapy-induced painful peripheral neuropathy. *Journal of the American Medical Association*, 309(13), 1359–1367.

Ellen, M., Campbell, G., Tofthgen, C., et al. (2014) Nursing knowledge, practice patterns and learning preferences regarding chemotherapy induced peripheral neuropathy. *Oncology Nursing Forum*, 41(6), 669–679.

Emmanouil, D. & Quock, R. (2007) Advances in understanding the actions of nitrous oxide. *Anesthesia Progress* 54(1), 9–18.

European Oncology Nursing Society (EONS) (2013) Breakthrough cancer pain guidelines 2013. EONS. Available at: https://www.cancernurse.eu/documents/EONSBreakthroughCancerPainGuidelines.pdf (Accessed: 17/4/2018)

Faddy, S.C. & Garlick, S.R. (2005) A systematic review of the safety of an algesia with 50% nitrous oxide: can lay responders use analgesic gases in the prehospital setting? *Emergency Medicine Journal*, 22(12), 901–906.

Fallon, M., Cherny, N.I. & Hanks, G. (2010) Opioid analgesia therapy. In: Doyle, D., Cherny, N.I., Christakis, N.A., Fallon, M., Kasasa, S. & Portenoy, R.K. (eds) *Oxford Textbook of Palliative Medicine*, 4th edn. Oxford: Oxford University Press, pp. 599–625.

Fallon, M.T. (2013). Neuropathic pain in cancer. *British Journal of Anaesthesia*, 111(1), 105–111.

Fallon M.T., Storey D.J., Krishan, A., et al. (2015) Cancer treatment-related neuropathic pain: proof of concept study with menthol – a TRPM8 agonist. *Supportive Care in Cancer*, 23(9), 2769–2777.

Farquhar-Smith, P. & Brown, M. (2016) Persistent Pain in Cancer Survivors: Pathogenesis and Treatment Options. International Association for the Study of Pain. *Pain Clinical Updates*, XXIV(4), 1–8. Available at: https://www.iasp-pain.org/PublicationsNews/NewsletterIssueWIP.aspx?ItemNumber=5705 (Accessed: 17/4/2018)

Farquhar-Smith, P. (2012) Chapter 5. Neuraxial (epidural and intrathecal) infusions I: Anatomy and commonly used drugs: mode of action, pharmacokinetics, side effects and evidence base for effectiveness. In: Hester, J., Sykes, N. & Peat, S. (eds) *Interventional Pain Control in Cancer Pain Management*. Oxford: Oxford University Press.

Farrell, A. & Rich, A. (2000) Analgesic use in patients with renal failure. *European Journal of Palliative Care*, 7(6), 201–205.

Filshie, J., & Thompson, J.W. (2009) Acupuncture. In: Hanks, G., Cherny, N.I., Christakis, N.A., Fallon, M., Kaasa, S. & Portenoy, R. (eds) *Oxford Textbook of Palliative Medicine*, 4th edn. New York: Oxford University Press.

Filshie J., White A., & Cummings, M. (2016) *Medical Acupuncture: A Western Scientific Approach*. Edinburgh: Elsevier.

Flatters, S.J. & Bennett, G.J. (2006) Studies of peripheral sensory nerves in paclitaxel induced painful peripheral neuropathy: evidence for mitochondrial dysfunction. *Pain*, 122, 245–257.

Forbes, G.M. & Collins, B.J. (2000) Nitrous oxide for colonoscopy: a randomized controlled study. *Gastrointestinal Endoscopy*, 51(3), 271–278.

Fotiadis, R.J., Badvie, S., Weston, M.D. & Allen-Mersh, T.G. (2004) Epidural analgesia in gastrointestinal surgery. *British Journal of Surgery*, 91(7), 828–841.

Fraise, A.P. & Bradley, T. (eds) (2009) *Ayliffe's Control of Healthcare-associated Infection: A Practical Handbook*, 5th edn. London: Hodder Arnold.

French, S.D., Cameron, M., Walker, B.F., Reggars, J.W. & Esterman, A.J. (2006) Superficial heat or cold for low back pain. *Cochrane Database of Systematic Reviews*, 1, CD004750.

Furler, L. (2013) Validity and reliability of the pain questionnaire "Brief Pain Inventory". A literature research. *Pflege Zeitschrift* 66(9), 546–550.

Gaiser, R. (2006) Postdural puncture headache. *Current Opinion in Anaesthesiology*, 19(3), 249–253.

Gannon, C. (1997) Clinical management. The use of methadone in the care of the dying. *European Journal of Palliative Care*, 4(5), 152–159.

Gardner-Nix, J.S. (1996) Oral methadone for managing chronic nonmalignant pain. *Journal of Pain and Symptom Management*, 11(5), 321–328.

Gelinas, C. & Arbour, C. (2014) Pain and pain management. In: Urden, L.D., Stacy, K.M. & Lough, M.E. (eds) *Critical Care Nursing: Diagnosis and Management*, 7th edn. St Louis, MO: Mosby Elsevier, pp. 143–169.

Godfrey, H. (2005) Understanding pain, part 1: physiology of pain. *British Journal of Nursing*, 14(16), 846–852.

Gogarten, W., Vandermeulen, E., Van Aken, H., et al. (2010) Regional anaesthesia and antithrombotic agents: recommendations of the European Society of Anaesthesiology. *Anaesthesiology*, 24(5), 573–580.

Grassin-Delyle, S., Naline, E., Faisy, C., et al. (2012) Intranasal drug delivery: an efficient and non-invasive route for systemic administration: focus on opioids. *Pharmacology and Therapeutics*, 134(3), 366–379.

Hall, J. (2000) Epidural analgesia management. *Nursing Times*, 96(28), 38–40.

Hanks, G., Cherny, N. & Fallon, M. (2004) Opioid analgesic therapy. In: Doyle, D. (ed.) *Oxford Textbook of Palliative Medicine*, 3rd edn. Oxford: Oxford University Press, pp. 316–342.

Harmer, M. & Davies, K.A. (1998) The effect of education, assessment and a standardised prescription on postoperative pain management. The value of clinical audit in the establishment of acute pain services. *Anaesthesia*, 53(5), 424–430.

Harrop-Griffiths, W., Cook, T., Gill, H., et al. (2013) Regional anaesthesia and patients with abnormalities of coagulation. The Association of Anaesthetists of Great Britain & Ireland The Obstetric Anaesthetists Association Regional Anaesthesia UK. *Anaesthesia*, 68(9), 966–972.

Hasuo, H., Ishihara, T., Kanbara, K. & Fukunaga, M. (2016) Myofacial trigger points in advanced cancer patients. *Indian Journal of Palliative Care*, 22(1), 80–84.

Hebl, J.R. (2006) The importance and implications of aseptic techniques during regional anesthesia. *Regional Anesthesia and Pain Medicine*, 31(4), 311–323.

Heiser, R.M., Chiles, K., Fudge, M. & Gray, S.E. (1997) The use of music during the immediate postoperative recovery period. *AORN Journal*, 65(4), 777–778, 781–785.

Heiskanen, T. & Kalso, E. (1997) Controlled-release oxycodone and morphine in cancer related pain. *Pain*, 73(1), 37–45.

Hershman, L., Lacchetti, C., Dworkin, R., et al. (2014) Prevention and Management of Chemotherapy-Induced Peripheral Neuropathy in Survivors of Adult Cancers: American Society of Clinical Oncology Clinical Practice Guideline. *Journal of Clinical Oncology*, 32, 1941–1967.

Hervik, J. & Mjaland, O. (2009) Acupuncture for the treatment of hot flushes in breast cancer patients. A randomized controlled trial. *Breast Cancer Research and Treatment*, 116(2), 311–316.

Higginson, I.J. (1998) Can professionals improve their assessments? *Journal of Pain and Symptom Management*, 15(3), 149–150.

Hjermstad, M.J., Fayers, P.M. & Haugen, D.F. (2011) Studies compare Numerical Rating Scales, Verbal Rating Scales and Visual Analogue Scales for assessment of pain intensity in adults: a systematic literature review. *Journal of Pain and Symptom Management*, 41, 1073–1093.

Hobbs, G.J. & Hodgkinson, V. (2003) Assessment, measurement, history and examination. In: Rowbotham, D.J. & Macintyre, P.E. (eds) *Acute Pain*. London: Arnold, pp. 93–112.

Horlocker, T.T. (2011) Regional anaesthesia in the patient receiving antithrombotic or thrombolytic therapy. *British Journal of Anaesthesia*, 107(Suppl 1), 196–106.

Horlocker, T.T., Wedel, D.J., Rowlingson, J.C. & Enneking, F.K. (2010) Regional anesthesia in the patient receiving antithrombotic or thrombolytic therapy: American Society of Regional Anesthesia and Pain Medicine Evidence-Based Guidelines (Third Edition). *Regional Anesthesia and Pain Medicine*, 35(1), 64–101.

Hu, C., Zhang, H., Wu, W., et al. (2015) Acupuncture for pain management in cancer: a systematic review and meta-analysis. *Evidence-Based Complementary and Alternative Medicine* 2016, 1720239.

Hurley, R., Cohen, S. & Wu, C. (2010) Acute pain in adults. In: Fishman, S., Ballantyne, J. & Rathmell, J. (eds) *Bonica's Management of Pain*, 4th edn. Philadelphia: Lippincott Williams & Wilkins.

Idvall, E., Hamrin, E., Sjostrom, B. & Unosson, M. (2002) Patient and nurse assessment of quality of care in postoperative pain management. *Quality and Safety in Health Care*, 11(4), 327–334.

International Association for the Study of Pain (IASP) (1994) *IASP Pain Terminology*. Available at: www.iasp-pain.org/taxonomy (Accessed: 17/4/2018)

International Association for the Study of Pain (IASP) (1996) Classification of chronic pain. *Pain*, 3(Suppl), 51–226.

International Association for the Study of Pain (IASP) (2009) Total Cancer Pain Factsheet- Global Year Against Cancer Pain. *International Association for the Study of Pain (IASP)*. Available at: www.iasp-pain.org/GlobalYear (Accessed: 17/4/2018)

ISO 80369-1:2010 (2010) Small-bore connectors for liquids and gases in healthcare applications – Part 1: General requirements. Available at: https://www.iso.org/standard/45976.html (Accessed: 17/4/2018)

ISO 80369-6:2016 (2016) Small-bore connectors for liquids and gases in healthcare applications – Part 6: Connectors for neuraxial applications. Available at: https://www.iso.org/standard/50734.html (Accessed: 17/4/2018)

Jain, S. (2014) Chapter 3. Neurolytic blocking agents. In: Sharma, M., Simpson, K.H., Bennett, M.I. & Gupta, S. (eds) *Practical Management of Complex Cancer Pain*. Oxford: Oxford University Press.

Jevtovic-Todorovic, V., Beals, J., Benshoff, N. & Olney, J.W. (2003) Prolonged exposure to inhalational anesthetic nitrous oxide kills neurons in adult rat brain. *Neuroscience*, 122, 609–616.

Johnson, M. & Martinson, M. (2007) Efficacy of electrical nerve stimulation for chronic musculoskeletal pain: a meta-analysis of randomized controlled trials. *Pain*, 130(1), 157–165.

Kane, C.M. & Bennett, M.I. (2015) Cancer induced bone pain. *BMJ*, 350, h315.

King, A. (1999) *King's Guide to TENS for Health Professionals: A Health Professionals' Guide to Transcutaneous Electrical Nerve Stimulation for the Treatment of Pain*. London: King's Medical.

King, S., Forbes, K., Hanks, G.W., Ferro, C.J. & Chambers, E.J. (2011) A systematic review of the use of opioid medication for those with moderate to severe cancer pain and renal impairment: a European Palliative Care Research Collaborative opioid guidelines project. *Palliative Medicine*, 25(5), 525–552.

Kinirons, B., Mimoz, O., Lafendi, L., Naas, T., Meunier, J. & Nordmann, P. (2001) Chlorhexidine versus povidone iodine in preventing colonization of continuous epidural catheters in children: a randomized, controlled trial. *Anesthesiology*, 94(2), 239–244.

Kitson, A. (1994) Post-operative pain management: a literature review. *Journal of Clinical Nursing*, 3(1), 7–18.

Kuroi, K. & Shimozuma, K. (2004) Neurotoxicity of taxanes: symptoms and quality of life assessment. *Breast Cancer Journal*, 11(1), 92–99.

Lang, S. & Patt, R. (2004) *The Complete Guide to Relieving Cancer Pain and Suffering*. New York: Oxford University Press, pp. 3–26.

Leng, G. (2013) Use of acupuncture in hospices and palliative care services in the UK. *Acupuncture in Medicine*, 31, 16–22.

Le Wendling, L. & Enneking, F.K. (2008) Continuous peripheral nerve blockade for postoperative analgesia. *Current Opinion in Anaesthesiology*, 2008, 21(5), 602–609.

Lim, J.T.N., Wong, E.T. & Aing, S.K.H. (2011) Is there a role for acupuncture in the symptoms management of patients receiving palliative care for cancer? A pilot study of 20 patients comparing acupuncture with nurse led supportive care. *Acupuncture in Medicine*, 29, 173–179.

Lim, S.N., Han, H.S., Lee, K.I., et al. (2015) A satisfaction survey on cancer pain management using a self-reporting pain assessment tool. *Journal of Palliative Medicine*, 18(3), 225–231.

Loveday, H.P., Wilson, J.A., Pratt, R.J., et al. (2014) epic3: National Evidence-Based Guidelines for Preventing Healthcare-Associated Infections in NHS Hospitals in England. *Journal of Hospital Infection*, 86S1, S1–S70.

Loveman, E. & Gale, A. (2000) Factors influencing nurses' inferences about patient pain. *British Journal of Nursing*, 9(6), 334–337.

Lynch, M.E. & Campbell, F. (2011) Cannabinoids for treatment of chronic non-cancer pain; a systematic review of randomized trials. *British Journal of Clinical Pharmacology*, 72(5), 735–744.

Macintyre, P.E. & Schug, S.A. (2015) *Acute Pain Management: A Practical Guide*, 4th edn. Boca Raton, FL: CRC Press.

Macintyre, P.E., Scott, D.A, Schug, S.A., Visser, E.J. & Walker, S.M. (eds) (2010) *Acute Pain Management: Scientific Evidence*, 3rd edn. Melbourne: ANZCA and FPM.

Mackintosh, C. & Elson, S. (2008) Chronic pain: clinical features, assessment and treatment. *Nursing Standard*, 23(95), 48–56.

Macpherson, H., Thomas, K., Wakters, S. & Fitter, M. (2001) The York acupuncture safety study: prospective survey of 34,000 treatments by traditional acupuncturist. *BMJ*, 323(7311), 486–487.

Majithia, N., Temkin, S., Ruddy, K.J., et al. (2016) National Cancer Institute-supported chemotherapy-induced peripheral neuropathy trials: outcomes and lesson. *Supportive Cancer in Care*, 24(3), 1439–1447.

Manikandan, R., Srirangam, S.J., Brown, S.C., O'Reilly, P.H. & Collins, G.N. (2003) Nitrous oxide vs periprostatic nerve block with 1% lidocaine during transrectal ultrasound guided biopsy of the prostate: a prospective, randomized, controlled trial. *Journal of Urology*, 170(5), 1881–1883.

Mann, E. (2008) Neuropathic pain: could nurses become more involved? *British Journal of Nursing*, 17(19), 1208–1213.

Mann, E. & Carr, E. (2006) *Pain Management*. Oxford: Blackwell Publishing.

Mantyh, P.W. (2014) Bone cancer pain: from mechanism to therapy. *Current Opinion in Supportive and Palliative Care*, 8(2), 83–90.

Maze, M. & Fujinaga, M. (2000) Recent advances in understanding the actions and toxicity of nitrous oxide. *Anaesthesia*, 55(4), 311–314.

McCaffery, M. & Beebe, A. (1989) Perspectives on pain. In: McCaffery, M. & Beebe, A. (eds) *Pain: Clinical Manual for Nursing Practice*. St Louis, MO: Mosby, pp. 1–5.

McCaffery, M. & Ferrell, B.R. (1997) Nurses' knowledge of pain assessment and management: how much progress have we made? *Journal of Pain and Symptom Management*, 14(3), 175–188.

McCaffery, M. & Pasero, C. (1999) *Pain Clinical Manual*, 2nd edn. St Louis, MO: Mosby.

McCaffery, M. & Robinson, E.S. (2002) Your patient is in pain – here's how you respond. *Nursing*, 32(10), 36–45.

McCaffrey, R. (1968) *Nursing Practice Theories Relating to Cognition, Bodily Pain and Man Environment.* Los Angeles, CA: University of California Los Angeles.

McCaffrey, R. (2000) *Nursing Management of the Patient with Pain*, 3rd edn. Philadelphia, PA: Lippincott Williams & Wilkins.

McQuay, H.J., Moore, A. & Justins, D. (1997) Treating acute pain in hospital. *BMJ*, 314(7093), 1531–1535.

Medicines and Healthcare Products Regulatory Agency (MHRA) (2005) Medical Device Alert Ref. MDA/2005/027. Heat patches or heat packs intended for pain relief. London: MHRA.

Mercadante, S. (1999) Problems of long-term spinal opioid treatment in advanced cancer patients. *Pain*, 79(1), 1–13.

Mimoz, O., Karim, A., Mercat, A., et al. (1999) Chlorhexidine compared with povidone-iodine as skin preparation before blood culture. A randomized, controlled trial. *Annals of Internal Medicine*, 131(11), 834–837.

Morley, J.S. & Makin, M.K. (1998) The use of methadone in cancer pain poorly responsive to other opioids. *Pain Reviews*, 5(1), 51–59.

Mucci-LoRusso, P., Berman, B.S., Silberstein, P.T., et al. (1998) Controlled-release oxycodone compared with controlled-release morphine in the treatment of cancer pain: a randomized, double-blind, parallel-group study. *European Journal of Pain*, 2(3), 239–249.

Nagashima, M., Ooshiro, M., Moriyama, A., et al. (2014) Efficacy and tolerability of controlled-release oxycodone for oxaliplatin-induced peripheral neuropathy and the extension of FOLFOX therapy in advanced colorectal cancer patients. *Supportive Care in Care*, 22(6), 1579–1584.

National Patient Safety Agency (NPSA) (2007) *The Fifth Report from the Patient Safety Observatory: Safer Care for the Acutely Ill Patient: Learning from Serious Incident.* London: NPSA. Available at: www.nrls.npsa.nhs.uk/resources/?entryid45=59828

National Patient Safety Agency (NPSA) (2009) *Safer Spinal (Intrathecal), Epidural and Regional Devices – Part B.* London: NPSA. Available at: www.nrls.npsa.nhs.uk/alerts/?entryid45=94529

Ngamkham, S., Vincent, C. & Funnegan, L., et al. (2012) The McGill Pain Questionnaire as a multidimensional measure in people with cancer: an integrative review. *Pain Management Nurse*, 13, 27–51.

NICE (2015) *Non-Steroidal Anti-Inflammatory Drugs.* London: NICE. Available at: https://www.nice.org.uk/advice/ktt13 (Accessed: 17/4/2018)

NICE (2016). *Palliative Care for Adults: Strong Opioids for Pain Relief.* May 2012, updated August 2016. London: NICE. Available at: https://www.nice.org.uk/guidance/cg140 (Accessed: 17/4/2018)

NICE (2017) *Neuropathic Pain in Adults: Pharmacological Management in Non-Specialist Settings.* CG173. London: NICE. Available at: https://www.nice.org.uk/guidance/cg173 (Accessed: 17/4/2018)

Nickel, F.T., Seifert, F., Lanz, S. & Maihofner, C. (2012) Mechanisms of neuropathic pain. *European Neuropsychopharmacology*, 22, 81–91.

Nursing & Midwifery Council (NMC) (2010) *Record Keeping: Guidance for Nurses and Midwives.* London: NMC. Available at: https://www.nmc.org.uk/standards/code/record-keeping (Accessed: 17/4/2018)

Nursing & Midwifery Council (NMC) (2015) *The Code: Professional Standards of Practice and Behaviour for Nurses and Midwives.* London: NMC. Available at: https://www.nmc.org.uk/globalassets/sitedocuments/nmc-publications/nmc-code.pdf (Accessed: 17/4/2018)

O'Neill, J. (2012) Chapter 7. Practical nursing management of epidural and intrathecal infusions. In: Hester, J., Sykes, N. & Peat, S. (eds) *Interventional Pain Control in Cancer Pain Management.* Oxford: Oxford University Press.

Orenius, T., Koskela, T., Koho, P., et al. (2013) Anxiety and depression are independent predictors of quality of life of patients with chronic musculoskeletal pain. *Journal of Health Psychology*, 18(2), 167–175.

O'Sullivan, I. & Benger, J. (2003) Nitrous oxide in emergency medicine. *Emergency Medicine Journal*, 20(3), 214–217.

Pargeon, K.L. & Hailey, B.J. (1999) Barriers to effective cancer pain management: a review of the literature. *Journal of Pain and Symptom Management*, 18(5), 358–368.

Parizkova, B. & George, S. (2009a) Regional anaesthesia and analgesia, Part 1: peripheral nerve blockade. In: Cox, F. (ed.) *Perioperative Pain Management.* Oxford: John Wiley & Sons.

Parizkova, B. & George, S. (2009b) Regional anaesthesia and analgesia, Part 2: central neural blockade. In: Cox, F. (ed.) *Perioperative Pain Management.* Oxford: John Wiley & Sons.

Park, J.E., Lee, M.S., Choi, J.Y., et al. (2010) Adverse events associated with acupuncture: a prospective survey. *Journal of Alternative and Complementary Medicine*, 16 (9), 959–963.

Parker, L. (2004) Infection control: maintaining the personal hygiene of patients and staff. *British Journal of Nursing*, 13(4), 474–478.

Parlow, J.L., Milne, B., Tod, D.A., Stewart, G.I., Griffiths, J.M. & Dudgeon, D.J. (2005) Self-administered nitrous oxide for the management of incident pain in terminally ill patients: a blinded case series. *Palliative Medicine*, 19(1), 3–8.

Pasero, C. & McCaffery, M. (2011) Intraspinal analgesia (epidural and intrathecal). In: *Pain Assessment and Pharmacologic Management.* St Louis, MO: Elsevier Mosby.

Peat, S. & Hester, J. (2012) Chapter 2. Difficult pain problems. In: Hester, J., Sykes, N. & Peat, S. (eds). *Interventional Pain Control in Cancer Pain Management.* Oxford: Oxford University Press.

Peat, S., Fai, K. & Hester, J. (2012) Chapter 8. Peripheral blocks, plexus blocks and intrathecal neurolysis. In: Hester, J., Sykes, N. & Peat, S (eds). *Interventional Pain Control in Cancer Pain Management.* Oxford: Oxford University Press.

Peate, I. & Lancaster, J. (2000) Safe use of medical gases in the clinical setting: practical tips. *British Journal of Nursing*, 9(4), 231–237.

Pickup, S. & Pagdin, J. (2000) Procedural pain: Entonox can help. *Paediatric Nursing*, 12(10), 33–37.

Portenoy, R.K. (2011) Treatment of cancer pain. *Lancet*, 377, 2236–2247.

Portenoy, R.K., Payne, R., Coluzzi, P., et al. (1999) Oral transmucosal fentanyl citrate (OTFC) for the treatment of breakthrough pain in cancer patients: a controlled dose titration study. *Pain*, 79(2–3), 303–312.

Postma, T.J, Aaronson, N.K., Heimans J.J., et al. (2005) The development of an EORTC quality of life questionnaire to assess chemotherapy-induced peripheral neuropathy: the QLQ-CIPN20. *European Journal of Cancer*, 41(8), 1135–1139.

Preston, R.M. (2005) Aseptic technique: evidence-based approach for patient safety. *British Journal of Nursing*, 14(10), 540–542, 544–546.

Proudfoot, C., Garry, E., Cottrell, D., Rosie, R., Fleetwood-Walker, S.M. & Mitchell, R. (2006) Analgesia mediated by the TRPM8 cold receptor in chronic neuropathic pain. *Current Biology*, 16, 1591–1650.

Raiman, J. (1986) Coping with pain. Pain relief – a two-way process. *Nursing Times*, 82(15), 24–28.

Rao, R.D., Michalak, J.C., Sloan, J.A., et al. (2007) Efficacy of gabapentin in the management of chemotherapy-induced peripheral neuropathy: a phase 3 randomized, double-blind, placebo-controlled, crossover trial (N00C3). *Cancer*, 110, 2110–2118.

Raphael, J., Ahmedzai, S., Hester, J. et al. (2010) Cancer pain: part 1: Pathophysiology; oncological, pharmacological, and psychological treatments: a perspective from the British Pain Society endorsed by the UK Association of Palliative Medicine and the Royal College of General Practitioners. *Pain Medicine*, 11(5), 742–764.

Rauch, R.L., Tark, M., Reyes, E., et al. (2009) Efficacy and long term tolerability of sublingual fentanyl oral disintegrating tablet in the treatment of breakthrough cancer pain. *Current Medical Research and Opinion*, 25(12), 2877–2885.

Ready, L. & Edwards, W. (1992) *Management of Acute Pain: A Practical Guide.* Seattle, WA: IASP Publications.

Reicin, A., Brown, J., Jove, M., et al. (2001) Efficacy of single-dose and multidose rofecoxib in the treatment of post-orthopedic surgery pain. *American Journal of Orthopedics*, 30(1), 40–48.

Reid, C. & Davies, A. (2004) The World Health Organization three-step analgesic ladder comes of age. *Palliative Medicine*, 18, 175–176.

Richman, J.M., Liu, S.S., Courpas, G., et al (2006) Does continuous peripheral nerve block provide superior pain control to opioids? A meta analysis. *Anesthesia and Analgesia*, 28(4), 279–288.

Riley, J. (2006) An overview of opioids in palliative care. *European Journal of Palliative Care*, 13(6), 230–233.

Riley, J. (2012) Conference Paper presentation. Morphine or oxycodone for cancer pain? A randomized controlled trial comparing response to first-line opioid and clinical efficacy of opioid switching. Norway: European Association of Palliative Care Research.

Ripamonti, C.I., Santini, E., Maranzano, E., et al. (2012) Management of cancer pain: ESMO Clinical Practice Guidelines. *Annals of Oncology* 23(Supplement 7), vii139–vii154.

Rockford, M. & DeRuyter, M. (2009) Perioperative epidural analgesia. In: Smith, H. (ed.) *Current Therapies in Pain*. Philadelphia, PA: Elsevier.

Romer, H.C. & Russell, G.N. (1998) A survey of the practice of thoracic epidural analgesia in the United Kingdom. *Anaesthesia*, 53(10), 1016–1022.

Romsing, J., Moiniche, S. & Dahl, J.B. (2002) Rectal and parenteral paracetamol, and paracetamol in combination with NSAIDs, for postoperative analgesia. *British Journal of Anaesthesia*, 88(2), 215–226.

Rosen, M.A. (2002) Nitrous oxide for relief of labor pain: a systematic review. *American Journal of Obstetrics and Gynecology*, 186(5 suppl), S110–S126.

Rowbotham, D.J. (2000) Non-steroidal anti-inflammatory drugs and paracetamol. In: Rowbotham, D.J. (ed.) *Chronic Pain*. London: Martin Dunitz, pp. 19–26.

Royal College of Anaesthetists (2006) Section 1. Key issues in developing new materials. In: Lack, J.A., Rollin, A.M., Thoms, G., White, L. & Williamson, C. (eds) *Raising the Standard: Information for Patients*, 2nd edn. London: Royal College of Anaesthetists, pp. 14–29.

Royal College of Anaesthetists (2010) *Best Practice in the Management of Epidural Analgesia in the Hospital Setting*. London: Royal College of Anaesthetists and Faculty of Pain Medicine.

Royse, C.F., Hall, J. & Royse, A.G. (2006) The 'mesentery' dressing for epidural catheter fixation. *Anaesthesia*, 61(7), 713.

Sagar S.M. & Capsulet, B.R. (2005) Integrative oncology for comprehensive cancer centers: definitions, scope and policy. *Current Oncology*, 12, 103–117.

Saunders, C.M. (1978) *The Management of Terminal Malignant Disease*. London: Edward Arnold.

Schofield, P. (2018) The assessment of pain in older people: UK National Guidelines. *Age and Ageing*, 47, (1)1, i1–i22. https://doi.org/10.1093/ageing/afx192

Schroeder, S., Mayer-Hamme, G. & Epplee, S. (2012) Acupuncture for chemotherapy-induced peripheral neuropathy (CIPN): A pilot study using neurography. *Acupuncture in Medicine*, 30 (1), 4–7.

Schug, S.A. & Chong, C. (2009) Pain management after ambulatory surgery. *Current Opinion in Anaesthesiology*, 22(6), 738–743.

Schwartz, S., Etropolski, M., Shapiro, D.Y., et al. (2011) Safety and efficacy of tapentadol ER in patients with painful diabetic peripheral neuropathy: results of a randomized-withdrawal, placebo-controlled trial. *Current Medical Research Opinion*, 27(91), 151–162.

Sharma, M. & Gupta, S. (2014) Chapter 7. Mesothelioma and chest wall pain. In: Sharma, M.L., Simpson, K.H., Bennett, M.I., Gupta, S. (eds) *Practical Management of Complex Cancer Pain*. Oxford: Oxford University Press.

Simpson, K.H. (2011) Interventional techniques for pain management in palliative care. *Medicine*, 39(11), 645–647.

Sindrup, S.H. & Jensen, T.S. (1999) Efficacy of pharmacological treatments of neuropathic pain: an update and effect related to mechanism of drug action. *Pain*, 83(3), 389–400.

Sloan, P.A. (2004) The evolving role of interventional pain management in oncology. *Journal of Supportive Oncology*, 2(6), 491–500, 503.

Smitt, P.S., Tsafka, A., teng-van de Zande, F., et al. (1998) Outcome and complications of epidural analgesia in patients with chronic cancer pain. *Cancer*, 83(9), 2015–2022.

Stannard, C.F. & Booth, S. (2004) Clinical pharmacology. In: Stannard, C.F. & Booth, S. (eds) *Churchill's Pocket Book of Pain*, 2nd edn. London: Elsevier Churchill Livingstone.

Tan, G., Jensen, M.P., Thornby, J.I. & Shanti, B.F. (2004) Validation of the Brief Pain Inventory for chronic nonmalignant pain. *Journal of Pain*, 5(2), 1331–1337.

Taverner, T. (2015) Neuropathic pain in people with cancer (part 2): pharmacological and non-pharmacological management. *International Journal of Palliative Care Nursing*, 21(8), 380–384.

Tofthagen, C. (2010) Patient perceptions associated with chemotherapy induced peripheral neuropathy (online exclusive). *Clinical Journal of Oncology Nursing*, 14, E22–E28.

Tofthagen, C., Visovsky, C.M. & Hopgood, R. (2013) Chemotherapy-induced peripheral neuropathy: an algorithm to guide nursing management. *Clinical Journal of Oncology Nursing*, 17(2), 138–144.

Tortora, G.J. & Derrickson, B.H. (2011) *Principles of Anatomy and Physiology*, 13th edn. Hoboken, NJ: John Wiley & Sons.

Towler, P., Molassiotis, A. & Brearley, S.G. (2013) What is the evidence for the use of acupuncture as an intervention for symptom management in cancer supportive and palliative care: an integrative overview of reviews. *Supportive Care Cancer*, 21(10), 2913–2923.

Trelle, S., Reichenbach S., Wandel S., et al. (2011) Cardiovascular safety of non-steroidal anti-inflammatory drugs: network meta-analysis. *BMJ*, 342, c7086.

Trojan, J., Saunders, B.P., Woloshynowych, M., Debinsky, H.S. & Williams, C.B. (1997) Immediate recovery of psychomotor function after patient-administered nitrous oxide/oxygen inhalation for colonoscopy. *Endoscopy*, 29(1), 17–22.

Twycross, R. & Wilcock, A. (2001) Chapter 2. Pain relief. In: *Symptom Management in Advanced Cancer*. Abingdon: Radcliffe Medical Press.

Twycross, R., Harcourt, J. & Bergl, S. (1996) A survey of pain in patients with advanced cancer. *Journal of Pain and Symptom Management*, 12(5), 273–282.

Twycross R., Wilcock A. & Howard P. (2014) *Palliative Care Formulary*. palliativedrugs.com.

Tzatha, E. & DeAngelis, L.M. (2016) Chemotherapy-induced peripheral neuropathy. *Oncology*, 30(3), 240–244.

Urban, D., Cherny, N. & Catane, R. (2010) The management of cancer pain in the elderly. *Oncology Hematology*, 73(2), 176–183.

Urdan, L.D., Stacy, K.M. & Lough, M.E. (2006) Pain and pain management. In: Urdan, L.D., Stacy, K.M. & Lough, M.E. (eds) *Thelan's Critical Care Nursing Diagnosis and Management*, 5th edn. St Louis, MO: Mosby Elsevier.

Vaajoki, A., Pietilä, A.M., Kankkunen, P. & Vehviläinen-Julkunen, K. (2012) Effects of listening to music on pain intensity and pain distress after surgery: an intervention. *Journal of Clinical Nursing*, 21(5–6), 708–717.

van den Beuken-van Everdingen, M.H., Hochstenbach, L.M., Joosten, E.A., Tjan-Heijnen, V.C. & Janssen, D.J. (2016) Update on prevalence of pain in patients with cancer: systematic review and meta-analysis. *Journal of Pain and Symptom Management*, 51(6), 1070–1090.e9.

Ventzel, L., Jensen, A.B., Jensen, A.R., Jensen, T.S. & Finnerup, N.B. (2016) Chemotherapy-induced pain and neuropathy: a prospective study in patients treated with adjuvant oxaliplatin or docetaxel. *Pain*, 157(3), 560–568.

Vondrackova, D., Leyendecker, P., Meissner, W., et al. (2008) Analgesic efficacy and safety of oxycodone in combination with naloxone as prolonged release tablets in patients with moderate to severe chronic pain. *Journal of Pain*, 9(12), 1144–1154.

Walker, S.M., Macintyre, P.E., Visser, E. & Scott, D. (2006) Acute pain management: current best evidence provides guide for improved practice. *Pain Medicine*, 7(1), 3–5.

Walker, V., Dicks, B. & Webb, P. (1987) Pain assessment charts in the management of chronic cancer pain. *Palliative Medicine*, 1(2), 111–116.

Wallace, M.S. (2002) Treatment options for refractory pain: the role of intrathecal therapy. *Neurology*, 59 (5 Suppl 2), S18–S24.

Weetman, C. & Allison, W. (2006) Use of epidural analgesia in post-operative pain management. *Nursing Standard*, 20(44), 54–64.

Wheatley, R.G., Schug, S.A. & Watson, D. (2001) Safety and efficacy of postoperative epidural analgesia. *British Journal of Anaesthesia*, 87(1), 47–61.

White, A., Cummings, M. & Filshie, J. (2008) *An Introduction to Western Medical Acupuncture*. Edinburgh: Churchill Livingstone Elsevier.

Wild, J.E., Grond, S., Kuperwasser, B., et al. (2010) Long-term safety and tolerability of tapentadol extended release for the management of chronic low back pain or osteoarthritis pain. *Pain Practice*, 10(5), 416–427.

Wong, R. & Sagar, S. (2006) Acupuncture treatment for chemotherapy induced peripheral neuropathy – case series. *Acupuncture in Medicine*, 24(2), 87–91.

World Health Organization (WHO) (1996) *Cancer Pain Relief*, 2nd edn (with a guide to opioid availability). Geneva: WHO.

Xiao, W.H. & Bennett, G.J. (2008) Chemotherapy-evoked neuropathic pain: abnormal spontaneous discharge in A-fiber and C-fiber primary afferent neurons and its suppression by acetyl-L-carnitine. *Pain*, 135, 262–270.

Zeppetella, G. (2011) Breakthrough pain in cancer patients. *Clinical Oncology (The Royal College of Radiologists)*, 23, 393–398.

Chapter 4

Administration of systemic anticancer therapies

Procedure guidelines

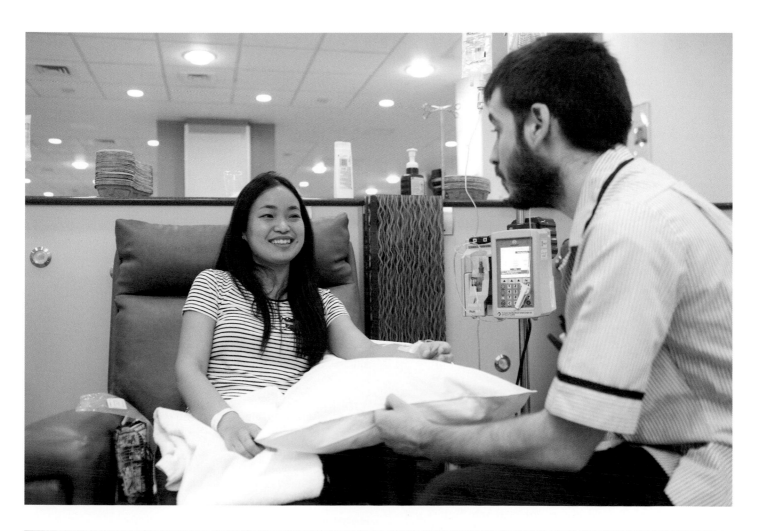

The Royal Marsden Manual of Cancer Nursing Procedures. Edited by Sara Lister and Lisa Dougherty, with Assistant Editor Louise McNamara.
© 2019 The Royal Marsden NHS Foundation Trust. Published 2019 by John Wiley & Sons, Ltd.

Overview

This chapter focuses upon the theoretical and practical aspects of administering chemotherapy. Procedure guidelines are included in the text as well as essential information provided in the tables and boxes. The use of the terms SACT and chemotherapy are used interchangeably throughout this chapter, SACT refers to any medication using any route that has direct anti-tumour activity including cytotoxic chemotherapy such as carboplatin, monoclonal antibodies and immunotherapy. SACT does not refer to hormonal medication or intrathecal chemotherapy (UKONS 2018).

Systemic anticancer treatment

Definition

Advances in knowledge relating to the functioning of the cancer cell have led to a greater understanding of the signalling pathways and molecular processes that allow a cancer cell to proliferate, resist attrition and invade other organs (Eggert 2018). Systemic anticancer therapy (SACT) encompasses both biological therapy (therapies that use the body's immune system to fight cancer or to lessen the side-effects that may be caused by some cancer treatments) and cytotoxic chemotherapy (a group of medicines containing chemicals directly toxic to cells, preventing their replication or growth and so active against cancer) (Scottish Government 2012).

Related theory

Cytotoxic drugs

The term 'cytotoxic', literally translated, means 'toxic to cells'. Hence cytotoxic drugs are those which kill cells (malignant or non-malignant). Chemotherapy works by disrupting cellular growth and causing damage to DNA, RNA and proteins (Dougherty and Bailey 2008, Skeel 2016). The aim of chemotherapy is to prevent cancer cells multiplying, invading or metastasizing, and optimizing survival (Skeel 2016).

All proliferating cells (normal cells and cancer cells) go through the same division cycle (Figure 4.1). The cell cycle is a series of phases through which cells must pass as they replicate (Dougherty and Bailey 2008). The DNA in a parent cell replicates and divides, producing two daughter cells.

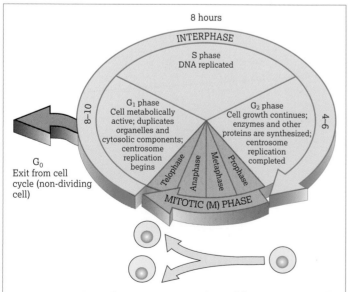

Figure 4.1 The cell cycle. *Source:* Adapted from Tortora and Derrickson (2009). Reproduced with permission of John Wiley & Sons.

- Following cell division or mitosis (M) (which occurs within an hour), cells enter the first gap or G phase, where cells prepare to synthesize DNA but where synthesis of RNA and protein occurs.
- The next phase, called the S phase or synthesis phase (which occurs within 10–20 hours), results in the cells doubling their DNA content. Many cytotoxic drugs work by disrupting the genetic codes during DNA synthesis.
- The second gap or G_2 phase (can last from 2 to 10 hours) is where the cell is preparing for division. DNA synthesis stops while RNA synthesis and protein synthesis continue in preparation for mitosis (Yarbro et al. 2016).
- Mitosis occurs in the final stage of the cell cycle, M phase, and can last from 30 to 90 minutes. At the end of this phase, cells either rejoin the cell cycle at G or enter the resting subphase G_0.

Cancer chemotherapy drugs tend to be administered in combination, which means that they can act upon different phases of the cell cycle, thus producing maximum cytotoxic effect. Many drugs are licensed for the treatment of cancer and most of these (with the exception of antihormonal drugs used to treat breast and prostate cancers) target rapidly dividing cells, either through the effects on DNA or factors involved in mitosis (Kelland 2005). A greater understanding of the molecular biology of both normal and cancer cells has resulted in significant developments in targeting mechanisms of tumour growth, invasion and metastasis.

Cancer immunology

This relates to the interactions between the immune system and cancer cells. The functioning of the immune system has an impact upon the development and management of cancer (Yarbro et al. 2016). The immune system functions as a result of different organs and tissues (bone marrow, spleen, thymus, circulatory and lymphatic system) working together to prevent infection. There are two types of immune response, based on their roles in response to an antigen: innate and adaptive (Polovich et al. 2014). The first response, which involves neutrophils, monocytes, macrophages and large granular lymphocytes, does not produce an immunological memory whereas the secondary adaptive response, involving lymphocytes, B cells and T cells, has a specific memory.

Cells in the immune system express proteins on the surface of the cell membrane which are referred to as markers or clusters of differentiation (CD) (Yarbro et al. 2016). These markers, such as CD4 and CD20, are used to create cell-specific therapy which is prevalent in the management of cancer.

Biological and molecular targeted therapy

Molecular targeted therapy (MTT) is a new aspect of cancer treatment that has resulted from the vast number of molecular and biological advances into the aetiology of cancer over the last few decades (Skeel 2016). These drugs have been developed to specifically target molecules that are uniquely or abnormally expressed within cancer cells whilst sparing normal cells. Once the targeted molecule has been switched off, the cancer cell is not able to develop a resistance to the therapeutic agent. There are two different classifications of MMT based upon each molecule's targeting strategy: function-directed therapy, which targets specific cellular pathways, and phenotype-directed therapy, which targets the unique phenotype of the cancer cell relying on non-specific mechanisms to kill the cancer cells (Skeel 2016). Epidermal growth factor receptors (EGFRs) are proteins that belong to the larger tyrosine kinase family. In a healthy cell, EGFRs allow cells to grow and divide, however too many receptors caused by a mutation or cancer allow the cancer cells to grow and divide. Tyrosine kinase inhibitors block EGFRs from working and therefore can slow or stop tumour growth. Examples of drugs that inhibit EGFRs are cetuximab, panitumumab, trastuzumab, pertuzumab and bevacizumab.

Hormone agents

The hormone agents that are used to treat cancer include steroids, oestrogens, progestins, androgens, corticoids and their synthetic derivatives, non-steroidal compounds with steroid or steroid-antagonist activity, aromatase inhibitors, hypothalamic–pituitary analogues and thyroid hormones (Toumeh and Skeel 2016).

Safe handling of hazardous drugs

Evidence-based approaches

There are hazards associated with many drugs but the highest risks are those associated with cytotoxic drugs because these chemicals can pose a risk to healthcare workers. Cytotoxic drug handling by nursing, pharmacy and other healthcare professionals is an occupational hazard (Weinstein and Hagle 2014). Cytotoxic drugs have been shown to be mutagenic, teratogenic and carcinogenic when given at therapeutic levels to animals and humans to destroy malignant cells (Weinstein and Hagle 2014).

Patients receive cytotoxic drugs over a period of months whereas healthcare workers are exposed to low levels of the drugs over a period of years, and risks from exposure need to be minimized at every opportunity (Polovich et al. 2014). The potential benefits of treatment for the patient outweigh the risk to them; healthcare workers have no benefit but are at risk of harm through exposure.

The American National Institute for Occupational Safety and Health (NIOSH 2014) described six characteristics of hazardous drugs:

- Carcinogenicity.
- Teratogenicity/developmental toxicity.
- Reproductive toxicity.
- Organ toxicity at low doses.
- Genotoxicity.

New drugs with structural and toxicity profiles that mimic those of existing drugs are regarded as hazardous, based on these criteria (NIOSH 2014).

In 2015, the International Agency for Research on Cancer (IARC) and the World Health Organization (WHO) re-evaluated over 1000 chemical drugs to examine their carcinogenic potential to humans which reconfirmed cytotoxic drugs as hazardous (BJN 2016).

Common routes of exposure for healthcare workers are:

- contact with skin or mucous membranes (e.g. through accidental spillage or splashing)
- inhalation: aerosol, vapours and particles
- ingestion: eating/drinking in clinical areas/contaminated residue on the hands reaching the mouth
- percutaneous injury: needlestick injury (less common).

The risk to health associated with exposure is measured by the time, dose and routes of exposure. Safe levels of exposure to hazardous agents cannot be determined because of the lack of a reliable monitoring method to measure risk, so personal protective equipment (PPE) is vital for the protection of healthcare workers (Polovich et al. 2014). Many studies have demonstrated that healthcare workers are exposed to cytotoxic drugs through drug residue on contaminated worksurfaces, vial surfaces and surfaces in drug administration areas (Polovich et al. 2014). Cytotoxic drugs can be absorbed through the skin (although with the majority of the compounds there is little or no absorption through intact skin; the exceptions are those which are lipid soluble) (Weinstein and Hagle 2014). Skin exposure can occur by contact with contaminated equipment used in preparing or administering the drugs or during the handling and disposal of waste. More than 60 studies have demonstrated the presence of cytotoxic drugs in the urine of nurses and pharmacy personnel who were routinely involved in the handling of cytotoxic drugs (Polovich et al. 2014). Some studies have reported measurable amounts of drugs in personnel who did not report handling them, which may suggest that exposure happened because of contaminated workplace surfaces (Friese et al. 2015).

It is imperative therefore that the risks of exposure are kept to a minimum and that the workplace has a Control of Substances Hazardous to Health (COSHH) risk assessment completed to assess the level of risk and ensure that control measures are in place (HSE 2017).

In 2016 the European Parliament released 'Preventing occupational exposure to cytotoxic and other hazardous drugs', which is a list of 11 recommendations relating to protecting healthcare personnel and reducing exposure to a minimum (European Policy Recommendations 2016). It also advises that actions should be taken in the hierarchical order of prevention as set out by the International Society of Oncology Pharmacy Practitioners (ISOPP) 2007 (BJN 2016):

- Engineering controls are related to biological safety cabinets, aseptic isolators and closed system transfer devices
- Administrative controls include education and training relating to all aspects of cytotoxic drug handling, disposal and management of spillage, competency assessment of the healthcare worker and PPE to be worn at all times when handling cytotoxics (BJN 2016)
- Workplace controls include ensuring that all procedures and practices are organized in a manner such that exposure and environmental contamination are minimized at every stage of the work flow pathway including disposal of waste
- Risks to personnel involved in the reconstitution and administration of cytotoxic drugs fall into three categories: acute effects, chronic effects and reproductive risks and systemic effects.

Acute effects

These are usually caused by direct contact with the skin, eyes and mucous membranes, for example dermatitis, inflammation of mucous membranes, excessive lacrimation, pigmentation, nausea, headaches, blistering (associated with mustine) and other miscellaneous, allergic reactions (Dranitsaris et al. 2005, European Policy Recommendations 2016, Weinstein and Hagle 2014).

Chronic effects and reproductive risks

Chronic effects may last for years and include damage to the bone marrow and kidney as well as effects on reproduction (European Policy Recommendations 2016). There is an association between the risk of cancer and handling cytotoxic drugs although it is difficult to quantify (Polovich et al. 2014).

Reproductive risks include menstrual dysfunction and infertility following exposure to cytotoxic drugs (European Policy Recommendations 2016, Polovich et al. 2014). Studies have suggested that serious long-term effects may result from exposure to cytotoxic drugs during pregnancy. Effects include miscarriages and stillbirths (Valanis et al. 1999), chromosomal abnormalities (Polovich et al. 2014), low birthweight and congenital abnormalities. However, when analysing the data, consideration needs to be given to the fact that most of the studies were conducted in the 1980s or based on staff exposure data from that time. During that period, PPE and safe working practices were not well established and therefore these data do not reflect current working practices.

The issue is of high importance to staff, and organizational procedures should be in place to minimize the risk of exposure to all staff at all times. A literature review by Gilani and Giridharan (2014) showed that the risk of handling cytotoxic drugs could be reduced if staff adhered to the standard safety precautions (BJN 2016). It has been suggested that nurses 'avoid working in high risk areas during the first 84 days of their pregnancy' and that standard safety precautions including PPE should be adhered to (Gilani and Giridharan 2014). The Health and Safety Executive has issued guidance for new and expectant mothers and states that because 'a safe level of exposure cannot be determined for these drugs, one should avoid exposure or reduce it to as low a level as possible' (HSE 2017).

Systemic effects

It has been shown that although alterations in cell structure have been detected, they appear to be transient and at a low level. Studies have shown that changes to the DNA can occur following occupational exposure to cytotoxic drugs. Researchers demonstrated that DNA strand breaks were higher in exposed nurses than in controls (Polovich et al. 2014). A comet assay was used by Yoshida et al. (2006) and revealed that a greater DNA tail length, which was due to the unravelling of genetic material, was present in nurses who routinely handled cytotoxic drugs as opposed to those who did not (Yoshida et al. 2006). Furthermore, chromosomal abnormalities in peripheral blood lymphocytes were identified in nurses and pharmacists who were handling alkylating agents (McDiarmid et al. 2010).

There is no legal obligation for employers to screen healthcare workers exposed to cytotoxic drugs; however, the Health and Safety Executive provides advice relating to the 'health surveillance cycle' which advocates that the employer should apply surveillance according to need (HSE 2017). Since occupational hazards of cytotoxic drugs pose a health risk for healthcare personnel, minimizing the risk of exposure by strict adherence to organizational policies is vital and the emphasis should be on clear guidelines to reduce occupational exposure to all staff at all times (BJN 2016, European Policy Recommendations 2016, Polovich et al. 2014).

Cytotoxic drugs may also have harmful short- or long-term systemic effects if inhaled or ingested during preparation or handling. These effects include light-headedness, dizziness, nausea, headache, rashes and skin discolouration and are normally associated with accidental spillage of the drugs during handling or with surface contamination (Polovich et al. 2014).

Legal and professional issues

The hazards of handling cytotoxic drugs are well recognized, along with the requirement to adhere to safety measures recommended to protect all staff who prepare, administer and handle cytotoxic drugs or waste products. The Control of Substances Hazardous to Health (COSHH) Regulations (HM Government 2002) were updated in 2017. The Health and Safety Executive (HSE 2017) has provided a document on the safe handling of cytotoxic drugs. National evidence-based guidelines have been implemented to reduce exposure, provide adequate protective equipment, ensure regular staff monitoring and provide effective written procedures for dealing with preparation, administration, disposal and dealing with spills and accidents. To limit exposure, cytotoxic drugs should be prepared only by skilled, knowledgeable and experienced healthcare professionals (Polovich et al. 2014, RCN 2016). A full risk assessment under the COSHH Regulations must be made by all departments and wards handling, preparing or administering cytotoxics (HSE 2017). The assessment should identify all appropriate procedures for the safety of staff.

Health surveillance

It has been suggested that organizations should provide health surveillance programmes for staff exposed to hazardous drugs and that they should be an integral part of health and safety in the workplace (European Policy Recommendations 2016, Nixon and Schulmeister 2009). Some organizations offer yearly health surveillance for staff directly involved in handling cytotoxics on a regular basis, for example certain staff working in pharmacy reconstitution units. Surveillance normally includes physical examinations, blood samples and history of exposure (HSE 2017). If no surveillance is offered, a risk assessment focusing upon exposure should be initiated (Box 4.1).

Pre-procedural considerations

Equipment

It is vital for healthcare personnel to use PPE while handling cytotoxic drugs. This includes consideration of the environment.

Box 4.1 Employers' obligations regarding safe handling of cytotoxic medications (HSE 2017)

Employers are obliged to:
- identify substances that are a hazard to staff and others who may be exposed
- manage how the drugs should be handled and what to do in the event of a spill or accident
- ensure that healthcare personnel have access to the ideal environment, protective clothing, policies and procedures, a system of monitoring and recording effects, and any necessary equipment such as spill kits.

The most effective means of minimizing the hazard is to arrange for all cytotoxic drugs to be prepared on a named patient basis by trained pharmacy staff in a specially equipped area. Chemotherapy should be reconstituted in a vertical class II or III biological safety cabinet with laminar flow or an isolator if drugs are prepared on the ward (Ferguson and Wright 2002, Weinstein and Hagle 2014, Wilkes 2018). Cabinets should be situated in a dedicated area with access restricted to trained or supervised personnel.

There is no doubt that the existence of a formal hospital policy for handling cytotoxic drugs has a positive influence on the use of PPE. Minimizing occupational exposure to hazardous drugs, and therefore reducing health risks for personnel, can only be achieved by strict adherence to policies and procedures regarding the safe handling of cytotoxic drugs (Polovich et al. 2014). Protective clothing should always be worn during all types of cytotoxic drug handling (HSE 2017). There are minimum requirements for the type and degree of protective clothing which are based on possible exposure and type of environment. However, even though cytotoxic exposure is known to be harmful, many healthcare workers do not comply with some PPE precautions. Studies have demonstrated that not all PPE is worn, with approximately 95% of healthcare workers reporting wearing gloves but less than 50% wearing gowns while administering chemotherapy (Polovich and Clark 2012). A study carried out by Polovich and Clark in 2012 demonstrated that circumstances in the workplace such as a high volume of patients per day were the reason that nurses did not wear PPE. Furthermore, managers cited that a lack of time was also a reason why nurses may not use PPE (Polovich and Clark 2012).

Gloves

Disposable gloves should be worn at all times and appear to be the only type of protective clothing that most practitioners consistently wear when handling cytotoxic drugs. Polovich and Clark (2012) state that 95% of nurses routinely wear gloves when handling hazardous materials. No type of glove is completely impermeable to every cytotoxic agent and there is no consensus as to which glove material offers the best protection (Weinstein and Hagle 2014). The key points to consider when selecting gloves are the main factors that affect permeation rates, including glove thickness, lipophilicity, the nature of the solvent in which the cytotoxic drug is dissolved and glove material composition (Ferguson and Wright 2002, Polovich et al. 2014). Using poor-quality low-cost gloves is neither safe nor cost-effective. The risk of allergic reactions to latex and powdered medical gloves has been well documented in recent years. The Health and Safety Executive (HSE 2018) has issued advice on the use of these types of gloves. Powder-free gloves should be used for handling cytotoxic drugs and should be inspected for any defects before use. Gloves should be changed after 30 minutes during each work session or at the end of a work session and immediately if contaminated with cytotoxic agent or punctured (Polovich 2016). The use of gloves made of other material, such as nitrile, provides protection when dealing with a cytotoxic spill. Double gloving is recommended when reconstituting cytotoxic drugs (Polovich et al. 2014, Polovich 2016, Weinstein and Hagle 2014).

Gowns

The literature supports the use of a disposable gown for both reconstitution and administration (HSE 2017). It has been suggested that a long-sleeved, non-absorbent gown made of a low-linting, low-permeability material such as Tyvek is used (Ferguson and Wright 2002, Weinstein and Hagle 2014). Gowns coated with polyethylene or vinyl offer the best protection (Polovich 2016). Gowns should have a solid front and a back closure as well as long sleeves and tight cuffs (Polovich et al. 2014, Weinstein and Hagle 2014). Gowns are designed for single use only and should not be hung up or reapplied once removed (Polovich 2016). This will prevent drug contamination of the environment as well as the worker's clothing. Armlets and plastic aprons can be used as a substitute for long-sleeved gowns during administration (HSE 2017).

Goggles

Goggles are used to protect the eyes from splashes and particles; they should fully cover the eyes of the handler. Goggles should meet BS EN 166 requirements and be worn whenever reconstituting chemotherapy where there is a possibility of splashing or dealing with a spill (Ferguson and Wright 2002, LCA 2014a, Polovich 2016).

Masks

These should be worn whenever there is a possibility of inhalation or if the drug is being prepared in an uncontrolled environment. Masks should conform to BS EN standard. The key factor regarding respiratory protective equipment is that it fits well and is sealed properly to the wearer's face. A range of different sizes of disposable masks should be made available to healthcare workers (Ferguson and Wright 2002). A suitable dust mask or particulate respirator with a FFP2 or FFP3 filter should be used (LCA 2014a).

Waste disposal

Sharps should be placed in a sharps bin compliant with waste management regulations to ensure incineration and to prevent laceration and/or inoculation during transit and disposal (DH 2013). The government guidance on safe management of healthcare waste (HTM) 07-01, which includes cytotoxic and cytostatic waste advice, should inform local healthcare policy (DH 2005). Cytotoxic waste is segregated into purple-lidded waste bins (DH 2013). Dry waste, intravenous administration sets and other contaminated material should be placed in the appropriate waste disposal bags. The practitioner should wear gloves and an apron when disposing of contaminated waste (DH 2012, Polovich et al. 2014).

Spillage

Spillage is when cytotoxic drugs are accidentally splashed, spilled or leaked onto a surface, equipment or a person's skin or mucous membranes. Procedure guideline 4.1 should be followed when managing a spillage. Prevention measures consist of careful connection of infusions using Luer-Lok equipment to reduce risk of disconnection and spiking infusion bags flat in a plastic tray (never spike a hanging bag).

Uncontrolled exposure may lead to symptoms which may be attributed to the effects of harmful levels of cytotoxic drugs, for example headache, dizziness, eye or skin irritation.

Procedure guideline 4.1   Cytotoxic spillage management

Essential equipment
- Two plastic overshoes
- Two disposable armlets
- Two clinical waste bags
- Two pairs of disposable non-sterile vinyl or nitrile gloves
- Goggles (non-disposable): EN 166-8
- Particulate respirator mask
- Plastic apron
- Long-sleeved gown
- Paper towels
- Plastic bucket
- Copy of spillage procedure

Pre-procedure

Action	Rationale
1 Act immediately. Assess the level of exposure of any individual and isolate them from the spill.	Any spillage may become a health hazard (Polovich et al. 2014, **C**).
2 Collect spillage kit.	It contains all necessary equipment (Polovich et al. 2014, **C**).
3 Put on both pairs of gloves, goggles and a gown and then a disposable plastic apron over the gown (see **Action figure 3**).	To provide personal protection. **E**
• If there is visible powder spill, put on a good-quality particulate respirator mask.	To prevent inhalation of powder. **E**
• If spillage is on the floor, put on overshoes.	For protection and to minimize the spread of contamination. **E**

Procedure

Action	Rationale
4 Wipe up powder spillage quickly with well-dampened paper towels, starting at the outer edge of the spill area and working in a circular motion towards the middle to contain spill (Weinstein and Hagle 2014), and dispose of the towels as 'high-risk' waste.	To prevent dispersal of powder. To prevent spread of contamination to a wider area. To protect others and ensure safe disposal by incineration (DH 2012, **C**; Weinstein and Hagle 2014, **E**).
5 Mop up liquids that have been spilled on a hard surface with paper towels, starting at the outer edge of the spill area and working in a circular motion towards the middle to contain spill (Ferguson and Wright 2002), and dispose of the towels as 'high-risk' waste.	To prevent spread of contamination to a wider area. To protect others and ensure safe disposal by incineration (DH 2012, **C**).

(continued)

Procedure guideline 4.1 Cytotoxic spillage management *(continued)*

Action	Rationale
6 Wash hard surfaces at least twice with copious amounts of cold, soapy water and dry with paper towels. The floor should then be given a routine clean as soon afterwards as possible. If spillage has occurred on a carpet, it will require cleaning as soon as possible.	To remove residual contamination. **E**
• If spillage is on clothing, remove it as soon as possible and treat as 'soiled linen'.	To decontaminate clothing without hazard to laundry staff. **E**
• If spillage has penetrated clothing, wash contaminated skin liberally with soap and cold water.	To decontaminate skin and prevent drug absorption. **E**
• If spillage is on bedlinen, put on gloves and an apron, change it immediately and treat as 'soiled linen'.	To protect the patient and the laundry staff. **E**
• If an accident or spillage involving direct skin contact occurs, the area should be washed thoroughly with soapy water as soon as possible. In the event of a cytotoxic splash to the eye, irrigate thoroughly with 0.9% sodium chloride or tap water for at least 15 minutes.	To decontaminate the area and minimize the risk of drug absorption and damage (Weinstein and Hagle 2014, **E**).

Post-procedure

7 Any accident or spillage by nursing staff involving direct skin contact with a cytotoxic drug must be reported to the occupational health department and manager as soon as possible after the first aid is performed and appropriate documentation completed (see Box 4.2).	To ensure that details of accidental contact are entered in the nurse's health record and appropriate follow-up is initiated (Polovich et al. 2014, **C**).

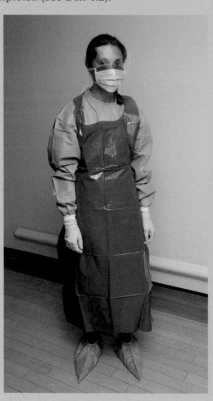

Action Figure 3 Protective clothing for spillage kit. *Source:* Dougherty and Lister (2011).

If this occurs it may be necessary to do the following:

a) Take six-monthly blood tests are taken, which include full blood count, urea and electrolytes and liver function tests.
b) Perform six-monthly urinalysis is performed to detect raised protein, presence of glucose, blood and bilirubin and any abnormal cytology.

If any abnormalities are present, the individual is referred to the occupational health doctor (Polovich 2016)

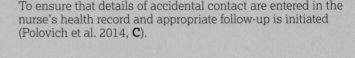

Box 4.2 Cytotoxic health surveillance

The Health and Safety Executive (2016) recommends:
• taking a detailed medical history of the individual
• maintaining an exposure record
• ensuring personal protective equipment is used
• ensuring control measures are in place.

Administration of cytotoxic medications by nurses

Legal and professional issues

The nurse is accountable to the public, patient, employer and profession. The Nursing & Midwifery Council (NMC) requires registrants to maintain and develop their knowledge and skill and to obtain help or supervision for any knowledge deficit (NMC 2015). It is important that the nurse understands the legal responsibilities of administering chemotherapy. Cytotoxic drugs can be administered via a variety of routes but, regardless of the route used, there are certain pre-administration principles that the nurse should apply. The nurse should remember that the administration of medicines is a collaborative process which involves the nurse, doctor and pharmacist (NMC 2010). Medicine administration is not solely a mechanistic task; it requires thought and exercising of professional judgement (NMC 2010). Furthermore, the nurse must operate within the limit of their competence (NMC 2015). Therefore, cytotoxic drugs should always be administered by a knowledgeable and skilled practitioner.

Competencies

Administering chemotherapy requires extensive knowledge and skill as well as practical experience (Wickham et al. 2006). To provide consistently safe, appropriate and high-quality patient care, the nurse must be assessed as being competent to administer chemotherapy. The National Chemotherapy Advisory Group (NCAG) has recognized the need for chemotherapy to be administered and managed by knowledgeable chemotherapy-trained nurses to ensure quality and safety (NCAG 2009). Individual hospitals and organizations provide educational input along with practical experience in administration of chemotherapy. The NCAG has highlighted the need for high-quality, continual professional development to maximize and provide safe and effective care. It also recommends that the National Peer Review Team audits cancer services and that subsequently areas such as nurse chemotherapy competencies should be self-assessed on a yearly basis (NCAG 2009).

National standards for safe administration of chemotherapy have been developed by the American Society of Clinical Oncology and the Oncology Nursing Society (ONS) in America, the aim of which was to improve patient safety (Neuss et al. 2016). The Royal College of Nursing has produced standards for infusion therapy and states that the nurse managing chemotherapy should have knowledge of and technical expertise in both administration and specific interventions associated with cytotoxic agents and have received education and training (RCN 2016). Standardizing education and practical guidelines for safe administration of chemotherapy reduces the risk of error. Having a comprehensive knowledge and skill base for administering chemotherapy also ensures that the nurse is fit for purpose (NMC 2010).

Competency documents, such as the UKONS Systemic Anticancer Therapy (SACT) Competency Passport (UKONS 2018), have been developed to ensure that the nurse has the required knowledge and skill to safely administer chemotherapy. Following a period of training, theoretical and practical competency needs to be demonstrated by the practitioner and recorded by the assessor. The competency is reaccredited annually. Competency frameworks and assessment tools are adopted within most organizations.

Non-medical prescribing of chemotherapy has been developed over the years, with many organizations having nurse-led chemotherapy prescription clinics as part of normal practice. The *Cancer Reform Strategy* (DH 2007) advocated nurse-led chemotherapy services for cancer patients to improve the patient experience and reduce waiting times. Improving efficiency of services for patients was echoed in the National Chemotherapy Advisory Board (DH 2009b) report which identified the need to improve the patient care experience by ensuring quality and safety. Nurse-led interventions, such as nurse-chemotherapy prescribing and assessments, are recognized as enhancing the chemotherapy care pathway for patients.

Consent

Patients have a fundamental and ethical right to determine what happens to their bodies, and consent is central to all aspects of healthcare delivery. When gaining valid consent, the nurse must be sure that the patient is a legally competent person and gives consent voluntarily after being fully informed of what they are consenting to (NMC 2015). Written consent must be obtained before chemotherapy is commenced and every time the patient is changed from one protocol/regimen to another. The National Chemotherapy Board released guidance related to the use of national regimen-specific chemotherapy consent forms which incorporates guidance on the process of providing information and gaining consent (NCB 2016). Information regarding the process of auditing consent compliance is also provided within the document. Electronic scanning of consent forms into the patient's medical record is advocated and utilized in many organizations. However, if the organization is not paperless, one copy of the consent form is kept in the medical notes while the other is given to the patient (NMC 2015).

Pre-procedural considerations

Specific patient preparations

Provision of information

The provision of patient information is an integral part of the care pathway. The patient should be fully informed of all the possible side-effects of chemotherapy, how to cope with any side-effects at home, types of supportive therapy they may receive, and where and how they are to receive the drugs (NCAG 2009, NMC 2010). Patients should then receive written information, which can be used to reinforce verbal explanation and will enable patients to spend time reading and formulating any questions about treatments (INS 2016, Scaramuzzo 2017). Patients should receive information leaflets explaining the rationale for the use of medications as well as the side-effects. Guidance based upon EU and national legislation regarding best practice requirements for patient information is provided by the Department of Health and should be used when formulating patient information leaflets (MHRA 2014).

The main aim of providing information is to help the patient and their family to gain control, reduce anxiety, improve compliance, develop realistic expectations, promote self-care, enhance participation and generate feelings of safety and security (Scaramuzzo 2017, van der Molen 2005). The nurse should consider barriers to effective communication, for example hearing difficulties, sight difficulties, culture and language barriers, and plan realistic interventions in respect of such barriers. Written information about side-effects of the treatment as well as healthcare professional contact numbers should be provided (DH 2007, NCAG 2009). Patient empowerment is essential in helping patients recognize and report side-effects, which commonly occur while they are at home. The use of a traffic light symptom-reporting tool can help the patient identify when they need to seek medical assistance (Oakley et al. 2016). A 24-hour contact number as well as advice on how to deal with emergencies should be included. Organizations should provide patients with chemotherapy alert cards that contain essential information for out-of-hours queries (NCB 2016). These alert cards should contain information about signs and symptoms that require medical intervention so that the patient is aware of when to seek advice. Many organizations advocate the use of patient-held diaries that contain information relating to symptoms and indicate to the patient which symptoms require telephone advice and which require urgent medical assistance. Empowering the patient to facilitate their own selfcare needs is vital in keeping the patient safe while they are receiving chemotherapy. A nurse-led holistic needs assessment prior to the initial chemotherapy consultation may help the patient and carer identify self-management requirements and encourage symptom reporting (NCB 2016). Many web-based information advisory and support groups such as Macmillan Cancer Support provide comprehensive information to help patients and carers understand the processes and side-effects related to chemotherapy administration.

Ascertaining whether the patient is fit for treatment

There are criteria that must be confirmed prior to administration of chemotherapy. For example, full blood count, electrolyte and renal function blood results are essential to:

- ensure that the patient is fit enough to receive the treatment; if any of the blood results are too low, then supportive therapy may be prescribed
- calculate the dose of drug, for example in the case of platinum-based drugs, ethylenediamine tetra-acetic acid (EDTA), or if 24-hour urine collection for creatinine is required (Polovich et al. 2014).

The Eastern Cooperative Oncology Group (ECOG) performance status should be recorded which shows the impact of chemotherapy upon the daily activities of the patient and thus is used to make decisions regarding dose reduction or delay in treatment (Oken et al. 1982).

Calculating body surface area

This is done by using the patient's height and weight and should be performed every time a cycle or dose of chemotherapy is given. The patient's height and weight should be recorded on the prescription chart, ideally by the person who performed the recording to avoid transcription errors. Electronic height and weight recording in the patient's notes which have integral mechanisms for prompting a double check if the weight changes by 10% help ensure corrective action is taken to adjust the dose of medication. Once the surface area is determined, this will be used to calculate the dose of a chemotherapy drug (Wilkes 2018).

Knowledge of the chemotherapy regimen

The nurse should have knowledge of the chemotherapy regimen to be checked or administered to maintain patient safety and prevent error (NMC 2010, Wickham et al. 2006). Prior to administering chemotherapy in the hospital setting, the NPSA guidance for safer practice should be adhered to, including the use of standardized patient wristbands that contain the core patient identifiers, all of which should be electronically generated (NPSA 2009). The patient's allergy status should be checked by the prescriber and checked again by the nurse prior to the administration of any drug at every medication intervention (NMC 2010). The prescription should be signed by the medical practitioner and verified by a pharmacist. Electronic prescribing and the use of computer-generated prescriptions may reduce the risk of medication error (BOPA 2015). It is recommended that two registered nurses check chemotherapy prior to administration. Independent 'double checking' involves:

1 the first check of prescription and medication carried out by one nurse, and the chart signed as 'first checker'; this can be carried out in the clinical room
2 the second check carried out by the nurse who will be administering the chemotherapy, immediately prior to administration beside the patient and signed on completion of the administration (LCA 2015a, Wilkes 2018).

Box 4.3 lists the five rights.

Intravenous administration of systemic anticancer therapy

Definition

This is the administration of SACT via a peripheral or central vein and is the route most commonly used (Polovich et al. 2014).

Evidence-based approaches

Rationale

Intravenous administration enables:

- rapid and reliable delivery of a cytotoxic drug to the tumour site
- rapid dilution of a drug, which reduces local irritation and the risk of tissue damage
- accurate titration of the drug to achieve the desired effect.

Methods of administration

Cytotoxic drugs may be administered as a direct bolus injection (Figure 4.2), a bolus via the side arm of a rapid infusion of 0.9% sodium chloride or a continuous infusion. The choice is dependent on (Wilkes 2018):

- the type of cytotoxic drug, for example etoposide is only given as an infusion
- pharmacological considerations, for example stability, need for dilution
- degree of venous irritation, for example vinorelbine is a highly irritant drug
- whether the drug is a vesicant
- the type of device *in situ*.

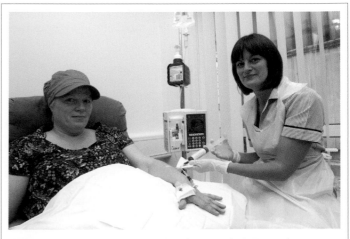

Figure 4.2 Chemotherapy bolus being administered.
Source: Dougherty and Lister (2011).

The advantage of the bolus injection is that the integrity of the vein and any early signs of extravasation can be observed more easily than during an infusion. However, bolus injections can increase the risk of venous irritation due to the constant contact of the drug with the intima of the vein, resulting in pain, which makes it difficult to differentiate between venous spasm and extravasation (Gabriel 2008). It could also lead to inappropriate rapid administration of the drug (Weinstein and Hagle 2014).

Bolus injections administered via the side arm of a rapid infusion of solution ensure greater dilution of potentially irritating drugs and enable rapid removal of the drug from the insertion site and smaller vessels. The disadvantages are that a small vein may not allow rapid flow of the infusate and this may result in the drug backing up the tubing, causing the practitioner to clamp the tubing while checking for blood return and flow rate of the infusate, therefore interrupting constant observation of the site (Gabriel 2008).

Adding the drug to an infusion bag allows for greater dilution, thus reducing the possibility of chemical irritation. Some drugs may only be administered as infusions owing to the type of side-effects associated with them (e.g. hypotension with etoposide) and long-term continuous infusions, for example of 5-fluorouracil (5-FU), may also be necessary to reduce the risk of side-effects such as diarrhoea. Patency and device position cannot be easily assessed and the longer the infusion, the greater the possibility of device dislodgement, extravasation or infiltration and general complications associated with the device (Weinstein and Hagle 2014).

Pre-procedural considerations

Equipment
SACT may be administered via a peripheral cannula or a central venous access device (CVAD). A peripheral cannula is used for bolus injections and short or intermittent infusions of both vesicant and non-vesicant drugs (Box 4.4). However, this device is associated with phlebitis and increased risk of extravasation (Gabriel 2008, INS 2006, Scales 2005). A central venous catheter is useful for patients with poor venous access, those at high risk of extravasation and those undergoing long-term, high-dose or continuous infusional chemotherapy (Gabriel 2008, Weinstein and Hagle 2014, Wilkes 2018). These devices are associated with infection and thrombosis (Dougherty 2006a).

For the peripheral route, a cannula may be used. The insertion site of choice should be the large veins of the forearm (cephalic or basilic) as these are easier to access, reduce the risk of chemical phlebitis and result in fewer problems if extravasation should occur (Weinstein and Hagle 2014). The next area

of choice would be the dorsum of the hand, then the wrist. The antecubital fossa should only be used as the last resort as it can limit movement and is associated with problems if extravasation occurs in this area (Gabriel 2008, Weinstein and Hagle 2014). The general rule is to start distally and proceed proximally where possible and also to alternate the arms (Weinstein and Hagle 2014) to ensure that the same veins are not being used and damaged by chemical and mechanical irritation (Dougherty 2008a, RCN 2016).

When using the peripheral intravenous route, the following principles should be adhered to.

- Patency should be checked at the start of administration by achieving a blood return and then flushing with 10 mL of 0.9% sodium chloride to ensure there is no resistance, swelling or pain. Blood return should then be checked after every 2–4 mL of a bolus drug is administered (Gabriel 2008, Weinstein and Hagle 2014).
- The site should be assessed for signs of phlebitis.
- The site should be observed when a bolus injection is administered, particularly of a vesicant drug, for signs of infiltration or extravasation.
- Certain vesicants must not be administered as infusions into a peripheral vein as the risk of extravasation and damage is greater than via the central venous route (Weinstein and Hagle 2014).

In addition, where possible, a new site should be used for vesicants, to ensure the vein is healthy and patent, although this may not always be possible. There are some controversial issues related to peripheral intravenous cytotoxic drug administration (Box 4.5).

Central venous access devices have the advantage of providing a more reliable form of vascular access (Table 4.1). This is because the problems associated with peripheral devices, such as phlebitis, venous irritation and pain, are eliminated as central venous access enables rapid dilution and circulation of the drug. However, extravasation can still occur because of catheter tip malposition, catheter malfunction, a damaged catheter, port needle dislodgement or fibrin sheath formation along the length of the catheter, faulty equipment, human error and system problems (Dougherty 2006a, Mayo 1998).

Vascular access devices are often inserted without an assessment of the suitability of the vein for the patient-intended therapy, which can result in repeated attempts at cannulation as well as device failure during treatment (Moureau et al. 2012). Complications related to poor choice of device and vein suitability such as

---

Box 4.4 Arguments for using either a larger- or smaller-gauge peripheral vascular access device

Larger
- Enables irritant drugs to reach general circulation quickly, without irritating peripheral veins.
- Administration time is decreased and therefore patient does not need to spend as much time in a stressful environment.

Smaller
- Less chance of puncturing the posterior vein wall.
- Less likely to cause trauma and result in scar formation.
- Less pain on needle insertion.
- Increased blood flow around small needle increases dilution of drug and reduces risk of chemical phlebitis.

Box 4.5 Controversial issues: use of antecubital fossa

For
- Larger veins permit rapid infusion of drug.
- Larger veins allow irritant drugs to reach general circulation more quickly and with less irritation than small veins.
- Easier to palpate and therefore increases successful insertion of device.

Against
- Mobility is restricted.
- Risk of extravasation is increased if patient tends to be mobile.
- Early recognition of extravasation is difficult due to the deep veins. This means there is less chance of observing swelling which could go undetected. The patient may also have a delayed reaction to pain.
- Damage can result in loss of structure and function, ulceration and fibrosis.

Table 4.1 Types of central venous access device (CVAD)

CVAD	Advantages	Disadvantages	Suggested for
PICC	• Ease of insertion • Ease of removal • Ease of access • Small catheter gauge	• Risk of infection and thrombosis • Self-care not possible	Short-term (<6 cycles) intermittent IV therapy and slow-rate continuous infusion, for example FEC or continuous 5-FU
Implanted port	• Low infection risk • Low maintenance • Improved body image • No restrictions on ADL	• Surgical insertion • Specialist equipment and skills required • Surgical removal	Long-term intermittent IV therapy (>6 months), for example trastuzumab
Skin-tunnelled catheter	• Low infection risk • Self-care possible • High flow rates	• Risk of thrombosis • Large catheter gauge • Surgical removal	Fluid-intensive and myelosuppressive therapy, for example leukaemic inductions

ADL, activities of daily living; FEC, 5-fluorouracil, epirubicin, cyclophosphamide; IV, intravenous; PICC, peripherally inserted central catheter.

occlusion, chemical phlebitis and infection can lead to a delay in the patient's treatment as well as causing unnecessary discomfort and pain for the patient. A vessel health preservation (VHP) framework was developed from the US version in the UK (Jackson et al. 2013); this focuses upon vein assessment, drug assessment, best vascular access device and regular evaluation of the device and therapy required (Hallam et al. 2016) (Figure 4.3). The use of the tool was positively evaluated by nurses who stated that it assisted in making vein assessments in clinical practice (Hallam et al. 2016). The tool has demonstrated improved success of insertion, improved patient outcomes as well as time saved through efficiency (Moureau and Carr 2018).

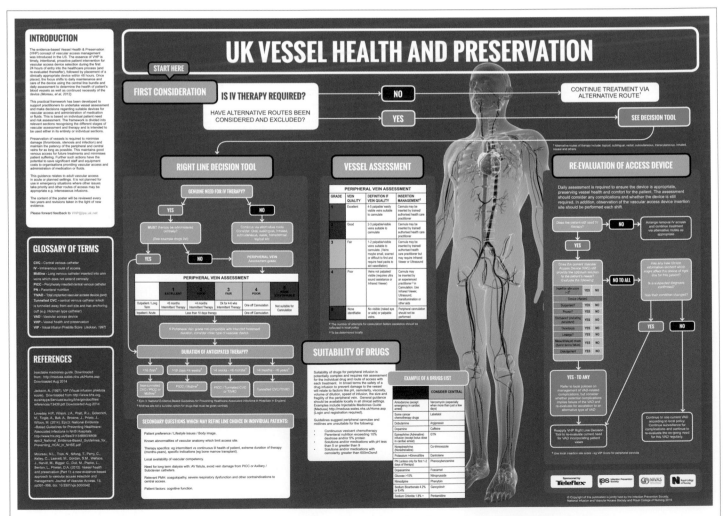

Figure 4.3 Vessel health poster. *Source:* Hallam et al. (2016). Reproduced with permission of Sage Publications.

Procedure guideline 4.2 Cytotoxic therapy: intravenous administration of cytotoxic drugs

Essential equipment
- Patient prescription chart
- Patient information literature
- Personal protective equipment
- Intravenous (IV) pack

Medicinal products
- Medication(s) in a plastic tray

Pre-procedure

Action	Rationale
1 Explain and discuss the procedure with the patient. Evaluate the patient's knowledge of cytotoxic therapy. If this knowledge appears to be inadequate, offer an explanation of the use, action, dose and potential side-effects of the drug or drugs involved.	To ensure that the patient understands the procedure and gives their valid consent. The patient has a right to information (NMC 2010, **C**; van der Molen 2005, **E**).
2 Check that the patient has given their consent and is fit to receive the treatment.	To ensure that the patient gives a valid informed consent and is fit for treatment (NMC 2015, **C**).
3 Put on gloves and an apron before commencing the procedure.	To protect the nurse from local contamination of skin or clothing (Polovich et al. 2014, **C**). *Note*: with careful handling technique this risk is minimal but splashes can occur when changing syringes or infusion containers.
4 Prepare the necessary equipment for a safe and aseptic administration procedure. This includes spiking initial chemotherapy infusion bags over a deep plastic tray in the clinical room.	To minimize the risk of local and/or systemic infection (Fraise and Bradley 2009, **E**). Patients are frequently immunosuppressed and at greater risk of hospital-acquired infection (Weinstein and Hagle 2014, **E**). To contain any splashes. **E**
5 Check that the prescription and medication have been first checked by another chemotherapy-competent nurse and then check that all details on the syringe or infusion container are correct when compared with the patient's prescription, before opening the sterile packaging.	To ensure the patient is given the correct drug that has been dispensed for them. To prevent wastage (NMC 2010, **C**).
6 Be aware of the immediate effects of the drug.	To observe the patient during administration for any known side-effects. To be prepared to manage any side-effects that occur (NMC 2010, **C**).
7 Take the medication and the prescription chart to the patient.	To prevent error and comply with professional guidelines (NMC 2010, **C**).
8 Check the patient's identity, drug, dose, route and timing of administration.	To ensure the medication is administered to the correct patient (NMC 2015, **C**).

Procedure

9 Ensure that an appropriate device has been inserted. Inspect the device site, and consult the patient about sensation around the site.	To detect any problems, for example phlebitis, which would render the device unusable (Dougherty 2006a, **E**; Lavery and Ingram 2010, **E**).
10 Check the patency of the vein for blood return and then flush using 0.9% sodium chloride.	To determine whether the vein will accommodate the extra fluid flow and irritant drugs and remain patent (Weinstein and Hagle 2014, **E**).
11 Ensure the syringe is attached carefully to the needle-free injection site of the administration set, extension set or injection cap.	To prevent disconnection and possible contamination (European Policy Recommendations 2016, **C**).
12 Secure a good connection by always using Luer-Lok syringes.	To prevent leakage or separation, which may occur due to pressure during administration, resulting in spray and contamination (European Policy Recommendations 2016, **C**).
13 Take care when removing the blind hub, changing syringes, and inserting the administration set spike when changing infusion bags (which must be done with the bag lying flat within a deep plastic tray).	To avoid leakage or splashes and contamination of the nurse or patient. To prevent mis-spiking the bag and puncturing it (European Policy Recommendations 2016, **C**).
14 Check the injection site or injection cap at the end of the procedure.	To ensure that there is no leakage (European Policy Recommendations 2016, **C**).
15 Act promptly by washing the area with soap and water if any contamination of an individual is noted.	To prevent any local skin reaction (itchiness, redness or inflammation of the skin). To prevent absorption via skin, mucous membranes, and so on (Polovich et al. 2014, **C**).

(continued)

Procedure guideline 4.2 Cytotoxic therapy: intravenous administration of cytotoxic drugs *(continued)*

Action	Rationale
16 Administer drugs in the correct order: antiemetics, then vesicant cytotoxic drugs, then all others.	To ensure that those agents likely to cause tissue damage are given when venous integrity is greatest, that is, at the beginning of the administration process (Gabriel 2008, **E**).
17 Ensure the correct administration rate.	To prevent 'speed shock'. To prevent extra pressure and irritation within the vein (Weinstein and Hagle 2014, **E**).
18 Observe the vein throughout for signs of infiltration or extravasation, for example swelling or leakage at the site of injection. Note the patient's comments about sensation at the site, for example pain.	To detect any problems at the earliest opportunity. To prevent any damage to soft tissue, and to enable the remainder of the drug(s) to be given correctly at another site. To enable prompt treatment to be given, thus minimizing local damage and possibly preserving venous access for future treatment (Polovich et al. 2014, **C**). (For further information see Methods for preventing extravasation.)
19 Flush the device with 5–10 mL 0.9% sodium chloride between drugs and after administration.	To prevent drug interaction. To prevent leakage of drug from the puncture site on removal of the device (Dougherty 2008a, **E**).
20 Be aware of the patient's comfort throughout the procedure.	To minimize trauma to the patient. To involve the patient in treatment and detect any side-effects and/or problems that may then be avoided at the next treatment. **E**

Post-procedure

21 Record details of the administration in the appropriate documents including start and stop times, infusion site and rates checks and any problems during administration.	To prevent any duplication of treatment and to provide a point of reference in the event of queries and adhere to professional guidelines (NMC 2015, **C**).

Complications

Extravasation

Definition

Extravasation literally means 'leaking into the tissues'; in relation to vesicants it describes a process that requires immediate action if local tissue damage is to be prevented (INS 2016, Polovich et al. 2014, Schulmeister 2009). A vesicant is any solution or medication (DNA or non-DNA binding) that causes the formation of blisters with subsequent tissue necrosis (INS 2016, Polovich et al. 2014).

Related theory

It is important to recognize and distinguish extravasation from an infiltration or flare reaction.

Infiltration refers to the leakage of non-vesicant solutions/medications into the surrounding tissues (INS 2016). It generally does not cause tissue necrosis but can result in long-term injury due to local inflammatory reactions or compression of the surrounding tissues (if a large volume infiltrates) which is known as compartment syndrome (Dougherty and Lister 2015, RCN 2016). Flare reaction is a local inflammatory reaction to an agent manifested by red tracking along the vein or red blotches but without pain (although the area may feel itchy) (Polovich et al. 2014, Wilkes 2018). It occurs in 3–6% of patients (How and Brown 1998). It is caused by a venous inflammatory response to histamine release, is characterized by redness and blotchiness and may result in the formation of small wheals, having a similar appearance to a nettle rash. It usually subsides in 30–60 minutes, with 86% resolving within 45 minutes (How and Brown 1998). Slowing the infusion rate may be helpful but it responds well within a few minutes to the application of a topical steroid (Schulmeister 2009, Weinstein and Hagle 2014).

Tissue damage following extravasation of vesicant drugs occurs for many reasons (Polovich et al. 2014, Schulmeister 2009):

- Whether the drugs bind to DNA or not:
  - DNA-binding vesicants (e.g. doxorubicin, epirubicin) bind to nucleic acids in the DNA of healthy cells, resulting in cell death. There is then cellular uptake of extracellular substances and this sets up a continuing cycle of tissue damage as the DNA-binding vesicant is retained and recirculated in the tissue, sometimes for a prolonged period (Goolsby and Lombardo 2006, Polovich et al. 2014, Schulmeister 2009).
  - Non-DNA binding vesicants (e.g. paclitaxel, vinca alkaloids) have an indirect rather than a direct effect on the cells. They are eventually metabolized in the tissue and then neutralized (more easily than DNA-binding vesicants) (Polovich et al. 2014).
- The concentration and amount of vesicant drug in the tissue.
- The location of the extravasation, for example hand, arm.
- Patient factors, for example older age, co-morbidities.

Evidence-based approaches

Extravasation is a well-recognized complication of intravenous (IV) chemotherapy administration, but in general is a condition that is often underdiagnosed, undertreated and under-reported (Stanley 2002). The incidence of extravasation is estimated to be between 0.5% and 6.0% of all cytotoxic drug administrations (Goolsby and Lombardo 2006, Kassner 2000, Khan and Holmes 2002, Lawson 2003, Masoorli 2003), with some estimates for peripheral extravasation between 23% and 25% (Roth 2003). CVADs have decreased the incidence of extravasation but it can still occur and the incidence is estimated to be up to 6% with ports (Masoorli 2003). However, whilst the incidence is lower, the severity of the injuries is far greater as detection tends to occur later (Kassner 2000, Polovich et al. 2014, Stanley 2002). Even when practitioners have many years of experience, extravasation of vesicant agents can occur and is an extremely stressful event, but is not in itself an act of negligence (Weinstein and Hagle 2014). Early detection and treatment are crucial if the consequences of an untreated or poorly managed extravasation are to be avoided (see Box 4.6 and Figure 4.4). These may include (Polovich et al. 2014):

- blistering (typically occurs 1–2 weeks post extravasation)
- peeling and sloughing of the skin (about 2 weeks post extravasation)
- tissue necrosis (2–3 weeks post extravasation) with resulting pain
- damage to tendons, nerves and joints
- functional and sensory impairment of affected area such as limb disfigurement
- loss of limb or breast.

Box 4.6 Considerations for the prevention of extravasation

- Monitoring the site.
- Location of the device.
- Patients at risk.
- Sequence of drugs.
- Types of devices.
- Method of administration.
- Skill of practitioner.
- Informing the patient.

These can all result in possible hospitalization and plastic surgery, delay in the treatment of disease and psychological distress for the patient.

Before administration of any vesicant drug, the nurse should know which agents are capable of producing tissue necrosis. Damage is usually caused because of the ability to bind to DNA, pH, osmolarity or vasoconstrictive nature of the drugs (Box 4.7). Drugs should not be reconstituted to give solutions that are higher in concentration than is recommended by the manufacturer, and the method of administration should be checked, for example infusion or injection. If there is any doubt, the drug data sheet should be consulted or the pharmacy department should be consulted if the information is insufficient, regarding action to take if a vesicant drug extravasates. Consideration should be given to the management of mixed vesicant drug extravasation in terms of which drug to treat with which antidote. For example, if drug A and drug B were in the same infusion and they required different antidotes but if drug A would cause more damage than drug B, the correct action would be to use antidote for drug A (How and Brown 1998).

Possible causes of extravasation are shown in Box 4.8.

Methods for preventing extravasation

The nurse's focus should be on safe intravenous technique and implementing strategies to minimize risk (Weinstein and Hagle 2014). These include the following strategies.

Patients at risk

Patients who are at increased risk of extravasation (Box 4.9) should be observed more closely.

Types of devices

The use of steel needles is associated with a greater risk of extravasation and should be discouraged; a plastic cannula should be used instead (INS 2016, Polovich et al. 2014, Rodrigues et al, 2012, Sauerland et al. 2006). Vesicants should be given via a newly established cannula wherever possible (Dougherty 2008a, Goolsby and Lombardo 2006) and consideration should be given to changing the cannula site after 24 hours (Wilkes 2018).

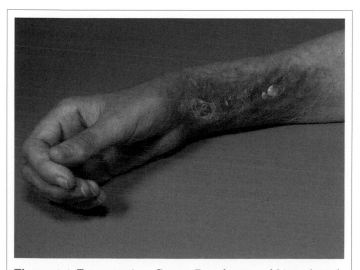

Figure 4.4 Extravasation. *Source:* Dougherty and Lister (2011).

Box 4.7 Examples of vesicant cytotoxic drugs in common use

Group A drugs
- Vinca alkaloids:
  - Vinblastine
  - Vindesine
  - Vinorelbine
  - Vincristine
  - Vinflunine
- Paclitaxel

Group B drugs
- Amsacrine
- Carmustine (concentrated solution)
- Dacarbazine (concentrated solution)
- Dactinomycin
- Daunorubicin
- Doxorubicin
- Epirubicin
- Idarubicin
- Amrubicin
- Actinomycin D
- Mitomycin C
- Mechlorethamine
- Streptozocin

Box 4.8 Possible causes of extravasation

Peripheral devices
- Vein wall puncture or trauma.
- Dislodgement of the cannula from the vein.
- Administration of a vesicant in a vein below a recent venepuncture or cannulation site (<24 hours).

Central venous access devices
- Perforation of the vein.
- Catheter leakage, rupture or fracture.
- Separation of the catheter from the portal body of an implanted port.
- Incomplete insertion of needle into an implanted port.
- Needle dislodgement from an implanted port.
- Fibrin sheath – leading to backflow of drug along the catheter from the insertion site.

Source: Adapted from Mayo (1998), Polovich et al. (2009), Schulmeister (1998).

Box 4.9 Patients at risk of extravasation

- Infants and young children.
- Elderly patients.
- Those who are unable to communicate, for example sedated, unconscious, confused, language issues.
- Those with chronic diseases, for example cancer, peripheral vascular disease, superior vena cava (SVC) syndrome, lymphoedema.
- Those on medications: anticoagulants, steroids.
- Those who have undergone repeated intravenous cannulation/ venepuncture.
- Those with fragile veins or who are thrombocytopenic.

Source: Boulanger et al. 2015, INS 2016, Polovich et al. 2014, Sauerland et al. 2006.

However, if the fluid runs freely, there is good blood return and there are no signs of erythema, pain or swelling at the site, there is no reason to inflict a second cannulation on the patient (Weinstein and Hagle 2014). Consideration should be given to a CVAD if peripheral access is difficult and a decision-making tool such as the one in Figure 4.3 (vessel health and preservation [VHP]) can assist with this (Hallam et al. 2016).

Location of the device

The most appropriate site for the location of a peripheral cannula is the forearm (INS 2016, Schrijvers 2003, Weinstein and Hagle 2014). However, a large straight vein over the dorsum of the hand is preferable to a smaller vein in the forearm (Weinstein and Hagle 2014). Siting over joints should be avoided as tissue damage in this area may limit joint movement in the future. It is also recommended that the antecubital fossa should never be used for the administration of vesicants because of the risk of damage to local structures such as nerves and tendons (Gabriel 2008, Weinstein and Hagle 2014). Avoid venepuncture sites in limbs with impaired circulation, sclerosis, thrombosis or scar formation. Also avoid cannulation below a recent venepuncture site (Goolsby and Lombardo 2006).

Sequence of drugs

Following the administration of any antiemetics, when administration of the cytotoxic drugs commences, vesicants should be given first (Goolsby and Lombardo 2006, Wilkes 2018). Box 4.10 outlines the reasons for this (Weinstein and Hagle 2014).

Methods of administration

Many vesicants must be given as a slow bolus injection, often via the side arm of a fast-running intravenous infusion of a compatible solution, for example doxorubicin or epirubicin via an infusion of 0.9% sodium chloride. If repeated infusions are to be given then a CVAD may be more appropriate (Stanley 2002, Weinstein and Hagle 2014).

Monitoring the site and early recognition of extravasation

Confirm venous patency by flushing with 0.9% sodium chloride solution with at least 5–10 mL prior to administration of vesicants and monitor frequently thereafter (Goolsby and Lombardo 2006, Weinstein and Hagle 2014). Checking blood return after every 2–5 mL is recommended but cannot be relied upon as the key sign when giving a bolus injection; monitor the site every 5–10

Box 4.10 Drug sequencing – rationale for administering vesicant drugs first or last

Vesicants first
- Vascular integrity decreases over time.
- Vein is most stable and least irritated at start of treatment.
- Initial assessment of vein patency is most accurate.
- Patient's awareness of changes more acute.

Vesicants last
- Vesicants are irritating and increase vein fragility.
- Venous spasm may occur and mask signs of extravasation.

Source: Adapted from Weinstein and Hagle (2014), Wilkes (2018).

minutes for any swelling (Weinstein and Hagle 2014). If a vesicant is administered as an infusion over less than 30 minutes the site should be constantly observed (Wilkes 2018).

It is important that the nurse does not rely on infusion pumps to alarm downstream occlusion and alert her/him to an infiltration or extravasation (Huber and Augustine 2009, INS 2016, Marders 2005) (see Table 4.2 and Box 4.11).

Legal and professional issues

Competencies

Nurses are now being named in malpractice allegations, and infiltration and extravasation injuries are an area for concern (Dougherty 2003, Masoorli 2003, Roth 2003, Weinstein and Hagle 2014). Therefore, it is vital that nurses have the correct level of knowledge and skills to perform the following (Dougherty 2008b, Goolsby and Lombardo 2006, Sauerland et al. 2006, Schrijvers 2003):

- correct choice of device and location
- the ability to use the most appropriate vasodilation techniques
- early recognition of infiltration/extravasation and ability to take prompt action.

Table 4.2 Nursing assessment of extravasation

Assessment parameter	Flare reaction	Venous irritation	Immediate manifestations, i.e. during drug administration	Delayed manifestations, i.e. from 24 hours after extravasation
Pain	None	Aching, throbbing sensation along vein and in the limb	Severe stinging or burning pain (not always present). This can last from minutes to hours and will eventually subside. Occurs during drug administration at the device site and surrounding areas	Can continue following extravasation or start within 48 hours. Pain may intensify over time
Redness	Immediate blotches or tracking along the vein. This will subside within 30–45 minutes with or without treatment (usually steroid cream)	Vein may become red or darkened	Not always present immediately: more likely to see blanching of the skin. As area becomes inflamed, redness will appear around the device site	Later occurrence
Swelling	Unlikely	Unlikely	May occur immediately but may not always be easy to identify immediately	Usually within 48 hours
Blood return	Usually present	Usually present but may require application of heat to improve blood return	Inability to obtain blood return (peripheral or central) but blood return may be present throughout	
Ulceration	Unlikely	Unlikely	Unlikely	Can occur within 48–96 hours but may take 3–4 weeks to develop
Others	Urticaria	None	Change in quality of the infusion or pressure on the syringe	Local tingling and sensory deficits

Box 4.11 Signs of extravasation

- The patient complains of burning, stinging pain or any other acute change at the injection site, although this is not always present (Wilkes 2018). This should be distinguished from a feeling of cold, which may occur with some drugs, or venous spasm which can be caused by irritation and is usually accompanied by pain described as an achiness or tightness (Wilkes 2018). Any change of sensation warrants further investigation (Goolsby and Lombardo 2006).
- Swelling is a common symptom (Polovich et al. 2014). Induration or leakage may also occur at the injection site. Swelling may not always be immediately obvious if the patient has the cannula sited in an area of deep subcutaneous fat, in a deep vein or if the leak is via the posterior vein wall (Dougherty 2008a).
- Blanching of the skin occurs (Comerford et al. 2002). Erythema can occur around the injection site but this is not usually present immediately (Wilkes 2018). It is important that this is distinguished from a flare reaction (Polovich et al. 2014).
- Blood return is one of the most misleading of all signs, particularly in relation to peripheral devices. In peripheral devices, if blood return is sluggish or absent, this may indicate lack of patency or incorrect position of the device. However, if no other signs are apparent, this should not be regarded as an indication of a non-patent vein, as a vein may not bleed back for a number of reasons. Extravasation may occur even in the event of good blood return as the device may still be in the vein but the leak may be in the posterior vein wall (Wilkes 2018). Any change in blood flow should be investigated (Weinstein and Hagle 2014, Wilkes 2018). In CVADs there should always be blood return. If this is absent, steps should be followed to verify correct tip and needle position or resolve a fibrin sheath (see Figure 4.5).
- A resistance is felt on the plunger of the syringe if drugs are given by bolus (Stanley 2002).
- There is absence of free flow when administration is by infusion, once other reasons have been excluded, for example position (Polovich et al. 2014, Stanley 2002).
- Leaking around the IV cannula or implanted port needle (Polovich et al. 2014).

Note: one or more of the above may be present. If extravasation is suspected or confirmed, the injection or infusion must be stopped immediately and action must be taken (INS 2016, Polovich et al. 2014, Weinstein and Hagle 2014).

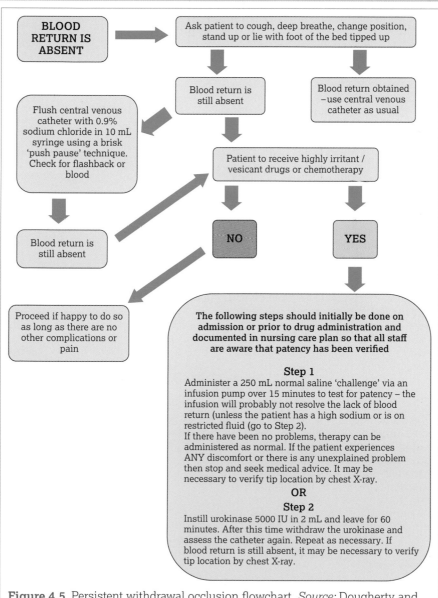

Figure 4.5 Persistent withdrawal occlusion flowchart. *Source:* Dougherty and Lister (2011).

Successful cannulation at the first attempt is ideal, as vesicants have been known to seep into tissues at a vein entry site of a previous cannulation (Gault and Challands 1997). This also includes accessing a port as it is vital that the correct selection of needle is made and that the device is secured adequately (Camp-Sorrell 2005).

Consent

Patients should be informed of the potential problems of administering vesicants and the possible consequences of extravasation (Polovich et al. 2014, Sauerland et al. 2006, Stanley 2002, Weinstein and Hagle 2014). Adequate information given to patients will ensure early recognition and co-operation as patients are the first to notice pain. The patient should be urged to report immediately any change in sensation such as burning or stinging (Goolsby and Lombardo 2006).

Pre-procedural considerations

Equipment

Extravasation kits

The use of extravasation kits has been recommended to provide immediate management (Khan and Holmes 2002). Kits should be assembled according to the needs of individual institutions. They should be kept in all areas where staff are regularly administering vesicant drugs, so that staff have immediate access to equipment (Gabriel 2008). The kit should be simple, to avoid confusion, but comprehensive enough to meet all reasonable needs (Wilkes 2018) (see Procedure guideline 4.3). Instructions should be clear and easy to follow, and the use of a flowchart enables staff to follow the management procedure in easy steps (Figure 4.6).

Decision-making tools have been developed both nationally (Figure 4.3) and locally (Figure 4.7) to address issues related to selecting the correct vascular access device (Vessel Health Preservation; Hallam et al. 2016) as well as grading extravasation (see Table 4.3) (INS 2016).

Pharmacological support

Many 'antidotes' are available but there is a lack of scientific evidence to demonstrate their value and so the role of antidotes is still not clear (Polovich et al. 2014). There appear to be two main methods: (i) localize and neutralize (using hyaluronidase) (CP Pharmaceuticals 1999); and (ii) spread and dilute (using an antidote) (Stanley 2002). Administration of injectable antidotes if not via the cannula is by the pincushion technique, that is, instilling small volumes around and over the areas affected using a small-gauge (25) needle towards the centre of a clock face. The procedure causes considerable discomfort to patients and, if large areas are to be tackled, analgesia should be considered (Stanley 2002).

Hyaluronidase

This is an enzyme which breaks down hyaluronic acid, a normal component of tissue 'cement', and helps to reduce or prevent tissue damage by allowing rapid (within 10 minutes) diffusion of the extravasated fluid and restoration of tissue permeability within 24–48 hours (Doellman et al. 2009, Few 1987, INS 2016). The usual dose is 1500 IU (Bertelli 1995). It should be injected within 1 hour of extravasation, ideally through the intravenous device *in situ*, to deliver the enzyme to the same tissue (Perez Fidalgo et al. 2012, Weinstein and Hagle 2014).

Note: Hyaluronidase increases the absorption of local anaesthetic. Therefore, if local anaesthetic has been applied to the area, for example Ametop gel prior to cannulation, within 6 hours of extravasation, then the patient should be monitored for signs and symptoms of systemic anaesthesia such as increased pulse rate and decreased respirations and the doctor informed immediately (Joint Formulary Committee 2018).

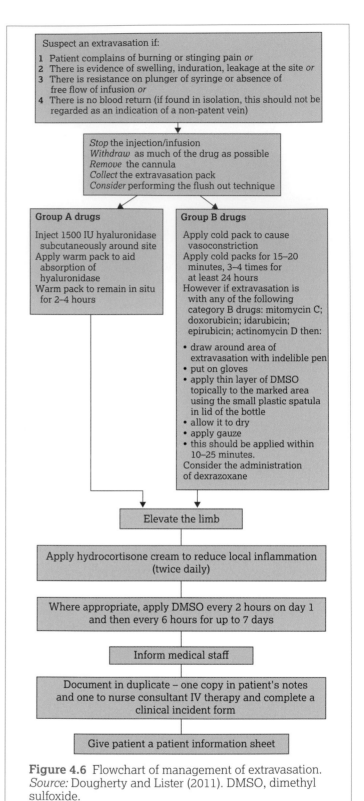

Figure 4.6 Flowchart of management of extravasation. *Source:* Dougherty and Lister (2011). DMSO, dimethyl sulfoxide.

Corticosteroids

These have long been advocated as a treatment for anthracycline extravasation in reducing inflammatory components, although inflammation is not a prominent feature of tissue necrosis (Camp-Sorrell 1998) and they appear to have little benefit. Data now discourage the use of locally injected corticosteroids as there is little evidence to support their use (Bertelli 1995, Gault and Challands 1997, Perez Fidalgo et al. 2012, Wickham et al. 2006). However,

**Any drug to be delivered by a continuous ambulatory drug delivery system
or TPN must be administered via central venous access.**

Patient Identification label	Date	
	Regimen	
	Planned length of treatment	

Vein assessment	Yes	No	
Absence of larger palpable veins			*Does the patient have accessible peripheral veins of sufficient quality suitable to provide the required level of venous access? Does your team have the necessary skill level to establish peripheral venous access for the patient at every visit?*
Extensive oedema/adipose tissue over forearms			
Inadequate venous fill of target veins			
Significant vein wall rigidity			
Significant cellulitis of forearm and/or upper arms			

Vein availability	Yes	No	
Axillary lymph node clearance			*Will the patient have accessible peripheral veins available for the proposed term of treatment (accounting for vein rotation and deterioration)?*
Upper limb/axilla/SVC venous thrombosis			
Extensive skin lesions - forearms			
Previous CVA			
Thrombo-phlebitis present			

VAD insertion and patency factors	Yes	No	
Fragile skin quality			*Is there an increased risk of cannula dislodgement, haematoma formation or thrombo-phlebitis for the patient with peripheral venous access? Is there an increased risk of infection for this patient e.g. long-term steroid therapy?*
Decreased platelets < 50 x 10^9/L			
Anticoagulant therapy i.e warfarin, aspirin, LMWH			
Anxiety/Needle phobia			

Factors affecting long-term venous access patency	Yes	No	
Vesicant and/or irritant therapy for > 6 cycles			*Will the patient be receiving therapy where intensive fluid management will be required (such as concentrated electrolytes)? Is there an increased risk of vein deterioration and thrombo-phlebitis in the patient? Would a skin-tunnelled catheter or implanted port offer a lower risk of site infection for the patient?*
Anticipated intensive IV therapy, i.e. blood products, electrolyte support, fluid support, multiple antimicrobial therapy			
Expected periods of sustained neutropenia (<0.5 x 10^9/L for > 7 days)			

Co-morbidities that may affect peripheral venous access	Yes	No	
Diabetes			*The effects of co-morbidities individual to the patient must be accounted when undertaking a venous access assessment. Would the patient be able to cope with the presence of a CVAD and notify the team appropriately to report adverse events?*
Peripheral vascular disease			
Raynaud's phenomenon			
Hypotension			
Other (please state):			
Other (please state):			

Practitioner recommended venous access device:	
Comments:	

Patient & practitioner agreed venous access device:	
Comments:	

Figure 4.7 Decision-making tool for vascular access device. *Source:* Dougherty and Lister (2015). CVAD, central venous access device; IV intravenous(ly); LMWH, low molecular weight heparin; SVC, superior vena cava; TPN, total parenteral nutrition.

(continued)

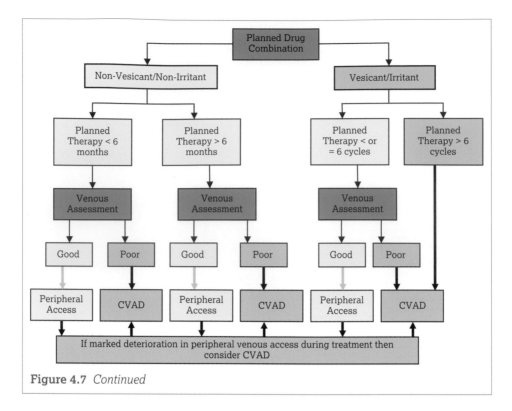

Figure 4.7 *Continued*

given as a cream, they can help to reduce local trauma and irritation (Stanley 2002).

Dimethyl sulfoxide (DMSO)

This is a topically applied solvent that may improve absorption of vesicants. It acts as a potent free radical scavenger that rapidly penetrates tissues and prevents DNA damage (Bertelli 1995, Doellman et al. 2009). Reports on the clinical use of topical DMSO show that it is effective and well tolerated in extravasation (Bertelli 1995). However, this is based on a high dose (99%) solution which is not always available (Pérez Fidalgo et al. 2012). Side-effects from DMSO include itching, erythema, mild burning and a characteristic breath odour (Bertelli 1995).

Dexrazoxane (Savene)

A topoisomerase II catalytic inhibitor, used clinically to minimize the cardiotoxicity of doxorubicin, dexrazoxane was first tested in animals (Langer et al. 2006) and then a small number of patients for its use in extravasation (Doroshow 2012). It is given IV as soon as possible after the extravasation and it appears to reduce the wound size and duration of tissue damage with anthracyclines. The triple dosage appears to be more effective than a single dose (El-Saghir et al. 2004, Langer et al. 2000). In two multicentre studies, it was shown that the administration of dexrazoxane reduced the need for surgical interventions, and late sequelae such as pain, fibrosis, atrophy and sensory disturbance were judged as mild (Doroshow 2012, Mouridsen et al. 2007).

A consensus group (Jackson 2006) developed recommendations for the use of dexrazoxane and these have been further adapted by the European Oncology Nursing Society (2007) which recommended that in anthracycline extravasations resulting from peripheral administration, the site expert or team should be consulted to determine whether the use of dexrazoxane is indicated. Absolute indications are if the peripherally extravasated volume exceeds 3–5 mL and in the event of a central venous access device extravasation (Langer 2008). Dexrazoxane is now recommended in many treatment algorithms for anthracycline extravasations (Gonzalez 2013, INS 2016, Pérez Fidalgo et al. 2012, Roe 2011, Vidall et al. 2013). See Figure 4.8.

Granulocyte-macrophage colony stimulating factor

Granulocyte-macrophage colony stimulating factor (GM-CSF) is a growth factor and is effective in accelerating wound healing and inducing formation of granulation tissue (El-Saghir et al. 2004, Ulutin et al. 2000).

Non-pharmacological support

Stopping infusion/injection and aspirating the drug

It appears that most authors agree that aspirating as much of the drug as possible, as soon as extravasation is suspected, is beneficial (Polovich et al. 2014, Rudolph and Larson 1987, Weinstein and Hagle 2014) and can help lower the concentration of the drug in the area (Goolsby and Lombardo 2006). However, withdrawal is only possible immediately during bolus injections, because if the drug was being delivered via an infusion this would need to be stopped and a syringe attached in an attempt to aspirate. Aspiration may be successful if extravasation presents as a raised blister, but may be unsuccessful if tissue is soft and soggy (CP Pharmaceuticals 1999, Stanley 2002). It may help to reduce the size of the lesion. In practice, it may achieve little and often distresses the patient (Gault and Challands 1997). The likelihood of withdrawing blood (as suggested by Ignoffo and Friedman [1980]) is small and the practitioner may waste valuable time attempting this which could lead to delay in the rest of the management procedure.

Removing the device

Some clinicians advocate that the peripheral vascular access device be left *in situ* to instil the antidote via the device and into the affected tissues (Kassner 2000, Stanley 2002, Weinstein and Hagle 2014). However, others recommend that the peripheral device should be removed to prevent any injected solution increasing the size of the affected area (CP Pharmaceuticals 1999, Rudolph and Larson 1987). There appears to be no research evidence to support either practice.

Application of hot or cold packs

Cooling appears to be a better choice, except for the vinca alkaloids and some non-cytotoxic drugs, than warming (Bertelli 1995, CP Pharmaceuticals 1999). Cold causes vasoconstriction, localizing

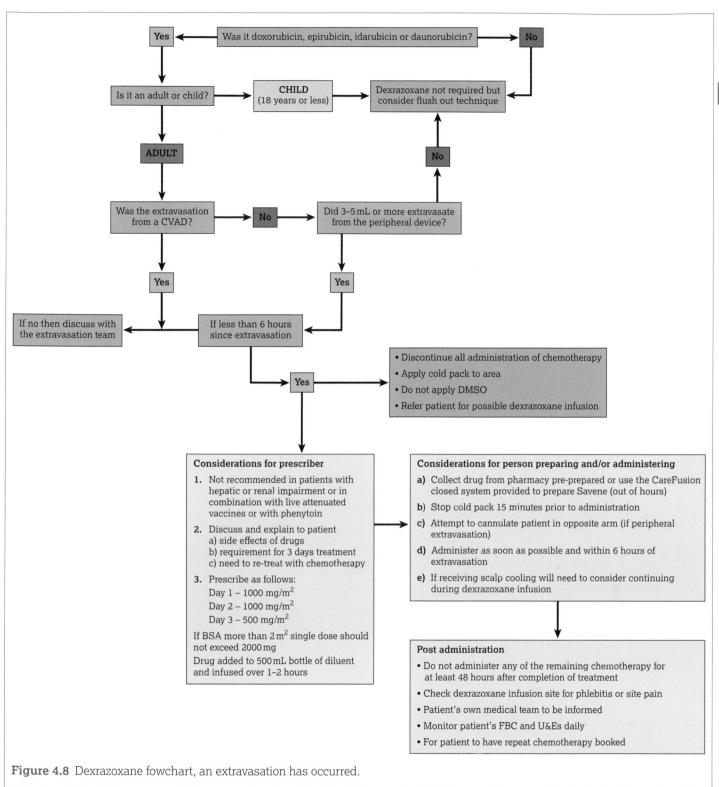

Figure 4.8 Dexrazoxane fowchart, an extravasation has occurred.

the medication in the tissues, and reduces inflammation, perhaps allowing time for local vascular and lymphatic systems to contain the drug (INS 2016). It should be applied for 15–20 minutes, 3–4 times a day for up to 3 days (Polovich et al. 2014, Wilkes 2018). Heat promotes blood flow and disperses medication through the tissues (Polovich et al. 2014, Weinstein and Hagle 2014). Increasing the blood flow also decreases local drug concentration, which

results in enhanced resolution of pain and reabsorption of a localized swelling.

Elevation of limb

This is recommended as it minimizes swelling (Rudolph and Larson 1987). This can be achieved by use of a Bradford sling but is usually recommended when the extravasation has occurred in the hand. Gentle movement should be encouraged to prevent adhesion of damaged areas to underlying tissue (Gabriel 2008, INS 2016).

Surgical techniques

It is now recognized that a plastic surgery consultation should be performed as part of the management procedure to remove the tissue containing the drug. Surgical intervention is recommended, especially if the lesion is greater than 2 cm, there is significant residual pain 1–2 weeks after extravasation, or there is minimal healing 2–3 weeks after injury despite local therapeutic measures (Goolsby and Lombardo 2006, Pérez Fidalgo et al. 2012). A liposuction cannula can be used to aspirate extravasated material and subcutaneous fat or a flush-out technique can remove extravasated drug without resorting to excision and skin grafting.

Flush-out technique

If there is little subcutaneous fat, then the saline flush-out technique is recommended, particularly if it can be done within the first 24 hours (Dionyssiou et al. 2011, Gault 1993). It has been suggested as a less traumatic and cheaper procedure than surgery. Only appropriately trained doctors or nurses may perform the flush-out technique for superficial peripheral extravasations where there is no visible skin damage or extensive swelling (Dougherty and Oakley 2011). A few small stab incisions are made and large volumes of 0.9% sodium chloride are administered which flush out the extravasated drug (Dougherty and Oakley 2011, Gault and Challands 1997); this is more successful if performed within 24 hours of extravasation (Dionyssiou et al. 2011) (see Procedure guideline 4.4).

Procedure guideline 4.3 Extravasation management: peripheral cannula

The procedure detailed was drawn up with the assistance of pharmacist and medical colleagues. It relates specifically to the management of extravasation of a drug from a peripheral cannula.

Essential equipment

- Gel pack × 2: one to be kept in the fridge and one available for heating (an electric heating blanket can be used while the pack is heating)
- 2 mL syringe × 1
- 25 G needle × 2
- Alcohol swabs
- Documentation forms

- Copy of extravasation management procedure
- Patient information leaflet

Medicinal products

- Hyaluronidase 1500 IU/2 mL sterile water
- Hydrocortisone cream 1% 15 g tube × 1
- Savene (dexrazoxane) (optional)

Procedure

Action	Rationale
1 Stop injection or infusion *immediately,* leaving the cannula in place.	To minimize local injury. To allow aspiration of the drug to be attempted (Polovich et al. 2014, **C**; RCN 2016, **C**).
2 If an infusion, wash hands and apply gloves. Then disconnect infusion, clean needle free connector and connect a syringe.	To gain access to the cannula to aspirate drug. **E**
3 Aspirate any residual drug from the device and suspected extravasation site.	To minimize local injury by removing as much drug as possible, but only attempt if appropriate. Subsequent damage is related to the volume of the extravasation, in addition to other factors (INS 2016, **C**; Polovich et al. 2014, **C**; RCN 2016, **C**).
4 Remove the cannula.	To prevent the device from being used for antidote administration (INS 2016, **C**; Rudolph and Larson 1987, **E**).
5 Consider contacting the extravasation team to find out if the flush-out technique would be appropriate (see Figure 4.6).	Flush-out is most effective if undertaken as soon as extravasation is suspected (Gault 1993, **E**).
6 Collect the extravasation pack and take it to the patient.	It contains all the equipment necessary for managing extravasation (Dougherty 2008a, **E**; Stanley 2002, **E**).
7 *Either:* For Group A drugs: • Draw up hyaluronidase 1500 IU in 1 mL water for injection and inject volumes of 0.1–0.2 mL subcutaneously at points of the compass around the circumference of the area of extravasation. • Apply warm pack. *Or:* For Group B drugs (except those listed below): • Apply cold pack or ice instantly. *Or:* If extravasation is with any of the following Group B drugs: mitomycin C, doxorubicin, idarubicin, epirubicin, actinomycin D, then: • Draw around the area of extravasation with indelible pen. • Put on gloves.	This is the recommended agent for Group A drugs. The warm pack speeds up absorption of the drug by the tissues (Bertelli 1995, **E**). To localize the area of extravasation, slow cell metabolism and decrease the area of tissue destruction. To reduce local pain (Polovich et al. 2014, **C**).

- Apply a thin layer of dimethyl sulfoxide (DMSO) topically to the marked area using the small plastic spatula in lid of the bottle. Allow it to dry.
- Apply gauze.
- This should be applied within 10–25 minutes.

Or:

If extravasation of doxorubicin, epirubicin, idarubicin or daunorubicin occurs (i.e. 5 mL or more peripherally or any volume from a central venous access device) then stop cold pack, do not apply DMSO and contact a member of the extravasation team to advise on use of dexrazoxane.

DMSO is the recommended agent for these anthracyclines and helps to reduce local tissue damage (Bertelli 1995, **E**).

Cooling and DMSO interfere with the efficacy of dexrazoxane and it should be administered as soon as possible after extravasation (El Saghir et al. 2004, Langer et al. 2000).

8	Where possible, elevate the extremity and/or encourage movement.	To minimize swelling and to prevent adhesion of damaged area to underlying tissue, which could result in restriction of movement or neuropathy (Wilkes 2018, **E**).

Post-procedure

9	Inform a member of the medical staff at the earliest opportunity and administer any other prescribed antidotes, for example dexrazoxane.	To enable actions differing from agreed policy to be taken if considered in the best interests of the patient. To notify the doctor of the need to prescribe any other drugs. **E**
10	Apply hydrocortisone cream 1% twice daily, and instruct the patient how to do this. Continue as long as erythema persists.	To reduce local inflammation and promote patient comfort (Stanley 2002, **E**).
11	Where appropriate, apply DMSO every 2 hours on day 1 and then every 6 hours for up to 7 days (patients will need to have this prescribed as a to take out (TTO) and continue treatment at home where necessary).	To help reduce local tissue damage (Bertelli 1995, **E**).
12	Heat packs (Group A drugs) should be reapplied after initial management for 2–4 hours. Cold packs (Group B drugs) should be applied for 15–20 minutes, 3–4 times a day for up to 3 days.	To localize the steroid effect in the area of extravasation. To reduce local pain and promote patient comfort (Bertelli 1995, **E**; Wilkes 2018, **E**).
13	Provide analgesia as required.	To promote patient comfort. To encourage movement of the limb as advised. **E**
14	Arrange to have a photograph of the area taken.	To have a baseline photograph of the area for later comparison. **E**
15	Document the following details, in duplicate, on the form provided. (a) Patient's name/number. (b) Ward/unit. (c) Date, time. (d) Signs and symptoms. (e) Cannulation site (on diagram). (f) Drug sequence. (g) Drug administration technique, that is, 'bolus' or infusion. (h) Approximate amount of the drug extravasated. (i) Diameter, length and width of the extravasation area. (j) Appearance of the area. (k) Step-by-step management with date and time of each step performed and medical officer notification. (l) Patient's complaints, comments, statements. (m) Indication that the patient information sheet has been given to the patient. (n) Follow-up section. (o) Whether photograph was taken. (p) If required, when patient referred to plastic surgeon. (q) Signature of the nurse.	To provide an immediate full record of all details of the incident that can be referred to if necessary. To provide a baseline for future observation and monitoring of patient's condition. To comply with NMC guidelines (INS 2016, **C**; NMC 2015, **C**; RCN 2016, **C**; Schulmeister 2009, **E**; Weinstein and Hagle 2014, **E**).
16	Explain to the patient that the site may remain sore for several days.	To reduce anxiety and ensure continued co-operation. **P, E**
17	Observe the area regularly for erythema, induration, blistering or necrosis. *Inpatients*: monitor daily. Where appropriate, take further photographs.	To detect any changes at the earliest possible moment (RCN 2016, **C**).
18	If blistering or tissue breakdown occurs, begin dressing techniques and seek advice regarding wound management.	To minimize the risk of a superimposed infection and sterile increase healing (Naylor 2005, **E**).

(continued)

Procedure guideline 4.3 Extravasation management: peripheral cannula *(continued)*

Action	Rationale
19 Depending on size of lesion, degree of pain, type of drug, refer to plastic surgeon.	To prevent further pain or other complications as chemically induced ulcers rarely heal spontaneously (Dougherty 2005, **E**; Polovich et al. 2014, **C**).
20 As part of the follow-up, all patients should receive written information explaining what has occurred, what management has been carried out, what they need to look for at the site and when to report any changes. For example, increased discomfort, peeling or blistering of the skin should be reported immediately.	To detect any changes as early as possible, and allow for a review of future management. This may include referral to a plastic surgeon (Gault and Challands 1997, **E**; Polovich et al. 2014, **C**; RCN 2016, **C**).

Procedure guideline 4.4 Extravasation: performing flush-out following an extravasation

This procedure would begin once the immediate management of extravasation had been performed; that is, stop infusion/injection, aspirate any drug if possible, apply appropriate pack and elevate limb.

Essential equipment
- Eye protection
- Disposable gown
- 20 mL Luer-Lok syringe × 1
- 10 mL Luer-Lok syringe × 1
- 5 mL Luer-Lok syringe × 1
- 25 G needle × 1
- 23 G needle × 3
- Disposable scalpel (size 11)
- Bandage
- Sterile pack (containing gauze, drapes/towels and gallipot)
- Sterile transparent dressing
- Sterile gloves
- Cleaning solution (2% chlorhexidine Chloraprep 3 mL)
- Blunt needle/18 G or 20 G cannula × 4
- Three-way tap with extension set
- Blank labels for syringes
- Solution administration set
- Sterile marker pen
- Plastic-backed towel (e.g. incontinence pad)

Medicinal products
- Lidocaine 1% 10 mL (kept at room temperature)
- Hyaluronidase 1500 IU and 2 mL water for injection
- Mepitel dressing
- 500 mL 0.9% sodium chloride infusion bag
- Bactericidal alcohol handrub
- Bactericidal soap

Pre-procedure

Action	Rationale
1 Explain the procedure and reason for performing it to the patient and gain written consent using pre-prepared consent form.	To ensure that the patient understands the procedure and gives their valid consent (NMC 2015, **C**).
2 Ascertain what emergency treatment has been carried out, for example was hyaluronidase administered?	To ensure that only required treatment is carried out; for example, if hyaluronidase has been given, no further dose should be administered as this could result in a sensitivity reaction. **E**
3 Assemble all the equipment necessary for the procedure.	To ensure that time is not wasted and the procedure goes smoothly without any unnecessary interruptions. **E**
4 Check all packaging before opening and preparing the equipment to be used.	To maintain asepsis throughout and check that no equipment is damaged or out of date (Fraise and Bradley 2009, **E**).
5 Carefully wash hands using bactericidal soap and water or bactericidal alcohol handrub before commencement and dry.	To minimize the risk of infection (DH 2007, **C**).
6 Place the patient's arm on the plastic-backed towel.	To prevent leakage of the flushed-out solution and possible contamination of the area with cytotoxic drugs. **E**
7 Apply disposable gown and eye protection.	To prevent possible contamination of practitioner with cytotoxic drugs. **E**
8 Open a pack, empty all equipment onto the pack and place a sterile dressing towel under the patient's arm.	To create a sterile working area. **E**
9 Wash hands using bactericidal soap and water.	To minimize the risk of infection (DH 2007, **C**; Fraise and Bradley 2009, **E**).

10	Apply sterile gloves.	To minimize the risk of infection (DH 2007, **C**; Fraise and Bradley 2009, **E**) and prevent contamination of the nurse.
11	Clean skin with 2% chlorhexidine and allow the area to dry.	To maintain asepsis and remove skin flora (DH 2007, **C**; Fraise and Bradley 2009, **E**).

Procedure

12	Draw up 1% lidocaine in 10 mL syringe and label.	To prepare for infiltration of area. **E**
13	Mix hyaluronidase with sterile water in a separate 5 mL syringe.	To ensure drug is reconstituted correctly (Joint Formulary Committee 2018, **C**).
14	Mark the area of extravasation with a sterile marker and indicate where the incisions will be made (**Action figure 14**).	To ensure the correct area is treated. **E**
15	Using a 25 G needle, make a small bleb at the lowest point of the marked area by inserting the needle intradermally and administering 0.1–2 mL of lidocaine slowly towards the four points of the compass. Allow it to take effect (**Action figure 15**).	To reduce any discomfort to the patient. **E**
16	Then, using a 23 G needle, infiltrate the marked area with lidocaine subdermally towards the four points of the compass. Check with the patient what kind of sensation they can feel, for example sharp or dull, before proceeding.	To ensure administration of anaesthetic to area and to ensure anaesthetic has taken effect. **E**
17	Attach a 23 G needle to the syringe of hyaluronidase and infiltrate the anaesthetized area at the four points of the compass.	This will facilitate the flush-out by loosening the tissues. **E**
18	Cut an opening in a transparent dressing that matches the size of the infiltrated area and apply to the patient's skin.	To protect the skin from the flushed out cytotoxic drugs. **E**
19	Attach the administration set, three-way tap and extension set to the bag of 0.9% sodium chloride and withdraw 20 mL via the tap.	To prepare the syringe and to enable continued access without having to open the system. **E**
20	Make at least four incisions at the four points of the compass using a size 11 scalpel by inserting the blade straight down to a depth of no more than 0.5 cm and one small incision to use for insertion of the cannula 20 (**Action figure 20**).	To prepare the area for flushing. The number of incisions will depend on the size of the area to be treated. To reduce risk of damage to tendons or other anatomical structures (Gault 1993, **E**).
21	Gently press on the area.	This alone may allow the fluid to escape (Gault 1993, **E**).
22	Insert the cannula through one of the incisions and push along tissues within the marked area (**Action figure 22**).	To free up tissues from skin and to aid advancement of cannula and flush (Gault 1993, **E**).

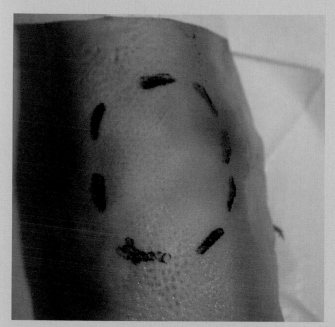

Action Figure 14 Mark the area of extravasation.

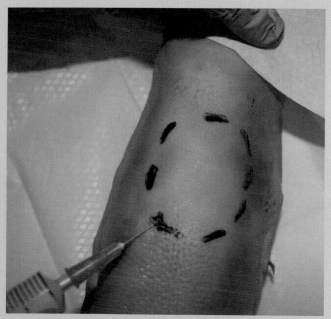

Action Figure 15 Administer lidocaine.

(continued)

Action	Rationale
23 Remove the stylet, dispose of in the sharps bin and attach the extension set to the cannula.	To facilitate the flushing. **E**
24 Flush the 0.9% sodium chloride through – it will exit out of the other incision holes. Pat with a sterile gauze swab, massaging and milking the area at the same time. The area will become puffy and swollen – this is normal (**Action figure 24**).	To commence the flushing procedure. To assist with removal of the extravasated drug (Gault 1993, **E**).

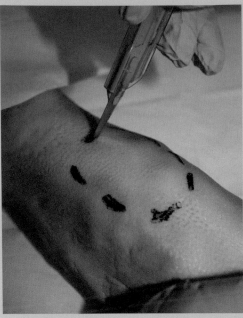

Action Figure 20 Make incisions at the four points of the compass and one small incision for insertion of the cannula.

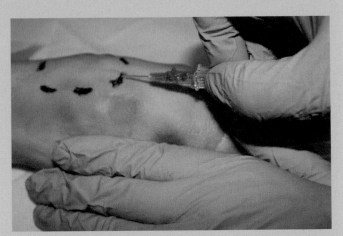

Action Figure 22 Insert the cannula.

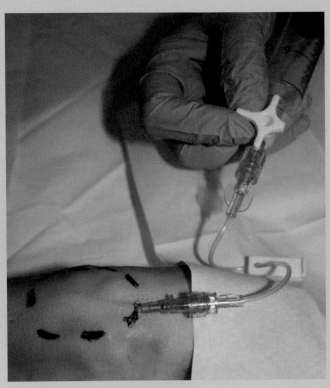

Action Figure 24 Flush with 0.9% sodium chloride.

25	Draw up more 0.9% sodium chloride and repeat the procedure using a minimum of 100 mL (up to 500 mL) of 0.9% sodium chloride.	To facilitate the flushing of the drug from the area (Gault 1993, **E**).
26	If 0.9% sodium chloride does not flow out of one incision, it may be necessary to remove the cannula from the original incision and insert a new cannula into another incision.	To ensure all areas are flushed. **E**

Post-procedure

27	Clean and dry the area although it will continue to leak.	To aid patient comfort. **E**
28	Apply a Mepitel dressing and a loose bandage (do not wrap tightly).	To reduce the risk of infection and to prevent compression of the skin. **E**
29	Elevate the limb so that the hand is level with the head until swelling has reduced.	To aid reduction of oedema. **E**
30	Discard waste in appropriate containers.	To ensure safe disposal in the correct containers and avoid laceration or injury of other staff. **E**
31	Document in the patient's medical and nursing notes and on the flush-out technique form.	To ensure adequate records and enable continued care of the patient (NMC 2015, **C**).
32	Discuss with medical colleagues the prescribing of oral antibiotics (flucloxacillin is recommended for reducing skin pathogens) and if necessary analgesia.	If the patient is neutropenic they may be more at risk of infection. To minimize pain and discomfort. **E**
33	Refer to a plastic surgeon if there are any problems during procedure or if there are any skin problems.	To ensure rapid access for further management. **E**
34	Have a photograph taken if possible.	To observe and document for any skin changes. **E**
35	Monitor and review within first 24 hours.	To observe and document for any skin changes or infection and provide immediate treatment. **E**
36	Dressing will need to be changed every 48 hours and should remain *in situ* for up to a week. The skin incisions will heal within 1–2 weeks.	To prevent risk of infection. **E**
37	Ensure the patient knows when and how to make contact if they have any problems once at home. Organize for the patient to return for dressing changes at the hospital or with the district nurses. Inform the patient to contact the hospital if: • the swelling does not reduce • they have pain • there is any tingling or numbness in the fingers or arm.	To ensure the patient receives immediate treatment should there be any problems post procedure. **E**

Post-procedural considerations

Ongoing care

Patient follow-up will depend upon the patient's needs and the degree of damage. Assessment should be carried out using a standardized tool (INS 2016) and include inspection and management of the area of extravasation, skin integrity, presence of pain and other symptoms such as mobility and sensation of the limb (see Table 4.3). If damage has occurred, it will be determined by the site, amount of drug, concentration of the agent and if it binds to DNA or not (Polovich et al. 2014). Blistering may occur within 24 hours (for example, with vinorelbine) or ulceration may occur over a period of days to weeks (for example, with epirubicin), and extravasation wounds may be

Table 4.3 Grading scale for monitoring extravasation

Grade	1	2	3	4	5
Skin colour	Normal	Pink	Red	Blanched area surrounded by red	Blackened
Skin integrity	Unbroken	Blistered	Superficial skin loss	Tissue loss and exposed subcutaneous tissue	Tissue loss and exposed bone/muscle with necrosis/crater
Skin temperature	Normal	Warm	Hot		
Oedema	Absent	Non-pitting	Pitting		
Mobility	Full	Slightly limited	Very limited	Immobile	
Pain		Grade using a scale of 0–10 where 0 = no pain and 10 = worst pain			
Temperature	Normal	Elevated (indicate actual temperature)			

Box 4.12 Key elements of vesicant extravasation documentation

- Date and time the extravasation occurred.
- Type and size of vascular access device.
- Length and gauge of needle (ports only).
- Location of device.
- Details of how patency was established before and during administration (description and quality of blood return).
- Number and location of all cannulation attempts.
- Vesicant administration method, for example bolus/infusion.
- Estimated amount of extravasated drug.
- Symptoms reported by the patient.
- Description of device site, for example swelling, redness and so on.
- Assessment of limb (where applicable) for range of movement.
- Immediate nursing interventions.
- Follow-up interventions.
- Patient information.

complicated by tissue ischaemia related to endothelial damage (Naylor 2005). The type of injury will dictate the type of dressing. Assessment of the wound should include position and size of the wound, amount and type of tissue present, amount and type of exudate, and extent and spread of erythema (Naylor 2005). If the flush-out technique has been undertaken then the incisions should be dressed using a dressing that allows the fluid to continue to leak from the site, for example Mepitel. It is also important to recognize the impact on the patient's psychological and situational dynamics that may diminish their quality of life (Gonzalez 2013).

Documentation

An extravasation must be reported and fully documented because it is an accident and the patient may require follow-up care (NMC 2010, RCN 2016). The Oncology Nursing Society has listed the key elements of vesicant extravasation documentation (Polovich et al. 2014) (see Box 4.12). Statistics on the incidence, degree, causes and corrective action should be monitored and analysed (Gonzalez 2013, INS 2016, Pérez Fidalgo et al. 2012). Finally, documentation may be required in the case of litigation, which is now on the increase (Doellman et al. 2009, Dougherty 2003, Masoorli 2003).

Education of patient and relevant others

Patients should always be informed when an extravasation has occurred and be given an explanation of what has happened and what management has been carried out (INS 2016, McCaffrey Boyle and Engelking 1995). An information sheet should be given to patients with instructions of what symptoms to look out for and when to contact the hospital during the follow-up period (Gabriel 2008).

Oral administration of systemic anticancer therapy

Definition

The term 'oral anticancer medicine' is used to refer to drugs with direct antitumour activity, administered via the oral route to cancer patients, including traditional cytotoxic chemotherapy (e.g. capecitabine, vinorelbine), small molecule treatments (e.g. imatinib, erlotinib) and teratogenic agents such as thalidomide. It does not include hormonal therapies such as tamoxifen or anastrazole (BOPA 2004, NPSA 2008a). See Table 4.4.

Table 4.4 Examples of oral anticancer medications

Drug class	Drug	Cancers for which drug is used
Alkylating agent	Busulfan	Leukaemia
	Chlorambucil	Leukaemia, lymphoma
	Cyclophosphamide	Leukaemia, lymphomas, many solid tumours
	Lomustine (CCNU)	Lymphoma
	Melphalan	Myeloma
	Temozolomide	Glioma (brain tumour)
Antimetabolites	Capecitabine	Breast, colorectal, upper gastrointestinal tract
	Fludarabine	Leukaemia
	Mercaptopurine	Leukaemia
	Methotrexate	Leukaemia, solid tumours
	Tegafur-uracil	Colorectal cancer
	Tioguanine	Leukaemia
Epipodophyllotoxins	Etoposide	Leukaemia, solid tumours (lung, testicular)
Tyrosine kinase inhibitors	Afatinib	Lung
	Ceritinib	Lung cancer
	Crizotinib	Lung cancer
	Dabrafenib	Melanoma
	Dasatinib	Chronic myeloid leukaemia
	Erlotinib	Lung cancer
	Gefitinib	Lung cancer
	Imatinib	Chronic myeloid leukaemia
	Lapatinib	Breast cancer
	Nilotinib	Chronic myeloid leukaemia
	Sorafenib	Renal and liver
	Sunitinib	Renal cancer, gastrointestinal stromal tumour
Antitumour antibiotics	Idarubicin	Leukaemia
Plant alkaloids	Vinorelbine	Lung and breast
Miscellaneous	Hydroxycarbamide	Leukaemia
	Lenalidomide	Myeloma
	Tretinoin	Leukaemia
	Thalidomide	Myeloma

Source: Adapted from Williamson (2008).

Evidence-based approaches

Rationale

The use of oral anticancer medications, while not new, has increased greatly in recent years. This increase is set to continue, with around 25% of all anticancer drugs in development being oral preparations (Bedell 2003, Szetela and Gibson 2007). This shift to oral anticancer medications has implications for nurses, who will focus less on drug administration and more on educating and monitoring patients (Kav et al. 2008, Szetela and Gibson 2007).

There are considerable advantages to administering anticancer medications via the oral route. The primary benefit is one of patient preference. The majority of patients (90%) would prefer to take oral anticancer medications as long as there was no reduced efficacy (Aisner 2007, Barefoot et al. 2009, Sharma and Saltz 2000). Patients prefer oral anticancer medication because of its ease and convenience; it allows them to take their medication in the comfort of their own home and is often associated with fewer or shorter hospital appointments (Barefoot et al. 2009, Bedell 2003, Winkeljohn 2007). Oral anticancer therapy is non-invasive, eliminating the need for IV access (Sharma and Saltz 2000, Wilkes 2018).

Some evidence suggests that oral anticancer therapy is more cost-effective. Although the cost of new oral medications may be high, the staff and equipment costs of IV administration can be greater. Therefore, the overall costs of administering oral anticancer therapy may be less (Holmberg and Zanni 2005). Oral anticancer medications are also often considered to be less toxic than those needing other routes of administration (Holmberg and Zanni 2005, Wilkes 2018). However, this view is not universally accepted (Birner et al. 2006, Sharma and Saltz 2000). Use of the oral route can be beneficial when chronic exposure to a drug is important, for example cell cycle-specific drugs (Scurr 2005).

There are several disadvantages associated with giving anticancer medications orally. Oral formulations are not suitable for all patients. Although most oral anticancer drugs are absorbed well if the gastrointestinal tract is functioning normally, many factors affecting cancer patients can alter absorption, making the oral route unreliable (Findlay et al. 2008, O'Neill and Twelves 2002). These include primary tumour, gastrointestinal (GI) surgery and concomitant medications. Side-effects of anticancer treatment such as diarrhoea or nausea and vomiting can also affect absorption (Goodin 2007, Scurr 2005, Sharma and Saltz 2000, Wilkes 2018).

Some patients may experience difficulty swallowing, which makes taking tablets or capsules problematic. Crushing or dissolving oral anticancer medications could result in changes to the tablets' disposition and effectiveness, and advice should be sought from an oncology pharmacist. Patients usually self-administer at home which can result in less monitoring and support from healthcare professionals (Kav et al. 2008). This can lead to poor adherence and under-reporting of side-effects (Barefoot et al. 2009). Patient adherence to anticancer treatment is important to maximize the chance of achieving the goals of therapy. However, there is a greater chance of patient non-adherence with oral anticancer medications than with parenteral therapy which tends to be administered under direct supervision in a healthcare setting. Fear of side-effects can lead patients to stop taking or reduce their dose of oral anticancer medications.

Conversely, patients may feel that their oral chemotherapy is not effective enough and increase their doses (Findlay et al. 2008, Ruddy et al. 2009). They may continue taking oral anticancer medications despite toxicity because they feel the treatment is helping and do not want it stopped (Szetela and Gibson 2007). Other factors that can affect adherence are the complexity of the treatment regimen, number and type of concomitant medications, cognitive impairment, treatment of asymptomatic disease, lack of insight into disease seriousness, lack of confidence in treatment and poor patient–provider relationships (Barefoot et al. 2009, Hartigan 2003, Holmberg and Zanni 2005, Viele 2007, Wilkes 2018, Winkeljohn 2007).

Pre-procedural considerations

Specific patient considerations

Education

Lack of individual adherence to self-administered medications is a common clinical problem and it is even more critical when the patient is taking oral chemotherapy. There are significant safety issues surrounding these medications and patient education is paramount. It is critical that patient education is thorough so the patient understands:

- why they are taking their tablets
- how many tablets to take, how often and for how long
- the potential side-effects of the treatment
- how to recognize toxicity
- what to do if they feel unwell.

For home-based therapy to be successful, it is vital that patients take an active part in their care.

The responsibility to recognize and report any side-effects rests with the patient. Therefore, patient education must emphasize recognition of early signs and symptoms and when to report problems. The role of pharmacy and nursing staff in educating the patient is paramount to ensure the safe handling and concordance to get the maximum benefit for the patient from their oral chemotherapy treatment. The London Cancer Alliance oral SACT counselling checklist forms the basis of oral chemotherapy counselling and is completed for every patient starting oral chemotherapy prior to cycle 1 (Table 4.5). Patients should be advised about all the safety aspects of handling oral chemotherapy, see Procedure guideline 4.5.

Before all subsequent cycles:

- Check that the patient understood the counselling checklist in Table 4.5 and repeat if necessary.
- Check that any side-effects experienced with their previous cycle were discussed with the patient's medical team.
- If a dose adjustment has been made, check that the patient is aware of why their dose has been changed and how many tablets/capsules they should now take.
- Check that the patient had no problems taking their previous cycle.
- Check that the patient understands how to take the treatment, by asking them to repeat back their instructions.

Patients with swallowing difficulties

Before advising patients to dissolve/open capsules or prepare for administration via feeding tubes, the patient must be assessed for the suitability of self-administering oral SACT. Swallowing difficulties or the inability to manipulate medicines may contribute to the decision whether to treat with SACT via the oral route. Alternatively, if the patient is unable to swallow solids or liquids, they may have a feeding tube. Examples of feeding tubes include:

- short-term: nasogastric (NG), nasoduodenal (ND), nasojejunal (NJ)
- long-term: gastrostomy and jejunostomy (surgically placed), and percutaneous endoscopic gastrostomy (PEG) – and percutaneous endoscopic jejunostomy (PEJ) (endoscopically placed) (see Dougherty and Lister [2015] *The Royal Marsden Manual of Clinical Nursing Procedures, Ninth Edition*: Chapter 8 Patient comfort and end-of-life care).

Table 4.5 Counselling checklist

Oral anticancer patient and carer education checklist	
Prior to first cycle	
This checklist must be completed with the patient/carer at the point of handing the medication to the patient either in conjunction with or following a pre-treatment consultation	Tick if discussed with the patient/carer
Instructions for taking	
Explain how and when to take the medicine including any treatment breaks	
If the patient is unable to swallow tablets or capsules or has a feeding tube, please refer to local chemotherapy/SACT treatment policy for information on how to dissolve or open capsules (if appropriate for the oral anticancer medicine)	
Missed doses can be taken if near to the scheduled time. Otherwise, do not try and catch up or double the next dose. Wait until the next dose is due	
In case of vomiting after taking a dose, do not repeat the dose and take the next dose at the normal time. If this occurs again, contact the chemotherapy team/24-hour advice line	
Check the patient is aware of side-effects and has received written information. Any side-effects should be reported to their chemotherapy nurse or doctor	
If the patient is taking any prescribed/over the counter medicine/supplement the patient should inform their medical team	
Return any unused oral anticancer medicine to the hospital pharmacy. Do not flush or throw them away (for high-cost drugs see counselling handbook)	
Storage and handling	
The oral anticancer medicine should not be handled by anyone who is pregnant or planning a pregnancy (unless taking on the advice of the medical team)	
If the carer is giving the anticancer medicine they should not handle the medicine directly but wear gloves or push the medicine out of the blister pack (if applicable) directly into a medicine pot	
Store the tablets/capsules in the container provided	
Store the tablets/capsules in a secure place, away from and out of sight of children	
Wash hands thoroughly after taking/giving the oral anticancer medicine	
Check the patient understands how to take the treatment, by asking them to repeat back their instructions	
Written information provided	
Taking an oral anticancer medicine patient information sheet	
Diary for taking oral anticancer medicine (if applicable)	
For swallowing difficulty only – give relevant factsheet if appropriate for the oral anticancer medicine and an oral anticancer pack with disposables (e.g. oral/enteral syringes)	
Dissolving oral anticancer tablets safely	
Opening oral anticancer capsules safely	
Giving an oral anticancer medicine through a feeding tube	
Giving an anticancer syringe by mouth	
Patient name	**Counselled by**
Hospital number	**Pharmacist/Pharmacy technician/ Nurse/Interpreter**
Signature and date	**Signature and date**

Source: LCA (2015a). Reproduced with permission of the London Cancer Alliance.

Table 4.6 details medicines that can be dissolved or opened and liquids/foods that can be used to mask the taste. All patients with swallowing difficulties should be provided with the relevant patient information factsheet (if applicable for the medicine) and an oral anticancer pack only after the pharmacist, pharmacy technician or nurse has talked through the procedure with the patient. There is a space on the relevant patient information factsheet to specify the suitable liquid/flavouring or food. Factsheets can be found in the oral SACT counselling handbook available at rmpartners.cancervanguard.nhs.uk.

Table 4.6 Oral anticancer administration table for patients with swallowing difficulties

Drug name Tablet (T) / capsule (C)	Can be:			Route PO/feeding tube	Comment
	Dissolved	Opened	Mixed with:		
Afatinib (T)	Yes		Non-carbonated water. No other liquids should be used	PO/enteral tube	Disperses in approximately 100 mL of non-carbonated drinking water. The tablet should be dropped into the water without crushing it, and stirred occasionally for up to 15 minutes until it is broken up into very small particles. The dispersion should be consumed immediately. Rinse glass with approximately 100 mL of water which should also be consumed. The dispersion can also be administered through a gastric tube
Axitinib (T)	Yes		Distilled/purified water	PO/enteral tube	Do *not* use tap/bottled water. 15 mL distilled/purified water should be used for enteral route. Use amber coloured syringe/container to disperse tablet – light sensitive. Ensure suspension is protected from light
Bosutinib (T)	No		See comment	PO	Film coated, immediate release tablets. Do not crush. Pfizer have not evaluated crushing, splitting, dissolving or feeding tube administration
Busulfan (T)	Yes		Water	PO/enteral tube	Disperses in 18 minutes. Liquid preparation available
Cabozantinib (C)		No	See comment	PO	This class of drugs – TKIs – and Cometriq® in particular is associated with increased likelihood of gastrointestinal bleeding and fistula formation. For this reason, opening the capsules cannot be recommended
Capecitabine (T)	Yes		Raspberry or blackcurrant juice (*not* citric juices)	PO/enteral tube	Disperses in 15 minutes in 200 mL lukewarm water (not hot)
Chlorambucil (T)	Yes		Water	PO/enteral tube	Disperses in 18 minutes. Tablets should not be divided
Crizotinib (T)	Yes		Water	PO/enteral tube	Allow capsule to disintegrate in 30 mL (2 tablespoons) boiling water, add 15 mL (1 tablespoon) room temperature water – consume immediately but ensure not boiling hot on drinking. A mint sweet before and after taking can help mask the taste
Cyclophosphamide (T)	Yes		Water	PO/enteral tube	Disperses in ~25 minutes. Liquid preparation available
Dabrafenib (C)		No	See comment	PO	Capsules should not be opened or crushed and should not be mixed with food or liquids due to chemical instability of dabrafenib
Dasatinib (T)	Yes		100% apple or 100% orange juice (*not* water)	PO/enteral tube	Disperses in 20 minutes in 30 mL volume and rinse with 15 mL. Resting of suspension increases bitterness – consume immediately after dispersion
Erlotinib (T)	Yes		Water, sweetened fruit juice (*not* grapefruit juice), or a sweet	PO/enteral tube	Disperses in 5–8 minutes
Etoposide (C)	No	No	Oral injection can be mixed with orange/apple juice/lemonade (*not* milk, grapefruit or cranberry juice)	PO/enteral tube	Use injection orally at 70% of oral dose. Prepared by aseptic unit (requires orange order form by pharmacist). Liquid preparation available
Everolimus (T)	Yes		Water (*not* milk or fruit juice)	PO/enteral tube	Disperses in 5–10 minutes in 30 mL

(continued)

Table 4.6 Oral anticancer administration table for patients with swallowing difficulties *(continued)*

| Drug name Tablet (T) / capsule (C) | Can be: | | | Route | |
	Dissolved	Opened	Mixed with:	PO/feeding tube	Comment
Fludarabine (T)	No		See comment	PO	Alternative IV route, refer to pharmacist/clinician
Gefitinib (T)	Yes		Water	PO/enteral tube	Disperses in 20 minutes
Hydroxycarbamide (C)	Yes		Water	PO	Siklos® tablets disperse immediately in 5 mL or capsules can be opened. Liquid preparation available
Ibrutinib (C)		No	See comment	PO	The capsules are hard and should not be opened, broken, or chewed
Idarubicin (C)	No	No	See comment	PO	Contents of idarubicin capsules are extremely irritating to tissues. Alternative IV route
Imatinib (T)	Yes		Water, apple juice	PO	Nil info enteral feeding
Isotretinoin (C)		Yes	Lukewarm milk or soft food, e.g. cottage cheese, yoghurt, chocolate mousse or oatmeal	PO/enteral tube	See patient information sheet. Enteral feeding – may need dose adjustment if given by this route (lower peak levels)
Lapatinib (T)	Yes		Water (*not* grapefruit juice)	PO/enteral tube	Disperses in 15 minutes
Lenalidomide (C)	No	No	See comment	PO	No info available, refer to pharmacist/clinician
Lomustine (C)		Yes	Milk, yoghurt, fromage frais, ice cream, pureed food	PO	Nil info enteral feeding. Do *not* mix with water or juice as this can cause stomach irritation
Melphalan (T)	Yes		Water	PO	Nil info enteral feeding. Best not to take with food due to reduction in bioavailability
Mercaptopurine (T)	Yes		Water	PO/enteral tube	Disperse in a syringe (oral/enteral). Liquid preparation available
Methotrexate (T)	Yes		Water	PO/enteral tube	Tablets disperse. Liquid preparation available
Mitotane (T)	No		High-fat food/dairy-based products, e.g. yoghurt, mousse	PO/enteral tube	Dilute dairy-based products containing crushed tablets in water for administration via enteral feeding tube. Liquid preparation available
Nilotinib (C)		Yes	Apple sauce (pureed apple)	PO	Only use apple sauce. Content of *one* capsule in *one* teaspoon of apple sauce only. Nil info on enteral feeding
Pazopanib (T)	No		See comment	PO	Crushing tablets significantly increases bioavailability and absorption (adverse events reported most frequently with crushed tablet administration included erythema, vomiting and fatigue). Refer to pharmacist/clinician
Pomalidomide (C)		No	See comment	PO	Hard gelatine capsules should not be opened or crushed. If powder from pomalidomide makes contact with the skin, the skin should be washed immediately and thoroughly with soap and water. If pomalidomide makes contact with mucous membranes, they should be thoroughly flushed with water
Ponatinib (T)	No		See comment	PO	Film-coated tablets should not be dissolved or crushed. Nil info on the safety and efficacy of crushed or broken tablets, or nasogastric tube administration
Procarbazine (C)		Yes	Water	PO/enteral tube	Powder is very irritant. Give immediately once dispersed as unstable. Liquid preparation available
Ruxolitinib (T)	No		See comment	PO	Tablets are uncoated, immediate release and should not be crushed. In addition, risk of drug exposure from dust/powder/bits of tablet if crushed. Contact medicines information

Drug name Tablet (T) / capsule (C)	Can be:		Mixed with:	Route PO/feeding tube	Comment
	Dissolved	Opened			
Sorafenib (T)	Yes		Water	PO	Disperses in 10 minutes. Nil info on enteral feeding
Sunitinib (C)		Yes	Apple sauce, yoghurt (saline if used for enteral feeding)	PO/enteral tube	Mix contents in a teaspoonful of apple sauce/yoghurt. For enteral feeding, disperse contents in 5 mL saline, and rinse with 5 mL. Some discolouration of the tube may remain, due to the strong orange colour of the sunitinib
Temozolomide (C)		Yes	Fruit juice (*not* grapefruit), apple sauce	PO/enteral tube	30 mL fruit juice for enteral route. Liquid preparation available
Teysuno (C)		No	Water	PO/enteral tube	Try commercial jelly products obtainable over-the-counter to aid swallowing of tablets (e.g. Pill Glide). Capsules dissolve in 50°C water
Thalidomide (C)		Yes	Semi-solid foods, e.g. apple sauce, ice cream. (Water for nasogastric)	PO/enteral tube	Disperses in water but not very water-soluble, therefore enteral tubes must be flushed well post dose to avoid blockage
Tioguanine (T)	Yes		Water (simple syrup, wild cherry syrup as flavouring)	PO	Do *not* stir tablets or shake the container; allow tablets to disperse naturally. Liquid preparation available. Nil info on enteral feeding. Tablets can be halved using dedicated tablet cutter
Topotecan (C)	No	No	See comment	PO	No information on opening capsules
Tretinoin (C)		Yes	Soya bean oil or lukewarm milk	PO/enteral tube	See patient information sheet
Vandetanib (T)	Yes		Water (*no* other liquid)	PO/enteral tube	Stir tablet until dispersed (approx. 10 minutes)
Vemurafenib (T)	No		See comment	PO	Tablets have low solubility and permeability. Due to hardness of tablets, crushing is difficult. Refer to pharmacist/clinician
Vinorelbine (C)		No	See comment	PO	Vinorelbine capsules must not be opened as they are carcinogenic, and the liquid is irritant to oesophagus. Alternative IV route
Vismodegib (C)		No	See comment	PO	The capsules must not be opened. Vismodegib has a low solubility in aqueous media

Source: LCA (2015). Reproduced with permission of the London Cancer Alliance.
IV, intravenous; PO, *per os* (by mouth); TKI, tyrosine kinase inhibitor.

Procedure guideline 4.5 Cytotoxic therapy: education for patients on oral cytotoxic drugs

Essential equipment
- Patient prescription chart
- Patient information literature

Medicinal products
- Medication(s) to be supplied to patient

Pre-procedure

Action	Rationale
1 Prior to the first cycle of treatment, check that the appropriate consent procedure has been completed.	To ensure that the patient gives valid informed consent for treatment (NMC 2015, **C**).
2 Evaluate the patient's knowledge of the oral anticancer medication(s) being administered. Explain the treatment plan to the patient and/or carer. Teaching should include verbal and up-to-date written information on the use, action, dose and potential side-effects of prescribed oral anticancer medication(s).	To ensure that the patient is fully informed and understands the aim of the treatment and potential adverse effects (DH 2009a, **C**; NMC 2010, **C**; NPSA 2008a, **C**; van der Molen 2005, **E**; Viele 2007, **E**).

(continued)

Procedure guideline 4.5 Cytotoxic therapy: education for patients on oral cytotoxic drugs *(continued)*

Procedure

Action	Rationale
3 Using the counselling checklist, educate patient and/or carer about oral anticancer treatment, including: (a) How to take their medication(s) (b) What dose to take (c) When to take their medication(s) and any breaks in treatment (d) What to do in the event of omitted doses (e) What to do if they vomit a dose (f) When to seek advice about adverse effects (g) When and who to contact in the event of an emergency (h) Use of personal protective equipment, safe handling and storage (i) Disposal of unused oral anticancer medication(s).	To ensure patients understand that they need to take the correct dose for maximum therapeutic effect. To ensure safety of patient and/or carers. In line with national and local policies (BOPA 2004, **C**; NECN 2017, **C**).
4 Before supplying oral anticancer medication(s) to patient, consult the prescription chart and ascertain that the following are correct: (a) Medication (b) Dose (c) Route (d) Dates and times of administration (e) Prescription is correct and legible (f) Signature of prescriber.	To ensure the patient is given the correct medications(s) and dose via the correct route at the correct times (NMC 2010, **C**). To protect the patient from harm (NMC 2015, **C**).
5 Check the patient's identity by asking them to state their full name and date of birth. If unable to verbally confirm details then check identity wristband against prescription chart.	To ensure the medication is supplied to the correct patient (NMC 2015, **C**).
6 Obtain a full medication history from the patient and check for potential allergies and drug interactions with oral anticancer medication(s).	To protect patient from harm (NMC 2015, **C**; Szetela and Gibson 2007, **E**). To prevent unwanted toxicity and therapeutic failure (Goodin 2007, **C**).
7 Assess the patient's ability to take oral anticancer medications in the dosage and form supplied. If any problems with taking medication(s) in prescribed form are identified, provide teaching and written information on crushing or dissolving oral anticancer medication(s) along with any necessary equipment.	To ensure patient can take prescribed treatment (BOPA 2004, **C**).

Post-procedure

Action	Rationale
8 Record and sign that medication(s) have been supplied on the appropriate section on the oral chemotherapy prescription chart.	To provide a written record that medication has been supplied to patient (NECN 2017, **C**; NMC 2015, **C**; NMC 2010: **C**).

Post-procedural considerations

Monitoring and follow-up of patients who have been prescribed oral anticancer medication(s) are vital (Oakley et al. 2010a). All patients should be fully assessed by a healthcare professional with specialist knowledge prior to each cycle. The following should be assessed and recorded.

- Adherence to prescribed therapy and the continued ability of the patient to manage treatment at home (BOPA 2004, Oakley et al. 2010a).
- Assessment of toxicity, including grade, duration and management (BOPA 2004, NECN 2017, Oakley et al. 2010a).
- Performance status of the patient (Oakley et al. 2010a).
- Dose modifications and/or cycle delays. Patients and carers need to be fully informed of any alterations to the dose of oral anticancer medication(s) or to the treatment schedule and the reasons for the changes. Ensure that any written instructions on taking medications are updated (BOPA 2004, NECN 2017, Oakley et al. 2010b).

The use of oral anticancer medication diary cards can assist the patient to record the doses of medication that have been taken and side-effects experienced (Hartigan 2003, Winkeljohn 2007).

Intramuscular and subcutaneous administration of cytotoxic drugs

Definition

- *Subcutaneous.* This is the administration of cytotoxic drugs by injection into the subcutaneous tissues. Subcutaneous injections deliver medications into the loose fat and connective tissue under the dermis. The subcutaneous route is used for slow, sustained absorption of medication (Downie et al. 2003).
- *Intramuscular.* This is the administration of cytotoxic drugs by injection into the deep muscle under the subcutaneous tissue. As the muscle is so vascular it aids the absorption of medication (Ostendorf 2012).

Evidence-based approaches

Rationale

Indications

Intramuscular and subcutaneous injections are a useful route:

- when administering therapy in the community
- for patient convenience
- when regular administration is required and journeys to the hospital are impractical, for example younger or elderly patients on maintenance therapy.

They are also useful if venous access is limited, although only small volumes (up to 2 mL) are recommended using this route (Downie et al. 2003, Polovich et al. 2014, Sewell et al. 2002). Cytotoxic and biological agents administered in this way include (Stanley 2002, Weinstein and Hagle 2014, Wilkes 2018):

- intramuscular:
  - methotrexate
  - bleomycin
  - cytosine arabinoside
  - L-asparaginase
  - ifosfamide
  - interferon
  - non-cytotoxic drugs
- subcutaneous:
  - colony-stimulating factor
  - trastuzumab
  - rituximab
  - denosumab
  - goserelin
  - fulvestrant.

Contraindications

Reasons for not administering cytotoxic drugs via the intramuscular or subcutaneous routes would include the following factors (Polovich et al. 2014):

- the irritant nature of the drugs and/or tissue damage
- possible incomplete absorption
- bleeding because of thrombocytopenia
- discomfort of regular injections.

Although the volume of drug and diluent handled is less than for the intravenous route, preparation and reconstitution of the agents should be commensurate with the information listed in the safe handling section. The use of safety needles to administer medications is recommended by the European Union directive on safe handling of sharps (EU 2010). The nurse should wear an apron and gloves during administration. Disposal of equipment and spillage should be dealt with in the same way as for any other cytotoxic medication. Where community nurses are to be responsible for administration, they must be supplied with adequate information when the patient is discharged and arrangements for cytotoxic waste collection should be in place.

Recommendations about administration should be followed carefully, for example deep intramuscular injection using a Z-track technique to prevent leakage onto the skin (Wilkes 2018) and rotation of sites to prevent local irritation developing. The skin should be cleaned with antiseptic prior to injection (Sansivero and Barton-Burke 2001) and the smallest needle used, the gauge of which will allow passage of the solution to minimize discomfort and scarring (Weinstein and Hagle 2014).

Procedure guideline 4.6 Cytotoxic therapy: intramuscular administration of cytotoxic drugs (Z-track)

Essential equipment

- Alcohol swab
- Needle
- Syringe containing prepared intramuscular (IM) medication
- Non-sterile gloves
- Plastic apron

Pre-procedure

Action	Rationale
1 Explain and discuss the procedure with the patient.	To ensure that the patient understands the procedure and gives their valid consent (Griffith et al. 2003, **E**; NMC 2015, **C**).
2 Consult the patient's prescription sheet, and ascertain the following: (a) Drug. (b) Dose. (c) Date and time of administration. (d) Route and method of administration. (e) Diluent as appropriate. (f) Validity of prescription. (g) Signature of doctor. (h) Allergy status.	To ensure that the patient is given the correct drug in the prescribed dose using the appropriate diluent and by the correct route (DH 2003, **C**; NMC 2010, **C**; NPSA 2008a, **C**).

Procedure

3 Assist the patient into the required position.	To allow access to the injection site and to ensure the designated muscle group is flexed and therefore relaxed (Workman 1999, **E**).
4 Put on apron and gloves.	To ensure the practitioner is protected from possible accidental exposure (Polovich 2016, **C**).

(continued)

Procedure guideline 4.6 Cytotoxic therapy: intramuscular administration of cytotoxic drugs (Z-track) *(continued)*

Action	Rationale
5 Remove the appropriate garment to expose the injection site.	To gain access for injection (Workman 1999, **E**).
6 Assess the injection site for signs of inflammation, oedema, infection and skin lesions.	To promote effectiveness of administration. To reduce the risk of infection (Workman 1999, **E**). To avoid skin lesions and avoid possible trauma to the patient (Elkin et al. 2007, **E**; Workman 1999, **E**).
7 Clean the injection site with a swab saturated with isopropyl alcohol 70% for 30 seconds and allow to dry for 30 seconds.	To reduce the number of pathogens introduced into the skin by the needle at the time of insertion. To prevent stinging sensation if alcohol is taken into the tissues upon needle entry (Hunter 2008, **E**; Workman 1999, **E**).
8 With the non-dominant hand, pull the skin 2–3 cm sideways or downwards from the injection site.	To displace the underlying subcutaneous tissues to slide over the underlying muscle by 1–2 cm (Antipuesto 2010, **E**; Hunter 2008, **E**).
9 Holding the syringe in the dominant hand like a dart, inform the patient and quickly plunge the needle at an angle of 90° into the skin until about 1 cm of the needle is left showing.	To ensure that the needle penetrates the muscle (Hunter 2008, **E**; Workman 1999, **E**).
10 Pull back the plunger. If no blood is aspirated, depress the plunger at approximately 1 mL every 10 seconds and inject the drug slowly. If blood appears, withdraw the needle completely, replace it and begin again. Explain to the patient what has occurred.	To confirm that the needle is in the correct position and not in a vein (Antipuesto 2010, **E**). This allows time for the muscle fibres to expand and absorb the solution (Hunter 2008, **E**; Workman 1999, **E**). To prevent pain and ensure even distribution of the drug (Ostendorf 2012, **E**).
11 Wait 10 seconds before withdrawing the needle.	To allow the medication to diffuse into the tissue (Antipuesto 2010, **E**).
12 Withdraw the needle rapidly and release the tension on the skin but do not massage the site.	This causes the tissues to return to their original position to create a disjointed pathway and seals the injection entry point to prevent medication from seeping into the subcutaneous tissues or from leaking out through the injection site (Antipuesto 2010, **E**).
13 Apply gentle pressure to any bleeding point and then apply a small plaster over the puncture site.	To prevent tissue injury and haematoma formation (Ostendorf 2012, **E**).
Post-procedure	
14 Ensure that all sharps and non-sharps waste are disposed of safely and in accordance with locally approved procedures, for example put sharps into sharps bin and syringes into cytotoxic clinical waste bag.	To ensure safe disposal and to avoid laceration or other injury to staff (DH 2009b, **C**).
15 Record the administration on appropriate charts.	To maintain accurate records, provide a point of reference in the event of any queries and prevent any duplication of treatment (NMC 2015, **C**; NPSA 2008a, **C**).

Topical application of cytotoxic drugs

Definition
Topical application is the application of cream or ointments containing cytotoxic agents for local effects (Potter 2011).

Evidence-based approaches

Rationale

Indications
Topical application is only suitable for superficial lesions and has been found to be useful in the treatment of cutaneous malignant lesions, for example cutaneous T-cell lymphomas, basal cell carcinoma, squamous cell carcinoma and Kaposi's sarcoma (Wilkes 2018).

Principles of care
Topical agents include mustine and 5-FU (Wilkes 2018). The most widely used is 5% 5-FU cream for the treatment of basal and squamous cell carcinomas. It is usually applied once or twice daily until significant penetration of the damaged or diseased skin can be achieved, and a typical response pattern has been observed. This can take up to 1–3 weeks when local erythema, blistering and ulceration occur. Once the affected skin starts sloughing, regranulization of normal tissue will begin to occur (Wilkes 2018).

Procedure guideline 4.7 Cytotoxic therapy: topical application of cytotoxic drugs

Essential equipment
- Clean non-sterile gloves
- Plastic apron
- Applicators
- Sterile topical swabs

Pre-procedure

Action	Rationale
1 Explain and discuss the procedure with the patient.	To ensure that the patient understands the procedure and gives their valid consent (Griffith et al. 2003, **E**; NMC 2010, **C**).
2 Check the patient's prescription chart against the chemotherapy medication.	To ensure that the patient is given the correct drug and dose (NMC 2015, **C**; NMC 2010, **C**).

Procedure

3 Close room door or curtains if appropriate.	To ensure patient privacy and dignity. **E**
4 Put on apron and gloves.	To ensure that the practitioner is protected from accidental spillage (Polovich 2016, **E**).
5 Assist the patient into the required position.	To allow access to the affected area of skin. **E**
6 Assess the condition of the skin and use aseptic technique if the skin is broken.	To prevent local or systemic infection (DH 2007, **C**; Fraise and Bradley 2009, **E**).
7 If the medication is to be rubbed into the skin, the preparation should be placed on a sterile topical swab.	To minimize the risk of cross-infection. To protect the nurse (DH 2007, **C**; Fraise and Bradley 2009, **E**).
8 If the preparation causes staining, advise the patient of this.	To ensure that adequate precautions are taken beforehand and to prevent unwanted stains (NMC 2010, **C**).
9 Use a sterile dressing if required.	To ensure the ointment remains in place (Chernecky et al. 2002, **E**).

Post-procedure

10 Ensure that all waste is discarded according to policy guidance.	To minimize the risk of exposure to hazardous waste (HSE 2017, **C**).
11 Record the administration on appropriate charts.	To maintain accurate records, provide a point of reference in the event of any queries and prevent any duplication of treatment (NMC 2015, **C**).

Considerations include safe handling when applying the cream by wearing gloves and using low-linting swabs or non-metal applicators (Weinstein and Hagle 2014, Wilkes 2018). It is important to protect the normal skin and avoid the eyes and other mucous membranes.

Post-procedural considerations

Ongoing care
The affected area should not be washed vigorously during treatment (Wilkes 2018). The area should be observed for any adverse reactions such as pain, pruritus and hyperpigmentation, which may result in discontinuation and subsequent dose reduction.

Intrathecal administration of cytotoxic drugs

Definition
Intrathecal administration is the administration of cytotoxic drugs into the central nervous system (CNS) via the cerebrospinal fluid. This is usually achieved using a lumbar puncture (Polovich et al. 2014, Stanley 2002, Wilkes 2018).

Related theory
Intrathecal administration is only appropriate for a limited number of drugs (Scurr 2005):

- thiotepa
- cytarabine
- methotrexate.

The advantage of this route is that it allows the direct access to the CNS of a drug that does not normally cross the blood–brain barrier in sufficient amounts and thus ensures constant levels of the drug in this area. The main disadvantage is that it requires a standard lumbar puncture before the drug can be injected, and this may need to be performed on a daily to weekly basis (Stanley 2002, Wilkes 2018). Although this can be quick and easy to perform, it can be distressing for the patient and could even result in CNS trauma and infection. It may also only reach the epidural or subdural spaces and therefore the concentrations in the ventricles may not be therapeutic (Wilkes 2018). However, central instillation of the drug into the ventricle can be achieved via an Ommaya reservoir (Figure 4.9), which is surgically implanted through the cranium (Sewell et al. 2002, Weinstein and Hagle 2014, Wilkes 2018). It carries more risks but provides permanent access and can be inserted under local or general anaesthetic (Sansivero and Barton-Burke 2001, Wilkes 2018). Doses of intraventricular drugs tend to be lower than those given intrathecally.

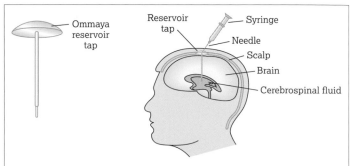

Figure 4.9 Ommaya reservoir. *Source:* Dougherty and Lister (2011).

Evidence-based approaches

Rationale

Indications

Intrathecal administration has proved to be of benefit in prophylactic treatment in cases of leukaemias and some lymphomas, where the CNS may provide a sanctuary site for tumour cells not reached during systemic chemotherapy (Wilkes 2018). It can also be used for metastasis to the brain or leptomeninges from solid tumours, lymphoma and leukaemia (Aiello-Laws and Rutlidge 2014).

Principles of care

The preparation of the drug must be performed using aseptic technique to reduce the risk of infection. The drug should be free from preservatives to reduce neurotoxicity. Cerebrospinal fluid removal and volumes of medications should not be more than 2 mL/min.

Legal and professional issues

Chemotherapy administered using this route has the potential to cause great harm (Sewell et al. 2002) and has been associated with the deaths of at least 13 patients since 1985. The risks of intrathecal chemotherapy have been well documented in *An Organization with a Memory* (DH 2000) and the government set a target to eliminate incidents of patients dying or being paralyzed by maladministered intrathecal injections by the end of 2001 (DH 2000). Two reports on injection errors (Toft 2001) gave rise to the publication of the national guidance for the safe administration of intrathecal chemotherapy.

Following the publication of the guidance, all UK trusts that undertake to administer intrathecal cytotoxic chemotherapy (ITC) must ensure safe practice guidelines have been introduced and that they are fully compliant with the *Updated National Guidance on the Safe Administration of Intrathecal Chemotherapy* (DH 2008). The key requirements of the guidance are noted in Box 4.13.

The chief executive must identify a 'designated lead' who in turn must ensure the appropriate induction, training and continuing professional development of designated personnel authorized to administer intrathecal chemotherapy. A register of these personnel must be kept along with details of certain competency-based tasks such as prescribing, dispensing, issuing, checking and administration. It is important to keep up to date with relevant safety alerts concerning intrathecal chemotherapy which may be issued by the Department of Health agencies such as the Medicines and Healthcare products Regulatory Agency (MHRA) or National Patient Safety Agency (NPSA).

Box 4.13 Summary – requirements of intrathecal guidance

- Only trained, designated personnel whose names are recorded on the appropriate intrathecal register are authorized to prescribe, dispense, check or administer intrathecal chemotherapy.
- All staff involved in the intrathecal chemotherapy process must undertake a formal competency-based induction programme that is appropriate to their role, and annual training must be provided for all professional staff to remain on the register.
- Staff involved with intrathecal chemotherapy must use this policy in conjunction with the national guidance HSC 2008/001 and the Rapid Response Report NPSA/2008/RRR004 relating to intravenous vinca alkaloid administration.
- Staff are given an annual date-expiring certificate on satisfactory completion of their training.
- Intrathecal chemotherapy must be prescribed by a consultant, associate specialist, specialist registrar, staff grade or ST3 grade doctor only and they must be on the register.
- Intrathecal chemotherapy drugs must be issued and received by designated staff only. Any such products not used must be returned to the pharmacy at the end of the intrathecal chemotherapy session.
- In adults, intravenous drugs must be administered *before* intrathecal drugs are issued (or once intravenous continuous infusions have been started).
- Children receiving intrathecal therapy under general anaesthetic will have their intrathecal treatment first in theatre. Intravenous drugs (excluding vinca alkaloids) may be given later in day care or on the ward, but never in theatre.
- Intrathecal chemotherapy should always be administered in a designated area, within normal working hours; out-of-hours administration must only occur in exceptional circumstances.
- Checks must be made by medical, nursing and pharmacy staff at relevant stages throughout the prescribing, preparation and administration process.
- This guidance predominantly relates to treatment given intrathecally, by lumbar puncture (i.e. via spinal injection) but is also relevant to intraventricular chemotherapy (i.e. via injection into the ventricles of the brain).

Such reports have highlighted concerns over the risk of neurological injury due to implantable drug pumps for intrathecal therapy (MHRA 2008) and the storage of vinca alkaloid minibags (NPSA 2008b).

Procedure guideline 4.8 Cytotoxic therapy: intraventricular administration of cytotoxic drugs via an intraventricular access device (Ommaya reservoir)

Essential equipment
- 25 G winged infusion devices or small non-coring needle
- Sterile dressing pack
- Cleaning solution
- Pre-prepared chemotherapy
- Three-way tap

Pre-procedure

Action	Procedure
1 Explain and discuss the procedure with the patient.	To ensure that the patient understands the procedure and gives their valid consent (Griffith et al. 2003, **E**; NMC 2010, **C**).

2 Consult the patient's prescription sheet, and ascertain the following: (a) Drug. (b) Dose. (c) Date and time of administration. (d) Route and method of administration. (e) Diluent as appropriate. (f) Validity of prescription. (g) Signature of doctor. (h) Allergy status.	To ensure that the patient is given the correct drug in the prescribed dose using the appropriate diluent and by the correct route (NPSA 2008a, **C**).
3 Position the patient comfortably.	To gain access to the site. **E**
4 Apply apron and necessary personal protective equipment, for example gloves, goggles.	To protect the practitioner from splashes and spills (HSE 2017, **C**; Polovich 2016, **E**; RCN 2016, **C**).
5 Wash hands with antibacterial soap.	To prevent contamination (Fraise and Bradley 2009, **E**).
6 Open sterile pack and pour antiseptic liquid into gallipot.	To prepare the area. **E**
7 Open intrathecal chemotherapy drugs by cutting plastic pack and place on sterile field.	To gain access to chemotherapy. **E**
8 Open non-coring winged infusion device and connect a three-way tap to the tubing.	To prepare the equipment. **E**
9 Clean hands with alcohol gel.	To prevent contamination (Fraise and Bradley 2009, **E**).

Procedure

10 Locate the reservoir by slightly depressing the dome several times. There should be free flow of CSF from the ventricle into the dome.	To ascertain where the reservoir is and that it is functional (RCN 2016, **C**).
11 Wash hands with antibacterial handwash and put on sterile gloves.	To prevent contamination (Fraise and Bradley 2009, **E**).
12 Prepare the skin by cleaning the site.	To minimize risk of infection (Fraise and Bradley 2009, **E**).
13 Using the 25 G needle, access the reservoir and remove a small amount of CSF equal to the amount of drug to be instilled.	To check free flow of CSF and patency of reservoir (RCN 2016, **C**).
14 Connect syringe containing chemotherapy to three-way tap and inject slowly. No resistance should be felt.	To maintain a closed system and administer medication (RCN 2016, **C**).
15 Compress and release the dome after all medication is given.	To facilitate medication administration and dispense the drug (RCN 2016, **C**).
16 The reservoir can now be flushed with the CSF removed at the start of the procedure. Do not flush with 0.9% sodium chloride or heparin.	Flushing is not required as CSF flows freely through the device (RCN 2016, **C**; **E**).
17 Remove the needle and apply pressure with gauze.	To prevent leakage of CSF or chemotherapy. **E**
18 Dispose of sharps and syringe in a purple-lidded sharps container.	To maintain a safe environment. **E**
19 Once CSF stops leaking, apply a small gauze dressing and tape.	To minimize risk of infection (Fraise and Bradley 2009, **E**).

Post-procedure

20 Assist patient in repositioning if required.	To maintain comfort. **E**
21 Dispose of equipment in appropriate waste bags.	To maintain a safe environment. **E**
22 Wash and dry hands.	To minimize risk of contamination (Fraise and Bradley 2009, **E**).
23 Document chemotherapy administration on the prescription chart.	To maintain records and for continuity of care (NMC 2015, **C**).
24 Monitor the patient for any side-effects of the drugs and check reservoir site for any leaks.	To recognize complications early and report to medical staff (RCN 2016, **C**).

Post-procedural considerations

It is important that the nurse monitors the patient for signs of discomfort and administers any analgesics required. Vital signs should be recorded regularly, at least every 1–2 hours initially and then 4 hourly. Observations should include signs of infection, headache and raised intracranial pressure (Scurr et al. 2005, Wilkes 2018). For more detail, please refer to Dougherty and Lister (2015) *The Royal Marsden Manual of Clinical Nursing Procedures, Ninth Edition*: Chapter 11 Observations.

Intrapleural instillation of cytotoxic drugs

Definition

Intrapleural instillation is the introduction of cytotoxic drugs, or other substances, into the pleural cavity.

Related theory

Pleural effusion is a common complication of malignant disease and may pose a considerable management problem. Installation should occur following drainage of an effusion to prevent or delay a recurrence caused by malignant cells, as after aspiration alone 60% of patients would present with pleural malignant recurrence (Wilkes 2018).

The most common neoplasms associated with the development of malignant pleural effusions are those of the (Wilkes 2018):

- breast
- lung
- gastrointestinal tract
- prostate
- ovary.

Such effusions can be very distressing to the patient, causing progressive discomfort, dyspnoea and death from respiratory insufficiency.

The alteration in normal anatomy due to the pressure of an effusion is illustrated in Figure 4.10. In health, less than 5 mL of transudate fluid is present between the visceral and parietal pleura. This fluid acts as a lubricant and hydraulic seal. Infections and malignancies disrupt this mechanism, often repeatedly. Patients may survive for months or years, therefore effective palliation is important in maintaining or improving their quality of life. Administering chemotherapy via this route may alleviate symptoms and also has the potential to deliver the drugs to a site of poor systemic penetration (Sewell et al. 2002). A study using intrapleural hypotonic cisplatin for malignant pleural effusion demonstrated encouraging results. Eighty patients were observed during the study, of whom 27 (34%) and 39 (49%) achieved a complete response and partial response respectively (Seto et al. 2006).

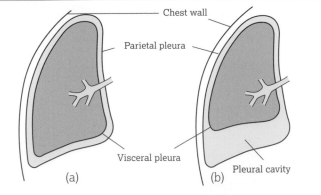

Figure 4.10 Lung anatomy. (a) Normal lung anatomy showing pleura. (b) Lung demonstrating presence of pleural effusion. *Source:* Dougherty and Lister (2011).

Evidence-based approaches

Principles of care

Several methods have been used to treat pleural effusions, including:

- surgical techniques, such as ablation of the pleural space
- radiotherapy
- systemic chemotherapy
- the insertion of a small-bore catheter and installation of a pleural shunt (Sewell et al. 2002) to deliver cytotoxic agents.

In addition, instillation of sclerosing agents into the pleural space has been reported to have highly variable success rates of 20–88% (Sewell et al. 2002). Cytology may show the presence of tumour cells in effusion fluid, but even when these are absent, instillation of drugs may be effective in preventing recurrence due to the inflammatory reaction which obliterates the pleural space.

Agents used have included talc, radioactive phosphorus, bacille Calmette–Guérin (BCG), tetracycline and, more recently, cytotoxic drugs. The drug most frequently instilled is bleomycin, but others include mitoxantrone, doxorubicin, mustine and thiotepa (Sewell et al. 2002, Wilkes 2018).

Pre-procedural considerations

Equipment

Improvements in equipment used, for example flexible cannulas or catheters, and lengthening of both the initial drainage period and that following instillation of the drug have contributed to increased patient comfort and greater effectiveness (Wilkes 2018). The insertion of small-bore percutaneously placed catheters or ports, as well as pleuroperitoneal shunts (Wilkes 2018), has been found to be useful for recurrent effusions.

Procedure guideline 4.9 Cytotoxic therapy: intrapleural instillation of cytotoxic drugs

Essential equipment

- Sterile chest drain pack containing gallipot, disposable towel, forceps, disposable scalpel and sterile low-linting gauze
- Suture material: silk
- Cleaning solution: chlorhexidine gluconate 0.5% in 70% alcohol
- Sterile gloves and gown
- Syringes: 2 × 10 mL

Medicinal products

- Local anaesthetic: lidocaine 1%
- Sterile water: 1 litre bottle
- Needles: 1 × 21 G, 1 × 23 G
- Chest drain: check appropriate size to be used for insertion
- Sterile dressing
- Tape
- Chest drain tubing
- Chest drain bottle
- Chest drain clamps × 2
- Low-vacuum suction pump, if required

Pre-procedure

Action	Rationale
1 Explain and discuss the procedure with the patient.	To ensure that the patient understands the procedure and gives their valid consent (NMC 2015, **C**).
2 Administer premedication to the patient if prescribed.	To relax the patient. **E**
3 Prepare the required equipment and cytotoxic drug. Wear protective clothing.	To ensure the procedure goes smoothly without interruption. To protect the practitioner from exposure (HSE 2017, **C**).

Procedure

Action	Rationale
4 Assist the doctor with the installation and provide support for the patient. Place the patient in a sitting position, leaning forward over a strong surface or table which is locked in position.	To increase the efficiency of the procedure and reduce discomfort for the patient (Shuey and Payne 2005, **E**).
5 At the end of the installation, clamp the drainage tube and leave for the desired period.	To prevent backflow of the drug (Weinstein and Hagle 2014, **E**).
6 Observe regularly for patient comfort. Administer analgesic as required.	To keep the patient comfortable and free from pain. **E**
7 Record the patient's respirations and colour at least every 15 minutes for 1 hour, then every hour until stable, then 4 hourly or as frequently as the patient's condition dictates. Record temperature at least 4 hourly.	To ensure there is no change in respiratory function following the procedure. **E** To observe for pyrexia, a common side-effect that may indicate a developing infection or a reaction to chemotherapy. **E** Administer antihistamine if required. **E**

Post-procedure

Action	Rationale
8 When ready to remove the drain, ensure the patient is in a comfortable position, and is aware of any limitations about movement.	To prevent discomfort or dislodgement of the drainage tube. **E**
9 Unclamp the chest tube.	To allow drainage of the drug instilled. **E**
10 Record the colour and amount of fluid drained.	To monitor the immediate effectiveness of therapy (NMC 2015, **C**).

Post-procedural considerations

Immediate care
The literature recommends that the patient should be turned regularly following instillation of the drug to facilitate its complete distribution over the pleural surfaces. The rationale for such turning is based on clinical observation and there is a lack of research comparing patients who are turned with those who are not.

Ongoing care
Local pleural pain and inflammation can last for 24–48 hours after instillation. Good symptom management should focus upon emesis control, adequate analgesia and emotional support and chest tube security to ensure patient comfort (Wilkes 2018).

Intravesical instillation of cytotoxic drugs

Definition
Intravesical instillation is the instillation of cytotoxic drugs directly into the bladder via a urinary catheter (Dougherty and Bailey 2008).

Related theory
Instillation of cytotoxic agents, and immunotherapy, into the bladder via a urinary catheter has been used for many years in selected cases and has proved to be an effective and simple method of controlling and treating superficial bladder cancer

(Washburn 2007). In measurable disease, average response rates are 60%. Approximately 30% of patients experience a complete response. Cytotoxic drugs found to be effective include (Washburn 2007):

- thiotepa
- mitomycin C
- doxorubicin
- epirubicin
- mitoxantrone
- BCG (non-cytotoxic).

Intravesical instillation allows a high concentration of drug to bathe the endothelium, which enables localized treatment of the tumour and limits the systemic absorption so toxicity is reduced. Systemic toxicity is a problem with thiotepa, but otherwise the main problems are local inflammation, pain, burning on urination, frequency and occasional haematuria. An aseptic technique must be maintained throughout the procedure to minimize the risk of urinary tract infection (Polovich 2016).

Evidence-based approaches

Rationale

Indications
- Intravesical instillation has been shown to be effective in the treatment of small, multiple, superficial, well-differentiated, non-invasive papillomatous carcinomas as high drug

concentrations can be achieved using this route because there is limited penetration of the drug into normal and malignant tissue.
- This method is only of benefit when treating small and superficial disease (Scurr 2005).
- It minimizes recurrence in patients with a history of multiple tumours known to readily seed locally (Stanley 2002).
- It also reduces cytotoxic exposure to patients and their carers because excretion of the drug is quicker than when administered systemically (Washburn 2007).

Pre-procedural considerations

Specific patient preparations

Instillation first involves the insertion of a urinary catheter, drainage of the bladder, then the instillation of the drug. This usually takes about 50–60 minutes. The drug is retained for 1–2 hours with frequent movement by the patient to disperse it through the bladder (Sewell et al. 2002, Wilkes 2018). Therapy may be repeated on alternating days for three doses or weekly for varying lengths of time (4–12 weeks).

Procedure guideline 4.10   Cytotoxic therapy: intravesical instillation of cytotoxic drugs

Essential equipment
- Urotainer containing prescribed drug in clinically clean tray (delivered from pharmacy reconstitution unit)
- Sterile gloves
- Disposable apron and eye protection
- Gate clip or equivalent clamp for catheter
- Catheter drainage bag, if catheter is to remain in position
- 10 or 20 mL sterile syringe
- Small dressing pack that includes a sterile field

Pre-procedure

Action	Rationale
1 Explain and discuss the procedure with the patient.	To ensure that the patient understands the procedure and gives their valid consent (NMC 2015, **C**).
2 Check the patient's full blood count, as instructed by the medical staff, and inform them of any deficit before administration.	Absorption of the drug through the bladder wall may cause some myelosuppression. However, there are differing opinions as to whether regular checks are necessary. **E**
3 Check all the details on the container of cytotoxic drug against the patient's prescription chart.	To minimize the risk of error and comply with legal requirements (NMC 2010, **C**).
4 Assemble all necessary equipment, including the cytotoxic drug container, and proceed to the patient.	To ensure that the instillation proceeds smoothly and without interruption. **E**
5 Screen the patient's bed/couch.	To ensure privacy during the procedure. **E**
6 Check that the patient's identity matches the patient's details on the prescription chart.	To ensure that the correct patient has been identified. To reduce the risk of error (NMC 2010, **C**).

Procedure

Action	Rationale
7 If the patient does not have a catheter *in situ*, then pass a catheter (see Dougherty and Lister [2015] *The Royal Marsden Manual of Clinical Nursing Procedures, Ninth Edition*: Chapter 5 Elimination).	To enable the medication to be administered. **E**
8 Ensure the bladder is empty of urine.	To prevent dilution of the drug. (Washburn 2007, **E**).
9 Put on gloves, apron and eye protection.	To protect the nurse from contact with the cytotoxic drugs. With correct technique, the risk of contamination is minimal but splashes can occur (Wilkes 2018, **E**).
10 Using aseptic technique and sterile gloves, place a receiver under the end of the catheter to catch any urine and disconnect the drainage bag.	To protect the patient from infection. To protect the nurse from drug spillage. To gain access to the catheter. To prevent urine from soiling the bed. **E**
11 Remove the cover from the urotainer, connect to the catheter and release the clamp on the urotainer.	To facilitate drug instillation. **E**
12 Using gravity to create pressure, instil the cytotoxic drug into the bladder. Gentle squeezing may be needed to assist this process.	Rapid instillation would be uncomfortable for the patient, especially if the bladder is small or scarred from previous treatment or disease. **E**
13 When the correct prescribed volume has been instilled, slide urotainer clamp over filling port.	To prevent drainage of drug from the bladder (Weinstein and Hagle 2014, **E**).
14 When the drug has been in the bladder for 1 hour, ask the patient to micturate or slide clamp across filling port and place receiver under connectors. Disconnect urotainer and connect new drainage bag.	One hour is the usual time specified for intravesical drugs to ensure the maximum therapeutic effect with minimum toxicity. To prevent contamination of bedlinen (Nixon and Schulmeister 2009). **E**

Post-procedure

15	If the catheter is to be removed, withdraw the water from the catheter balloon (if appropriate – some catheters do not have a balloon) using the sterile syringe and remove the catheter using gentle traction. Dispose of equipment into clinical waste bag and seal.	The catheter may not be required for continued urinary drainage, and may have been inserted to facilitate drug administration, particularly in the outpatient department. The risk of infection is greater if the catheter remains *in situ* (Weinstein and Hagle 2014, **E**).
16	The patient should be made aware that their urine may be cloudy. Instruct the patient to report any discomfort or inability to pass urine immediately to ward staff or general practitioner/ district nurse, or to telephone the hospital if anxious.	To detect and resolve any problems at the earliest moment. To reduce anxiety experienced by the patient. **E**
17	Record the administration of the medication in the patient's records.	To ensure that medication and interventions are recorded (NMC 2010, **E**).

Problem-solving table 4.1 Prevention and resolution (Procedure guideline 4.10)

Problem	Cause	Prevention	Action
No drainage of urine when the catheter is inserted.	Bladder is empty or the catheter is in the wrong place, for example in the urethra or in a false track. False tracks may develop after repeated cystoscopy or bladder surgery.	Ensure experienced nurses catheterize the patient and check notes for any previous difficulties with insertion or false tracks.	Do not inflate the balloon but tape the catheter to the skin to keep it in position. Check when the patient last micturated. Encourage the patient to drink a few glasses of fluid. Do not give the drug until urine flow is seen or correct positioning of the catheter is established. Inform a doctor if no urine has drained during the next 30 minutes.
No drainage of urine when catheter unclamped.	Blocked with clots or debris.	May not be possible to prevent.	Check the position of the catheter and perform bladder lavage if necessary.
Patient has pain during instillation of the drug or while the drug is in the bladder.	Following resection of mucosa, the bladder can become acutely sensitive to irritants, thus causing painful spasm, resulting in possible expulsion of the cytotoxic agent.	Administer analgesics pre procedure. Help to keep the patient as calm and comfortable as possible.	Allow the drug to drain out and/or stop instillation if the pain is severe. Inform a doctor. Administer Entonox if appropriate (see Chapter 3) and have analgesics prescribed for subsequent administration.
Patient is unable to retain the requisite drug volume in the bladder for the time required.	Low bladder capacity; weak sphincter muscles or unstable detrusor muscle causing uncontrolled bladder contractions.	May not be able to prevent.	The nurse should record the actual duration of the drug in the bladder and inform a doctor if the patient is unable to retain the drug in the bladder.
Patient is unable to pass urine following removal of catheter.	Anxiety; poor bladder tone or prostatism.	Reassure patient and encourage fluids prior to removal.	The nurse should provide comfort and reassurance to the patient and encourage the patient to drink fluids.

Post-procedural considerations

Education of patient and relevant others
The patient should be provided with information about the amount of movement required, but if an outpatient, the journey home is usually sufficient to coat the bladder mucosa. An increase in oral intake while the treatment is being given will increase the dilution of medication required, ensure that there is sufficient washing out of the bladder and reduce the likelihood of local irritation or difficulty in urination due to debris from the tumour (Wilkes 2018).

Patients should be instructed in good personal hygiene such as washing hands and genitalia thoroughly after voiding, and the toilet should be flushed once after voiding or twice if it is a low-flushing toilet (Wilkes 2018). With BCG, the patient should be taught to bleach the toilet and leave it for 15 minutes before flushing with the toilet lid down (Wilkes 2018).

Complications

Haematuria
This can occur within 24–48 hours as a direct consequence of the trauma of catheterization or the loosening of blood clots following cystoscopy by fluid injected into the bladder. The patient needs to be monitored for signs of clot retention, shock, haemorrhage or fluid retention and any complications should be reported to the medical team. The patient should be encouraged to drink plenty of fluids to help reduce the risk of clot formation.

Leakage
Another complication can be leakage from around the catheter following administration of the drug. This may be caused by the catheter slipping out of the bladder or bladder spasm caused by the drug itself. It is therefore important that the nurse checks the position of the catheter regularly and informs the doctor if leakage

persists. Any leakage should be washed thoroughly using protective personal equipment. The patient's skin should be protected by wrapping sterile topical swabs around the catheter and promoting strict personal hygiene (Wilkes 2018).

Intraperitoneal instillation of cytotoxic drugs

Definition

Intraperitoneal administration is the introduction of cytotoxic drugs into the peritoneal space to prevent or delay a recurrence (Wilkes 2018).

Related theory

The peritoneal space is semi-permeable, allowing high concentrations of a drug to be achieved at the site of the tumour throughout the peritoneal space, but with lower concentrations entering the bloodstream, thus reducing the toxicity (Sewell et al. 2002). In this way, increased dosages of drug can be delivered to the tumour site than could be delivered systemically.

Large volumes of fluid containing chemotherapy agents should be administered intermittently. The chemotherapy agents used include (Sewell et al. 2002):

- cisplatin
- carboplatin
- bleomycin
- paclitaxel
- mitoxantrone
- mitomycin C
- 5-FU.

Evidence-based approaches

Rationale

Indications

Treatment failures of primary malignant tumours of the colon and rectum as well as ovary occur most frequently as regional disease. Extensive tumours may be present intra-abdominally without evidence of disease at other sites in the body. In view of this, chemotherapy treatment given intraperitoneally has been shown to be effective in treating locally recurrent ovarian and colon cancer (Sewell et al. 2002, Wilkes 2018).

Methods of accessing the peritoneal space

There are three methods of accessing the peritoneal space.

1 Intermittent placement of a temporary indwelling catheter into the peritoneal cavity. This is used for a short time such as for symptom relief or palliation.
2 Placement of an external catheter such as a Tenckhoff. This is surgically placed through the anterior abdominal wall and the catheter exits through the skin on the abdomen. This is the most widely used method. The Tenckhoff catheter has the advantages of allowing a high flow rate (2 litres in 10–15 minutes) and allowing for manipulation to dislodge fibrin deposits (Wilkes 2018). Problems include occlusion, infection, leakage around the catheter and body image problems.
3 Placement of an implantable peritoneal port. The port is internal with no care required when not accessed and therefore has a lower rate of infection and may be more acceptable to the patient. However, ports tend to provide a slower flow rate than a catheter (Wilkes 2018).

Procedure guideline 4.11 Cytotoxic therapy: intraperitoneal instillation of cytotoxic drugs

Essential equipment
- Sterile gloves
- Disposable apron and goggles
- Y-tube irrigation set

Medicinal products
- Syringe or infusion bag containing prescribed drug in clinically clean tray (delivered from pharmacy reconstitution unit)
- Gate clip or equivalent clamp for catheter
- Catheter drainage bag, if catheter is to remain in position
- Small dressing pack containing sterile field

Pre-procedure

Action	Rationale
1 Explain and discuss the procedure with the patient.	To ensure that the patient understands the procedure and gives their valid consent (NMC 2015, **C**).
2 Administer premedication to the patient if prescribed.	To ensure the patient is relaxed during the procedure. **E**
3 Check all the details on the container of the cytotoxic drug against the patient's prescription chart.	To minimize the risk of error and comply with legal requirements (NMC 2010, **C**).
4 Assemble all necessary equipment, including the cytotoxic drug container, and proceed to the patient.	To ensure that the instillation proceeds smoothly and without interruption. **E**

Procedure

5 Prior to instillation, pre-warm the infusion to body temperature.	To prevent cramping (Wilkes 2018, **E**).
6 Use a Y-tube irrigation set. The catheter is attached by this Y-tube to a bottle of dialysate and a drainage bag.	To ensure minimum intervention in draining the peritoneal cavity. **E**
7 Instil fluid at the prescribed rate, usually 1–2 litres over 10–15 minutes, but can be extended to 30–60 minutes.	To ensure the correct instillation at the correct rate (NMC 2010, **C**; Wilkes 2018, **E**).
8 Document administration on the prescription chart.	To record administration (NMC 2010, **C**).
9 Wait for the prescribed period after administration prior to draining off excess fluid. This may be from 1 to 3 hours.	To ensure fluid has coated all parts of peritoneal cavity. **E**

10	Observe regularly for patient comfort and intervene as appropriate. If the patient experiences any discomfort or pain, administer prescribed analgesia.	To keep patient comfortable and pain free. **E**
11	Record temperature 4 hourly.	To observe for pyrexia, a common side-effect that may indicate a developing infection or a reaction to chemotherapy. **E**
12	Unclamp the drainage tube and, where necessary, flush the port or pump using appropriate flushing solution. The catheter may be removed after drainage is complete.	To allow drainage of the drug. **E**

Post-procedure

13	Record accurate fluid balance.	To maintain accurate records (NMC 2015, **C**).

Problem-solving table 4.2 Prevention and resolution (Procedure guideline 4.11)

Problem	Cause	Prevention	Action
Abdominal pain or discomfort.	Peritoneal irritation following placement of catheter. Incomplete drainage of the dialysate solution.		Observe for a reaction and treat symptomatically.
	Failure to warm dialysate solution to body temperature.	Warm the dialysate fluid.	Ensure that solution is warmed and procedure is followed.
	Chemical peritonitis resulting from chemotherapeutic agent.		Observe for any signs of discomfort and treat symptomatically.
Leakage from around the catheter following administration of the drug.	Peritoneum is not intact or catheter is not entirely within the peritoneal cavity.	Check that the catheter is in the correct place before administration.	Strict aseptic technique required. Dressings to be changed frequently. When skin around the catheter has healed, there should be no further leakage.

Post-procedural considerations

To ensure safe disposal of waste, it is important that if there is leakage around the drainage site or a drainage bag is attached, nurses must remember that the fluid may still contain the cytotoxic drug and should therefore take the same precautions as when handling any cytotoxic waste.

Complications

General complications of intraperitoneal chemotherapy include respiratory distress, abdominal pain and distension, discomfort and diarrhoea (all of which result in increased abdominal pressure) (Wilkes 2018). Other problems include mechanical difficulties with the catheter (inflow and outflow obstructions), electrolyte imbalance and peritonitis caused by chemical irritation of the peritoneal space or by infection or both. Intraperitoneal chemotherapy is usually tolerated well by patients and provides a safe and effective treatment in the management of peritoneal disease (Weinstein and Hagle 2014).

Intra-arterial administration of cytotoxic drugs

Definition

Intra-arterial administration is the delivery of a cytotoxic drug to the tumour site by catheterization of the artery providing the blood supply to the affected organ. This allows a high concentration of drug to be delivered (Weinstein and Hagle 2014).

Related theory

The advantage of the intra-arterial route is that it facilitates the delivery of high concentrations of drug to the primary or secondary tumour mass (Sewell et al. 2002). A reduction in systemic circulating levels of drugs has been shown to occur in many circumstances,

resulting in a corresponding reduction in side-effects to the patient (Wilkes 2018). The cytotoxic drugs used vary with the histology and site of the tumour. All of the following have been administered via the intra-arterial route (Weinstein and Hagle 2014):

- actinomycin D
- BCNU (carmustine)
- bleomycin
- cisplatin
- doxorubicin
- 5-FU
- 5-FUDR
- methotrexate
- melphalan
- mitomycin C
- vincristine.

The main disadvantage of this route is that very high levels of drug in a perfused organ may result in excessive tissue damage (Sewell et al. 2002).

Evidence-based approaches

Rationale

The tumour site determines which artery will be used to deliver the chemotherapy because it is the artery supplying the tumour that is cannulated. The most common route is the hepatic artery (Weinstein and Hagle 2014).

Indications

Intra-arterial chemotherapy has been used to treat a variety of malignancies at many different sites. These include:

- head and neck lesions
- liver metastases from colorectal cancer

- sarcomas/melanomas of upper and lower limb (including isolated limb perfusion)
- carcinoma of the stomach
- carcinoma of the breast
- carcinoma of the cervix.

Methods of infusion

Two main methods are used for arterial infusional chemotherapy: external and internal.

The external method

This involves radiographic placement of an arterial catheter and attachment to an external infusion pump (Wilkes 2018). Temporary catheter placement is used for short-term therapies, that is, from hours up to 5 days. Therapy can be given intermittently for several courses. This method is unsuitable for long-term use (6 months or longer) as it is uncomfortable, inconvenient and expensive, although a subcutaneous implanted port increases the patient's comfort and freedom (Wilkes 2018).

Once the catheter is in place and secured, cytotoxic drugs may be administered by:

- injection, using a syringe
- small-volume infusion, using a syringe pump.
- large-volume infusion, using a volumetric pump.

Internal or implantable methods

These involve the surgical placement of a totally implantable pump and appear to have a lower complication rate than the external method. The catheter is inserted into an appropriate artery and attached to the pump, which is filled with chemotherapy. This approach is more frequently used for colorectal cancer metastases to the liver.

Confirmation that the artery supplies the desired area can be achieved by instillation of yellow fluorescent dye if the tumour site is visible, or contrast medium if an internal organ such as the liver is the target area.

All delivery systems must provide adequate pressure to combat arterial pressure, that is, 300 mmHg (Wilkes 2018). The majority of infusion pumps meet this requirement. Patient education is very important as the patient may have to maintain the implantable pump and be able to recognize any complications or malfunctions.

Principles of care

The catheter is inserted in theatre or in the X-ray department and its position checked at that time. The catheter is then secured and an occlusive dressing applied. This should *not* be touched as it is essential that the catheter is *not* displaced. A three- or one-way tap is connected to the catheter and it is at this point that all manipulations take place. An extension set should be connected to this at the time of insertion or on return to the ward to prevent unnecessary handling near the skin exit site. The system will consist of catheter, tap, extension set, administration set and infusion device.

Legal and professional issues

Consent

Insertion of the catheter is an operative procedure and consent must be obtained. Adequate explanation to the patient is essential, especially what to expect on return to the ward.

Procedure guideline 4.12   Intra-arterial administration of cytotoxic drugs

Essential equipment

- Sterile dressing pack
- Infusion pump containing the prescribed drug in a clinically clean tray (delivered from pharmacy reconstitution unit)
- Disposable gown and gloves
- Luer-Lok extension set with clamp
- Three-way tap

Pre-procedure

Action	Rationale
1 Explain and discuss the procedure with the patient.	To ensure that the patient understands the procedure and gives their valid consent (Griffith et al. 2003, **E**; NMC 2010, **C**).
2 Check the patient's prescription chart.	To ensure that the patient is given the correct drug and dose (NMC 2010b, **C**).

Procedure

Action	Rationale
3 Close room door or curtains if appropriate.	To ensure patient privacy and dignity. **E**
4 Assist the patient into the required position.	To allow access to the arterial device. **E**
5 Check confirmation of patency with the medical and radiological team as necessary.	To confirm patency and to ensure that the catheter is in the correct position (Wilkes 2018, **E**).
6 Use aseptic technique at all manipulations.	To minimize the risk of cross-infection (Wilkes 2018, **E**).
7 Attach the medication to the extension set, ensuring that the equipment is securely connected.	To minimize risk of air entry to the device or artery (Wilkes 2018, **E**).
8 Administer chemotherapy.	To ensure the patient receives therapy as prescribed. **E**
9 Ensure that the dressing is secure.	To prevent dislodgement of the catheter (Wilkes 2018, **E**).

Post-procedure

Action	Rationale
10 Record the administration on the appropriate charts.	To maintain accurate records, provide a point of reference in the event of any queries and prevent any duplication of treatment (NMC 2015, **C**; NPSA 2008a, **C**).
11 Observe for signs of bleeding.	To prevent haemorrhage (Wilkes 2018, **E**).

Problem-solving table 4.3 Prevention and resolution (Procedure guideline 4.12)

Problem	Cause	Prevention	Action
Displacement of the catheter.	Dressing disturbed.	Do not disturb the dressing. Ensure that the dressing and all equipment are connected securely and monitor the site regularly.	If bleeding occurs, pressure should be applied immediately and a member of the medical staff contacted.
	Excessive movement by patient.	Instruct the patient on the amount of movement permitted. Check catheter position daily.	

Post-procedural considerations

Immediate care

The dressing must not be touched but should be observed regularly for signs of bleeding. All Luer-Lok connections should be checked to prevent exsanguination, air embolism or disconnection under pressure. Any bleeding should be reported immediately to the medical staff, including the radiologist (Allwood et al. 2002).

Ongoing care

The catheter must be clamped securely or switched off, closing the tap *in situ* before any equipment changes. A positive pressure greater than arterial pressure must always be maintained. When chemotherapy is not being infused, the flushing solution must be used to maintain patency. This should be via a syringe or syringe pump during transfer between wards or departments, or via a syringe pump or infusion pump in the ward (when a nurse escort may be necessary). It should be delivered at the minimum rate sufficient to combat arterial pressure and maintain patency, approximately 3–5 mL per hour or 10 drops per minute, depending on the device used. If a specialist delivery system is used, the manufacturer's instructions should be followed.

The position of the catheter may be checked daily by X-ray; this will be performed on the ward. Fluoroscopy and instillation of dye are other methods of confirming position. At the end of treatment, the patency of the arterial catheter should be maintained using an appropriate flushing solution until a decision has been made about removal. Instructions for this and the amount of heparin to be used should be prescribed in advance to enable the nurse to initiate the procedure when appropriate. Before removal, the tap may be switched off and the catheter allowed to clot. The catheter should be removed by a doctor and firm pressure applied for at least 5 minutes or until all bleeding has ceased. A dressing should be applied to the site. Pressure dressings are not indicated if bleeding has ceased as they can obscure the formation of a haematoma.

Education of the patient and relevant others

The patient must be instructed on how often they can move and mobilize. This may vary depending on the site of the catheter. Assistance may be needed to maintain personal hygiene and relieve pressure to prevent the development of pressure ulcers on all points of contact.

Complications

Arterial occlusion and thrombosis

The literature indicates that thrombosis occurs in over 40% of arteries catheterized for over 48 hours. However, this is dependent on the vessel used. Most catheters used for chemotherapy delivery pose no problem and will remain patent for the treatment period. However, a thrombus may embolize, causing vascular insufficiency or distal or central embolism (Weinstein and Hagle 2014). When occlusion occurs due to thrombus formation or spasm, blood flow is usually maintained by the collateral circulation until the vessel recovers. Presence of a pulse and the colour of the area should be checked daily or a Doppler flow meter may be used (Yarbro et al. 2018). Any abnormality should be reported to the medical staff and radiologist. The catheter should be removed by the doctor using firm, steady traction, to prevent dislodging any thrombus present. The condition of the patient and the limb/area should be observed carefully at the time that vital signs are measured.

Damage to the artery, arteriovenous fistula, aneurysm formation

The incidence of these is low and the likelihood of problems occurring can be minimized by gentle handling of the catheter and immobilization of the limb/area as soon as appropriate (Weinstein and Hagle 2014).

Chemical hepatitis and biliary sclerosis

The occurrence of these will be evident from elevated liver enzymes. Therefore, monitoring of liver function tests is important. Any elevation is usually transient (Weinstein and Hagle 2014).

Exsanguination/air embolism

The seriousness of an air embolus depends on the siting of the arterial catheter and whether it is a direct route to the carotid artery and so to the brain. Luer-Lok connections must be used throughout the pathway. These should be checked at regular intervals and continuous flow maintained. Care must be taken when changing equipment to prevent blood loss occurring, or air entering the catheter, for example shutting off the tap and firm clamping, if necessary.

Infection due to poor aseptic technique

Strict aseptic technique must be maintained for all procedures and manipulations of the arterial catheter (Weinstein and Hagle 2014).

Extravasation of the medication and failure of the medication to reach the target

Although these are both rare, they may occur because of incorrect placement of the catheter. If there is any doubt concerning the placement of the catheter, the doctor and radiologist should be notified because extravasation of the medication may lead to ulceration and necrosis (Weinstein and Hagle 2014).

Side-effects of chemotherapy

The systemic side-effects of chemotherapy vary for every individual and are influenced by the drug or combination of drugs that the patient is receiving (Yarbro et al. 2018). The essential prerequisite of chemotherapy delivery is a comprehensive medical or nursing assessment of the patient in order to ascertain fitness for treatment. The assessment also allows the determination of response to therapy (i.e. tumour markers) and regulation of the dose of drugs in relation to toxicity (Dougherty and Bailey 2008). Using tools such as a chemotherapy symptom assessment scale (CSAS) can enhance the accuracy of reporting the symptoms experienced by the patient while receiving chemotherapy, which can have a positive impact upon the nursing and medical interventions offered. Such tools are essentially a patient-held record of symptoms following chemotherapy and reflect the extent to which the symptoms impact upon the daily life of the patient.

The patient produces the record at each cycle of chemotherapy and the information is used to plan interventions to suit their individual needs. Patients require information relating to their chemotherapy treatment as well as information regarding possible side-effects and how to manage them (Roe and Lennan 2014).

Haematological side-effects

Bone marrow suppression

Myelosuppression is one of the most common dose-limiting side-effects of chemotherapy (Schulmeister 2009). All chemotherapy has an effect on the bone marrow, resulting in a reduction in white blood cells, red blood cells and platelets. Myelosuppression that causes bleeding or infection can be life-threatening. Colony-stimulating factors (CSFs) enhance granulocyte production and shorten the nadir (the point at which the lowest blood count is reached after chemotherapy) (Schulmeister 2009).

Leucopenia

Leucopenia is classified as a lower than normal number of white blood cells in the bloodstream. White blood cells are often categorized as granulocytes and agranulocytes. Granulocytes include neutrophils, which have a lifespan of 6 hours to a few days; eosinophils, which have a lifespan of 8–12 days; and basophils, which have a lifespan of a few hours to few days. CSFs such as filgrastim and pegfilgrastim can be used to manage neutropenia, a condition in which the number of neutrophils in the bloodstream is decreased, impairing the body's ability to fight infection (Campbell 2005).

Anaemia

The lifespan of a red blood cell is 120 days. A patient is considered anaemic if the haemoglobin level is lower than 8 g/dL (Weinstein and Hagle 2014). Patients with anaemia may be asymptomatic or may manifest symptoms such as headache, light-headedness, shortness of breath, fatigue or pallor of skin and nail beds. A blood transfusion will help raise the haemoglobin level. One unit of red blood cells can raise the haemoglobin by 1 g/dL (Schulmeister 2009). Erythropoietin can be used to stimulate red blood cell production (Weinstein and Hagle 2014).

Thrombocytopenia

Thrombocytopenia is classified as a lower than normal number of platelets in the bloodstream. A normal range for the platelet count is $150–400 \times 10^9$/L. The risk of bleeding increases if the platelet count reduces to 100×10^9/L (Schulmeister 2009). Signs and symptoms of thrombocytopenia include bruising, petechiae, bleeding from the gums and nose, and haemorrhage in the central nervous system or gastrointestinal tract (Dougherty and Bailey 2008). Risk of bleeding is considered severe when the platelet count reaches 20×10^9/L. Activities that carry a high risk, such as contact sports, should be avoided since they can cause injury and subsequent bleeding. Patients should be encouraged to report signs of spontaneous bruising, nosebleeds, bleeding gums and bloody stools (Weinstein and Hagle 2014). A low platelet count can delay the continuation of chemotherapy. Platelet transfusions can be given in order to manage thrombocytopenia.

Fatigue

Fatigue has been defined as an overwhelming sense of exhaustion and inability to perform physical or mental work that is not relieved by rest (Weinstein and Hagle 2014). It is a common side-effect of chemotherapy (60% of patients) and is often not recognized, reported or treated (Schwartz 2007). Fatigue can also be a result of anaemia, infection, dehydration, electrolyte imbalances and poor nutritional status (see Chapter 8, Living with and beyond cancer). Interventions are focused upon conserving energy, resting or sleeping for short periods of time, and alternating periods of rest with activity in order to build up the body to maintain levels of functionality (Dougherty and Bailey 2008).

Gastrointestinal side-effects

Nausea and vomiting

Nausea and vomiting are two of the most common and distressing side-effects of chemotherapy (Schulmeister 2009). Approximately 70–80% of all cancer patients receiving chemotherapy experience vomiting (Weinstein and Hagle 2014). Chemotherapy-induced nausea and vomiting can be described as acute (occurring within 2 hours and lasting up to 24 hours), delayed (occurring 24 hours after chemotherapy administration) and anticipatory (happening before and during chemotherapy administration, often as a result of conditioning from stimuli associated with the chemotherapy process or environment) (Dougherty and Bailey 2008). Factors predisposing to nausea and vomiting include age and gender: younger patients experience more nausea and vomiting than older patients, and females more than males.

The emetic potential of chemotherapy drugs can be classified as low, moderate or high (MASCC 2011, NCCN 2018). Guidelines on the use of antiemetic drugs to control chemotherapy-induced nausea should be used to prevent, treat and manage patients' symptoms (London Cancer New Drugs Group 2016). When choosing the antiemetic medication consideration needs to be given to the emetogenic potential of the individual drugs within the regimen; treatment may include corticosteroids and 5-HT3 inhibitors.

Successful management of nausea and vomiting combines pharmacological intervention with non-pharmacological strategies. Antiemetic guidelines are available in most treatment centres, and antiemetics should be commenced prior to treatment and continued throughout the emetic activity of the chemotherapy drug used (Weinstein and Hagle 2014). Non-pharmacological interventions such as acupressure have been reported to relieve nausea. Acupressure works on the principle of pressure being applied to the P6 (pericardium) pressure point. The pressure point is located on the inner aspect of the wrist and the pressure band disc is placed three fingers' width from the wrist crease between the two tendons (Figure 4.11). Although it has been suggested that nausea can be relieved within the first 24 hours following chemotherapy, the pressure bands do not appear to have any impact upon vomiting (Dougherty and Bailey 2008).

Taste changes/anorexia

Patients receiving chemotherapy can experience changes in taste as well as loss of appetite. Foods that the patient is used to eating can taste very different following chemotherapy (Weinstein and Hagle 2014). It is therefore important to ensure that a nutritional assessment forms part of the patient's care plan and that strategies are adopted to maximize nutritional well-being. Many patients complain of a bitter or metallic taste and can be advised to experiment with different flavours and spices, the aim of which

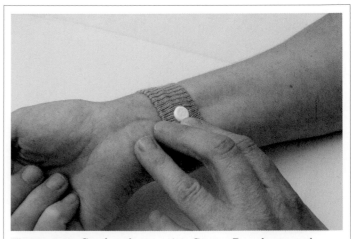

Figure 4.11 Sea-bands on wrist. *Source:* Dougherty and Lister (2011).

is to stimulate the taste buds, making the mouth feel more comfortable (Schulmeister 2009). Plastic utensils can help reduce the metallic taste. Generally, patients find that cold food as opposed to hot is more palatable and that having meals served on glass rather than plastic helps reduce odours (Bernhardson et al. 2009).

Odours from cooking can have a negative impact upon the desire to eat; advise the patient to avoid areas where food is being prepared. Appetite stimulants can be prescribed if necessary in an attempt to maintain a healthy diet. Nutritional supplements such as protein drinks, protein powders and soft foods may be required (Schulmeister 2009).

Constipation

Constipation is the passing of hard, dry stools, causing difficulty in defaecation (Weinstein and Hagle 2014). The severity of the problem can range from mild discomfort to paralytic ileus (Schulmeister 2009). There are many causes of constipation including side-effects of medication, hypercalcaemia, dehydration, immobility and dietary deficiencies. Chemotherapy agents such as vinca alkaloids (vincristine, vinblastine) commonly cause constipation secondary to autonomic nerve dysfunction (Dougherty and Bailey 2008).

Prevention of constipation should be part of the medical and nursing assessment of the patient, and prophylactic laxatives, lubricants or stimulants should be used. Education about prevention interventions is important and the patient should be instructed to increase their dietary intake of fresh fruits, vegetables and fibre. Patients should be encouraged to drink 2–3 litres of fluid a day and to avoid cheese, eggs and starches (Weinstein and Hagle 2014). Physical activity stimulates peristalsis, so patients can be encouraged to be as mobile as possible. They should also be encouraged to defaecate immediately upon feeling the urge to do so and not to wait (Weinstein and Hagle 2014). See Chapter 7, Acute oncology.

Diarrhoea

The function of the colon is to absorb fluid. When this does not happen, diarrhoea ensues. Diarrhoea is the abnormal passage of three or more loose or watery stools in a 24-hour period and is often accompanied by abdominal cramps (Schulmeister 2009). There are many causes of diarrhoea including post-operative intestinal resection, *Clostridium difficile* and other intestinal infections. Chemotherapy agents such as 5-FU, capecitabine, docetaxel, doxorubicin and methotrexate can cause diarrhoea (Dougherty and Bailey 2008).

Nursing interventions should focus on the early detection of the problem and patients should be encouraged to report symptoms promptly. Normal bowel activity should be assessed as well as the frequency of the diarrhoea and the patient's oral intake over a 24-hour period. Patients require a minimum of 2 litres of fluid in a 24-hour period because electrolytes are lost as a consequence of diarrhoea (Schulmeister 2009). Potassium is the most significant electrolyte to be reduced and the patient should be encouraged to eat potassium-rich foods (Weinstein and Hagle 2014). Intravenous fluid replacement as well as antimotility agents can be used in severe cases. A high-calorie, high-protein and low-residue diet is recommended (Dougherty and Bailey 2008). See Chapter 7, Acute oncology. Other agents such as EGFR tyrosine kinase inhibitors (e.g. erlotinib, gefitinib and lapatinib) are associated with severe diarrhoea (Camp-Sorrell 2018). The diarrhoea is the result of the inhibitor activating on T-cell immune response in which many different effects can occur including colitis (Camp-Sorrell 2018).

Adverse drug reactions

It is essential that the allergy status of the patient is known and recorded in the patient's notes as failure to do so can have catastrophic results (DH 2003). All healthcare professionals have a responsibility to ensure that the allergy status of the patient has been assessed and recorded correctly, which should happen at every intervention. It is known that the use of taxanes is associated with a high risk of hypersensitivity and local policies should be adopted to manage any adverse drug reaction. The risk of allergic reactions can be reduced by administering hydrocortisone and chlorphenamine prior to administration of SACT and many organizations have a protocol to manage such reactions. Symptoms of a reaction are flushing, dizziness, restlessness, breathlessness, chest pain, tachycardia, hypertension, nausea or abdominal pain. Such reactions will normally resolve with the administration of antihistamines and corticosteroids as described above. Reactions are often classed by a grading system of severity and should always be documented in the patient's clinical notes. To manage severe or reoccurring sensitivities that do not respond to hydrocortisone and chlorphenamine, a desensitization programme that involves delivering the total drug in smaller infusion doses over a longer period of time can help.

Neurotoxicity

Neurotoxicity as a result of chemotherapy occurs when the CNS, peripheral nervous system, cranial nerves or a combination of all three are damaged either directly or indirectly. The damage may be transient, however some patients will experience permanent neurological deficits (Camp-Sorrell 2018). The severity of toxicities is related to the dose of chemotherapy. Neurotoxicity may manifest in different and unpredictable ways and diagnosis is confirmed by the patient's reporting of the symptoms as well as a physical neurological examination (Camp-Sorrell 2018). Chemotherapy agents such as platinum, vinca alkaloids and taxanes are known to cause peripheral neuropathy. Chemotherapy-induced peripheral neuropathy is caused by inflammation, degeneration or injury of the peripheral nerve fibres and requires a dose reduction to alleviate the symptoms (Camp-Sorrell 2018). Oxaliplatin is known to cause peripheral sensory neuropathy, which is exacerbated by cold air, cold drinks and touching cold surfaces. During or at the end of the infusion of oxaliplatin patients can experience pharyngolaryngeal dysaesthesia, hoarseness, dyspnoea or a tight sensation at the back of the throat. Patients are encouraged to protect themselves from the cold during the winter months with a thick scarf to cover the neck and mouth and gloves to help to prevent the symptoms.

High doses of methotrexate can cause encephalopathy resulting in blurred vision, lethargy and confusion, which normally resolves once the drug is stopped (Camp-Sorrell 2018). Seizures and cranial nerve and motor dysfunction have been associated with the use of ifosfamide; symptoms resolve within 48–72 hours once the therapy has ceased (Camp-Sorrell 2018). Methylene blue (MB) can be given for ifosfamide-induced encephalitis, although there is little conclusive evidence to support its use. It is thought to act as an electron acceptor to prevent the formation of chloroacetaldehyde. Without MB treatment, the reported recovery time from encephalopathy ranges from 2 to 29 days, but published studies show that the time to recovery from encephalopathy with MB varies from 10 minutes to 8 days (LCA 2014b).

A neurotoxicity which is becoming recognized is posterior reversible encephalopathy syndrome (PRES) which is associated with the administration of cisplatin, rituximab, bevacizumab and immunosuppressive therapy such as tacrolimus (Camp-Sorrell 2018). The symptoms are headaches, focal neurological and visual changes, encephalopathy and seizures (Polovich et al. 2014). Diagnosis of PRES is confirmed by MRI of the brain, where symmetrical subcortical white and grey matter lesions can be seen. PRES is reversible and the management of the condition is a reduction or withholding of the causative agent (Camp-Sorrell 2018).

Mucositis/stomatitis

Mucositis

Mucositis is the general term used to describe the painful inflammation and ulceration of the mucous membranes of the gastrointestinal tract by the cytotoxic effects of chemotherapy (Camp-Sorrell 2018). The growth patterns, replacement and functions of mucous membranes are similar and as such any part of the gastrointestinal tract can be adversely affected by chemotherapy. There is rapid renewal of the epithelial cells in the gastrointestinal tract to enable replenishment of cells that are lost during the natural process of eating. Chemotherapy-induced mucositis occurs when the mucosal cells are damaged and not able to repair quickly enough to replenish normal cell loss (Camp-Sorrell 2018).

Stomatitis

Chemotherapy-induced oral complications can be acute or chronic and healing of the oral mucosa is a complex process (Wilkes 2018). Acute complications include mucosal inflammation and ulceration, infection and bleeding (Wilkes 2018). The risk of developing stomatitis is dependent upon the type of chemotherapy, dose and schedule (Wilkes 2018). The majority of patients will develop some degree of chemotherapy-related stomatitis; risk factors include poor oral hygiene and dental health, poor nutrition, tobacco and alcohol use and acidic or spicy foods (Camp-Sorrell 2018). Younger patients are thought to be more at more risk due to their increased epithelial mitotic rate (Camp-Sorrell 2018).

A baseline oral cavity assessment should be performed before chemotherapy treatment begins and at each chemotherapy visit thereafter (Wilkes 2018). Patients should be given advice regarding oral hygiene and intervention strategies to help reduce or eliminate complications (Camp-Sorrell 2018).

Nephrotoxicity/haemorrhagic cystitis

Nephrotoxicity is caused when chemotherapy damages the proximal tubule epithelial cells of the kidney leading to acute tubular necrosis (Naughton 2008). Many chemotherapy drugs are metabolized and excreted by the kidneys; others such as cisplatin are excreted unchanged (Camp-Sorrell 2018, Wilkes 2018). Tumour lysis syndrome (TLS) is a condition caused by high levels of potassium, phosphorus and uric acid being released into the bloodstream. TLS is an oncological emergency because of the life-threatening complications of hypocalcaemia, hyperkalaemia, hyperuricaemia and hyperphosphataemia (Vioral 2018). Treatment includes hydration with 2–3 litres of sodium chloride or 5% dextrose to stimulate diuresis and administration of allopurinol. Rasburicase is recommended for patients who are at high risk of TLS; this drug can reduce uric acid levels within 4 hours (Polovich et al. 2014).

The dosage of chemotherapy drugs may be reduced in patients with pre-existing renal disease or if there are signs of early renal toxicity during the chemotherapy treatment schedule (Wilkes 2018). The risk of renal toxicity in elderly patients is higher as they have a lower total body water and glomerular filtration rate (Wilkes 2018). Assessment of renal function should continue throughout chemotherapy treatment. The role of the nurse is pivotal in terms of managing fluid replacement and monitoring urinary output (Wilkes 2018).

Haemorrhagic cystitis is inflammation of the mucosal surface of the bladder and/or ureters with associated haematuria (Polovich et al. 2014). It can present as microscopic haematuria or frank bleeding requiring instillation of sclerosing agents (Wilkes 2018). The risk of haemorrhagic cystitis relates to acrolein, which is a liver metabolite of cyclophosphamide and ifosfamide. Acrolein binds to the bladder mucosa causing ulceration, inflammation, necrosis and haemorrhage. Early diagnosis is vital for bladder preservation. If therapy is not stopped, up to 55% of patients continue to experience persistent symptoms (Wilkes 2018). Protecting the bladder from the harmful effects of acrolein can be achieved by administering mesna. Haemorrhagic cystitis is associated with other chemotherapy agents including paclitaxel and gemcitabine. Bladder preservation focuses on hydration, frequent voiding, mesna administration and diuresis (Wilkes 2018).

Cardiotoxicity

The effects of cardiotoxicity can be acute or chronic. Acute effects usually manifest as transient electrocardiogram changes, resolve without serious complications and occur in 10% of patients receiving chemotherapy; chronic effects manifest weeks or months following chemotherapy and manifest as non-reversible cardiomyopathy (Camp-Sorrell 2018). Chronic effects present as biventricular congestive heart failure with symptoms such as dyspnoea, non-productive cough and pedal oedema (Camp-Sorrell 2018). These symptoms tend to gradually deteriorate and are associated with a 60% mortality (Camp-Sorrell 2108).

Anthracyclines cause chronic cardiotoxicity by damaging the cardiac myocyte cells and cumulative doses should not exceed what is referred to as a 'lifetime dose'. The risk of acute and chronic cardiotoxicity of anthracyclines is increased in patients with pre-existing cardiac disease, hypertension, mediastinal radiation or exposure to other cardiotoxic agents (Camp-Sorrell 2018). Chemoprotectants such as dexrazoxane can be used as they have the ability to protect cardiac tissue by blocking damage to myocytes (Camp-Sorrell 2108).

Pulmonary toxicity

Pulmonary toxicity caused by chemotherapy can range from reversible short-term effects to permanent fibrosis and irreversible damage (Barber and Gant 2011). The initial damage occurs in the endothelial cells, producing an inflammatory type reaction which results in drug-induced pneumonitis (Wilkes 2018). Chronic disorders occur months to years following exposure to chemotherapy and are usually irreversible (Wilkes 2018). Clinical presentation of pulmonary toxicity ranges from mild to progressive, unproductive cough, bilateral basal rales, tachypnoea and low-grade fever (Wilkes 2018). Chemotherapy drugs such as bleomycin are well known to cause pulmonary toxicity. It is therefore important to monitor and detect pulmonary toxicity as soon as possible to enable interventions such as adjusting the dose of chemotherapy to prevent further damage (Wilkes 2018).

Hepatotoxicity

A range of hepatotoxicity conditions are caused by chemotherapy, occurring because of unforeseen or idiosyncratic reactions (Wilkes 2018). Symptoms present 1–4 weeks after chemotherapy administration and occur more frequently following multiple treatments. Damage seems to manifest in the parenchymal cells of the liver causing obstruction to hepatic blood flow and consequent fatty change, cholestasis, hepatitis, hepatocellular necrosis and veno-occlusive disease (Wilkes 2018). Assessment includes liver function tests, abdominal examination and visual inspection for jaundice, petechiae, skin rash and ecchymosis (Khalili et al. 2009). Although hepatic toxicity is uncommon it can have serious consequences ranging from a short duration of altered liver function tests to permanent cirrhosis. Therefore, careful monitoring of liver function throughout chemotherapy treatment is imperative to detect changes and prevent further problems (Wilkes 2018).

Skin toxicities

Chemotherapy has the potential to cause skin reactions including dryness, erythema and discolouration (hyperpigmentation), which can have a significant emotional impact upon the patient (Camp-Sorrell 2018). Hyperpigmentation is thought to be caused by the drug or a metabolic by-product stimulating the production of melanin. EGFR antagonist drugs have resulted in dry skin, rashes and pruritus (Camp-Sorrell 2018). The rash from EGFR inhibitors is commonly pustular in nature and is described as a form of acne that can affect the face, scalp and chest (Camp-Sorrell 2018). Treatment includes the use of over-the-counter moisturizing creams as well as oral antibiotics.

Alopecia

Definition

Chemotherapy-induced alopecia is the temporary loss of all body hair (Dougherty 2005).

Anatomy and physiology

In the bulb at the base of the follicle, the actual hair is produced by cells in the hair matrix zone, where the dermal papilla provides nutrients and growth factors to these cells. Keratinocytes in the hair matrix zone begin to rapidly divide and a keratinized hair emerges with a thin outer cuticle and a thick cortex (Janssen 2007). The hair follicle goes through three growth phases. Anagen is a phase of intensive growth and hair shaft production, which may last as long as 7 years. The hair follicle then enters the catagen phase (involution) in which the old hair shaft is broken down and a new hair follicle is formed. This lasts 2–3 weeks and is followed by the telogen phase (resting) which lasts 2–3 months before an intermediate regrowing state starts and new hair follicles are produced.

Chemotherapy affects rapidly growing keratinocytes in the hair matrix zone in anagen hair follicles and a decrease in the diameter of the hair bulb can be seen 4–6 days after administration of a single dose (Olsen 2003). Not all the hair follicles have the same rhythm of cycling; as approximately 90% of hair follicles are in a phase of growth at any given time, the resulting hair loss can be rapid and extensive (Janssen 2007).

Related theory

Alopecia is a common consequence of many chemotherapeutic regimens and is one of the most devastating effects of cancer chemotherapy (Choi et al. 2014, McGowan 2013, Pickard-Holley 1995, Power and Condon 2008, Williams et al. 1999). In a study of breast cancer survivors who completed a psychophysical scaling method, hair loss was ranked in the top five distressing side-effects of chemotherapy (Mulders et al. 2008, van den Hurk et al. 2012b), while Mols et al. (2009) found that the hair loss associated with chemotherapy was a source of distress for patients and was rated in the three most troublesome side-effects of treatment along with nausea and vomiting. Chemotherapy-induced alopecia adversely affects psychosocial functioning and quality of life (Choi et al. 2014, Hesketh et al. 2004, Lemieux et al. 2008, Rosman 2004; Young and Arif 2016). It has been identified as such a devastating prospect that some patients may refuse to accept treatment or choose regimens with less favourable outcomes (Boehmke and Dickerson 2005, Browall et al. 2006, Hesketh et al. 2004, Roe 2014, Rosenblatt 2006, Williams et al. 1999). Hair loss can also result in changes to the patient's body image (Freedman 1994, Gallagher 1996, Williams et al. 1999) which may not be reversed by the regrowth of hair (Munstedt et al. 1997).

Prevention of chemotherapy-induced alopecia

Several techniques have been tested to prevent chemotherapy-induced hair loss, the first being scalp tourniquets. These were used to minimize the contact the drug had with the hair follicles by occluding, using pressure, the superficial blood vessels supplying the scalp (Maxwell 1980). However, while some investigators found scalp tourniquets effective, others reported this method to be time-consuming, uncomfortable or ineffective (Parker 1987). Research findings indicate that scalp hypothermia (cooling) may be simpler, less traumatic and more effective as a means of preventing alopecia when compared with the scalp tourniquet (David and Speechley 1987).

It has been documented that men and women experience similar concerns about body image when they have experienced chemotherapy-induced hair loss, although women tended to speak about hair loss from the head and face (above the eyeline) while men spoke of losing hair from wider body surfaces (Hilton et al. 2008). Healthcare professionals must therefore be mindful that scalp cooling should be offered to patients as determined by the chemotherapy regimen and not the gender of the patient (Hilton et al. 2008).

In a study in which patients receiving chemotherapy for breast cancer who underwent scalp cooling were given questionnaires to complete before chemotherapy, after 3 weeks of treatment and 6 months after completion, the burden of scalp cooling was rated as low, suggesting that nursing staff must be aware of how distressing the matter of hair loss can be for patients, and scalp cooling should be offered wherever possible (Mols et al. 2009). Patients have been shown to be satisfied with scalp cooling when they experienced little hair loss and felt that it had been successful;

where it was not 100% successful it still reduced the patient's need to wear a wig or head covering (van den Hurk 2013a). Physicians tend to underestimate the impact of hair loss on patients so it may be up to the nurse to provide information on scalp cooling (Mulders et al. 2008, Rosman 2004).

Scalp cooling is a method of preventing chemotherapy-induced alopecia. It works in three ways (Batchelor 2001, Bulow et al. 1985):

1 reducing perfusion of hair follicles by vasoconstriction, thus limiting the amount of exposure to chemotherapy (an intradermal scalp temperature of 30°C decreases scalp blood flow by 25%)
2 reducing temperature-dependent cellular uptake of chemotherapy
3 reducing intrafollicular metabolic rate (Betticher et al. 2013).

The rationale is based on characteristics of hair growth, the effect of cytotoxic drugs on hair follicles, physiological changes in scalp circulation and pharmacokinetics (Keller and Blausey 1988). Ninety percent of all scalp hair is in an active phase of growth, characterized by significant mitotic activity; this means the hair bulb is especially sensitive to chemotherapeutic agents (Parker 1987). Scalp hypothermia produces changes in the scalp circulation by causing vasoconstriction of superficial vessels. Decreased blood flow to the scalp reduces the amount of the drug reaching the hair follicles and thus minimizes damage to the scalp hair (Kennedy et al. 1983, Parker 1987). Its success is also related to the metabolic effects of cooling, that is, slowing the metabolic rate (Bulow et al. 1985), and it also appears that the degree of hair loss is temperature dependent.

In order to prevent alopecia, the temperature of the scalp must be reduced to at least 24°C but preferably 22°C (Ekwall et al. 2013, Gregory et al. 1982). Caps have to be kept in a freezer in order to reach temperatures of −18 to −20°C (Anderson et al. 1981, Giaccone et al. 1988, Kennedy et al. 1983). Then, when the cap is placed on the head, the scalp temperature will drop from 37°C to 23–24°C within the first 15 minutes (Guy et al. 1982, Tollenaar et al. 1994). For this reason a preinjection scalp cooling time of 20–30 minutes is said to be required (Anderson et al. 1981, Giaccone et al. 1988, Kennedy et al. 1983, Middleton et al. 1985, Robinson et al. 1987, Satterwhite and Zimm 1984). Janssen (2007) studied the link between heat transfer in the human head and the transport of doxorubicin. This led to the development of a population-based computational model for scalp cooling which included doses of doxorubicin of 60–70 mg, lowering skin temperature to 17–18°C, leaving the cap on for the total infusion time plus 1 hour and having a haircut to reduce thermal resistance between head and cap, all of which provided the most effective scalp cooling. Daanen et al. (2015) found that slight cooling of patients with an elevated body temperature during scalp cooling contributed to the decrease in scalp temperatures and may improve the prevention of hair loss.

Scalp cooling has been used in an attempt to reduce hair loss with palliative whole-brain radiotherapy. However, a pilot study (Shah et al. 2000) found that all patients still lost their hair and there was evidence that the cold cap application increased the dose of radiotherapy to the scalp; this is supported by van den Hurk et al. (2015).

There have also been biological methods of preventing hair loss which have focused on promoting hair growth or protecting the hair follicles (Batchelor 2001). For example:

- minoxidil 2% topical solution applied twice a day (Shapiro and Price 1998, Yang and Thai 2015)
- topical topitriol (Hidalgo et al. 1999)
- application of a steroid 5-alpha reductase inhibitor (Uno and Kurata 1993)
- immunosuppressive immunophilin ligands such as ciclosporin (Maurer et al. 1997), immunomodulators, AS101 (Sredni et al. 1996), CDK2 inhibitors (Davis et al. 2001) and P53 (a mediator of cellular response which is essential for chemotherapy-induced hair loss) (Botchkarev et al. 2000)
- hair follicle targeted preparations (Chung et al. 2013, Haslam et al. 2013).

Evidence-based approaches

Rationale

Indications

All patients with solid tumours receiving doxorubicin, epirubicin, docetaxel or paclitaxel as a single agent or in combination should be offered scalp cooling.

Contraindications

Scalp cooling should not be offered to patients (Dougherty 2005):

- with haematological disease, unless the consultant feels it is appropriate to offer scalp cooling on the basis of quality of life
- who are receiving drugs that cause hair loss, for example vincristine, where there is no research or evidence of the effectiveness of scalp cooling
- who have already received a first course of chemotherapy that may induce hair loss but who were not offered or declined scalp cooling.

Principles of care

Scalp cooling

The effectiveness of scalp cooling has been demonstrated satisfactorily with doxorubicin, epirubicin, docetaxel and paclitaxel (Cigler et al. 2015, Dean et al. 1979, Katsimbri et al. 2000, Lemenager et al. 1995, Robinson et al. 1987, van den Hurk et al. 2012a). Patients receiving other cytotoxic drugs that may cause alopecia, such as vindesine and vincristine, have undergone the procedure, although there are insufficient data to evaluate its effectiveness with these drugs.

Doxorubicin is commonly used in cancer chemotherapy and has a uniquely short half-life of approximately 30 minutes (compared with other drugs such as cyclophosphamide, which has a plasma half-life of over 6 hours) (Priestman 1989). This factor makes prophylactic scalp cooling feasible because it need only be utilized during peak plasma levels (Cline 1984). This is particularly important because doxorubicin results in a consistently high incidence of alopecia (80–90% of all patients), often leading to total hair loss (Dean et al. 1983). The involvement of doxorubicin, whether used alone or in combination, is a feature of most of the reported scalp-cooling studies. In some studies there was less success in maintaining hair with increasing doses of doxorubicin and/or liver metastases (David and Speechley 1987, Dean et al. 1983), but this may be resolved by extending the time the cap remains in place following chemotherapy administration.

Scalp cooling has also been used during the administration of epirubicin, as a single agent, with good results (Robinson et al. 1987), although doses may influence outcomes (Adams et al. 1992). Subsequent studies have investigated combination regimens containing epirubicin and other drugs such as cyclophosphamide and 5-FU, with results of mild to moderate hair loss. However, when intravenous cyclophosphamide is added to anthracycline, the success rate is reduced from 80% of patients keeping most of their hair to about 50–60% of patients (David and Speechley 1987, Middleton et al. 1985). Some authors have therefore concluded that, when combinations of cyclophosphamide and anthracyclines are given, scalp cooling has no place at all (Tollenaar et al. 1994). The group of drugs known as the taxanes also has the unfortunate side-effect of total alopecia; however, there is now evidence that scalp cooling in patients receiving docetaxel and paclitaxel can prevent complete hair loss (Betticher et al. 2013, Katsimbri et al. 2000, Komen et al. 2013, Lemenager et al. 1995, 1997, Macduff et al. 2003, van den Hurk et al. 2012a).

Recommended cooling times have varied between studies and manufacturers. The common times are 15–30 minutes pre chemotherapy and then 45 minutes to 1 hour post anthracycline chemotherapy and 30–45 minutes post docetaxel administration (van den Hurk et al. 2012a).

Scalp cooling requires the consultant's permission as the procedure may protect micrometastases in the scalp from chemotherapy, especially where there is the possibility of circulating cancer cells, for example in cases of leukaemia and lymphoma (Witman et al. 1981). Despite this, scalp cooling has been used successfully in patients with relapsed lymphoma (Purohit 1992). Dean et al. (1983), drawing on evidence from 7800 women with breast cancer, found that only two experienced recurrence of disease on the scalp, suggesting that the risk of scalp metastases was minimal. They concluded that scalp cooling should not be contraindicated and could be used routinely with a wide variety of solid tumours. Nevertheless, patients with advanced metastatic disease have been found to develop scalp metastases during scalp cooling and Middleton et al. (1985) argued strongly against the use of scalp cooling in this group. Other studies have found no scalp metastases at follow-up (Ron et al. 1997). Lemieux et al. (2008) found the incidence of scalp metastases was low and no case presented as an isolated site of relapse. However, the potential risk of scalp metastases, albeit remote, should be addressed and demands discussion by healthcare professionals and patients (Batchelor 2001, Peck et al. 2000).

The issues relating to scalp metastases are controversial (Serrurier et al. 2012). This dilemma, along with the media coverage regarding preventive measures for chemotherapy-induced alopecia (Carr 1998, Kendell 2001), has led some practitioners to question whether scalp cooling should be offered. However, Lemieux et al. (2015) found no impact on overall survival in women with breast cancer who had received scalp cooling, and van den Hurk et al. (2013b) showed the incidence of scalp skin metastases to be very low with no difference between those who had scalp cooling (0.04%) and those did not (0.03–3%).

Patients have highlighted how they feel about hair loss (Carr 1998) and the need to provide more comfortable and effective scalp cooling in all cancer units and centres (Wilson 1994). In addition, an extensive review of the literature concluded that scalp cooling was effective and should be offered to all patients for whom it was appropriate (Batchelor 2001, Crowe et al. 1998, van den Hurk et al. 2014). This was supported by the views of many nurses who felt that the use of scalp cooling with chemotherapy protocols that are associated with hair loss can effectively prevent alopecia and result in improved quality of life for patients (Lemenager 1998, Young 2013). Patients also feel it is worthwhile to undergo scalp cooling regardless of how successful it is (Dougherty 2006b). However, although scalp cooling contributes to well-being in patients in whom it is successful, it can cause additional distress when patients lose their hair despite scalp cooling and so additional support may be required for those patients in whom scalp cooling is not successful (van den Hurk et al. 2010).

Limitations of scalp-cooling studies

Despite the large number of studies on scalp cooling, they are difficult to compare with one another owing to the many variables: different types of scalp-cooling caps, varying methods of applying the caps, different chemotherapy regimens, tools for assessment of hair loss (although Vleut et al. [2013] have developed a hair mass index obtained by cross-section trichometry) and who performs the assessment. Also, sample numbers are often small and few studies are randomized or have a control group (Dougherty 2006b, Grevelman and Breed 2005). This results in difficulties when making decisions related to selection of scalp-cooling systems, discussing the risk of scalp metastases, or even whether to offer scalp cooling at all (Breed 2004, Christodoulou et al. 2002, Grevelman and Breed 2005, Randall and Ream 2005).

Anticipated patient outcomes

The success of all these methods of preventing hair loss varies and the amount of hair loss experienced by the patient is dependent on many factors.

- Involvement of the liver with metastatic disease leads to elevated plasma levels of doxorubicin for a longer period. Impaired liver function can reduce success rates for scalp cooling

(Shin et al. 2015). Early studies seemed to indicate that extension of the cooling period did not improve the results (Satterwhite and Zimm 1984) whereas others have found that longer cooling times in general improve success rates (Massey 2004). Other factors that might influence success include comorbidities, menopausal status, nicotine abuse, medications and original hair density (Schaffrin-Nabe et al. 2015).

- Inadequate cooling because of exceptionally thick hair may lead to partial loss. It has been demonstrated that maximum cooling occurs 20 minutes after the cap has been placed in position.
- The weight of the cap (as well as the temperature) may be a factor, as this ensures that the contact is maintained over the complete scalp (Hunt et al. 1982).
- Success does not appear to be dose dependent, as was first thought (David and Speechley 1987, Dougherty 2006b).
- It seems likely that when anthracyclines are used in combination with other drugs that cause alopecia (e.g. etoposide and cyclophosphamide) the success rate is not as high as with anthracyclines alone (Middleton et al. 1985). It has also been found that the type of anthracycline used will affect success rates as hair loss is greater with doxorubicin and cyclophosphamide than with epirubicin and cyclophosphamide (Dougherty 2006b).

Legal and professional issues

Consent

Patients must give consent for the procedure but must first be fully informed about the nature and length of the procedure, the chances of success and, where appropriate, the risk of scalp metastases (Peck et al. 2000). Scalp cooling can be a long and uncomfortable procedure and should not be offered unless it is beneficial or the patient insists on undergoing the procedure. Peerbooms et al. (2015) found that not all patients are offered scalp cooling due to doubts from healthcare professionals regarding its efficacy and safety. Patients must also be informed that they may discontinue the procedure at any time if they find it too physically or psychologically traumatic (Tierney 1987) or if they fail to retain hair.

Research shows that scalp cooling can be very distressing (Tierney 1989), although patients still find it a worthwhile procedure to undergo regardless of whether it is successful and many would have it again if necessary (Dougherty 1996, 2006b). It has also been shown that the severity and distress associated with hair loss may be less for those who use scalp cooling (Protiere et al. 2002).

Pre-procedural considerations

Equipment

Most of the studies that used an ice cap method of scalp cooling used a 'home-made' or a commercial cap (Anderson et al. 1981, David and Speechley 1987, Dean et al. 1983, Lemenager et al. 1997).

Home-made caps

Initially scalp cooling was achieved using crushed ice in plastic bags (Dean et al. 1979). A study of the efficacy of using a moulded prefrozen ice cap hand-made from cryogel bags was conducted at the Royal Marsden Hospital (Anderson et al. 1981, David and Speechley 1987).

Cryogel caps

The first commercial cap (Kold Kap) was successful in reducing hair loss, particularly with higher doses of doxorubicin (Dean et al. 1983). A three-layer cap (inner cotton, middle cryogel, outer lamb's wool) was also reported to prevent total hair loss (Howard and Stenner 1983). However, Wheelock et al. (1984) found that most patients suffered from severe hair loss even with the use of the Kold Kap. The most recent work has involved the use of cryogel caps such as the Chemocap and Penguin caps, which have been used for patients receiving single agents and combinations of anthracyclines (Christodoulou et al. 2002, Kargar et al. 2011, Katsimbri et al. 2000, Peck et al. 2000) as well as docetaxel (Lemenager et al. 1995, 1997).

A large (170 patients) randomized study comparing Chemocap with the gel pack method found no statistical difference in efficacy between the two caps but Chemocap was shown to be more

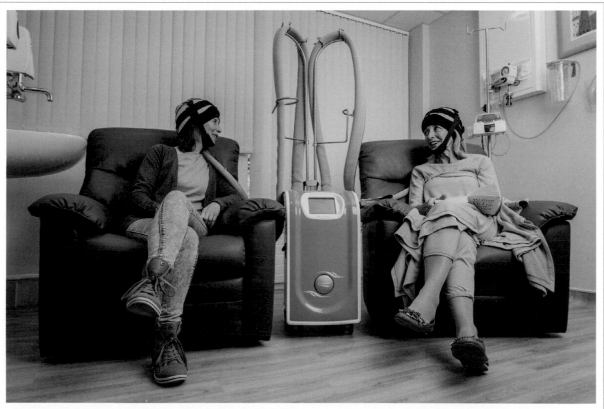

Figure 4.12 Paxman machine. *Source:* Photo courtesy of Paxman Coolers Ltd (www.paxmanscalpcooling.com)

comfortable and offered a better fit, as well as being easier to use (Dougherty 2006b).

Scalp-cooling machines

Attempts have been made to produce an alternative type of cap that would improve the effectiveness of scalp cooling, in particular to ensure a sufficiently low and constant reduction in scalp temperature that would endure during the entire procedure. Two types of scalp-cooling machine have been designed.

1 The use of refrigerated air passed over the patient's scalp via a hair-drying helmet was reported to be beneficial in over 50% of patients, with 16 out of 26 experiencing no hair loss, four experiencing slight loss and six requiring a wig (Symonds et al. 1986). However, other authors found that the system was only successful at lower doses of epirubicin (Adams et al. 1992).

2 In refrigerated cooling systems a liquid coolant is pumped via a cap and maintains a more reliable temperature. Guy et al. (1982) reported encouraging results when the Thermocirculator was first introduced, although Tollenaar et al. (1994) found that when used with patients receiving fluorouracil, epirubicin and cyclophosphamide (FEC), there was still a 50% chance of total alopecia occurring. Scalp-cooling machines, for example Paxman, Dignitana or Penguin, appear to provide a more comfortable and effective system (Betticher et al. 2013, Henricksen and Jensen 2003, Massey 2004, Ridderheim et al. 2003, Rugo et al. 2012, Serrurier et al. 2012, Spaëth et al. 2008, Uzzell et al. 2017) (Figures 4.12 and 4.13).

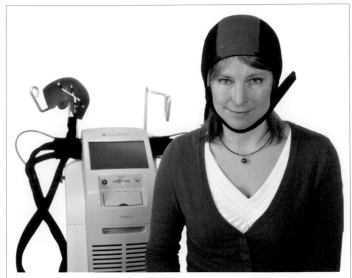

Figure 4.13 Dignitana machine. *Source:* Photo courtesy of Dignitana (www.dignicap.com)

Procedure guideline 4.13   Scalp cooling

Essential equipment

- A scalp-cooling cap
- Overcap
- Skin protection, for example gauze, cotton wool pads
- Comfortable chair (recliner) or bed
- Extra pillows and blankets as required
- Equipment to wet and condition patient's hair as determined by manufacturer's instructions

Pre-procedure

Action	Rationale
1 Before beginning, it is important to explain and discuss the procedure fully with the patient. Explain that the coldest and most uncomfortable time is the first 15 minutes after the cap has been applied. The patient should understand that the scalp cooling can be discontinued at any time and that it will not jeopardize the chemotherapy.	To ensure that the patient understands the procedure and what the success rate is likely to be depending on the type of chemotherapy regimen they are receiving (Dougherty 2006b, **R2b**). Patients who have undergone scalp cooling highlighted this as important knowledge to share when first undergoing the procedure (Dougherty 2006b, **R2b**). To ensure that the patient gives their valid consent and knows that if the scalp cooling does not work, they can obtain a wig (NMC 2015, **C**).

Procedure

Action	Rationale
2 Check that the machine has been cooled to the recommended temperature.	To ensure the coolant will be circulated at the correct temperature to be effective (manufacturer's recommendations, **C**).
3 Ascertain the correct cap size for the patient by ensuring that the manufacturer's recommendations relating to cap size are followed. Good cap fitting includes ensuring the cap is touching the crown of the head and that there is a tight fit around the entire hairline.	To ensure the cap is in close contact with the scalp (manufacturer's recommendations, **C**).
4 If necessary, wet hair or comb through conditioner.	To ensure there is adequate cooling over the head including all the hair roots. **E**
5 Place the cap on the patient's head, making sure it fits closely and covers the whole hairline.	To ensure the cap is in close contact with the scalp (manufacturer's recommendations, **C**).
6 Apply the overcap to the patient's head.	To ensure even and close contact of the cap to the scalp (Dougherty 2006b, **R2b**).

7	Place protection in any areas where the cap touches the skin.	To prevent cold injury and improve the patient's comfort. **E, P**
8	Place a pillow behind the patient's head if required.	To provide support for the patient's head and neck and to reduce the effect of the heaviness of the cap (**P**; Dougherty 1996, **R2b**).
9	Offer the patient the use of a blanket.	To provide the patient with some protection against the feeling of cold (**P**; Dougherty 1996, **R2b**).
10	Leave the patient for at least 15 minutes before injection of the drug.	To obtain initial cooling of the scalp (Dougherty 2006b, **R2b**; Hunt et al. 1982, **R4**; Lemenager et al. 1997, **R2b**; manufacturer's recommendations, **C**).
11	Administer the drug by intravenous injection as per prescription.	To administer treatment as appropriate. **E**
12	The cap must be on continuously for the recommended times (although the patient may detach themselves for a short period if they need to go to the toilet).	To maintain adequate cooling (Dougherty 2006b, **R2b**; Hunt et al. 1982, **R4**; Lemenager et al. 1997, **R2b**).
13	On completion of drug administration (i.e. the one likely to cause alopecia, for example epirubicin), leave the patient for the allocated time depending on the drug and where appropriate according to the manufacturer's recommendations.	To maintain cooling until the plasma levels of drug have fallen (Dougherty 2006b, **R2b**; Hunt et al. 1982, **R4**; Janssen 2007, **R2b**; Lemenager et al. 1997, **R2b**).
14	When sufficient time has elapsed, remove the cap.	To prevent damage to the scalp and hair. **E, P**

Post-procedure

15	Encourage the patient to rest, if desired.	To prevent the patient feeling faint when the cap is lifted off the head. **P, E**
16	Allow the patient to wash and dry their hair before leaving department	To ensure patient comfort. **E**
17	Wash or wipe the cap with detergent wipes, dry and store on cardboard insert or according to manufacturer's instructions.	To minimize cross-infection and to maintain shape (DH 2007, **C**).
18	Ensure the patient is given a patient information booklet on how to care for hair and manage hair loss.	To reinforce verbal information given during the procedure. **E, P**

Problem-solving table 4.4 Prevention and resolution (Procedure guideline 4.13)

Problem	Cause	Prevention	Action
Inadequate cooling.	Poorly fitting cap. Cap not sufficiently cooled.	Select correct size of cap for each individual patient.	Check that the cap fits and is the correct size and that the hair roots are covered.
		Follow the procedure correctly.	Check the cap has been cooled to the correct temperature.
Excess cooling.	Thin hair.	Use plenty of gauze between the cap and scalp.	Apply more gauze. If it is still painful then discontinue the procedure.
Complaints of headache.	Weight and coldness of cap.	Warn patient of weight and cold sensation. Provide physical support to the neck and shoulders and blankets as required.	Provide more support and warmth. Reassure the patient that it will ease off as cooling continues.
Distressed patient.	Claustrophobia.	Discuss with the patient and allow them to try the cap on before starting the procedure.	Support and reassure the patient. If necessary, remove the cap.
	Ice phobia.	Discuss with the patient and allow them to try the cap on before starting the procedure.	Be aware of this possible problem; encourage the patient to discuss their feelings.
Hair loss.	Scalp cooling was not successful.	Use correct size of cap and cool for the recommended time.	Offer the patient the opportunity to discontinue the scalp cooling. Make arrangements for the patient to see the appliance officer and obtain a wig. Discuss care of hair and scalp and give the patient an information booklet.

Post-procedural considerations

Immediate care

It is important to ensure that if a patient fails to retain hair or decides not to undergo scalp cooling, adequate time is spent helping the patient to adapt to the hair loss physically, psychologically and socially. It is recommended that nursing interventions be directed towards helping the patient and family to adapt to alopecia by using patient education, available resources and supportive listening (Pickard-Holley 1995). This can be partly achieved by ensuring that the patient sees the surgical appliance officer as soon as possible, to obtain a wig that can be matched to the patient's desired hair style and colour.

Ongoing care

Advice can be given on hair care such as the type of shampoo. There is a misconception that a mild shampoo such as baby shampoo is best, but this kind of shampoo is alkaline and it is recommended that a neutral pH shampoo be used (Dougherty 2005, 2006b). Using a wide-toothed comb can prevent pulling on hair but the patient should not be afraid to comb their hair daily (Dougherty 2006b). Patients should be advised to avoid anything that can dry out their hair such as using hair dryers on a hot setting, curlers and so on, or using chemicals such as perming lotions or hair dyes, and they should seek advice from a hairdresser. Finally, the patient should be given advice about the use of head coverings such as hats, turbans and scarves. All verbal information should be reinforced with a hair care information booklet (Batchelor 2001, Pickard-Holley 1995).

Complications

Patients have reported adverse effects during and following treatment such as headaches, claustrophobia, dizziness and ice phobias (Dougherty 2006b, Mols et al. 2009, Rosman 2004). Nurses need to understand the meaning that hair loss has for the patient. Alopecia can cause depression, loss of self-confidence and humiliation: it is a very visible sign of cancer. Patients who have relapsed and are undergoing further chemotherapy that causes alopecia may find the loss of hair a second time to be more devastating (Gallagher 1996).

Clinical research

Nurses are increasingly involved in cancer research and the following text is a brief introduction to clinical research in cancer care as it relates to clinical research nurses.

Definitions (ICH 1996, NIHR 2017a b, RCN 2017)

- *Clinical trial.* A clinical trial is a structured research process to investigate the safety, tolerability and efficacy of a medicinal product in human subjects or to investigate safety of medical devices in human subjects or to compare new medical approaches to a standard and routinely available process.
- *GCP: Good clinical practice.* A set of internationally recognized ethical and scientific quality requirements which must be observed for designing, conducting, recording and reporting clinical trials that involve the participation of human subjects (ICH 1996).
- *IB: Investigator's brochure.* A comprehensive document detailing information about an IMP (investigational medicinal product). It is designed to provide the investigator with IMP information necessary for the management of the study conduct and study participants' safety throughout the clinical trial.
- *ICF: Informed consent form.* A specific consent document that includes details of a study participant's consent to participate in a clinical trial.
- *ICH: International Council for Harmonisation of Technical Requirements for Pharmaceuticals for Human Use.* It aims to achieve greater harmonization worldwide to ensure that safe, effective and high-quality medicines are developed and registered in the most resource-efficient manner, by providing guidelines to conduct clinical trials.
- *IMP: Investigational medicinal product.* A pharmaceutical form of an active substance or placebo being tested or used as a reference in a clinical trial, including products already with a marketing authorization but used or assembled (formulated or packaged) in a way different from the authorized form, or when used for an unauthorized indication, or when used to gain further information about the authorized form.
- *PIS: Patient information sheet.* A document explaining in detail all relevant study information to assist the potential study participants in understanding the expectations and requirements of participation in a clinical trial.
- *Protocol.* A document that describes the objectives, design, methodology, statistical considerations, and organization of a clinical trial. A protocol provides an overview of the schedule of events, IMP doses, safety information about the study drug, clinical trial duration, etc.

Related theory

Phases of clinical trials

Clinical trials are conducted in a series of stages, commonly referred to as phases. Each phase is designed to answer a specific research question (NIHR 2017a). Table 4.7 provides an overview of the various clinical trial phases and their objectives.

Life cycle of a clinical trial

Clinical trials are intensely monitored by appropriate regulatory authorities. There are national regulatory bodies that govern the conduct of clinical trials. The Medicines and Healthcare products Regulatory Agency (MHRA) and Health Research Authority (HRA) in the UK, the Food and Drug Administration (FDA) in the United States and the European Medicines Agency (EMA) in European

Table 4.7 An overview of clinical trial phases

	Objective	Participants	Duration
Phase I	To establish safety of an IMP	20–80	Few months – 2 years
	To establish maximum tolerated dose of an IMP		
Phase II	To establish the efficacy of an IMP	100–250	2–3 years
Phase III	To confirm efficacy of an IMP	1000–3000	2–4 years
	To monitor side-effects of an IMP		
	To compare IMP with commonly used treatments		
	To collect all relevant information that will allow IMP to be used safely in an clinical environment		
Phase IV	To study long-term effects of an IMP	500–1000+	1–4+ years
	To study cost-effectiveness of an IMP		

Source: Adapted from NIHR Clinical trials toolkit (NIHR 2017a).
IMP, investigational medicinal product.

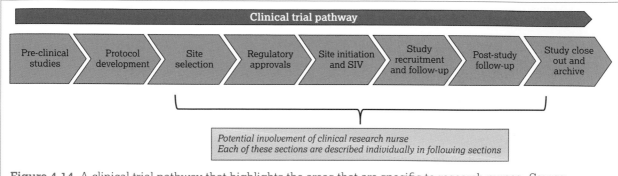

Figure 4.14 A clinical trial pathway that highlights the areas that are specific to research nurses. *Source:* Adapted from NIHR clinical trials toolkit (NIHR 2017a).

countries are a few examples. All studies involving a medical or therapeutic intervention in patients must be approved by a supervising regulatory and ethics committee before permission is granted to run the trial. The clinical trials must be conducted in accordance with ICH-GCP and in line with national regulatory standards. Following regulatory approvals, there are multiple steps involved in conducting a clinical trial, requiring input from a variety of expert groups. The study participation sites, patients and study data are monitored throughout the study period. Clinical trials can be audited or inspected by the study sponsor or by the regulatory authorities at any time. See Figure 4.14 (ICH 1996, NIHR 2017a).

Site selection

The study sponsors usually get in touch with the potential participating sites and would seek information to ensure the site has appropriate facilities to participate in the study of interest. A research nurse may be involved in liaising with the sponsor at this stage and the research nurse may be asked to review the study synopsis. See Figure 4.15 (NIHR 2017a).

Regulatory approvals and standard documents

The approvals to initiate any clinical trial vary from country to country. In general, each clinical trial site will have a study co-ordinator who liaises with the study sponsor to facilitate the regulatory processes and ensures that all approvals are obtained prior to opening the site to run the trial. See Box 4.14 (NIHR 2017a).

The study nurse or study co-ordinator will be provided with a set of documents prior to the start of the study. Depending on the responsibilities assigned by the principal investigator, it is important for the research nurse to go through these documents and understand the processes involved in the study. See Box 4.15 (NIHR 2017b).

It is good practice for the research nurse to develop a checklist and review the research protocol in advance. For a typical list of items that will need to be reviewed see Box 4.16 (NIHR 2017a). If any clarity is needed the research nurse should liaise with the study sponsor at the earliest possible opportunity.

Site initiation visit (SIV)

Once all the approvals are in place, the study sponsor will arrange a visit to the site to train the site team and also meet with all the study team members. During the visit, the sponsor will provide all study-related documents to the site including the standard

- Study staff
  - Experience of study investigator
  - Staff resources to support the conduct of study
  - CVs of key study team members
- Facilities
  - Pharmacy facilities for IMP storage and IMP prescription
  - Internal laboratory facilities to carry out study specific assessments
  - Internal facilities to carry out study procedures such as scans, ECGs, biopsies
  - Hospital safety management processes during patient emergencies
  - Appropriate participant treatment areas
  - Internal operating procedures and governance structure to conduct clinical trials
- Study feasibility
  - Potential patient population who could be eligible to study participation
  - Concurrent participation in any competing studies, which may affect recruitment
  - Willingness to participate in the study
- Regulatory processes at site
  - Regulatory requirement at site level
  - Institutional review timelines
  - Clinical trial contract agreement processes and timelines
- Site visit
  - Tour of the facilities
  - Meeting with key study staff

Figure 4.15 Information requested from study sponsor. *Source:* Adapted from NIHR (2017a).

Box 4.14 List of approvals required prior to start of the study

- Approval from national governing bodies (e.g., MHRA, EMA, FDA, etc.)
- Approval from ethics committee (NRES, IRB, etc.)
- Approvals from any other governing bodies as per national guidelines (e.g., ARSAC, GTAC in the UK)
- Approval from the institution to conduct the study

Source: Adapted from NIHR Clinical trials toolkit (NIHR 2017a).

Box 4.15 General documents that are usually circulated by the study sponsor

- Clinical study protocol
- Investigator's brochure
- Patient information sheet and informed consent form
- GP letter
- Lab manual
- Imaging manual
- User guides where applicable
- Tools to capture data from patients
- Any other document that needs to be used for the study

Source: Adapted from NIHR research design service (NIHR 2017b).

Box 4.16 Research nurse checklist

- Visit schedules
  - Logistics for study participants
  - Overlapping visits
  - Assessments to be carried out at each visit
  - Available window period
  - Expected commitments from study participants to comply with schedules
  - Expected duration of stay at the hospital during the visits
  - Participants' needs in terms of travel, support of overnight stay
  - Liaison with support services if there are any stringent schedules to be followed
- Contact details of study team, sponsor, and medical monitor
- Details of serious adverse event reporting and emergency contact details
- Emergency unblinding procedures in a double-blind study
- Study data collection tools
  - Drug compliance work sheets
  - Patient reported outcomes
  - Patient diary cards
  - Data collection tools

Source: Adapted from NIHR research design service (NIHR 2017b).

investigator's file. Site staff should receive GCP training as well as training in study inclusion and exclusion criteria, study process and safety reporting criteria. The site is activated once it confirms the receipt of all study materials.

The research nurse should prepare data collection tools and nursing guides as this will primarily support day-to-day management of the studies.

Data collection tools

It is good practice to develop appropriate data collection methods for the study. The research nurse may prepare a form to collect study data so that all data required for the study are appropriately captured in the form. These forms could be specific to each visit. General data collection tools could be prepared for screening, cycle 1, cycle 2, etc. See Box 4.17 and Figure 4.16 (NIHR 2017b).

Nursing guide

The nursing guide is an internal site document that is like a handbook for the research nurse. It is again good practice to prepare a nursing guide for the study. The nursing guide will contain information on the visit schedules, what to do in case of emergency, safety information about the study drug, essential contact, etc. The objective is that, should the study-specific nurse

Box 4.17 A toolkit to consider when reviewing a protocol during the site initiation visit

Investigational medicinal product (IMP)

Oral IMP
- If oral, is it easy to differentiate drug strengths, i.e. different shaped bottles or different shaped/coloured drugs, tablets/liquid?
- What is the dosing regimen length of cycle?
- Storage of the drug – fridge, room temperature.
- Are there food restrictions (fed or fasted)?
- Are there fasting requirements for the drug pre and post dose?
- Clarify fasting time for drug: if longer than 4 hours what is the rationale?
- Can the drug dosing time be changed, i.e. brought forward if patient was dosed late on cycle 1/day 1 (dosing time will always be out of sync on clinic days on BD dosing; do you skip a dose and single dose jump back to original time of drug)?
- Drug compliance – check if diary card is required.
- How long is a drug holiday?
- What percentage of drug intake to ensure patient is evaluable? Is it just cycle 1 or cycle 1 plus cycle 2?

Intravenous IMP
- If it is an IV drug, how long is the infusion?
- Length of infusion.
- Is it a vesicant?
- Can it be given peripherally or via central access?
- What is the regimen: dosing, days, length of cycle?
- Storage: room temperature or refrigerate, protect from light, special administration set?
- Do they want serial numbers of the IV pump used?
- Flushing instructions, clarify end of infusion.
- Post-dose assessments.

Trial sampling
- Find out if there is a window for safety bloods, i.e. ± 2 days for cycle 1/day 1 visits.
- Visit logistics, look at all the assessment time points and check if they can fit into the department's week, i.e. do any pharmacokinetics (PKs) fall on a weekend?
- Are there windows for sampling time points? This is critical as flexibility on the time points is required.
- Will it need to start on a specific day to fit in all assessments?
- Out of hours physical examinations and samples, i.e. processing of samples such as lipase or insulin when the labs are closed and physical examinations when the ward doctors are not available.
- Has the patient had biopsies – if so when, are they feasible (clarify post-dose biopsy, ask for windows in days not hours if possible)?
- Pharmacodynamics (PD) sampling. Who will this impact: local (ICR), central?
- Order of sampling when a few due at a specific time point, e.g. ECG, PK, PD then observations.
- Clarify fasting times for bloods, i.e. does patient fast for safety bloods, on which days, how long for?

Logistics
- How many overnight stays (or admissions) and how long for?
- Is it feasible/achievable/acceptable for the patient?
- Can frequency of visits be reduced after cycle 3?
- Extra costs, e.g. hotel stay, taxi, etc.
- Know side-effects; provide algorithms to manage these, especially for out of hours.

Source: Adapted from NIHR research design service (2017b).

Initials ---------------	Screening	Trial -----------------------------			
		Date		Time	Initials
Consent					
Study specific informed consent		/ /		:	
Histologic confirmation of indolent B-cell lymphoma (FL, MZL, or SLL)		/ /		:	
Medical history, demographics		/ /		:	
Cancer history	**Yes/No (Please indicate)**	/ /		:	
Follicular lymphoma international prognostic index score		/ /		:	
Comments:					
Biopsy					
Trial consent given for biopsy	**Yes/No (Please indicate)**	/ /		:	
Does patient have archival tissue?	**Yes/No (Please indicate)**	/ /			
Biopsy (biopsy site)		/ /		:	
Scans					
CT scan / MRI scan *(T.A.P)*		/ /		:	
(CT scans of chest, abdomen and pelvis)		/ /		:	
Bone scan *(if clinically indicated)*		/ /		:	
Time of scan _____					
Vitals signs					
		/ /		:	
	Height		cm		
	Weight		kg		
	Temp		°C		
	HR/pulse		bpm		
	RR		per min		
	Oxygen saturation		%		
	BP	/	mmHg		
	NEWS				
12 lead ECG (trial specific or unit machine)		/ /		:	
Questionnaires	**Questionnaires are required at all cycles**				
Quality of life (QOL) (EQ-5D)		/ /		:	

Figure 4.16 An example of a screening study data collection tool. *Source:* Adapted from NIHR research design service (NIHR 2017b).

(continued)

Comments:							
Blood samples							
<u>Central laboratory</u>							
Pharmacokinetic blood sample collection		/	/		:		
Serum and plasma biomarkers		/	/		:		
Immunophenotyping evaluations (e.g B/T-lymphocyte panel)		/	/		:		
Archival tumour tissue		/	/		:		
Optional pharmacogenomic blood sample		/	/		:		
Optional tumour tissue biopsy		/	/		:		
<u>Local laboratory</u>							
Haematology		/	/		:		
FBC, DIFF and RETIC							
Coagulation		/	/		:		
PT, PTT and INR							
Biochemistry		/	/		:		
U&E, LFT, Ca, LDH, Mg, Glu, GGT, urate, Cl & other: CO2, PO4, AST, ALT, ALP, Direct bilirubin, Total bilirubin, lipase, amylase							
Hepatitis serology		/	/		:		
CMV/EBV serology or viral load		/	/		:		
HIV testing		/	/		:		
Serum pregnancy test		/	/		:		
If not applicable, please give a reason		☐		Male			
☐	Female post menopausal	☐	Female surgically sterile				
MRSA screening *(Swab)*		/	/		:		
Urinalysis		/	/		:		
	Specific gravity						
	pH						
	Glucose						
	Blood						
	Ketones						
	Protein						
Comments:							

Figure 4.16 *Continued*

Doctor	No specific PE form; PE required at screening and on every cycle							
Physical examination	(Please complete PE form)	/	/					
Con medications	(Please complete con med form)	/	/					
Con procedures		/	/					
Assess AEs/SAEs	(Please complete AE form)	/	/					
Tumour assessment	(Please complete tumour assessment form)	/	/					
ECOG performance status (PS 0 to 5)					/	/		
Smoking status	Never smoked / Ex smoker / Current smoker							
	If ex smoker, please record approximate stopped				Date:	/	/	
	If patient ever smoked record approximate number of cigarettes per day					/	/	
Alcohol status	Does patient drink alcohol Yes		/	No				
	If yes, could it interfere in the trial Yes		/	No				
Patient eligibility:		Yes ☐	No ☐					
	Name: _____							
	Signature: _____			Date:				
Comments:								

Figure 4.16 *Continued*

not be available, any research nurse could get help from the nursing guide and act on immediate needs for the study participant. See Box 4.18.

Study recruitment and follow-up
As soon as the site is activated, the research nurse can begin handing out study PIS-ICFs to potential patients. The study cycle has defined steps which are listed below.

Patient selection
This is the first stage for the study participants, in which the specific clinical trial would be discussed with the patient in detail. The research nurse may be expected to go through databases to identify potential patients or liaise with other units within the hospital to raise awareness of the study. The potential participant would be referred to a clinical trial clinic where a clinician will go through the PIS-ICF with patients. Following this discussion, a research nurse will also discuss the study with patients, primarily addressing the logistics of the study and explaining to patients the commitments required to participate in the study. A research nurse will also gather background clinical history and assess the patient's well-being in order to understand if the patient is suitable for trial participation.

Further to initial discussion, follow-up conversations may be held over the phone or face to face with potential participants, to ensure they are fully informed about the study and the study drug/device (NIHR 2017a).

Screening
Once a patient expresses interest in participating in the study, screening processes can begin. Initially the participant's written consent is taken on the study-specific PIS-ICF, following which screening procedures will be carried out as per the schedule of events in the protocol. The screening process may take a few days to a month, based on the nature of the assessments required. A clinician and the research nurse will monitor patients and complete the study-specific inclusion/exclusion checklist (see Figure 4.17). The participant will need to meet all the criteria as per the checklist prior to confirming that he/she is eligible to participate in the study (NIHR 2017a).

Registration
If a potential patient successfully passes screening, he/she will be registered (or randomized if required) to the study, from which point a specific batch of study medication would be assigned to the participant.

Box 4.18 An example of a locally developed nursing guide

Contact numbers for the local team involved in the trial, together with contact details for the sponsor's trial-related team
- Principal investigator
- Clinical fellows
- Clinical trial coordinator
- Lead nurse
- Data manager
- Study trial monitor
- Technical support team if applicable

Background information on the trial drug (in brief)
- Class of compound
- Mode of action
- Summary of pre-clinical data
- Summary of clinical trial data
- Expected side-effects
- Rationale for study
- Potential drug-related toxicities

Drug administration requirements and restrictions
- Dietary requirements and restrictions
- Dosing schedule
- Route of administration
- Formulation
- Important contraindications with reference to the protocol

Fasting times should be clarified
- Fasting for bloods Routine e.g. glucose
- Trial bloods
- Fasting for drug Pre-dose fast e.g. 10 hours
- Post-dose fast, e.g. 2 hours
- Total hours of fasting prior to dose

Trial-specific assessment and sampling procedures and management, including, but not limited to:
- Pharmacokinetic samples
- Pharmacodynamics samples
- Trial-specific blood test sampling (safety bloods, e.g. tumour markers)
- Holter management
- ECG specifications
- Telemetry guidelines

Study treatment

The procedures would be followed as per the schedule of events and a research nurse will be involved in:

- collection of observations
- ECGs
- performing a physical examination
- collection of adverse events
- collection of concomitant medication details
- providing drug infusion/review of drug compliance
- continuous monitoring of the study participant during the study.

The research nurse will also need to alert the clinician should any untoward or unexpected events occur. A follow-up telephone call may be required if the participant is unwell. Overall, the research nurse not only collects study-specific data but also provides holistic care to study participants.

Study discontinuation

If the clinician has evidence to confirm that the participant is no longer receiving benefit from the study drug, the participant will be taken off the study. However, he/she is followed up for a minimum of 30 days to ensure there are no adverse events resulting from study participation.

Post-study follow-up

The follow-up period may vary from study to study and some studies may require monthly/3 monthly follow-up processes until death. Some studies may require more frequent telephone calls with participants and may also involve data collection over the phone.

Study close out and study archive

Once all participants are off study and all study data has been collected, the study can be closed. The regulatory authorities and the study site will need to be informed about study closure and all study documents must be archived for 25 years or as stated by national guidelines.

During the study, the research nurse is expected to continuously monitor participants and ensure they are safe. In addition, it is also the responsibility of a research nurse to adhere to study protocol. It can sometimes be challenging to maintain compliance and support participants' well-being. At all times, the research nurse must keep clinicians and the study PI informed about the participants' status. Where required, the research nurse should provide appropriate support to participants, educate them to maintain drug compliance and provide guidance on following patient-reported outcomes. Effective communication with participants and the study team is an absolute requirement from a research nurse. In addition, a research nurse should document all events and activities so that there is a full audit train of study activities (ICH 1996, NIHR 2017a).

Other important activities in a clinical trial

Study monitoring and audit

Any research study will be monitored by the sponsor or sponsor's representatives (they are sometimes called clinical research associates). A study monitor will primarily verify source data and ensure the data are credible and evaluable. Based on the nature of the study, the monitoring plan may contain 100% source verification or partial source verification. A monitor will also review if study processes have been followed appropriately and there are no deviations from the study. If there are any deviations, site staff will be asked to report these deviations. A monitor will also ensure all participants have appropriately consented to the study and all site staff are following GCP guidelines.

A monitor may wish to have a short meeting with the research nurse during the visits to resolve any queries that may arise. Frequency of monitoring may vary from study to study, but at the end of each monitoring visit there will be a monitoring report which needs to be reviewed and filed in the investigator's site file.

The study may also be audited by an external auditor or inspected by a regulatory authority.

Standard operating procedures

Each clinical trial site will have its own standard operating procedures (SOPs) to standardize and harmonize the operational aspects of clinical trials. The process of consenting, reporting of serious adverse events, maintenance of study documents, out of hours contact process for study participants, etc., are some of the examples which should be covered by SOPs. It is important for the research nurse to be familiar with all SOPs as at the time of audits/inspections the site may be asked to produce their SOPs for review.

Safety reporting

Any clinical trial will have a process for reporting any adverse event (AE) to the study sponsor. GCP provides classification for adverse events, which a research nurse must be aware of. If an adverse event become serious, it is termed a serious adverse event (SAE) which needs to be reported to the study sponsor as soon as possible or within 24 hours of the clinician being made aware of it. The study protocol will have details of the SAE reporting guidelines. Although it is the clinician who makes the decision about whether an AE is upgraded to an SAE, the research nurse is also duty bound to report any untoward event to the study team so

Patient baseline number: _____

Patients must meet all I/E criteria to be eligible for the study.

If you provide a "No" response to any criteria below the patient is not <u>currently</u> eligible for the study

Yes	No	Inclusion criteria
☐	☐	Be willing and able to provide written informed consent/assent for the trial.
☐	☐	Be ≥18 years of age on day of signing informed consent.
☐	☐	*For the purposes of this study, neoadjuvant and/or adjuvant chemotherapy regimens do not count as a prior line of therapy* Have a histologically or cytologically-documented, advanced (metastatic and/or unresectable) solid tumour that is incurable and for which prior standard first-line treatment has failed. Patients must have progressed on or be intolerant to therapies that are known to provide clinical benefit. There is no limit to the number of prior treatment regimens.
☐	☐	Have one of the following advanced (unresectable and/or metastatic) tumour types: (A) Anal squamous cell carcinoma (B) Biliary adenocarcinoma (gallbladder or biliary tree (intrahepatic or extrahepatic cholangiocarcinoma) except ampulla of vater cancers (C) Neuroendocrine tumours (well- and moderately-differentiated), of the lung, appendix, small intestine, colon, rectum, or pancreas) (D) Endometrial carcinoma (sarcomas and mesenchymal tumours are excluded) (E) Cervical squamous cell carcinoma (F) Vulvar squamous cell carcinoma (G) Small cell lung carcinoma (H) Mesothelioma (malignant pleural mesothelioma) (I) Thyroid carcinoma (papillary or follicular subtypes) (J) Salivary gland carcinoma,(sarcomas and mesenchymal tumours are excluded) (K) Any other advanced solid tumour (except CRC), which is MSI-H.
☐	☐	Have submitted an evaluable tissue sample for biomarker analysis from a tumour lesion not previously irradiated (exceptions may be considered after Sponsor consultation). The tumour tissue submitted for analysis must be from a single tumour tissue specimen and of sufficient quantity and quality to allow assessment of ALL required primary biomarkers *Note: SUBJECTS IN GROUPS A-J WILL NOT BE ELIGIBLE UNLESS ALL THREE PRIMARY BIOMARKERS (TUMOUR PD-L1 EXPRESSION, GEP SCORE, and MSI-H STATUS) CAN BE ASSESSED USING TISSUE FROM THE SAME SINGLE TUMOUR SPECIMEN*
☐	☐	**If enrolment in Groups A-J has moved to biomarker enrichment**, have a tumour that is <u>positive</u> for one or more of the pre-specified primary biomarker(s), as assessed by the central laboratory. These enrichment biomarkers may be PD-L1 expression by IHC (at a percentage to be prespecified), a positive tumour RNA GEP score (at a prespecified cut-off), and/or tumour MSI-H
☐	☐	Have measurable disease based on RECIST 1.1 as determined by central review. Tumour lesions situated in a previously irradiated area are considered measurable if progression has been demonstrated in such lesions.
☐	☐	Have a performance status of 0 or 1 on the ECOG performance scale.
☐	☐	Patient must have **adequate organ function** as indicated by following laboratory values:

System		Laboratory value
Hematological	Absolute neutrophil count (ANC)	≥ 1500 µL
	Platelets	≥ 100 000 µL
	Haemoglobin	≥ 9 g/dL **OR** ≥5.6 mmol/L, without recent transfusion
Renal	Creatinine OR Measured or calculated creatinine clearance (CrCl)[a] (GFR can also be used in place of creatinine or CrCl) [a]Creatinine clearance should be calculated per institutional standard	≤1.5 × upper limit of normal (ULN) **OR** ≥60 mL/min for subjects with creatinine levels >1.5 × institutional ULN

Figure 4.17 An example of a locally developed patient inclusion/exclusion checklist.

Hepatic	Total bilirubin	≤1.5 × ULN **OR** Direct bilirubin ≤ ULN for subjects with total bilirubin levels >1.5 × ULN
	AST (SGOT) and ALT (SGPT)	≤2.5 × ULN, **OR** ≤5 × ULN for subjects with liver metastases
Coagulation	International normalized ratio (INR) or Prothrombin Time (PT)	≤1.5 × ULN unless the subject is receiving anticoagulant therapy as long as PT or PTT is within therapeutic range of intended use of anticoagulants
	Activated partial thromboplastin time (aPTT)	≤1.5 × ULN unless the subject is receiving anticoagulant therapy as long as PT or PTT is within therapeutic range of intended use of anticoagulants

☐	☐	Female subject of childbearing potential should have a negative urine or serum pregnancy test within 72 hours prior to receiving the first dose of study medication. If the urine test is positive or cannot be confirmed as negative, a serum pregnancy test will be required.
☐	☐	Female subjects of childbearing potential should be willing to use two methods of birth control or be surgically sterile, or abstain from heterosexual activity for the course of the study for 120 days after the last dose of study medication. Subjects of childbearing potential are those who have not been surgically sterilized or have not been free from menses for > 1 year. Please see Section 5.7.2 of the Protocol for a list of acceptable birth control methods. **OR** Male subjects should agree to use an adequate method of contraception starting with the first dose of study therapy for 120 days after the last dose of study therapy.
☐	☐	Subject may also provide consent/assent for Future Biomedical Research. The subject may participate in the main trial without participating in Future Biomedical Research.

If you provide a 'Yes' response to any criteria below the patient is not currently eligible for the study

Yes	No	Exclusion criteria
☐	☐	Is currently participating or has participated in a study of an investigational agent or using an investigational device within 4 weeks prior to the first dose of trial treatment. If yes, patient may be placed on the watch list for later eligibility
☐	☐	Has a diagnosis of immunodeficiency or is receiving systemic steroid therapy or any other form of immunosuppressive therapy within 7 days prior to the first dose of trial treatment. The use of physiological doses of corticosteroids may be approved after consultation with the Sponsor. If yes, patient may be placed on the watch list for later eligibility
☐	☐	Has an active autoimmune disease that has required systemic treatment in past 2 years (i.e. with use of disease modifying agents, corticosteroids or immunosuppressive drugs). Replacement therapy (e.g. thyroxine, insulin, or physiological corticosteroid replacement therapy for adrenal or pituitary insufficiency, etc.) is not considered a form of systemic treatment.
☐	☐	Has had a prior anti-cancer monoclonal antibody (mAb) within 4 weeks prior to study Day 1 or who has not recovered (i.e. ≤ Grade 1 or at baseline) from adverse events due to agents administered more than 4 weeks earlier. If yes, patient may be placed on the watch list for later eligibility
☐	☐	Has had prior chemotherapy, targeted small molecule therapy, or radiation therapy within 2 weeks prior to study Day 1 or who has not recovered (i.e. ≤ Grade 1 or at baseline) from adverse events due to a previously administered agent. *Note: Subjects with ≤ Grade 2 neuropathy or ≤ Grade 2 alopecia are an exception to this criterion and may qualify for the study.* *Note: If subject received major surgery, they must have recovered adequately from the toxicity and/or complications from the intervention prior to starting therapy.* If yes, patient may be placed on the watch list for later eligibility
☐	☐	Has a known additional malignancy that is progressing or requires active treatment. Exceptions include basal cell carcinoma of the skin, squamous cell carcinoma of the skin that has undergone potentially curative therapy or *in situ* cervical cancer.
☐	☐	Has radiographically detectable (even if asymptomatic and/or previously treated) central nervous system (CNS) metastases and/or carcinomatous meningitis. Brain imaging at screening is required. Subjects with previously treated brain metastases may participate provided these brain metastases are stable (without evidence of progression by imaging over a period of at least 4 weeks and any neurological symptoms have returned to baseline), they have no evidence of new or enlarging brain metastases (confirmed by imaging within 28 days of the first dose of trial treatment), and they are not using steroids for at least 7 days prior to trial treatment. This exception does not include carcinomatous meningitis which is excluded regardless of clinical stability.

Figure 4.17 *Continued*

☐	☐	Has evidence of active non-infectious pneumonitis.
☐	☐	Has an active infection requiring systemic therapy.
☐	☐	Has a history or current evidence of any condition, therapy, or laboratory abnormality that might confound the results of the trial, interfere with the subject's participation for the full duration of the trial, or is not in the best interest of the subject to participate, in the opinion of the treating investigator.
☐	☐	Has known psychiatric or substance abuse disorders that would interfere with cooperation with the requirements of the trial.
☐	☐	Is pregnant or breastfeeding, or expecting to conceive or father children within the projected duration of the trial, starting with the screening visit to 120 days after the last dose of trial treatment.
☐	☐	Has received prior therapy with an anti-PD-1, anti-PD-L1, or anti-PD-L2 agent.
☐	☐	Has a known history of human immunodeficiency virus (HIV) (HIV 1/2 antibodies).
☐	☐	Has known active hepatitis B (e.g. HBsAg reactive) or hepatitis C (e.g. HCV RNA [qualitative] is detected).
☐	☐	Has received a live vaccine within 30 days of planned start of study therapy. *Note: Seasonal influenza vaccines for injection are generally inactivated flu vaccines and are allowed; however intranasal influenza vaccines (e.g. Flu-Mist®) are live attenuated vaccines, and are not allowed.* If yes, patient may be placed on the watch list for later eligibility

Figure 4.17 *Continued*

that the event is appropriately captured and the participant's well-being is maintained. The research nurse may also be involved in collecting additional SAE information from the study participant/family/local hospital (ICH 1996, NIHR 2017a).

References

Adams, L., Lawson, N., Maxted, K.J. & Symonds, R.P. (1992) The prevention of hair loss from chemotherapy by the use of cold-air scalp-cooling. *European Journal of Cancer Care*, 1(5), 16–19.

Aiello-Lawes, L. & Rutlidge, D.N. (2014) In: Polovich, M., Olsen, M., LeFebvre, K. (eds) *Chemotherapy and Biotherapy Guidelines and Recommendations for Practice. Administration Considerations*, 4th edn. Pittsburgh, PA: Oncology Nursing Society, p. 123.

Aisner, J. (2007) Overview of the changing paradigm in cancer treatment: oral chemotherapy. *American Journal of Health-System Pharmacy*, 64(9 Suppl 5), S4–S7.

Allwood, M.C., Wright, P. & Stanley, A. (eds) (2002) *The Cytotoxics Handbook*, 4th edn. Oxford: Radcliffe Medical Press.

Anderson, J.E., Hunt, J.M. & Smith, I.E. (1981) Prevention of doxorubicin-induced alopecia by scalp cooling in patients with advanced breast cancer. *BMJ*, 282(6262), 423–424.

Antipuesto, D.J. (2010) Z Track Method. Nursing Crib. Available at: http://nursingcrib.com/nursing-notes-reviewer/fundamentals-of-nursing/z-track-method/ (Accessed: 1/4/2018)

Barber, N.A. & Gant, A.K. (2011) Pulmonary toxicities from targeted therapies: a review. *Targeted Oncology*, 6(4), 235–243.

Barefoot, J., Bletcher, C.S. & Emery, R. (2009) Keeping pace with oral chemotherapy. *Oncology Issues*, 24(3), 36–39.

Batchelor, D. (2001) Hair and cancer chemotherapy: consequences and nursing care – a literature study. *European Journal of Cancer Care*, 10(3), 147–163.

Bedell, C.H. (2003) A changing paradigm for cancer treatment: the advent of new oral chemotherapy agents. *Clinical Journal of Oncology Nursing*, 7(6 Suppl), 5–9.

Bernhardson, B., Tishelman, C. & Rutqvist, L.E. (2009) Taste and smell changes in patients receiving cancer chemotherapy: distress, impact on daily life and self care strategies. *Cancer Nursing*, 32(1), 45–54.

Bertelli, G. (1995) Prevention and management of extravasation of cytotoxic drugs. *Drug Safety*, 12(4), 245–255.

Betticher, D.C., Delmore, G., Breitenstein, U., et al. (2013) Efficacy and tolerability of 2 scalp cooling systems for the prevention of alopecia associated with docetaxel treatment. *Supportive Care in Cancer*, 21(9), 2565–2573.

Birner, A.M., Bedell, M.K., Avery, J.T. & Ernstoff, M.S. (2006) Program to support safe administration of oral chemotherapy. *Journal of Oncology Practice*, 2(1), 5–6.

Boehmke, M.M. & Dickerson, S.S. (2005) Symptom, symptom experiences, and symptom distress encountered by women with breast cancer undergoing current treatment modalities. *Cancer Nursing*, 28(5), 382–389.

BOPA (2004) Position statement on safe practice and the pharmaceutical care of patients receiving oral anticancer chemotherapy, in *British National Formulary*. London: Pharmaceutical Press.

BOPA (2015) Standards for Reducing Risks Associated with e-Prescribing Systems for chemotherapy. British Oncology Pharmacy Association. Available at: http://www.bopawebsite.org/sites/default/files/publications/Standards_reducing_risks_associated_ePrescribing_systems_chemo2015.pdf (Accessed: 7/5/2018)

Botchkarev, V.A., Komarova, E.A., Siebenhaar, F. et al. (2000) p53 is essential for chemotherapy-induced hair loss. *Cancer Research*, 60(18), 5002–5006.

Boulanger, J., Ducharme, A., Dufour, A., Fortier, S., Almanric, K.; Comité de l'évolution de la pratique des soins pharmaceutiques (CEPSP); Comité de l'évolution des pratiques en oncologie (CEPO) (2015) Management of the extravasation of anti-neoplastic agents. *Supportive Care in Cancer*, 23(5), 1459–1471.

Breed, W.P. (2004) What is wrong with the 30-year-old practice of scalp cooling for the prevention of chemotherapy-induced hair loss? *Supportive Care in Cancer*, 12 (1), 3–5.

British Journal of Nursing (BJN) (2016) Be compliant, protect each other and stay safe: avoiding accidental exposure to cytotoxic drugs. *British Journal of Nursing*, 24(16), S1–56.

Browall, M., Gaston-Johansson, F. & Danielson, E. (2006) Post-menopausal women with breast cancer: their experiences of the chemotherapy treatment period. *Cancer Nursing*, 29(1), 34–42.

Bulow, J., Friberg, L., Gaardsting, O. & Hansen, M. (1985) Frontal subcutaneous blood flow, and epi- and subcutaneous temperatures during scalp cooling in normal man. *Scandinavian Journal of Clinical and Laboratory Investigation*, 45(6), 505–508.

Campbell, K. (2005) Blood cells. Part three–granulocytes and monocytes. *Nursing Times*, 101(42), 26–27.

Camp-Sorrell, D. (1998) Developing extravasation protocols and monitoring outcomes. *Journal of Intravenous Nursing*, 21(4), 232–239.

Camp-Sorrell, D. (2005) *Oncology Nursing Society Access Device Guidelines: Recommendations for Nursing Practice and Education*. Pittsburgh, PA: Oncology Nursing Society.

Camp-Sorrell, D. (2018) In: Yarbro, C.H., Wujcik, D., Holmes Gobel, B. (eds) *Cancer Nursing. Principles and Practice*, 8th edn. Burlington, MA: Jones & Bartlett Learning, Chapter 16, p. 515.

Carr, K. (1998) How I survived the fall out. *You Magazine, Mail on Sunday*, 10 May, pp. 61–67.

Chernecky, C., Butler, S.W., Graham, P. & Infortuna, H. (2002) *Drug Calculations and Drug Administration*. Philadelphia: W.B. Saunders.

Choi, E.K., Kim, I.R., Chang, O., et al. (2014) Impact of chemotherapy induced alopecia distress on body image, psychosocial well-being, and depression in breast cancer patients. *Psychooncology*, 23(10), 1103–1110.

Christodoulou, C., Klouvas, G., Efstathiou, E., et al. (2002) Effectiveness of the MSC cold cap system in the prevention of chemotherapy-induced alopecia. *Oncology*, 62(2), 97–102.

Chung, S., Low, S.K., Zembutsu, H., et al. (2013) A genome-wide association study of chemotherapy-induced alopecia in breast cancer patients. Pyschooncology in breast cancer patients. *Breast Cancer Res*, 15(5), R81.

Cigler, T., Isseroff, D., Fiederlein, B., et al. (2015) Efficacy of scalp cooling in preventing chemotherapy induced alopecia in breast cancer patients receiving adjuvant doctaxel and cyclophosphamide chemotherapy. *Clinical Breast Cancer*, 15(5), 332–334.

Cline, B.W. (1984) Prevention of chemotherapy-induced alopecia: a review of the literature. *Cancer Nursing*, 7(3), 221–228.

Comerford, K., Eggenberger, T. & Robinson, K. (2002) Chemotherapy infusions. In: *Intravenous Therapy Made Incredibly Easy*. Philadelphia: Springhouse Publishing.

CP Pharmaceuticals (1999) *How Quickly Could you Act?* Wrexham: CP Pharmaceuticals.

Crowe, M., Kendrick, M. & Woods, S. (1998) Is scalp cooling a procedure that should be offered to patients receiving alopecia induced chemotherapy for solid tumours? Proceedings of the 10th International Conference on Cancer Nursing, Jerusalem.

Daanen, H.A., Peerbooms, M., van den Hurk, C.J., et al. (2015) Core temperature affects scalp skin temperature during scalp cooling. *Journal of Dermatology*, 54(8), 916–921.

David, J. & Speechley, V. (1987) Scalp cooling to prevent alopecia. *Nursing Times*, 83(32), 36–37.

Davis, S.T., Benson, B.G., Bramson, H.N., et al. (2001) Prevention of chemotherapy-induced alopecia in rats by CDK inhibitors. *Science*, 291(5501), 134–137.

Dean, J.C., Salmon, S.E. & Griffith, K.S. (1979) Prevention of doxorubicin-induced hair loss with scalp hypothermia. *New England Journal of Medicine*, 301(26), 1427–1429.

Dean, J.C., Griffith, K.S., Cetas, T.C., et al. (1983) Scalp hypothermia: a comparison of ice packs and the Kold Kap in the prevention of doxorubicin-induced alopecia. *Journal of Clinical Oncology*, 1(1), 33–37.

DH (2000) *An Organisation with a Memory*. London: Department of Health. Available at: http://webarchive.nationalarchives.gov.uk/20130105144251/http://www.dh.gov.uk/prod_consum_dh/groups/dh_digitalassets/@dh/@en/documents/digitalasset/dh_4065086.pdf (Accessed: 8/5/2018)

DH (2003) *Building a Safer NHS for Patients: Improving Medication Safety*. London: Department of Health.

DH (2005) *Hazardous Waste (England) Regulations*. London: Department of Health.

DH (2007) *Cancer Reform Strategy*. London: Department of Health. Available at: https://www.nhs.uk/NHSEngland/NSF/Documents/Cancer%20Reform%20Strategy.pdf (Accessed: 8/5/2018)

DH (2008) Updated national guidance on the safe administration of intrathecal chemotherapy. Available at: http://webarchive.nationalarchives.gov.uk/20121003015138/http://www.dh.gov.uk/en/Publicationsandstatistics/Lettersandcirculars/Healthservicecirculars/DH_086870 (Accessed: 8/5/2018)

DH (2009a) *Reference Guide to Consent for Examination or Treatment*, 2nd edn. London: Department of Health. Available at: https://www.gov.uk/government/publications/reference-guide-to-consent-for-examination-or-treatment-second-edition (Accessed: 1/4/2018)

DH (2009b) *The Operating Framework Enabling High Quality Care Throughout the NHS*. London: Department of Health.

DH (2013) Safe management of healthcare waste. Health Technical Memorandum. HTM 07.01 Available at: https://www.gov.uk/government/publications/guidance-on-the-safe-management-of-healthcare-waste (Accessed: 7/5/2018)

Dionyssiou, D., Chantes, A., Gravvanis, A., et al. (2011) The wash-out technique in the management of delayed presentations of extravasation injuries. *Journal of Hand Surgery*, 36(1), 66–69.

Doellman, D., Hadaway, L., Bowe-Geddes, L.A., et al. (2009) Infiltration and extravasation: update on prevention and management. *Journal of Infusion Nursing*, 32(4), 203–211.

Doroshow, J.H. (2012) Dexrazoxane for the prevention of cardiac toxicity and treatment of extravasation injury from the anthracycline antibiotics. *Current Pharmaceutical Biotechnology*, 13(10), 1949–1956.

Dougherty, L. (1996) Scalp cooling to prevent hair loss in chemotherapy. *Professional Nurse*, 11(8), 507–509.

Dougherty, L. (2003) The expert witness: working within the legal system of the United Kingdom. *Journal of Vascular Access Devices*, 8(2), 29–35.

Dougherty, L. (2005) Alopecia. In: Brighton, D. & Wood, M. (eds) *The Royal Marsden Hospital Handbook of Cancer Chemotherapy: A Guide for the Multidisciplinary Team*. Edinburgh: Elsevier Churchill Livingstone, pp. 197–200.

Dougherty, L. (2006a) *Central Venous Access Devices: Care and Management*. Oxford: Blackwell Publishing.

Dougherty, L. (2006b) Comparing methods to prevent chemotherapy-induced alopecia. *Cancer Nursing Practice*, 5(6), 25–31.

Dougherty, L. (2008a) IV therapy: recognizing the differences between infiltration and extravasation. *British Journal of Nursing*, 17(14), 896, 898–901.

Dougherty, L. (2008b) Obtaining peripheral access. In: Dougherty, L. & Lamb, J. (eds) *Intravenous Therapy in Nursing Practice*, 2nd edn. Oxford: Blackwell Publishing.

Dougherty, L. & Bailey, C. (2008) Chemotherapy. In: Corner, J. & Bailey, C. (eds) *Cancer Nursing Care in Context*. Oxford: Wiley-Blackwell.

Dougherty, L. & Lister, S. (eds) (2011) *The Royal Marsden Hospital Manual of Clinical Nursing Procedures*, 8th edn. Oxford: Wiley-Blackwell.

Dougherty, L. & Lister, S. (eds) (2015) *The Royal Marsden Hospital Manual of Clinical Nursing Procedures*, 9th edn. Oxford: Wiley-Blackwell.

Dougherty, L. & Oakley, C. (2011) Advanced practice in the management of extravasation. *Cancer Nursing Practice*, 10(5), 16–18.

Downie, G., MacKenzie, J. & Williams, A. (2003) Medicine management. In: Downie, G., Mackenzie, J. & Williams, A. (eds) *Pharmacology and Medicines Management for Nurses*, 3rd edn. London: Churchill Livingstone, pp.49–91.

Dranitsaris, G., Johnston, M., Poirier, S. et al. (2005) Are health care providers who work with cancer drugs at an increased risk for toxic events? A systematic review and meta-analysis of the literature. *Journal of Oncology Pharmacy Practice*, 11(2), 69–78.

Eggert, J.A. (2018) Biology of cancer. In: Yarbro, C.H., Wujcik, D., Holmes Gobel, B. (eds) *Cancer Nursing. Principles and Practice*, 8th edn. Burlington, MA: Jones & Bartlett Learning.

Ekwall, E.M., Nygren, L.M., Gustafsson, A.O. & Sorbe, B.G. (2013) Determination of the most effective cooling temperature for the prevention of chemotherapy-induced alopecia. *Molecular and Clinical Oncology*, 1(6), 1065–1071.

Elkin, M.K., Perry, A.G. & Potter, P.A. (2007) *Nursing Interventions and Clinical Skills*, 4th edn. St Louis, MO: Mosby.

El-Saghir, N., Otrock, Z., Mufarrij, A., et al. (2004) Dexrazoxane for anthracycline extravasation and GM-CSF for skin ulceration and wound healing. *Lancet Oncology*, 5(5), 320–321.

EU (2010) *Directive 2010/32/EU – Prevention from Sharp Injuries in the Hospital and Healthcare Sector*. Available at: www.osha.europa.eu/en/legislation/directives/sector-specific-and-worker-related-provisions/osh-directives/council-directive-2010-32-eu-prevention-from-sharps-injuries-in-the-hospital-and-healthcare-sector (Accessed: 1/4/2018)

European Oncology Nursing Society (2007) *Extravasation Guidelines: Guidelines Implementation Toolkit*. Brussels: European Oncology Nursing Society.

European Policy Recommendations (2016) Preventing occupational exposure to cytotoxic and other hazardous drugs. Available at: www.europeanbiosafetynetwork.eu (Accessed: 1/4/2018)

Ferguson, L. & Wright, P. (2002) Health and safety aspects of cytotoxics services. In: Allwood, M. & Stanley, A. (eds) *The Cytotoxics Handbook*, 4th edn. Oxford: Radcliffe Medical Press, pp. 35–62.

Few, B.J. (1987) Hyaluronidase for treating intravenous extravasations. *MCN: The American Journal of Maternal Child Nursing*, 12(1), 23–24.

Findlay, M., von Minckwitz, G. & Wardley, A. (2008) Effective oral chemotherapy for breast cancer: pillars of strength. *Annals of Oncology*, 19(2), 212–222.

Fraise, A.P. & Bradley, T. (eds) (2009) *Ayliffe's Control of Healthcare-associated Infection: A Practical Handbook*, 5th edn. London: Hodder Arnold.

Freedman, T.G. (1994) Social and cultural dimensions of hair loss in women treated for breast cancer. *Cancer Nursing*, 17(4), 334–341.

Friese, C.R., McArdle, C., Zhau, T., et al. (2015) Antineoplastic drug exposure in an ambulatory setting: a pilot study. *Cancer Nurse*, 38(2), 111–117.

Gabriel, J. (2008) Safe administration of intravenous cytotoxic drugs. In: Dougherty L. & Lamb J. (eds) *Intravenous Therapy in Nursing Practice*, 2nd edn. Oxford: Blackwell Publishing, pp. 461–494.

Gallagher, J. (1996) Women's experiences of hair loss associated with chemotherapy – longitudinal perspective. Ninth International Conference on Cancer Nursing, Brighton.

Gault, D. (1993) Extravasation injuries. *British Journal of Plastic Surgery*, 46(2), 91–96.

Gault, D. & Challands, J. (1997) Extravasation of drugs. *Anaesthesia Review*, 13, 223–241.

Giaccone, G., Di Giulio, F., Morandini, M.P. & Calciati, A. (1988) Scalp hypothermia in the prevention of doxorubicin-induced hair loss. *Cancer Nursing*, 11(3), 170–173.

Gilani, S. & Giridharan, S. (2014) Is it safe for pregnant health-care professionals to handle cytotoxic drugs? A review of the literature and recommendations. *ecancermedicalscience* 8, 418.

Gonzalez, T. (2013) Chemotherapy extravasations: prevention, identification, management, and documentation. *Clinical Journal of Oncology Nursing*, 17(1), 61–66.

Goodin, S. (2007) *Safe Handling of Oral Chemo Agents in Community Settings*. https://www.pharmacytimes.com/publications/issue/2007/2007-09/2007-09-6789.

Goolsby, T.V. & Lombardo F.A. (2006) Extravasation of chemotherapeutic agents: prevention and treatment. *Seminars in Oncology*, 33(1), 139–143.

Gregory, R.P., Cooke, T., Middleton, J., et al. (1982) Prevention of doxorubicin-induced alopecia by scalp hypothermia: relation to degree of cooling. *BMJ*, 284(6330), 1674.

Grevelman, E.G. & Breed, W.P. (2005) Prevention of chemotherapy-induced hair loss by scalp cooling. *Annals of Oncology*, 16(3), 352–358.

Griffith, R., Griffiths, H. & Jordan, S. (2003) Administration of medicines. Part 1: The law and nursing. *Nursing Standard*, 18(2), 47–53.

Guy, R., Shah, S., Parker, H. & Geddes, D. (1982) Scalp cooling by thermocirculator. *Lancet*, 1(8278), 937–938.

Hallam, C., Weston, V., Denton, A., et al. (2016) Development of the UK Vessel Health and Preservation (VHP) framework: a multi-organisational collaborative. *Journal of Infection Prevention*, 17(2), 65–72.

Hartigan, K. (2003) Patient education: the cornerstone of successful oral chemotherapy treatment. *Clinical Journal of Oncology Nursing*, 7(6 Suppl), 21–24.

Haslam, I.S., Pitre, A., Schuetz, J.D. & Paus, R. (2013) Protection against chemotherapy-induced alopecia: targeting ATP binding cassette transporters in the hair follicle? *Trends in Pharmacological Sciences*, 34(11), 599–604.

Henricksen, T. & Jensen, B.K. (2003) Advanced computerised cold cap for preventing chemotherapy induced alopecia. Paper presented at ECCO, Copenhagen, 21–25th September.

Hesketh, P.J., Batchelor, D., Golant, M., et al. (2004) Chemotherapy-induced alopecia: psychosocial impact and therapeutic approaches. *Supportive Care in Cancer*, 12(8), 543–549.

Hidalgo, M., Rinaldi, D., Medina, G., et al. (1999) A phase I trial of topical topitriol (calcitriol, 1,25-dihydroxyvitamin D3) to prevent chemotherapy-induced alopecia. *Anti-Cancer Drugs*, 10(4), 393–395.

Hilton, S., Hunt, K., Emslie, C., et al. (2008) Have men been overlooked? A comparison of young men and women's experiences of chemotherapy-induced alopecia. *Psychooncology*, 17(6), 577–583.

HM Government (2002) *The Control of Substances Hazardous to Health Regulations 2002*. London: Stationery Office. Available at: http://www.legislation.gov.uk/uksi/2002/2677/contents/made (Accessed: 7/5/2018)

Holmberg, M. & Zanni, G.R. (2005) Bring hope home with oral antineoplastic agents. *Pharmacy Times*, 71(3), 103–111.

How, C. & Brown, J. (1998) Extravasation of cytotoxic chemotherapy from peripheral veins. *European Journal of Oncology Nursing*, 2(1), 51–59.

Howard, N. & Stenner, R.W. (1983) An improved "ice-cap" to prevent alopecia caused by adriamycin (doxorubicin). *British Journal of Radiology*, 56(672), 963–964.

HSE (2017) Safe handling of cytotoxic drugs in the workplace. Available at: www.hse.gov.uk/healthservices/safe-use-cytotoxic-drugs.htm (Accessed: 1/4/2018)

HSE (2018) Latex allergies in health and social care. Available at: http://www.hse.gov.uk/healthservices/latex/ (Accessed: 7/5/2018)

Huber, C. & Augustine, A. (2009) IV infusion alarms: don't wait for the beep. *American Journal of Nursing*, 109(4), 32–33.

Hunt, J.M., Anderson, J.E. & Smith, I.E. (1982) Scalp hypothermia to prevent adriamycin-induced hair loss. *Cancer Nursing*, 5(1), 25–31.

Hunter, J. (2008) Intramuscular injection techniques. *Art and Science*, 22(24), 35–40.

ICH (1996) ICH Harmonised Tripartite Guideline. Guideline For Good Clinical Practice E6(R1). Step 4. Available at: https://www.ich.org/fileadmin/Public_Web_Site/ICH_Products/Guidelines/Efficacy/E6/E6_R1_Guideline.pdf (Accessed: 1/4/2018)

Ignoffo, R.J. & Friedman, M.A. (1980) Therapy of local toxicities caused by extravasation of cancer chemotherapeutic drugs. *Cancer Treatment Reviews*, 7(1), 17–27.

Infusion Nurses Society (INS) (2006) Infusion nursing standards of practice. *Journal of Infusion Nursing*, 29(1), Suppl, S1–S92.

Infusion Nurses Society (INS) (2016) Infusion Therapy Standards of Practice. *Journal of Infusion Nursing*, 39(1S), S1–159.

Institute for Safe Medication Practices (ISMP) (2007) The five rights: A Destination Without A Map. ISMP Medication Safety Alert Jan 25 2007. Institute for Safe Medication Practices. Available at: https://www.ncbi.nlm.nih.gov/pmc/articles/PMC2957754/pdf/ptj35_10p542.pdf (Accessed: 8/5/2018)

Jackson, G. (2006) *Consensus Opinion on the Use of Dexrazoxane (Savene) in the Treatment of Anthracycline Extravasation*. UK: Topotarget.

Jackson, T., Hallam, C., Corner, T. & Hill, S. (2013) Vascular access – right line, right patient, right time every choice matters. *British Journal of Nursing*, 22(8), S24–S27.

Janssen, F.P.E.M. (2007) Modelling physiological and biochemical aspects of scalp cooling. Unpublished thesis.

Kargar, M., Sarvestani, R.S., Khojasteh, H.N. & Heidari, M.T. (2011) Efficacy of penguin cap as scalp cooling system for prevention of alopecia in patients undergoing chemotherapy. *Journal of Advanced Nursing*, 67(11), 2473–2477.

Kassner, E. (2000) Evaluation and treatment of chemotherapy extravasation injuries. *Journal of Pediatric Oncology Nursing*, 17(3), 135–148.

Katsimbri, P., Bamias, A. & Pavlidis, N. (2000) Prevention of chemotherapy-induced alopecia using an effective scalp cooling system. *European Journal of Cancer*, 36(6), 766–771.

Kav, S., Johnson, J., Rittenberg, C., et al. (2008) Role of the nurse in patient education and follow-up of people receiving oral chemotherapy treatment: an international survey. *Supportive Care in Cancer*, 16(9), 1075–1083.

Kelland, L. (2005) Cancer cell biology, drug action and resistance. In: Brighton, D. & Wood, M. (eds) *The Royal Marsden Hospital Handbook of Cancer Chemotherapy: A Guide for the Multidisciplinary Team*. Edinburgh: Elsevier Churchill Livingstone, pp.3–15.

Keller, J.F. & Blausey, L.A. (1988) Nursing issues and management in chemotherapy-induced alopecia. *Oncology Nursing Forum*, 15(5), 603–607.

Kendell, P. (2001) Magic gel that helps cancer patients hold onto their hair. *Daily Mail*, 6 January, p. 19.

Kennedy, M., Packard, R., Grant, M. et al. (1983) The effects of using Chemocap on occurrence of chemotherapy-induced alopecia. *Oncology Nursing Forum*, 10(1), 19–24.

Khalili, M., Liao, C.E., & Nguten, T. (2009) Liver disease. In: Hammer, G.D. & McPhee, S.J. (eds) *Pathophysiology of Disease: An Introduction to Clinical Medicine*. New York: Lange Medical Books/McGraw-Hill.

Khan, M.S. & Holmes, J.D. (2002) Reducing the morbidity from extravasation injuries. *Annals of Plastic Surgery*, 48(6), 628–632; discussion 632.

Komen, M.M., Smorenburg, C.H., van den Hurk, C.J. & Nortier, J.W. (2013) Factors influencing the effectiveness of scalp cooling in the prevention of chemotherapy induced alopecia. *Oncologist*, 18(7), 885–891.

Langer, S. (2008) Treatment of anthracycline extravasation from centrally inserted venous catheters. *Oncology Reviews*, 2(2), 114–116.

Langer, S.W., Sehested, M. & Jensen, P.B. (2000) Treatment of anthracycline extravasation with dexrazoxane. *Clinical Cancer Research*, 6(9), 3680–3686.

Langer, S.W., Thougaard, A.V., Sehested, M. & Jensen, P.B. (2006) Treatment of anthracycline extravasation in mice with dexrazoxane with or without DMSO and hydrocortisone. *Cancer Chemotherapy and Pharmacology*, 57(1), 125–128.

Lavery, I. & Ingram, P. (2006) Prevention of infection in peripheral intravenous devices. *Nursing Standard*, 20(49), 49–56.

Lawson, T. (2003) A legal perspective on CVC-related extravasation. *Journal of Vascular Access Devices*, 8(1), 25–27.

Lemenager, M. (1998) Alopecia induced by chemotherapy – a controllable side-effect. *Oncology Nursing Today*, 3(2), 18–20.

Lemenager, M., Genouville, C., Bessa, E.H. & Bonneterre, J. (1995) Docetaxel-induced alopecia can be prevented. *Lancet*, 346(8971), 371–372.

Lemenager, M., Lecomte, S., Bonneterre, M.E. et al. (1997) Effectiveness of cold cap in the prevention of docetaxel-induced alopecia. *European Journal of Cancer*, 33(2), 297–300.

Lemieux, J., Maunsell, E. & Provencher, L. (2008) Chemotherapy-induced alopecia and effects on quality of life among women with breast cancer: a literature review. *Psychooncology*, 17(4), 317–328.

Lemieux, J., Provencher, L., Perron, L., et al. (2015) No effect of scalp cooling on survival among women with breast cancer. *Breast Cancer Research and Treatment*, 149(1), 263–268.

London Cancer Alliance (LCA) (2014a) Systemic Anti Cancer Treatment, Safe Handling and Drug Treatment. Knowledge and Skills Workbook 2014. Available at: http://www.londoncanceralliance.nhs.uk/media/95620/lca_sact_workbook_june_2014.pdf (Accessed: 7/5/2018)

London Cancer Alliance (LCA) (2014b) Guidelines for the Use of Methylene Blue for the Treatment and Prophylaxis of Ifosfamide-Induced Encephalitis. Available at: http://www.londoncancer.org/media/75878/London-Cancer-Methylene-Blue-Guideline-v1.pdf (Accessed: 1/4/2018)

London Cancer Alliance (LCA) (2015a) *Pan London Guidelines for the Safe Prescribing, Handling and Administration of Systemic Anti-Cancer Treatment Drugs*. https://www.pharmacytimes.com/publications/issue/2007/2007-09/2007-09-6789.

London Cancer Alliance (LCA) (2015b) Oral Systemic AntiCancer Therapies (SACT) Counselling Handbook for Pharmacy and Nursing Staff. Available at: http://www.londoncanceralliance.nhs.uk/media/122917/lca-oral-sact-counselling-handbook-amended-march-2016.pdf (Accessed: 7/5/2018)

London Cancer New Drugs Group (2016) *Antiemetic Guidelines for Adult Patients Receiving Chemotherapy and Radiotherapy*. London: London Cancer and London Cancer Alliance.

Macduff, C., Mackenzie, T., Hutcheon, A., et al. (2003) The effectiveness of scalp cooling in preventing alopecia for patients receiving epirubicin and docetaxel. *European Journal of Cancer Care*, 12 (2), 154–161.

Marders, J. (2005) Sounding the alarm for i.v. infiltration. *Nursing*, 35(4), 18, 20.

MASCC: Multinational Association for Supportive Care in Cancer (2011) MASCC Antiemetic Guidelines. Available at: http://www.mascc.org/antiemetic-guidelines (Accessed: 1/4/2018)

Masoorli, S. (2003) Extravasation injuries associated with the use of central vascular access devices. *Journal of Vascular Access Devices*, 8(1), 21–23.

Massey, C.S. (2004) A multicentre study to determine the efficacy and patient acceptability of the Paxman Scalp Cooler to prevent hair loss in patients receiving chemotherapy. *European Journal of Oncology Nursing*, 8(2), 121–130.

Maurer, M., Handjiski, B. & Paus, R. (1997) Hair growth modulation by topical immunophilin ligands: induction of anagen, inhibition of massive catagen development, and relative protection from chemotherapy-induced alopecia. *American Journal of Pathology*, 150(4), 1433–1441.

Maxwell, M.B. (1980) Scalp tourniquets for chemotherapy-induced alopecia. *American Journal of Nursing*, 80(5), 900–903.

Mayo, D.J. (1998) Fibrin sheath formation and chemotherapy extravasation: a case report. *Supportive Care in Cancer*, 6(1), 51–56.

McCaffrey Boyle, D. & Engelking, C. (1995) Vesicant extravasation: myths and realities. *Oncology Nursing Forum*, 22(1), 57–67.

McDiarmid, M.A., Oliver, M.S., Roth, T.S., Rogers, B. & Escalante, C. (2010) Chromosome 5 and 7 abnormalities in oncology personnel handling anticancer drugs. *Journal of Occupational and Environmental Medicine*, 52(10), 1028–1034.

McGowan, D. (2013) Chemo induced hair loss: prevention of a distressing side effect, *British Journal of Nursing*, 22(10), S12.

Medicines and Healthcare products Regulatory Agency (MHRA) (2008) *Implantable Drug Pumps for Intrathecal Therapy. All Manufacturers: MDA/2008/038*. London: Medicines and Healthcare products Regulatory Agency. Available at: http://webarchive.nationalarchives.gov.uk/20141205205054/http://www.mhra.gov.uk/Publications/Safety-warnings/MedicalDeviceAlerts/CON018012 (Accessed: 7/5/2018)

Medicines and Healthcare products Regulatory Agency (MHRA) (2014) *Best Practice Guidance on Patient Information Leaflets*. London: Medicines and Healthcare Regulatory Agency. Available at: www.gov.uk/government/publications/best-practice-guidance-on-patient-information-leaflets (Accessed: 1/4/2018)

Middleton, J., Franks, D., Buchanan, R.B., et al. (1985) Failure of scalp hypothermia to prevent hair loss when cyclophosphamide is added to doxorubicin and vincristine. *Cancer Treatment Reports*, 69(4), 373–375.

Mols, F., Van Den Hurk, C.J., Vingerhoets, A.J. & Breed, W.P. (2009) Scalp cooling to prevent chemotherapy-induced hair loss: practical and clinical considerations. *Supportive Care in Cancer*, 17(2), 181–189.

Moureau, N.L. & Carr, P.J. (2018) Vessel Health and Preservation: a model and clinical pathway for using vascular access devices. *British Journal of Nursing*, 27(8), S28–S35.

Moureau, N.L., Trick, N., Nifong, T., et al. (2012) Vessel health and preservation (Part 1): a new evidence-based approach to vascular access selection and management. *Journal of Vascular Access*, 13(3), 351–356.

Mouridsen, H.T., Langer, S.W., Buter, J., et al. (2007) Treatment of anthracycline extravasation with Savene (dexrazoxane): results from two prospective clinical multicentre studies. *Annals of Oncology*, 18(3), 546–550.

Mulders, M., Vingerhoets, A. & Breed, W. (2008) The impact of cancer and chemotherapy: perceptual similarities and differences between cancer patients, nurses and physicians. *European Journal of Oncology Nursing*, 12(2), 97–102.

Munstedt, K., Manthey, N., Sachsse, S. & Vahrson, H. (1997) Changes in self-concept and body image during alopecia induced cancer chemotherapy. *Supportive Care in Cancer*, 5(2), 139–143.

National Chemotherapy Advisory Group (NCAG) (2009) *Chemotherapy Services in England: Ensuring Quality and Safety*. London: National Chemotherapy Advisory Group.

National Chemotherapy Board (NCB) (2016) Consent forms for SACT (Systemic Anti-Cancer Therapy). Guidance Issued by the National Chemotherapy Board May 2016. Available at: www.cruk.org/sact_consent (Accessed: 1/4/2018)

National Comprehensive Cancer Network (NCCN) (2018) NCCN Clinical practice guidelines in oncology. Available at: https://www.nccn.org/professionals/physician_gls/default.aspx (Accessed: 1/5/2018)

National Institute for Occupational Safety and Health (NIOSH) (2016) NIOSH List of Antineoplastic and Other Hazardous Drugs in Healthcare Settings, 2016. DHHS (NIOSH) Publication No. 2016-161. Available at: https://www.cdc.gov/niosh/topics/antineoplastic/pdf/hazardous-drugs-list_2016-161.pdf (Accessed: 1/5/2018)

National Patient Safety Agency (NPSA) (2008a) The National Patient Safety Agency's rapid response report. *Oncology Nursing*, 11(3), 387–395.

National Patient Safety Agency (NPSA) (2008b) *Vinca alkaloid minibags (adult/adolescent units): NPSA/2008/RRR004*. London: National Patient Safety Agency. Available at: www.nrls.npsa.nhs.uk/resources/?EntryId45=59890 (Accessed: 1/4/2018)

National Patient Safety Agency (NPSA) (2009) *Standardising Wristbands Improves Patient Safety*. London: National Patient Safety Agency. Available at: http://www.nrls.npsa.nhs.uk/resources/?entryid45=59824 (Accessed: 8/5/2018)

Naughton, C.A. (2008) Drug-induced nephrotoxicity. *American Family Physician*, 78(6), 743–750.

Naylor, W. (2005) Extravasation of wounds; aetiology and management. In: Brighton, D. & Wood, M. (eds) *The Royal Marsden Hospital Handbook of Cancer Chemotherapy: A Guide for the Multidisciplinary Team.* Edinburgh: Elsevier Churchill Livingstone, pp.109–112.

Neuss, M.N., Gilmore, T.R., Belderson, K.M., et al. (2016) 2016 Updated American Society of Clinical Oncology/Oncology Nursing Society Chemotherapy Administration Safety Standards, Including Standards for Pediatric Oncology. *Oncology Nursing Forum*, 44(1), A1–A13.

NICE (2015) *Medicines Optimisation: The Safe and Effective use of Medicines to Enable the Best Possible Outcomes.* NICE Guideline [NG5] Published date: March 2015. Available at: https://www.nice.org.uk/guidance/ng5 (Accessed: 1/4/2018)

NIHR (2017a) Clinical trials routemap toolkit. Available at: http://www.ct-toolkit.ac.uk/routemap/ (Accessed: 1/4/2018).

NIHR (2017b) Research design service. Available at: https://www.nihr.ac.uk/about-us/how-we-are-managed/our-structure/research/research-design-service/ (Accessed: 7/5/2018)

Nixon, S. & Schulmeister, L. (2009) Safe handling of hazardous drugs: are you protected? *Clinical Journal of Oncology Nursing*, 13(4), 433–439.

NMC (2010) *Standards for Medicines Management.* London: Nursing & Midwifery Council.

NMC (2015) *The Code: Standards of Conduct, Performance and Ethics for Nurses and Midwives.* London: Nursing & Midwifery Council.

North of England Cancer Network (NECN) (2017) *Standards for the Safe Use of Oral Anticancer Medicines.* Available at: http://www.necn.nhs.uk/wp-content/uploads/2012/11/NECN-Oral-Anticancer-medicine-Policy-version-1.6.pdf (Accessed: 7/5/2018)

Oakley, C., Lennan, E., Roe, H., Craven, O., Harrold, K. & Vidall, C. (2010a) Safe practice and nursing care of patients receiving oral anticancer medicines: a position statement from UKONS. *ecancermedicalscience*, 4, 117.

Oakley, C., Johnson, J. & Ream, E. (2010b) Developing an intervention for cancer patients prescribed oral chemotherapy. *European Journal of Cancer Care*, 19, 21–28.

Oakley, C., Chambers P., Board, R., et al. (2016) Good Practice Guideline: Promoting Early Identification of Systemic Anti-Cancer Therapies Side Effects: Two Approaches. *Cancer Nursing Practice*, 15(9), 19–22.

Oken, M., Creech, R., Tormey, D., et al. (1982) Toxicity and response criteria of the Eastern Cooperative Oncology Group. *American Journal of Clinical Oncology*, 5, 649–655.

Olsen, E.A. (2003) Current and novel methods for assessing efficacy of hair growth promoters in pattern hair loss. *Journal of the American Academy of Dermatology*, 48(2 supplement), 253–262.

O'Neill, V.J. & Twelves, C.J. (2002) Oral cancer treatment: developments in chemotherapy and beyond. *British Journal of Cancer*, 87, 933–937.

Ostendorf, W. (2012) Preparation for safe medication administration. In: Perry, A.G., Potter, P.A. & Elkin, M.K. (eds) *Nursing Interventions & Clinical Skills*, 5th edn. St Louis, MO: Elsevier, pp.486–583.

Parker, R. (1987) The effectiveness of scalp hypothermia in preventing cyclophosphamide-induced alopecia. *Oncology Nursing Forum*, 14(6), 49–53.

Peck, H.J., Mitchell, H. & Stewart, A.L. (2000) Evaluating the efficacy of scalp cooling using the Penguin cold cap system to reduce alopecia in patients undergoing chemotherapy for breast cancer. *European Journal of Oncology Nursing*, 4(4), 246–248.

Peerbooms, M., van den Hurk, C.J. & Breed, W.P. (2015) Familiarity, opinions, experiences and knowledge about scalp cooling: a Dutch survey among breast cancer patients and oncological professionals. *Asia Pacific Journal of Oncology Nursing*, 2(1), 35–41.

Pérez Fidalgo, J.A., García Fabregat, L., Cervantes, A., et al., on behalf of the ESMO Guidelines Working Group (2012) Management of chemotherapy extravasation: ESMO–EONS Clinical Practice Guidelines. *Annals of Oncology*, 23(suppl 7), vii167–vii173.

Pickard-Holley, S. (1995) The symptom experience of alopecia. *Seminars in Oncology Nursing*, 11(4), 235–238.

Polovich, M. (2016) Minimizing occupational exposure to antineoplastic agents. *Journal of Infusion Nursing*, 39(5), 307–313.

Polovich, M. & Clark, P. (2012) Factors influencing oncology nurses' use of hazardous drug safe-handling precautions. *Oncology Nursing Forum*, 39(3), E299–E309.

Polovich, M., Olsen, M. & LeFebvre, K. (eds) (2014) *Chemotherapy and Biotherapy Guidelines and Recommendations for Practice*, 4th edn. Pittsburgh, PA: Oncology Nursing Society, Chapter 9.

Potter, P.A. (2011) Administration of nonparenteral medications. In: Perry, A.G., Potter, P.A. & Elkin, M.K. (eds) *Nursing Interventions & Clinical Skills*, 5th edn. St Louis, MO: Elsevier, pp.501–540.

Power, S. & Condon, C. (2008) Chemotherapy induced alopecia: a phenomenological study. *Cancer Nursing Practice*, 7(7), 44–47.

Priestman, T.J. (1989) *Cancer Chemotherapy: An Introduction*, 3rd edn. London: Springer-Verlag.

Protiere, C., Evans, K., Camerlo, J., et al. (2002) Efficacy and tolerance of a scalp-cooling system for prevention of hair loss and the experience of breast cancer patients treated by adjuvant chemotherapy. *Supportive Care in Cancer*, 10(7), 529–537.

Purohit, O.P. (1992) A 6 week chemotherapy regimen for relapsed lymphoma efficacy results and the influence of scalp cooling. *Annals of Oncology*, 3(5 supp), 126.

Randall, J. & Ream, E. (2005) Hair loss with chemotherapy: at a loss over its management? *European Journal of Cancer Care*, 14(3), 223–231.

RCN (2016) *Standards for Infusion Therapy*, 4th edn. London: Royal College of Nursing.

RCN (2017) Using and doing research: a novice's guide. Available at: https://www.rcn.org.uk/library/subject-guides/using-and-doing-research-a-novices-guide. (Accessed: 1/4/2018)

Ridderheim, M., Bjurberg, M. & Gustavsson, A. (2003) Scalp hypothermia to prevent chemotherapy-induced alopecia is effective and safe: a pilot study of a new digitized scalp-cooling system used in 74 patients. *Supportive Care in Cancer*, 11(6), 371–377.

Robinson, M.H., Jones, A.C. & Durrant, K.D. (1987) Effectiveness of scalp cooling in reducing alopecia caused by epirubicin treatment of advanced breast cancer. *Cancer Treatment Reports*, 71(10), 913–914.

Rodrigues, C.C., Guilherme, C., Lobo da Costa, M., Jr. & Campos de Carvalho, E. (2012) Risk factors for vascular trauma during antineoplastic chemotherapy: contributions of the use of relative risk. *Acta Paulista de Enfermagem*, 25(3), 448–452.

Roe, H. (2011) Anthracycline extravasations: prevention and management. *British Journal of Nursing*, 20(17), S18–S22.

Roe, H. (2014) Scalp cooling: management option for chemotherapy induced alopecia. *British Journal of Nursing*, 23(16), S4–S11.

Roe, H. & Lennan, E. (2014) Role of nurses in the assessment and mangement of chemotherapy-related side effects in cancer patients. *Nursing: Research and Reviews*, 4, 103–115.

Ron, I.G., Kalmus, Y., Kalmus, Z., et al. (1997) Scalp cooling in the prevention of alopecia in patients receiving depilating chemotherapy. *Supportive Care in Cancer*, 5(2), 136–138.

Rosenblatt, L. (2006) Being the monster: women's narratives of body and self after treatment for breast cancer. *Medical Humanities*, 32(1), 53–56.

Rosman, S. (2004) Cancer and stigma: experience of patients with chemotherapy-induced alopecia. *Patient Education and Counseling*, 52(3), 333–339.

Roth, D. (2003) Extravasation injuries of peripheral veins: a basis for litigation. *Journal of Vascular Access Devices*, 8(1), 13–20.

Ruddy, K., Mayer, E. & Partridge, A. (2009) Patient adherence and persistence with oral anticancer treatment. *CA: Cancer Journal for Clinicians*, 59, 56–66.

Rudolph, R. & Larson, D.L. (1987) Etiology and treatment of chemotherapeutic agent extravasation injuries: a review. *Journal of Clinical Oncology*, 5(7), 1116–1126.

Rugo, H., Serrurier, K.M., Melisko, M., et al. (2012) Use of the DigniCap System to prevent hair loss in women receiving chemotherapy (CTX) for Stage 1 breast cancer (BC). *Cancer Research*, 72(24 Suppl), 2–12.

Sansivero, G. & Barton-Burke, M. (2001) Chemotherapy administration: general principles for vascular access. In: Barton-Burke, M., Wilkes, G.M. & Ingwersen, K. (eds) *Cancer Chemotherapy: A Nursing Process Approach*, 3rd edn. Sudbury, MA: Jones and Bartlett, pp.645–670.

Satterwhite, B. & Zimm, S. (1984) The use of scalp hypothermia in the prevention of doxorubicin-induced hair loss. *Cancer*, 54(1), 34–37.

Sauerland, C., Engelking, C., Wickham, R. & Corbi, D. (2006) Vesicant extravasation part I: mechanisms, pathogenesis, and nursing care to reduce risk. *Oncology Nursing Forum*, 33(6), 1134–1142.

Scales, K. (2005) Vascular access: a guide to peripheral venous cannulation. *Nursing Standard*, 19(49), 48–52.

Scaramuzzo, L. (2017) Patient education. In: Newton, S., Hickey, M., & Brant, J.M. (eds) *Mosby's Oncology Nursing Advisor: A Comprehensive Guide to Clinical Practice*. St Louis: Elsevier, pp.436–442.

Schaffrin-Nabe, D. Schmitz, I., Josten-Nabe, A., von Hehn, U. & Voigtmann, R. (2015) The influence of various parameters on the success of sensor-controlled scalp cooling in preventing chemotherapy-induced alopecia. *Oncology Research and Treatment*, 38(10), 489–495.

Schrijvers, D.L. (2003) Extravasation: a dreaded complication of chemotherapy. *Annals of Oncology*, 14(Suppl 3), iii26–iii30.

Schulmeister, L. (1998) A complication of vascular access device insertion. A case study and review of subsequent legal action. *Journal of Intravenous Nursing*, 21(4), 197–202.

Schulmeister, L. (2009) Antineoplastic therapy. In: *Infusion Therapy and Transfusion Medicine*. Basel: S. Karger AG, pp.366–367.

Schwartz, A.L. (2007) Understanding and treating cancer-related fatigue. *Oncology*, 21(11 suppl), 30–34.

Scottish Government (2012) [Revised] Guidance for the safe delivery of systemic anti-cancer therapy, CEL 30. Available at: http://www.sehd.scot.nhs.uk/mels/CEL2012_30.pdf (Accessed: 8/5/2018)

Scurr, M. (2005) Combination chemotherapy and chemotherapy principles. In: Brighton D. & Wood M. (eds) *The Royal Marsden Hospital Handbook of Cancer Chemotherapy: A Guide for the Multidisciplinary Team*. Edinburgh: Elsevier Churchill Livingstone, pp.17–29.

Serrurier, K.M., Melisko, M.E., Glencer, A., Esserman, L.J. & Rugo, H.S. (2012) Efficacy and safety of scalp cooling treatment for alopecia prevention in women receiving chemotherapy (CTX) for breast cancer (BC). *Cancer Research Meeting Abstracts*, 72(24a), 725–726. Available at: http://cancerres.aacrjournals.org/content/72/24_Supplement/P2-12-12 (Accessed: 8/5/2018)

Seto, T., Ushijima, S., Yamamoto, H., et al. (2006) Intrapleural hypotonic cisplatin treatment for malignant pleural effusion in 80 patients with non-small-cell lung cancer: a multi-institutional phase II trial. *British Journal of Cancer*, 95(6), 717–721.

Sewell, G., Summerhayes, M. & Stanley, A. (2002) Administration of chemotherapy. In: Allwood, M., Stanley, A. & Wright, P. (eds) *The Cytotoxics Handbook*, 4th edn. Oxford: Radcliffe Medical Press, pp.85–115.

Shah, N., Groom, N., Jackson, S., et al. (2000) A pilot study to assess the feasibility of prior scalp cooling with palliative whole brain radiotherapy. *British Journal of Radiology*, 73(869), 514–516.

Shapiro, J. & Price, V.H. (1998) Hair regrowth. Therapeutic agents. *Dermatologic Clinics*, 16(2), 341–356.

Sharma, S. & Saltz, L.B. (2000) Oral chemotherapeutic agents for colorectal cancer. *Oncologist*, 5(2), 99–107.

Shin, H., Jo, S.J., Kim, D.H., Kwon, O. & Myung, S.K. (2015) Efficacy of interventions for prevention of chemotherapy-induced alopecia: a systematic review and meta-analysis. *International Journal of Cancer*, 136(5), E442–E454.

Shuey, K. & Payne, Y. (2005). Administration considerations. In: Polovich, M., Olsen, M. & LeFebvre, K. (eds) *Chemotherapy and Biotherapy Guidelines and Recommendations for Practice*. Pittsburgh, PA: Oncology Nursing Society, p.125.

Skeel, R. (2016) Biologic and pharmacologic basis of cancer chemotherapy. In: Khleif, S., Rixe, O. & Skeel, R. (eds) *Skeel's Handbook of Cancer Therapy*, 9th edn. Philadelphia, AP: Wolters Kluwer, p.2.

Spaëth, D., Luporsi, E., Coudert, B., et al. (2008) Efficacy and safety of cooling helmets for the prevention of chemotherapy induced alopecia: a prospective study of 911 patients. Paper presented at ASCO, Chicago, May 30–June 3.

Sredni, B., Xu, R.H., Albeck, M., et al. (1996) The protective role of the immunomodulator AS101 against chemotherapy-induced alopecia studies on human and animal models. *International Journal of Cancer*, 65(1), 97–103.

Stanley, A. (2002) Managing complications of chemotherapy administration. In: Allwood, M., Stanley, A. & Wright, P. (eds) *The Cytotoxics Handbook*, 4th edn. Oxford: Radcliffe Medical Press, pp.119–192.

Symonds, R.P., McCormick, C.V. & Maxted, K.J. (1986) Adriamycin alopecia prevented by cold air scalp cooling. *American Journal of Clinical Oncology*, 9(5), 454–457.

Szetela, A.B. & Gibson, D.E. (2007) How the new oral antineoplastics affect nursing practice: capecitabine serves to illustrate. *American Journal of Nursing*, 107(12), 40–48.

Tierney, A.J. (1987) Preventing chemotherapy-induced alopecia in cancer patients: is scalp cooling worthwhile? *Journal of Advanced Nursing*, 12(3), 303–310.

Tierney, A.J. (1989) *A Study to Inform Nursing Support of Patients Coping with Chemotherapy for Breast Cancer*. Edinburgh: Department of Nursing Studies, University of Edinburgh.

Toft, B. (2001) External Inquiry into the adverse incident that occurred at Queen's Medical Centre, Nottingham, 4th January 2001. London: Department of Health. Available at: http://webarchive.national-archives.gov.uk/20120524040348/http://www.dh.gov.uk/prod_consum_dh/groups/dh_digitalassets/@dh/@en/documents/digitalasset/dh_4082098.pdf (Accessed: 7/5/2018)

Tollenaar, R.A., Liefers, G.J., Repelaer van Driel, O.J. & van de Velde, C.J. (1994) Scalp cooling has no place in the prevention of alopecia in adjuvant chemotherapy for breast cancer. *European Journal of Cancer*, 30A(10), 1448–1453.

Tortora, G.J. & Derrickson, B. (2009) *Principles of Anatomy and Physiology*, 12th edn. Hoboken, NJ: John Wiley.

Toumeh, A. & Skeel, R. (2016) Classification, use and toxicity of clinically useful chemotherapy and molecular targeted therapy. In: Khleif, S., Rixe, O. & Skeel, R. (eds) *Skeel's Handbook of Cancer Therapy*, 9th edn. Philadelphia, PA: Wolters Kluwer, p.667.

UK Oncology Nursing Society (UKONS) (2018) *Systemic Anti-cancer Therapy (SACT) Competency Passport. Oral, Intravenous, Subcutaneous and Intramuscular SACT Administration for Adult Patients*. Available at: www.ukons.org/downloads/home.

Ulutin, H.C., Guden, M., Dede, M. & Pak, Y. (2000) Comparison of granulocyte-colony, stimulating factor and granulocyte macrophage-colony stimulating factor in the treatment of chemotherapy extravasation ulcers. *European Journal of Gynaecological Oncology*, 21(6), 613–615.

Uno, H. & Kurata, S. (1993) Chemical agents and peptides affect hair growth. *Journal of Investigative Dermatology*, 101(1 Suppl), 143S–147S.

Valanis, B., Vollmer, W.M. & Steele, P. (1999) Occupational exposure to antineoplastic agents: self-reported miscarriages and stillbirths among nurses and pharmacists. *Journal of Occupational and Environmental Medicine*, 41(8), 632–638.

Van den Hurk, C.J.G., Mols, F., Vingerhoets, J.J.M. & Breed, W.P.M. (2010) Impact of alopecia and scalp cooling on the well being of breast cancer patients. *Psychooncology*, 19(7), 701–709.

Van den Hurk, C.J.G., Breed, W.P.M. & Nortier, J.W.R. (2012a) Short post infusion scalp cooling time in the prevention of docetaxel induced alopecia. *Supportive Care in Cancer*, 20(12), 3255–3260.

Van den Hurk, C.J., Peerbooms, M., van de Poll-Franse, L.V., Nortier, J.W., Coebergh, J.W. & Breed, W.P. (2012b) Scalp cooling for hair preservation and associated characteristics in 1411 chemotherapy patients – results of the Dutch Scalp Cooling Registry. *Acta Oncologica*, 51(4), 497–504.

Van den Hurk, C.J.G., van den Akker-van Marle, M.E., Breed, W.P., van de Poll-Franse, L.V., Nortier, J.W. & Coebergh, J.W. (2013a) Impact of scalp cooling on chemotherapy induced alopecia: wig use and hair growth of patients with cancer. *European Journal of Oncology Nursing*, 17(5), 536–540.

Van den Hurk, C.J.G., van de Poll-Franse, L.V., Breed, W.P., Coebergh, J.W. & Nortier, J.W. (2013b) Scalp cooling to prevent alopecia after chemotherapy can be considered safe in patients with breast cancer. *Breast*, 22(5), 1001–1004.

Van den Hurk, C.J., van den Akker-van Marle, M.E., Breed, W.P., van de Poll-Franse, L.V., Nortier, J.W. & Coebergh, J.W. (2014) Cost-effectiveness analysis of scalp cooling to reduce chemotherapy-induced alopecia. *Acta Oncologica*, 53, 80–87.

Van den Hurk, C., de Beer, F., Dries, W., et al. (2015) No prevention of radiotherapy-induced alopecia by scalp cooling. *Radiotherapy and Oncology*, 117(1), 193–194.

Van der Molen, B. (2005) Patient information and education. In: Brighton, D. & Wood, M. (eds) *The Royal Marsden Hospital Handbook of Cancer Chemotherapy: A Guide for the Multidisciplinary Team*. Edinburgh: Elsevier Churchill Livingstone, pp.49–59.

Vidall, C., Roe, H., Dougherty, L. & Harrold, K. (2013) Dexrazoxane: a management option for anthracycline extravasations. *British Journal of Nursing*, 22(17), S6–S12.

Viele, C.S. (2007) Managing oral chemotherapy: the healthcare practitioner's role. *American Journal of Health-System Pharmacy*, 64(9 Suppl 5), S25–S32.

Vioral, A. (2018) In: Yarbro, C.H., Wujcik, D., Holmes Gobel, B. (eds) *Cancer Nursing. Principles and Practice*, 8th edn. Burlington, MA: Jones & Bartlett Learning, Chapter 44.

Vleut, R.E., van Poppel, J.E., Dercksen, M.W., Peerbooms, M., Houterman, S. & Breed, W.P. (2013) Hair mass index obtained by cross-section trichometry: an objective and clinically useful parameter to quantify hair in chemotherapy-induced alopecia. *Supportive Care in Cancer*, 21(7), 1807–1814.

Washburn, D.J. (2007) Intravesical antineoplastic therapy following transurethral resection of bladder tumors: nursing implications from the operating room to discharge. *Clinical Journal of Oncology Nursing*, 11(4), 553–559.

Weinstein, S. & Hagle, M.E. (2014) *Plumer's Principles and Practice of Intravenous Therapy*, 9th edn. Philadelphia, PA: Lippincott Williams and Wilkins, Chapter 19.

Wheelock, J.B., Myers, M.B., Krebs, H.B. & Goplerud, D.R. (1984) Ineffectiveness of scalp hypothermia in the prevention of alopecia in patients treated with doxorubicin and cisplatin combinations. *Cancer Treatment Reports*, 68(11), 1387–1388.

Wickham, R., Engelking, C., Sauerland, C. & Corbi, D. (2006) Vesicant extravasation part II: Evidence-based management and continuing controversies. *Oncology Nursing Forum*, 33(6), 1143–1150.

Wilkes, G.M. (2018) In: Yarbro, C.H., Wujcik, D., Holmes Gobel, B. (eds) *Cancer Nursing. Principles and Practice*, 8th edn. Burlington, MA: Jones & Bartlett Learning, Chapter 15.

Williams, J., Wood, C. & Cunningham-Warburton, P. (1999) A narrative study of chemotherapy-induced alopecia. *Oncology Nursing Forum*, 26(9), 1463–1468.

Williamson, S. (2008) Management of oral anti-cancer therapies. *Pharmaceutical Journal*, 281, 399–402.

Wilson, C. (1994) The ice cap that could help save your hair. *Daily Mail*, September 20th, pp.36–37.

Winkeljohn, D.L. (2007) Oral chemotherapy medications: the need for a nurse's touch. *Clinical Journal of Oncology Nursing*, 11(6), 793–796.

Witman, G., Cadman, E. & Chen, M. (1981) Misuse of scalp hypothermia. *Cancer Treatment Reports*, 65(5–6), 507–508.

Workman, B. (1999) Safe injection techniques. *Nursing Standard*, 13(39), 47–53.

Yang, X. & Thai, K.E. (2015) Treatment of permanent chemotherapy-induced alopecia with low dose oral minoxidil. *The Australasian Journal of Dermatology*, 57, 10.1111/ajd.12350.

Yarbro, C.H., Wujcik, D., Holmes Gobel, B. (eds) (2018) *Cancer Nursing. Principles and Practice*, 8th edn. Burlington, MA: Jones & Bartlett Learning.

Yoshida, J., Kosaka, H., Tomika, K. & Kumagai, S. (2006) Genotoxic risks to nurses from contamination of the work environment with antineoplastic drugs in Japan. *Journal of Occupational Health*, 48, 517–522.

Young, A. (2013) Chemotherapy induced alopecia: a cool to action. *British Journal of Nursing*, 22(11), 608.

Young, A. & Arif, A. (2016) The use of scalp cooling for chemotherapy induced hair loss. *British Journal of Nursing*, 25(10), S22–S27.

Chapter 5
Radionuclide therapy

Procedure guidelines

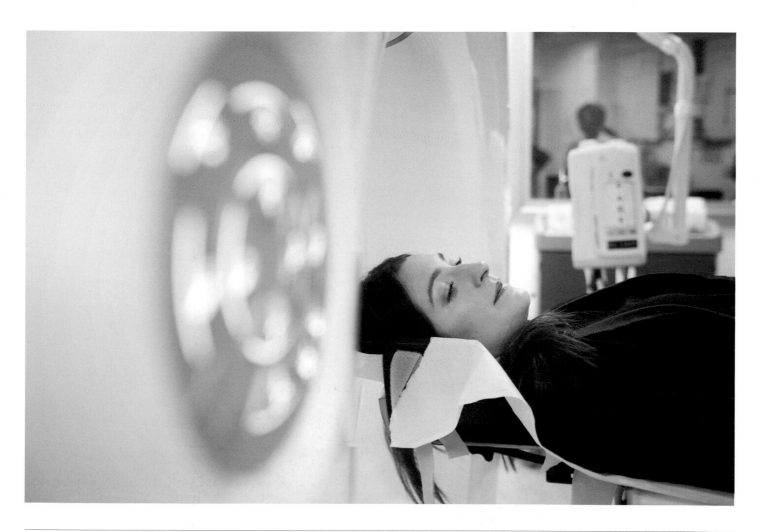

The Royal Marsden Manual of Cancer Nursing Procedures. Edited by Sara Lister and Lisa Dougherty, with Assistant Editor Louise McNamara.
© 2019 The Royal Marsden NHS Foundation Trust. Published 2019 by John Wiley & Sons, Ltd.

Overview

Radiation is capable of being beneficial and harmful; it is therefore essential that every effort is made to minimize the harmful effects of therapeutic radiation whilst maximizing its benefits (Darby 1999). This chapter provides specific detailed information on the principles of nursing care in relation to radioisotopes in the clinical setting. This will enable staff to apply best practice principles when caring for patients, and facilitate the education and support of other healthcare professionals and visitors.

Radiation

Definition

Radiation occurs when energy is emitted or generated as either waves or particles (known as electromagnetic or particulate radiation). Radioactivity is a natural phenomenon in which unstable atoms emit radiation. In stable atoms ionizing radiation is produced through excitation, ionization and nuclear disintegration. Radiography is the practice of using X-rays to produce an image on film (Ionising Radiations Regulations 1999).

Related theory

Every minute of our lives we are exposed to radiation from natural and artificial sources.

(Ionising Radiations Regulations 1999)

Naturally occurring radiation comprises radiation from outer space (known as cosmic radiation), from the ground and from the air (referred to as radon). Small amounts of naturally occurring radiation are also present in the food we eat. Natural radiation accounts for 85.5% of the total radiation received by the UK population. This belongs to a class of radiation known as electromagnetic radiation which transports energy through space in the form of electric and magnetic waves. Electromagnetic radiation is encountered in our day-to-day lives; in fact, life as we know it would not be possible without electromagnetic radiation.

Electromagnetic radiation provides radio and television signals, microwaves, visible light, X-rays and gamma rays. It is well known that, as well as providing many benefits, there are potentially serious health effects associated with electromagnetic radiation. The nature of these effects varies depending on which part of the spectrum the radiation belongs to. Radiation may also be encountered in the form of particles, rather than waves. Particulate radiation is capable of producing ionization and can therefore produce biological effects. The radiation particles most commonly used in hospitals are streams of electrons, known as beta radiation.

Artificial sources of radiation, including medical exposures, discharges from industrial premises and fall-out from atomic weapons testing, make up the remaining 14.5% of the radiation received by the population. Of these, medical exposures are the largest contributor.

Radiation is capable of disrupting the chemical balance in the cell by damaging the DNA. This is caused by the introduction of free radicals – atoms/molecules with unpaired electrons (HPA 2010) – that may lead to cell death or cancer at some time in the future. Therefore, substantial emphasis is placed on reducing the amount of radiation given during medical exposures.

Radiation is used in treating malignant disease and includes: X-rays produced artificially by electron bombardment of a metal target; gamma rays (a natural emission in the nuclear decay of radioisotopes), sometimes referred to as 'photon' radiation; and beta particles (capable of ionization). These are distinguishable from electromagnetic radiation by their characteristic of carrying a negative electrical charge. Beta particles result when a neutron within the nucleus disintegrates to form a proton and an electron. The electron is ejected from the nucleus, producing beta radiation (IPEM/RCN 2002).

Radiation used in nuclear medicine, in laboratory tests and for certain types of radiotherapy treatments is emitted by specific radioactive materials. In a process known as radioactive decay, the amount of radiation emitted by a radioactive material diminishes continuously over time until the material no longer produces radiation.

The time taken for the radioactivity in a radioactive material to be halved is known as the half-life. Different materials have different half-lives, ranging from a few seconds or minutes to many years. Most radioactive materials used within hospitals have relatively short half-lives and so diminish to insignificant levels within a few hours or a few days (HPA 2010).

Radioactive material may be encountered in solid (sealed), liquid or gaseous form (unsealed). Liquid or gaseous radioactive materials have the important advantage that they can be used *in vivo* to study metabolic processes. As radioactive materials emit radiation in all directions, they are usually kept in lead containers for safety.

Ionizing radiation is the term used to describe energetic particles (e.g. alpha, beta) or electromagnetic waves with a wavelength of no more than 100 nanometres because they are capable of producing ions by ejecting electrons from their atoms (DH 2016).

Radioisotopes are measured in becquerels (Bq). A becquerel is the Système International (SI) unit of activity and is 1 disintegration per second:

$$k \text{ (kilo)} = 1 \times 10^3$$
$$M \text{ (mega)} = 1 \times 10^6, \text{ e.g. megabecquerel (MBq)}$$
$$G \text{ (giga)} = 1 \times 10^9$$

The half-life of a radioactive substance is the time taken for it to decay to half its original number of radioactive atoms (Bomford 2002a). The sensitive target appears to be DNA in the nucleus of the cell. The ionizing radiation passes through the cells and tissues, and the dose of radiation received is measured in terms of energy absorbed. The unit of absorbed dose is known as a gray:

$$100 \text{ centigray (cGy)} = 1 \text{ gray (Gy)}$$

For the purposes of radiation protection for staff and patients, the dose calculated to the whole body must be known. *Whereas the absorbed dose is measured in grays, the dose to the whole body is measured in sieverts.* For example, staff over 18 years of age who are not pregnant must wear a monitoring badge to monitor their individual exposure to radiation. There is an annual dose limit of 20 millisieverts (mSv), but the dose to staff should be kept below 6 mSv (DH 2016). In practice, any person being exposed to over 5 mSv in the UK will be a classified worker (IRMER 2000).

Radiation protection

Evidence-based approaches

Rationale

Radiation protection is based on three principles.

1 *Justification:* no practice should be adopted unless its introduction produces a net benefit.
2 *Optimization:* all exposure shall be as low as reasonably practicable (ALARP).
3 *Limitation:* the dose equivalent to staff and members of the public shall not exceed the dose limits (1 mSv annually).

The requirements for procedures involving unsealed sources include the following.

- Those administering radioactive material must hold an approved Administration of Radioactive Substances Advisory Committee (ARSAC) certificate for each radionuclide they intend to use.
- Administration of therapeutic and diagnostic radioactive substances can only be carried out in centres with appropriate facilities (Cormack et al. 1998).
- Therapeutic unsealed sources generate a significant amount of liquid radioactive waste, from showers and toilets. The amount of radioactive waste that enters the sewage system is governed by local regulations. Multiple holding tank systems can be employed where waste can be held to allow decay to occur before being released into the main waste drainage system (Leung and Nikolic 1998).
- Risk assessments must be carried out prior to work with ionizing radiation, to ensure risks are properly controlled (Pearson et al. 2001).
- All controlled areas will have warning notices to restrict entry.
- All controlled and supervised areas have local rules and systems of work, summarizing the arrangements for controlling work with ionizing radiation. The radiation protection supervisor ensures that the local rules are followed.
- Visitors are restricted. Doses received by relatives/friends of patients undergoing treatment or examination with ionizing radiation are restricted to the doses allowed to members of the public unless they are classified as 'comforters and carers', when different rules and restrictions will apply.
- Exposure is controlled using time, distance and shielding.
- Personal protective clothing including gloves, aprons and overshoes must be used to limit the risk of contamination (Ionising Radiations Regulations 1999, IRMER 2000).
- Procedures are in place for reporting incidents (RIDDOR 1995).
- Adequate training is provided and only trained staff can work unsupervised.
- Pregnant staff or staff who are breastfeeding *cannot* enter the controlled area.
- Quality assurance initiatives must be undertaken; these include clinical audit of procedures and standards.

Legal and professional issues

Regulations

Radiation regulations are an essential component designed to protect healthcare workers. It is law that all organizations involved in a procedure using ionizing and non-ionizing radiation must adhere to radiation regulations.

The International Commission on Radiological Protection (ICRP) oversees radiation safety. The Health Protection Agency (HPA) has statutory responsibility for advising UK government departments as well as other professional groups such as the Institute of Physics and Engineering in Medicine (IPEM) on radiation protection and regulation.

Box 5.1 describes the legal Acts that all organizations must adhere to when providing diagnostic and therapeutic unsealed and sealed source radioisotopes.

Pre-procedural considerations

Within a controlled area

The entrance to the controlled area must be marked with a warning sign. Information is displayed to indicate the following.

- The radioactive material and activity administered.
- That only essential nursing procedures should be carried out and unnecessary time must not be spent near the patient while the sign is displayed.

Box 5.1 Legal Acts and guidance governing the use of radioactive materials

The Radioactive Substances Act 1993
Controls the use and disposal of radioactive materials in hospitals and elsewhere, and is enforced by the Environment Agency via a system of licensing and inspection.

Pregnancy and Work in Diagnostic Imaging. Report of a Joint Working Party of the Royal College of Radiologists and British Institute of Radiology, 1992
This report provides a summary of present knowledge on radiation effects in the fetus and recommends the steps to be taken when a member of staff declares she is pregnant.

Health and Safety at Work Act 1974
- Provides the umbrella for all safety-related legislation.
- Regulates safety in the workplace.
- Puts the responsibility for safety on the employer, for example the health authority, trust board or chief executive.
- Enforced by inspectors of the Health and Safety Executive who can prosecute for contravention of regulations and serve improvement and enforcement notices.
- Provides for health and safety representatives.

Ionising Radiations Regulations, SI 3232, 1999
- Regulates all radiation work from dental X-rays to nuclear power stations.
- Covers dose limitation and management systems for radiation safety including local rules, appointment of advisers and supervisors.

Approved Code of Practice, 'Work with Ionizing Radiation', 2000
- 'Approved' by the Health and Safety Commission.
- Gives acceptable methods of complying with legal requirements.
- Should be followed unless there is good reason to use alternatives.

Ionising Radiation (Medical Exposure) Regulations, SI 1059, 2000
- Employers are responsible for the radiation safety of patients.
- Staff must be competent and properly trained to undertake their role in any process that exposes patients to radiation.
- Expert advice must be sought from a medical physicist.
- Patient doses must be justifiable.

Medical and Dental Guidance Notes
- A good practice guide on all aspects of ionizing radiation protection in the clinical environment.
- Practical guide to safe practice.
- No legal status.

Appropriate barriers, that is lead shields, should be placed at the entrance to:

- prevent inadvertent entry by unauthorized personnel
- reduce radiation exposure to staff and visitors.

Patients treated with unsealed radioactive sources should be confined to their rooms. The exception would be for special medical or nursing procedures when they must be accompanied by suitably trained staff (e.g. when having a whole-body I-131 scan post treatment).

Decon 90™ should be available in a controlled area. Decon 90™ is an approved solution for neutralizing radiopharmaceuticals in the event of a spillage. The solution should be diluted according to manufacturer's instructions or be available as ready-to-use wipes. Once the spillage area has been initially wiped with absorbent paper/pads, Decon 90™ is used to clean the surface. The area is then monitored to check for radiation contamination. The process should be repeated until the contamination has been reduced to a safe level (DH 2016). In the event of any spillage medical physics should be notified immediately to assess and advise.

Equipment

Thermoluminescent dosimeter (TLD)

A TLD measures a person's exposure to radiation and must be worn always when on duty (see Figure 1.5). A digital dosimeter should be used when ongoing immediate dose records are required.

Use of a contamination monitor

Waste and equipment must be monitored before being removed from any controlled area where patients have received or are receiving unsealed or sealed sources. This monitoring will establish if contamination has occurred or a sealed source is present amongst the items being removed (Hart 2006).

Before using a contamination monitor (see Figure 1.6 and Figure 5.1) it is important to check that the monitor's batteries are fully charged; the background reading on the monitor must then be noted before undertaking the monitoring. The background must be reasonably low (normally less than 10 counts per second) otherwise it will be difficult to detect small levels of radioactivity present on the item being monitored. If the background reading immediately outside the treatment room is found to be high, it will be necessary to monitor the items further away where the background is lower.

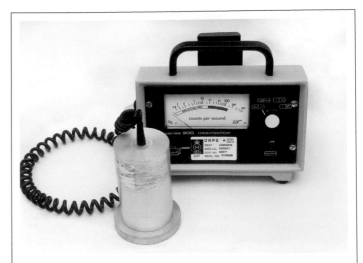

Figure 5.1 Hand-held contamination monitor. *Source:* Dougherty and Lister (2011).

Items should be monitored by passing the monitor's probe over each item while watching for fluctuations in the count rate. If an item is found to be contaminated (indicated by a sustained increase in count rate), it should either be returned to a safe location in the treatment room or set aside in a designated area while help is sought from the medical physics department (Bomford 2002a).

Procedure guideline 5.1	**Radiation protection: major spillage of radioactive body fluids through incontinence and/or vomiting**

Essential equipment: spillage kit
- Absorbent pads/paper
- Gloves
- Overshoes
- Apron and/or gown
- (COSHH) radiation waste bag
- Radiation warning tape
- Hand-held radiation monitor

Optional equipment
- Decon 90™, an approved solution for neutralizing isotopes

Procedure

Action	Rationale
1 Put on the protective clothing found in the spillage kit and immediately cover the spillage with absorbent material.	To absorb contamination and to contain the area of spillage (DH 2016, **C**).
2 Inform the medical physics department immediately.	So that the medical physics department can advise on radiation protection as soon as possible, to ensure local policy is adhered to (DH 2016, **C**).
3 If medical physics department staff are not immediately available, use a radiation monitor to assess the extent of the spillage.	To define extent of contamination and determine what further measures need to be taken (DH 2016, **C**).
4 Any waste that cannot be flushed down the toilet or macerated must be placed in a black polythene bag with a radiation label and the medical physics staff informed.	To prevent contamination of the environment (DH 2016, **C**).
5 Follow the advice of the medical physics department staff in clearing the spillage using the designated spillage kit.	To prevent spread of contamination (DH 2016, **C**).

Procedure guideline 5.2 Radiation protection: contamination of bare hands by radioactive body fluids

Essential equipment
- Soap and water
- Hand-held radiation monitor

Optional equipment
- Decon 90™, an approved solution for neutralizing isotopes

Procedure

Action	Rationale
1 Wash hands in warm soapy water, paying special attention to the areas around the fingernails, between the fingers and on the outer edges of the hands. Continue washing and monitoring hands until contamination is below the permissible limits indicated by local monitoring protocols.	To remove radioactive material from any areas where it might be trapped (PHE 2014, **C**).
2 If the skin is broken in a contamination accident, wash thoroughly under running water, opening the edges of the cut. This should be continued until medical physics staff can demonstrate that no residual radioactivity remains in the wound.	To stimulate bleeding and permit thorough flushing of the cut. **E**

Procedure guideline 5.3 Radiation protection: death of a patient who has received unsealed radioactive source therapy

Essential equipment
- Absorbent pads/paper
- Gloves
- Overshoes
- Apron and/or gown
- (COSHH) radiation waste bag
- Radiation warning tape
- Hand-held radiation monitor

Optional equipment
- Decon 90™, an approved solution for neutralizing isotopes

Procedure

Action	Rationale
1 Inform the medical physics department immediately.	So that the medical physics department staff can begin making the necessary arrangements for removal of the body to the mortuary (DH 2016, **C**).
2 Two nurses wearing gloves, plastic aprons or gown, and overshoes should perform Last Offices as per local policies. Any vomit, blood, faeces or urine must be cleaned from the body.	To avoid contamination with body fluids. Minimal handling of the body reduces the risk of contamination. **E**
3 The body should be totally enclosed in a plastic body bag.	To avoid contamination of the porters and the mortuary staff (DH 2016, **C**).
4 Transfer of the body should be arranged with the medical physics department.	The medical physics department will supervise the transfer of the body. **E**

Procedure guideline 5.4 Radiation protection: cardiac arrest of a patient who has received unsealed radioactive source therapy

Essential equipment
- Absorbent pads/paper
- Gloves
- Overshoes
- Apron and/or gown
- (COSHH) radiation waste bag
- Radiation warning tape
- Hand-held radiation monitor

Optional equipment
- Decon 90™, an approved solution for neutralizing isotopes

(continued)

Procedure guideline 5.4 Radiation protection: cardiac arrest of a patient who has received unsealed radioactive source therapy *(continued)*

Procedure

Action	Rationale
1 The switchboard must be told to inform the medical physics department as soon as possible after alerting the emergency resuscitation team.	So that the medical physics department can advise on radiation protection as soon as possible (DH 2016, **C**).
2 Start resuscitation as per UKRC guidelines. All areas must be supplied with an Ambu-bag for this purpose.	Mouth-to-mouth contact could result in contamination of the resuscitator (DH 2016, **C**).
3 Overshoes, gloves and apron or gowns must be put on as soon as is practicably possible.	To minimize personal contamination (DH 2016, **C**; PHE 2014, **C**).
4 All emergency equipment must be monitored and decontaminated as necessary before being returned to general use.	To prevent contaminated equipment leaving the controlled area (DH 2016, **C**).

Procedure guideline 5.5 Radiation protection: evacuation due to fire of patients who have received unsealed radioactive source therapy

Procedure

Action	Rationale
1 Every effort should be made to contact the medical physics department without compromising the patient's safety.	To help in the evacuation of patients treated with iodine-131 (DH 2016, **C**).
2 Following evacuation, patients treated with iodine-131 should be kept at a distance from other patients and staff.	To minimize exposure of others to radiation (DH 2016, **C**).

Post-procedural considerations

Ongoing care

Contamination control

When using unsealed sources, it is important to guard against contamination of both personnel and the hospital environment by the correct use of protective gloves, plastic aprons or gowns, and overshoes (DH 2016). The patient's body fluids are highly radioactive, especially in the days immediately after a radioactive substance has been administered. Any action that is likely to cause contamination of personnel, for example the application of cosmetics, eating, drinking or smoking when the healthcare worker's hands are contaminated with radioactivity, is prohibited.

In an emergency, the safety and medical care of the patient must take precedence over any potential radiation hazards to staff. Written radiation safety instructions must be available in all radiation areas where an emergency may arise. These instructions must contain a detailed description of how to manage a patient in the event of a medical emergency and the action required in other emergency situations, such as fire. The course of action in an emergency procedure depends on local circumstances and the nature of the emergency.

An incident occurring within the first 24 hours of a radioactive substance being administered is obviously a greater hazard than a similar incident on the day of discharge. Movement of the patient to other wards or areas, for example X-ray or the critical care unit (CCU), must only be undertaken following the medical physics department's advice.

Incident procedure

If an accident or incident has occurred or if one is suspected, the immediate priority is to ensure the safety of patients, staff and visitors and to take whatever action is practicable to prevent further damage or injury (see Procedure guideline 5.1).

As soon as immediate care has been provided, all accidents, untoward incidents and near misses, irrespective of severity, must be reported on an incident report form. Proactive and reactive risk management processes are important. These processes should identify areas of potentially higher risk or allow lessons to be learnt from past incidents and accidents. This will allow the implementation of appropriate action plans to reduce the probability and/or severity of an incident occurring or recurring.

Legal and professional issues of radiopharmaceuticals

Radiopharmaceuticals are legally categorized as prescription-only medicines (POMs), and, in addition to the standard legislation surrounding the administration of such drugs, are subject to regulations related to their radioactive content. In the UK, a statutory committee called the Administration of Radioactive Substances Advisory Committee (ARSAC) was established to give ionizing radiation advice to health ministers and to manage the certification process for administration of radiopharmaceuticals. This committee issues certificates that authorize individuals to administer radiopharmaceuticals to patients. It also lists the maximum permissible doses of radioactivity that may be administered to adult patients, and appropriately reduced adult doses for children, according to a child's bodyweight or body surface area (HPA 2006).

Unsealed source therapy

Definition

Unsealed source therapy or radionuclide therapy uses the same principles as diagnostic nuclear medicine procedures (see Chapter 1). There will be a vector (a pharmaceutical that will recognize the tumour or target organ) and an isotope (see Table 5.1). Depending on the half-life of the radiopharmaceutical, the therapy can be given in both outpatient and inpatient settings.

Evidence-based approaches

Rationale

Unsealed source therapy is complex because, in addition to the external hazard, there is an internal hazard from contamination arising from contact with the radiopharmaceutical itself or with the patient's body fluids.

Once a patient has been given a radioactive material, they become radioactive themselves, how much and for how long being dependent on the type and amount of radioactive material used.

The safety of all staff caring for these patients can be assured by implementing very detailed nuclear medicine and physics protocols and procedures.

Legal and professional issues

Patient preparation and consent

Every therapeutic use of radiation has an inherent risk. Awareness of the risk is essential for all staff who have to obtain informed consent from their patients (Picano 2004). A survey of patients and family members of patients receiving radioactive iodine found that many experienced psychological distress and few received adequate help (Fitch and McGrath 2003). Therefore, careful preparation of the patient before the administration of unsealed source therapy is essential.

Patients and relatives should be educated (Skalla et al. 2004) about the principles of radiation protection and the procedures with which the patient must comply while in isolation; this is part of the consent process. Psychosocial and physical needs must be addressed, requiring a collaborative approach between patients and nurses (Stajduhar et al. 2000). It is important to identify potential anxieties before administration while the nurse can reassure the patient and is unconstrained by time limits. Fully

Table 5.1 Therapeutic treatments

Radioactive material	In/outpatient	Condition	Route of administration	Notes
Iodine-131 sodium iodide	Outpatient treatment	Thyrotoxicosis	Oral (capsule or drink)	Most of the radioactive iodine is concentrated in the thyroid, but a substantial amount will be present in the urine and blood. Lesser quantities will be found in the patient's faeces, sweat, saliva and seminal fluid. The patient should receive an instruction document listing the precautions necessary to safeguard others. The patient may be infirm or incontinent and therefore admitted for treatment
Iodine-131 sodium iodide	Inpatient treatment	Thyroid cancer	Oral (capsule or drink)	Large administered dose therefore more significant risks. The patient is usually isolated in a special suite
Iodine-131 mIBG	Inpatient treatment	Neuroblastoma	IV via infusion pump	As above
Strontium-89	Outpatient treatment	Bone metastases	IV	The patient may be admitted to a ward within a short period of time following treatment, for example upon deterioration of their condition
Samarium-153	Outpatient treatment	Bone metastases	IV	Patients should be advised to drink plenty of fluids prior to treatment, and urine should be collected for at least 6 hours post treatment
Indium-111 octreotide	Inpatient treatment	GI cancer and neuroendocrine cancer	IV	Patients are always isolated following treatment, often in specially shielded rooms
Rhenium-186	Outpatient treatment	Prostate cancer	IV bolus	Radiation protection guidance is given to patients post procedure as per local policies
Radium-223	Outpatient treatment	Prostate cancer	IV bolus	Radiation protection guidance is given to patients post procedure as per local policies

GI, gastrointestinal; IV, intravenous; mIBG, iodine-123-metaiodobenzylguanidine.

prepared, knowledgeable patients and visitors are the key to radiation safety and contamination control (Stajduhar et al. 2000, Thompson 2001). Incidents and accidents are less likely to occur if the patient fully understands the reasons for the restrictions. The name and telephone number of the 'key worker', usually a clinical nurse specialist, is essential for patients before, during and after treatment (DH 2016, NICE 2005).

All patients are required to sign a consent form agreeing to treatment, following a full explanation from the treating clinician. This is to comply with medical, ethical and legal requirements and local hospital policy. Consent is usually obtained in the outpatient clinic before ordering the radioactive material. The patient must also agree to stay in hospital until the medical physics department advises that the level of radioactivity permits discharge (ICRP 2004).

Pre-procedural considerations

Equipment

Equipment in the room should be kept to a minimum. It must be checked to ensure that it is in working order, as maintenance staff will only be allowed into the room in exceptional circumstances.

Bedlinen and disposable items (gloves, aprons, overshoes, cutlery and crockery) should be kept in a utility room or anteroom along with the patient's treatment chart and a radiation monitor.

Protective floor covering

Plastic-backed absorbent paper, kept in place by adhesive tape, is used to retain accidental urine spills or splashes on the floor immediately surrounding the toilet. Each patient is assessed to decide whether further floor covering is necessary; for example, catheterized patients will require floor covering below the catheter bag.

Specific patient preparations

Although the patient will have been assessed in the outpatient department, it is important that all patients are reassessed on admission for their suitability for treatment. *In particular, the needs of a debilitated patient must be assessed to ensure that appropriate nursing care can be provided within the time constraints.* A review of a patient who was quadriplegic, doubly incontinent and unable to swallow found that nurses could provide appropriate care while following the recommended radiation protection restrictions (Williams and Woodward 2005). Multidisciplinary co-ordination of care is required in such complex cases.

Before the administration of any unsealed sources, any symptoms of diarrhoea or constipation must be resolved. Diarrhoea could result in contamination of the treatment area. Constipation not only inhibits the elimination of radioactivity but also could obscure radiological investigations, for example scanning. All investigations, including blood tests, must be undertaken before administration of diagnostic and therapeutic unsealed sources. If essential specimens need to be processed after administration, the specimen and the request card must be labelled with a radiation warning sticker. The laboratories must follow their standard operating procedures for processing and disposal of these specimens.

Personal items

Nurses should be sensitive to the psychological implications for patients of being labelled 'radioactive' and confined in isolation. Although patients may want to bring some personal belongings with them, they should be advised to keep these to a minimum, as items may become contaminated and need to be stored until radioactivity has decayed. Patients can be supplied with disposable slippers and be offered hospital nightwear. This is not essential and patients may feel more comfortable wearing their own personal clothing. Clothing and other items will be checked prior to discharge for contamination and instructions provided by the medical physics department as per IRMER 2000 guidelines.

Procedure guideline 5.6 Unsealed source therapy: entering and leaving the room of a patient who has received an unsealed radioactive source

Essential equipment
- Gloves
- Apron or gown
- Overshoes
- Clinical waste bag
- Soap and water

Pre-procedure

Action	Rationale
1 Collect digital dosimeter, record reading before entering and on leaving room.	A digital dosimeter provides an ongoing and immediate indication of the amount of exposure received (Ionising Radiations Regulations 1999, **C**).

Procedure

On entering:

2 Put on disposable gloves.	To prevent contamination of the hands (PHE 2014, **C**).
3 Put on disposable overshoes.	To prevent spread of contamination outside the treatment area (PHE 2014, **C**).
4 Put on a suitable protective plastic apron or gown: (a) long-sleeved cotton gown, for example for lifting patient (b) disposable plastic apron, for example for dealing with vomit or incontinence.	To protect against low levels of contamination, for example from the patient's skin (PHE 2014, **C**). To protect against high levels of contamination (PHE 2014, **C**).
5 Plan work before entering the controlled area and then work quickly and efficiently, keeping within the time allowance stated.	To minimize radiation exposure, as consistent with good nursing care (Ionising Radiations Regulations 1999, **C**).

On leaving:

Action	Rationale
6 Remove overshoes, taking care not to touch the shoes worn underneath.	Overshoes are removed first while gloves are still being worn to prevent the spread of contamination to hands or the floor outside the room. **E**
7 Remove the plastic apron by holding the front of the apron and breaking the neck and waist ties.	To prevent transfer of contamination from the gloves onto the uniform below. **E**
8 Remove gloves by peeling them off the hands, taking care not to touch the outside surfaces with bare hands, and discard them in the clinical waste bag provided.	To prevent transfer of contamination from the gloves' outer surfaces to the hands. **E**
9 Wash hands thoroughly using soap and water.	To remove any contamination (HSE 2003b, **C**).

Post-procedure

Action	Rationale
10 Use the radiation monitor each time when leaving the room and monitor for contamination of the hands, feet and clothing. If contamination has occurred, inform the medical physics department immediately and follow the decontamination procedure. The medical physics department will advise if further whole-body monitoring is required.	To ensure that the nurse is not contaminated (Ionising Radiations Regulations 1999, **C**).

Procedure guideline 5.7   Unsealed source therapy: iodine-131 (oral capsule/liquid): administration

Essential equipment
- Radioactive source
- Straw
- Water

Pre-procedure

Action	Rationale
1 Explain and discuss the procedure with the patient.	To ensure that the patient understands the procedure and gives their valid consent (O'Dwyer et al. 2003, **R1b**).
2 Check administrative documents, confirm that consent has been given and that pregnancy status has been recorded (must be negative to proceed with procedure).	Safe administration of radiopharmaceutical medicine (DH 2016, **C**; NMC 2010, **C**).

Procedure

Action	Rationale
3 Administer a prophylactic antiemetic 30 minutes before scheduled administration of the dose.	To reduce the risk of nausea and/or vomiting after ingestion of a radioactive source. **E**
4 Check that the preparation of the room and the patient is complete. Ensure that any surplus items have been removed.	To prevent contamination of extraneous equipment. **E**
5 Assist the patient to remove dentures/bridges, if dose is administered in liquid form.	To prevent radioactive material being trapped behind dental plates. **E**
6 Allow the patient to swallow the capsule or drink the iodine-131 through a straw, physically directed by an authorized member of staff.	Drinking through a straw reduces the amount of radioactive material left around the mouth. To comply with ARSAC regulations (HPA 2006, **C**).
7 Offer the patient a cold drink of water to rinse out the mouth and then swallow. Assist the patient to replace dentures.	To remove any iodine-131 from inside the mouth. **E**

Post-procedure

Action	Rationale
8 Ensure that the medical physics staff place the radiation warning sign at the entrance to the therapy room.	To identify the room as a controlled area (DH 2016, **C**).

Procedure guideline 5.8   Unsealed source therapy: iodine-131 mIBG treatment: patient care

Essential equipment
- A selection of needles and syringes
- Alcohol wipes
- Syringe shields
- Tape and gauze swabs
- Documentation for isotope to be administered

(continued)

Procedure guideline 5.8   Unsealed source therapy: iodine-131 mIBG treatment: patient care *(continued)*

Pre-procedure

Action	Rationale
1 Explain and discuss the procedure with the patient and/or parents if the patient is a child.	To ensure that the patient and/or parents understand the procedure and give their consent (O'Dwyer et al. 2003, **R1b**).
2 Apply a vital signs monitor with a variable time setting mode to the patient that will be visible to staff from outside the room.	Following the administration of mIBG, a transient rise in blood pressure and pulse rate may occur (Brophy et al. 2004, **E**).
3 Check that the patient has a patent vascular access device *in situ*, usually a cannula or, for children, a central venous access device.	To ensure administration of mIBG. **E**

Procedure

Action	Rationale
4 The nurse or doctor will set up the iodine-131 mIBG infusion and administer as prescribed.	To ensure safe administration of iodine-131 mIBG (DH 2016, **C**).
5 During the procedure, monitor blood pressure and pulse rate at 5-minute intervals during the infusion. (a) Monitor whole-body retention measurements at regular intervals as directed by the medical physics department. (b) After the procedure monitoring can be reduced to 4 hourly if the patient is clinically stable.	To detect and monitor any change to blood pressure and pulse rate. Alter rate according to changes as prescribed by clinician. **E** This may vary according to department policies. **E**

Post-procedural considerations

Ongoing care

Encourage the patient to shower frequently, at least once a day, and to wash their hands thoroughly after each possible contact with bodily fluids, for example cleaning teeth or going to the toilet. The patient should regularly remove any dentures and clean them under running water and remove any contact lenses and rinse in their usual cleaning fluid. All these actions will reduce any radioactivity from the skin or mucous membranes. The nurse should encourage the patient to maintain a fluid intake of between 2 and 3 litres per day to increase the urinary output and elimination of radioactivity from the bladder (Thompson 2001). The patient should have their own personal toilet facilities and flush the toilet twice after use to reduce contamination of others and of the environment as the urine of patients treated with iodine-131 is initially highly radioactive (Thompson 2001).

Bedbound patients should be catheterized before the dose is given and the bag emptied every 4–6 hours or more frequently if necessary to reduce the radiation level in the room. If the patient requires a bedpan or urinal, this item must be kept solely for this patient's use. The bedpan or urinal must be handled carefully and the contents disposed of in the patient's toilet (and flushed twice). The bedpan or urinal may be washed in the bedpan washer but sealed in a plastic bag for the journey to and from the sluice.

If leakage occurs from injection sites, wound sites and so on, the nurse should contact the medical staff and the physics department immediately. Any contact with the dressing should be carried out with long-handled forceps and gloves (HSE 2003a, b). All used linen must be deposited in a special bag provided for this purpose and must be monitored for contamination before going to the laundry.

Collection of laboratory specimens should, if possible, be deferred. If collections are unavoidable, a radiation warning sticker must be attached to the specimen and request card and the specimen delivered to the laboratory following consultations with the physics department in order to reduce the risk of contamination of the laboratory and its staff (Vialard-Miguel et al. 2005).

Only disposable crockery and cutlery should be used to present meals to patients as china crockery and cutlery may become contaminated. Uneaten food and disposable cutlery and crockery are disposed of in a macerator and all fruit stones and fish and meat bones should be removed from the diet to prevent blocking the macerator.

Guidance for visitors

Visitors must not enter radiation treatment areas unless special training and arrangements have been agreed in order to minimize the exposure of visitors to radiation (DH 2016). Visiting time during the first day following administration of an unsealed source should be limited as advised by the medical physicist because the patient is highly radioactive during this period (Ionising Radiations Regulations 1999).

On subsequent days, visiting is unlimited, providing visitors remain outside the room behind the lead screens, the exception being parents caring for young children who will need to be authorized by the medical physics department. Physical contact with the patient or bedlinen is not allowed as protective clothing is not available to visitors. Children under 16 years of age and pregnant women are discouraged from visiting to ensure that radiation exposure of children and the unborn child is kept as low as practicable (DH 2016).

Discharge of patient

A patient should not be discharged from hospital until the radiation activity retained has fallen below recommended levels (DH 2016, HPA 2006). This level will depend on several factors, including:

- mode of transport on leaving hospital
- journey time involved
- personal circumstances, for example young children or pregnant women at home.

Patients will be assessed individually for radiation clearance by the medical physics department before discharge. The treating physician will then be advised of the results of the assessment. Advice will be given to patients on issues such as return to work and visits to public places. On discharge, patients will be given appropriate written information in the form of an instruction card/

leaflet carrying details of the precautions to be taken. This varies according to local policies. The card/leaflet must be signed by the patient or parent of a child, the treating clinician or the medical physics staff.

It must be emphasized that this information must be carried and the instructions followed until the latest date shown so that, for instance, staff would be alerted should the patient be readmitted to a hospital setting. Additional verbal instructions may be necessary (IRMER 2000).

Cleaning the treatment room

During occupancy of the treatment room by the patient, cleaning of the room is kept to a minimum and should be supervised by the medical physics staff. After the patient is discharged, the monitoring and any necessary decontamination of the room will be arranged by the physics department. They will then inform the relevant personnel when this has been completed. *Only then may the room be entered and thoroughly cleaned* (DH 2000).

Sealed source therapy

Radioactive isotopes used as sealed sources for brachytherapy emit both beta and gamma radiation.

Definition

Brachytherapy is the term used for intracavity treatment in which radioisotope sources are placed in pre-existing body cavities such as the uterine cavity or vagina, or for interstitial treatment in which radioisotope sources are inserted directly into the tissues using tubes or needles or inserted into a gland, such as prostate seeds (Hoskin and Coyle 2005).

Sealed source therapy is complex because of the variation in sources and delivery systems used to administer radiation treatment. The main difference between sealed source and unsealed source treatment is the absence of contaminated bodily fluids. The hazard is therefore external radioactive sources.

Related theory

Specific isotopes used to treat malignant tumours

Iodine-125 used in prostate cancer

Seeds of iodine-125 have replaced those of gold-198, the half-life of iodine-125 being approximately 60 days. Some therapists believe that there is a radio-biological advantage to this long half-life in treating slow-growing tumours such as carcinoma of the prostate (Blank et al. 2000). The iodine-125 seeds are inserted into the tissue that is to be irradiated, for example the prostate gland, utilizing ultrasound guidance or an image intensifier control. The procedure requires the patient to have a general anaesthetic for the seeds to be inserted.

As the energy of the gamma-ray emission from iodine-125 is very low compared with that of gold-198, large numbers of seeds are required. This means that more precautions must be taken in order to achieve a regular geometrical arrangement to ensure satisfactory distribution of the dose (Stock et al. 2000). Implantation of iodine-125 is now a well-established procedure and an increasing number of patients throughout the world are treated in this manner (Anglesio et al. 2005, NICE 2005).

There are known complications from this form of treatment including incontinence, obstructive urinary symptoms, rectal symptoms and sexual dysfunction. The impotence rate has been reported at between 10% and 15%, much lower when compared with 45% of those patients undergoing radical prostatectomy (NICE 2005).

Zelefsky's (2006) study found that quality of life was initially worse during the first 4 weeks following iodine-125 treatment but returned to baseline values 1 year after the implants were inserted.

It is therefore of great importance that the patient understands the uncertainties of iodine-125 seed therapy and the possible alternative treatment options. The consent process should ensure that the patient is fully informed of:

- the rationale for the procedure
- the potential short-term and delayed side-effects of the procedure
- the alternative options
- the results of the treatment.

It is also important that the patient understands that it is unclear how the procedure affects general health or the chance of the cancer returning in the long term (Wust et al. 2004). The patient should be followed up and monitored as per local clinical guidance (NICE 2005).

Iridium-192 used in head and neck cancer

Iridium-192 is a radioisotope which is used in the form of pins or wires in interstitial therapy (Fung 2002). The half-life is 74.2 days and iridium is used because of the low energy of its gamma emission compared with caesium. This simplifies radiation protection issues. Iridium-192 is available in the form of a platinum–iridium alloy thin flexible wire. The active platinum–iridium alloy core of the wire is encased in a sheath of platinum 10 μm thick, which screens out the beta radiation from the iridium-192.

This high-activity source of iridium is used in a high dose-rate remote afterloading system, reducing the amount of radiation to which staff are exposed. Iridium-192 is used under the following circumstances:

- as a treatment for small primary lesions, for example tongue or breast lesions (Lapeyre et al. 2004)
- as a 'boost' dose after external radiotherapy for larger primary tumours or where nodes are also involved (Grabenbauer et al. 2001)
- to treat recurrence (Nutting et al. 2006).

Iridium-192 hair pin and single pin types of implants (see Figure 5.2) are usually used intraorally and are slotted into tissue using steel guides to obtain accurate alignment. Radiological examination is used to check the position of the guides before the

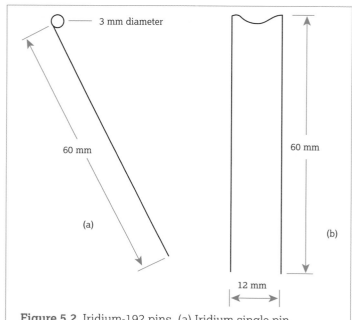

Figure 5.2 Iridium-192 pins. (a) Iridium single pin. (b) Iridium hair pin. *Source:* Dougherty and Lister (2011).

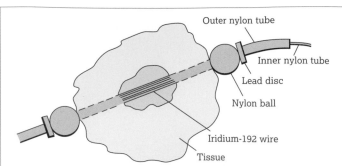

Figure 5.3 Iridium-192 wire in polythene cannula. Typical assembly in tissue. *Source:* Dougherty and Lister (2011).

iridium is inserted and the pins are held in place by sutures. Physicists are normally responsible for calculating how long a radioactive implant is to stay in place, usually about 6 days depending on the size of the tumour. Removal is carried out in theatre by appropriately trained clinical staff. Iridium-192 wires are usually used for head and neck, breast, vulval or perineal lesions (see Figure 5.3). Polythene or metal cannulas are inserted under a general anaesthetic, and in the case of breast lesions, both ends of each tube protrude through the skin. Correct alignment is established often with the aid of a Perspex template which fits over the breast and holds the metal cannulas in the correct alignment or, in the case of vulval or perineal insertions, one end of the tube protrudes. For alignment of the sources to be achieved, a Perspex template and vaginal obturator are used.

Iridium-192 interstitial brachytherapy can be used to treat locally advanced or recurrent tumours. Interstitial brachytherapy is a suitable alternative to standard intracavity brachytherapy where the treatment may be considered unsuitable because the dose distribution may be suboptimal (Agrawal et al. 2005).

The device itself consists of two acrylic cylinders and an acrylic template with an array of holes that serve as guides for trocars and a cover plate (Figure 5.4). The cylinders are usually placed in the vagina but can also be used in the rectum for rectal tumours. They are then fastened to the template, so that a fixed geometric relationship between the tumour volume and normal structures, that is bladder and rectum, is produced. This ensures that the source placement is preserved throughout the course of the implantation. The iridium wire is then manually afterloaded and held in place with a crimped washer to prevent movement of the source during treatment (see Figure 5.3).

The tiny size of the high-activity iridium-192 source in high dose-rate machines may allow some interstitial brachytherapy to be given as a few treatments of several minutes each, in contrast to the single treatment of many hours' duration that is necessary with low-activity iridium wire (Hart 2006).

Clinical oncologists are responsible for calculating how long a radioactive implant should stay in place, usually 3–6 days depending on the size of the tumour. Removal of these implants is usually carried out in the ward area. The procedures deliver a dose that is higher than can be achieved by external beam radiation alone, improving organ preservation rates and reducing acute and late side-effects (Karakoyun-Celik et al. 2005).

In a study by Budrukkar et al. (2001) evaluating the long-term efficacy and safety of transperineal interstitial implants for advanced pelvic malignancy, it was found that treatment offered a 5- and 10-year disease-free survival of 48% for patients aged 45 years and less, and an 80% disease-free survival in patients aged over 45 years.

Nursing care is similar to the care that patients receive for intracavity brachytherapy, with side-effects similar to those seen in 'afterloading' techniques. According to Syed et al. (2002) these side-effects are considered to be acceptable. Late effects of this type of treatment, specifically fistula formation and bowel complications that may require surgery, have been documented (Nag et al. 2002).

Caesium-137 used in head and neck cancer and gynaecological cancers

Caesium-137 is a radioisotope that can be used in the form of interstitial implants or in intracavity applicators, allowing a highly conformal dose of radioactivity to be delivered directly to the site of the cancer (Karakoyun-Celik et al. 2005). The most common malignancies treated by the use of radioactive applicators are tumours of the female genital tract (Kucera et al. 2001). Intracavity applicators are used to deliver a high dose to the region of the cervix, the paracervical tissue, the upper part of the vagina and the uterine body. Caesium has a half-life of 30 years and has largely replaced radium as a source for various brachytherapy treatments.

Oral implants of caesium-137 are 'needle-like' implants that are inserted directly into the tissue surrounding the tumour. They are a fairly common treatment for early lesions of the cheek, lip and anterior two-thirds of the tongue (Leborgne et al. 2002, Nutting et al. 2006). Oral implants have the advantage of allowing preservation of the structure and function of the tongue whilst avoiding the toxicity of external beam radiotherapy to the oral mucosa (Wadsley et al. 2003). If there is known or suspected bone involvement, in the mandible for example, the alternative external beam treatment will be given.

Caesium-137 sources (see Figure 5.5) are inserted in theatre under a general anaesthetic and placed individually in a predetermined pattern so that the implant covers the whole growth with a safety margin of at least 1 cm. Each individual needle is positioned by pushers so that its eye, through which silk is threaded, is just visible beneath the mucosal surface. Each silk is then stitched to the tongue with a single suture, and when all the needles have been inserted the silks are counted and gathered together. They are then threaded through a piece of rubber to prevent friction and trauma to the mouth. The silks are then strapped to the cheek to prevent any needle being swallowed should it work loose. Small beads are attached to the ends of the

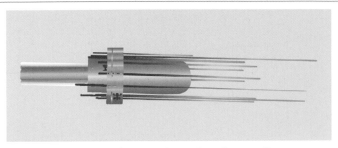

Figure 5.4 Interstitial perineal template device. *Source:* Dougherty and Lister (2011).

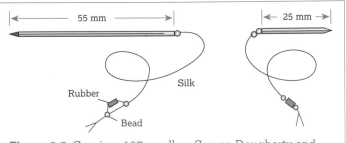

Figure 5.5 Caesium-137 needles. *Source:* Dougherty and Lister (2011).

threads to facilitate counting the needles. X-rays are always taken to check the positions of the needles and to enable estimation of the dose distribution (Takacsi-Nagy et al. 2001).

Evidence-based approaches

Methods of application

Intracavity applicators and interstitial implants

The application of sources varies according to the source and delivery method. Small sealed sources inserted into the body may take the form of:

- intracavity applicators, where sources are placed in natural cavities and usually held in place by packing
- interstitial implants, where sources are inserted directly into the tumour-bearing tissue (Hoskin and Coyle 2005).

Intracavity applicators and interstitial implants can be used in three forms.

1 The source is *preloaded in the applicator* before it is placed in the patient for a fixed length of time, for example caesium-137 needles and iridium-192 hair pins.
2 *Permanent insertion* in the case of iodine-125 seeds which, once inserted, would be difficult to remove. The available data show that, except in the case where the patient's partner is pregnant at the time of implantation, no restrictions are required once the patient is discharged home. Written information must be given to the patient on discharge which must include the following.
   - Possibility of triggering certain types of security radiation monitors.
   - Altered fertility, which is dependent on diagnosis, previous treatment, age, and type of brachytherapy offered.
   - The implant should be discussed if surgery is a possibility in the future.
   - Specific instruction should be available if the patient dies and cremation is required (ICRP 2005).
   - During hospital stay, all urine must be checked to ensure no seed has become dislodged; if this occurs, the loose seed should be placed in a lead pot with long-handled forceps. Any seed in a catheter bag should also be saved and placed into a lead pot and collected by the Hospital Radiation Protection Service, which is generally the medical physics department.
3 *Afterloading systems.* The applicator is placed in position and the radioactive source is inserted when the position of the applicator and the condition of the patient are satisfactory. Insertion of the sealed source can be undertaken manually in the case of iridium-192 wires or by remote control in the case of the low dose-rate 'Selectron' and high dose-rate 'micro-Selectron' machines, which are mainly used in the gynaecological setting. The proportions of radioisotope, initially radium and latterly caesium-137, within the intrauterine tube and the vaginal ovoids (oval intracavity applicators inserted into the vagina) are calculated to give a constant dose rate to a geometrical point A when using different lengths of intrauterine tube and different sizes of vaginal ovoids.

Types of gynaecological brachytherapy applicators

Manchester applicator

Manchester applicators (Figure 5.6a) in their original form were live sources enclosed in intrauterine tubes of varying lengths and vaginal applicators (ovoids) of varying sizes. The applicators were inserted under general anaesthetic and held in place by a gauze pack and were modified for either manual or remote afterloading for low or high dose rates with the principle of the three-applicator system remaining. Removal of the applicators and live sources is carried out on the ward.

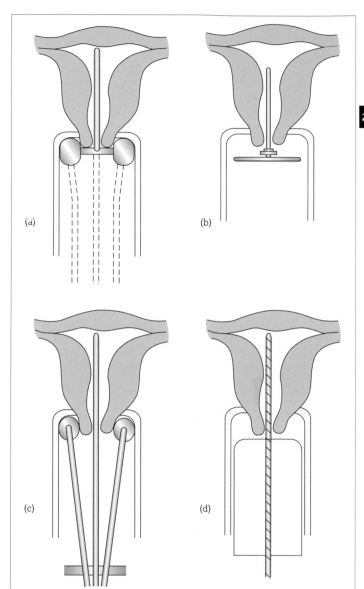

Figure 5.6 Gynaecological caesium applicators. Arrangement of brachytherapy sources in the uterus and vagina for treatment of cervical carcinoma. Sources may be active or, more usually these days, afterloaded into applicators along catheters protruding from the vagina. (a) Manchester applicator. (b) Modified Stockholm applicator. (c) Fletcher applicator. (d) Dobbie applicator. *Source:* Dougherty and Lister (2011).

Stockholm applicator

This is used for carcinoma of the uterine body or cervix. Usually a uterine tube and two vaginal packets are inserted. Occasionally, if the vaginal vault is small, one packet is omitted or replaced by a vaginal tube. The radioactive material is held in place with a proflavine-soaked gauze pack left *in situ* for approximately 22 hours. Tubes and packets have strings attached for removal and colour-coded beads indicate which should be removed first (Bomford 2002b).

Modified Stockholm applicator

This is used for carcinoma of the uterine body and cervix; it consists of a uterine tube and a square box which connect together by a point and a hole. The vagina is then packed with proflavine-soaked gauze pack and the applicator is left *in situ* for approximately 20 hours; the box is removed first (Bomford 2002b). See Figure 5.6b.

Fletcher applicator

This is used for carcinoma of the corpus or cervix, with the patient needing to have a fairly capacious vaginal vault. Hollow applicators, a uterine tube and two vaginal ovoids are inserted in theatre and afterloaded with the radioactive sources on the ward by the radiotherapist. The apparatus is held in place with a proflavine pack; long ends project through the vulva so that afterloading can be carried out. No strings are needed for this procedure, with insertions usually left in place for 60–72 hours (Bomford 2002b). See Figure 5.6c.

Dobbie applicator

This is used for irradiation of the whole vagina. It is a Perspex cylindrical applicator with radioactive sources in the centre and is inserted into the vagina and sutured in place to the vulva. It can be used with low or high dose rate sources with strings attached to the applicator for removal (Bomford 2002b). See Figure 5.6d.

Manual afterloading systems for treatment of gynaecological malignancies

The basis of 'afterloading brachytherapy' is that the applicators are placed within the cervix and vaginal fornices and the sources may then be inserted manually or by remote control. The radiation source is only introduced when the applicator's position has been checked as correct by specific imaging techniques and the patient is comfortable and is in a designated protected environment (Hoskin and Coyle 2005).

These rules ensure that the correct source has been inserted into the correct applicator for the programmed length of time. They also allow the dose rate of brachytherapy to be increased. Classically, the dose rate with the 'Manchester system' was approximately 50 cGy per hour to point A. With modern engineering methods, caesium-137 pellets can be produced which will allow a dose rate of between 150 and 200 cGy per hour to point A. Many systems now use sources that allow a higher than standard dose rate to be delivered, with the added advantage of reducing treatment time for the patient (Kuipers et al. 2001).

Manual afterloading systems are now largely being replaced by remote systems, but are still used in a few hospitals where services are still developing. The plastic applicator tubes follow the pattern of the 'Manchester system' with an intrauterine tube and two vaginal ovoids. The plastic tubes are designed to be disposed of after a single use. The tubes are inserted under general anaesthetic. X-rays are taken to confirm that the 'inactive' sources are in the correct position.

As with the classic 'Manchester system', there are varying lengths of intrauterine tube and sizes of ovoids. With X-ray confirmation and dosimetry calculated, the radioactive caesium-137 sources are introduced using long-handled forceps; once in place, a silver metal cap is screwed over the end of the plastic tube to hold the sources securely. Manual afterloading does not permit the use of high-activity sources for reasons of staff safety and treatment may last many hours or even several days. When treatment is complete, the caps are removed from the tubes and the sources are withdrawn and placed immediately in a lead storage vessel. The plastic applicator tubes are then removed.

It is particularly important to observe for displacement or extrusion of the applicator tubes over the long treatment times. It is customary to mark the thigh level with the end of the applicator tubes and to compare this alignment at regular intervals as the treatment progresses. The silver metal caps must be monitored regularly to assess for loosening or displacement (Bomford 2002b).

Remote afterloading

Remote systems have the advantage of complete protection of staff but the disadvantage of high cost and the need for interlocking mechanisms (Bomford 2002b).

Remote-controlled afterloading machines transfer active sources from a radiation-proof 'safe' to the patient only when all safety checks are completed (Hoskin and Coyle 2005). There are two types of delivery machine: one with a low dose rate (LDR), termed a Selectron, and a high dose rate (HDR) machine termed a micro-Selectron. Both machines are used generally in the treatment of gynaecological cancers and in some cases may also be useful in the treatment of bronchial, oesophageal and other intraluminal carcinomas (Tessa et al. 2005, Ung et al. 2006).

Low dose rate (LDR) Selectron unit

The Selectron unit comprises a lead-shielded safe, containing caesium-137 sources in the form of small spherical pellets, and a microprocessor, keyboard, display unit and printer (see Figure 5.7). Leading from the unit are either three or six flexible plastic transfer tubes corresponding to numbered treatment channels; each tube ends in a fragile plastic catheter which is inserted into the appropriately numbered applicator and secured by a coupling device. The unit has a supply of compressed air and it is air pressure that the system uses to transfer the sources from the safe within the unit to the applicators along the connecting tubes.

Operation of the unit is initiated from a remote-control unit situated outside the protected treatment area (Hoskin and Coyle 2005). The Selectron provides an accurate and safe method of radiotherapy treatment for cancers of the cervix, uterus and upper part of the vagina.

The advantages of the LDR Selectron system are as follows:

- Remote afterloading eliminates contact with radioactive material and protects personnel. The unit is switched off each time someone enters the patient's room, and only once all staff leave the room will the unit be switched back on. The unit will automatically return the radioactive pellets into the applicators, and the treatment that was temporarily discontinued will be recommenced (Hart 2006).
- It allows highly accurate dosimetry.

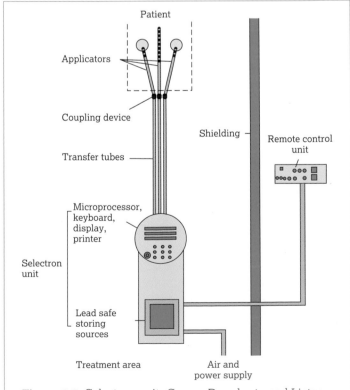

Figure 5.7 Selectron unit. *Source:* Dougherty and Lister (2011).

- The activity of the caesium-137 sources is such (up to 1.5 GBq) that treatment times for patients are considerably shorter than with conventional techniques.

Patients have hollow, lightweight stainless steel applicators positioned in the operating theatre under a general anaesthetic. These are usually modified Manchester or Fletcher type applicators consisting of a uterine tube and two vaginal ovoids held in place with proflavine-soaked vaginal packing. A urinary catheter is inserted in theatre at the same time to reduce urinary retention and the risk of the sources becoming dislodged by the patient when micturating. Accurate positioning of the applicators is confirmed by taking X-rays with dummy sources *in situ* and the optimum source configuration is selected, taking account of individual anatomical variations.

The Selectron unit is then programmed by the physicist. For each treatment channel being used, active source pellets are interspersed with inactive stainless steel spacer pellets to achieve the desired dose distribution (Hoskin and Coyle 2005). The treatment time required to reach the prescribed dose is also entered; with a six-channel Selectron, it is possible to treat two patients with three applicators each simultaneously. The radiotherapist/clinical oncologist is responsible for connecting the transfer tubes to the applicators. The transfer tubes are led over a bed bracket which supports the weight of the tubes and prevents traction being applied to the applicators inside the patient. If the wrong catheter is connected to the applicator, the system will fail to operate.

Operating the Selectron

Treatment is commenced by activation of the remote-control unit when all staff have left the treatment area. While treatment is in progress, it can be interrupted and restarted from the remote-control unit by pressing the stop and start buttons. The display panel indicates which channels are being used for treatment and which are unused, with red and green lights respectively. The time of the longest treatment is displayed on the panel and a telephone intercom system allows for communication with the patient without the need to interrupt treatment (Hoskin and Coyle 2005).

Interrupting the treatment is done by pressing the green stop button, which results in the radioactive sources being withdrawn into the Selectron unit and stops the treatment timer. This then allows nursing staff to enter the treatment area in safety and give care to the patient. Pressing the red start button transfers the sources back into the applicators and restarts the treatment timer; the red lights demonstrate that the channels are operating again satisfactorily. The system has built-in safety features so that in the event of a failure in the system, treatment stops automatically and an audible and visual alarm at the remote-control unit is instigated. This alerts staff to a problem, indicating whether this is a fault related to the air or power supply, the sources or the timer.

In some hospitals, an optional nurse station display unit is installed with similar alarm indicators which emit audible signals when treatment has been interrupted. This helps to prevent treatment being inadvertently interrupted for long periods. The Selectron records all breaks in treatment and these are shown on the print-out from the unit itself together with any programming or system fault. These appear as an error code and can be identified by reference to the Selectron user's manual.

At the end of the treatment time, all sources will be withdrawn automatically from the applicators back into the Selectron unit. If two patients are being treated simultaneously, termination of the treatment of one patient may be some time before that of the other. This means the timer will register the longer treatment time, but the indicator lights for the channels used for the first patient will have changed from red to green.

Additional safety features include a door switch facility to retract sources immediately if the door to the treatment area is opened when treatment is in progress, and/or Geiger dose meters visible when entering the treatment area and approaching the patient, which indicate when there are radioactive sources either in the patient or in the connecting tubes.

High dose rate (HDR) micro-Selectron unit

The operating principles of the HDR micro-Selectron are similar to those of the LDR Selectron. LDR Selectron applicators are afterloaded with active sources interspersed with inactive spacers to produce the correct isodose pattern. HDR micro-Selectron machines, on the other hand, achieve the desired isodose pattern with a single iridium-192 source that moves within the applicators and stops at preset positions for pre-determined dwell times.

The HDR micro-Selectron delivers radiation at approximately 100 times the rate of the LDR Selectron and treatment times are therefore much shorter, with the added advantage of applicators with a smaller diameter which can be put in place under local anaesthetic in the outpatient department. This is a suitable alternative for patients who may not be able to tolerate the demands of LDR (Hoskin and Coyle 2005).

Once in position, the micro-Selectron intracavity applicators are fixed to the treatment couch by means of an adjustable clamp; movement of the applicators is minimal and dosimetry calculations accurately represent actual treatment. In addition, more constant and reproducible geometry of source positioning is possible (Jones et al. 1999). Treatment protocols generally consist of two treatments but can involve as many as five. Following explanation and support for the patient, the procedure is carried out under local anaesthetic (Faithfull and Wells 2003); for the first treatment, a urinary catheter is passed and the balloon is inflated with dilute contrast medium. A check X-ray is taken once the applicator tubes are in place to collect information which is fed into the Selectron planning computer to calculate the treatment time (Hoskin and Coyle 2005).

The HDR micro-Selectron follows the same principles for programming and treatment as the LDR Selectron; when treatment is complete, the applicators and catheter are removed and the patient is free to go home after they have passed urine. A case report on patients undergoing treatment with the HDR micro-Selectron for gynaecological cancer suggested that they found the experience to be acceptable (Tan et al. 2004).

Adequate preparation and information sharing about this treatment is essential, as time spent preparing the patient for brachytherapy treatment makes them better equipped to make informed decisions related to their care (Faithfull and Wells 2003, Wallace et al. 2006). Poorly prepared patients are more anxious and less able to follow instructions and can be less tolerant of the implant procedure (Montgomery et al. 1999). An assessment of patients' physical and emotional needs must be made prior to each treatment to identify whether any aspect of the treatment is problematic (Faithfull and Wells 2003).

The advantages of HDR micro-Selectron brachytherapy are as follows.

- Shorter treatment time reduces variations in the patient's position and allows more accurate dosimetry (Jones et al. 1999).
- Treatment lasts only minutes, minimizing the need for immobilization; this reduces discomfort and the risk of complications associated with bedrest.
- Treatment can be offered on an outpatient basis with a consequent reduction in cost.
- It is an alternative to the LDR Selectron and may be more suitable for some patients.
- Complication rates are comparable with low-dose brachytherapy (Wong et al. 2003).

Legal and professional issues

Patient preparation and consent

Every therapeutic use of radiation has an inherent risk. Awareness of the risk is essential for all staff who must obtain informed consent from their patients (Picano 2004).

Information about radiation therapy should be given to patients and carers when therapy is first discussed to allay fears and misconceptions about radiotherapy. Verbal information should be reinforced with written material to prepare the patient, reduce anxiety and promote coping (Faithfull and Wells 2003). A contact name and telephone number of the 'key worker', usually a clinical nurse specialist, is essential for patients before, during and after treatment with sealed source brachytherapy (DH 2016, NICE 2005).

All patients require a thorough nursing assessment to assess their suitability for the treatment, ensuring that they are able to comply with the demands of the treatment and associated radiation protection measures.

Any doubt regarding physical or psychological concerns or problems can then be discussed with the patient and their medical team. Prior assessment allows for action to be taken, either to improve the patient's general condition so they are suitable for treatment, or to postpone or cancel the radioactive sealed source therapy in favour of a more suitable treatment option (Velji and Fitch 2001). Information for this group is divided into three main categories: (i) disease and treatment; (ii) short- and long-term side-effects from the treatment; and (iii) sexuality and sexual health (Faithfull and White 2008).

Pre-procedural considerations for gynaecological brachytherapy

Equipment

Equipment should be kept to a minimum. It must be checked to ensure that it is in working order, as maintenance staff will only be allowed into the room in exceptional circumstances.

Bedlinen and disposable items (e.g. gloves, aprons, catheter packs, sanitary towels) should be kept in a utility room or anteroom along with the patient's treatment chart and a radiation monitor.

Specific patient preparations

The patient is usually admitted 12–48 hours before the procedure so that any pre-anaesthetic investigations may be performed. Full bowel preparation with a low-residue diet will reduce the chance of the patient having a bowel action while the sources are in place to help reduce the risk of sources being dislodged. If patients present with pre-existing diarrhoea caused by previous radiotherapy on admission, regular antidiarrhoea medication should be prescribed and administered before and during the application of the sources. A full explanation should be given about the method and mode of treatment, possible side-effects, radiation protection issues and obtaining informed consent. The patient should be encouraged to have a bath before any pre-medication is administered.

LDR brachytherapy often follows 5 weeks of external beam radiotherapy (EBRT) to the pelvis (Petereit et al. 1998). Patients may embark on treatment already experiencing many symptoms, which are likely to include radiation-induced enteritis, nausea, fatigue, pain and skin reactions. Management of these symptoms is essential to ensure the safe and effective use of LDR brachytherapy.

Prior to the procedure, patients should also be prepared for the number of applicators to be inserted, dependent on previous treatment. A urinary catheter will be inserted because of the restriction around movement during the treatment. Small but significant aspects to highlight to the patient at this pre-assessment meeting include the noises made by the Selectron system, especially when sources are being transferred in and out of the applicators, that connection to the Selectron unit is with flexible plastic tubes, and informing all patients that this treatment will only enable them to lie in a semi-recumbent position.

A maximum of two pillows can be used to support the head whilst maintaining the pelvis in roughly the same position, ensuring no significant movement of the applicators. Where practicable, the patient should be closely monitored during treatment using closed-circuit television camera, telephone and/or intercom access for the patient as well as a nurse call system; all provide further reassurance for patients undergoing this treatment.

Personal items

Nurses should be sensitive to the psychological implications for patients confined in isolation and receiving radiation treatment. Although patients may want to bring some personal belongings with them, they should be advised to keep these to a minimum.

Procedure guideline 5.9   Sealed source therapy: caesium sources (manual or afterloading): patient care

Essential equipment
- Gloves and apron

Procedure

Action	Rationale
1 On return from theatre, the following should be checked: • Sanitary towel	To contain any blood loss from the procedure and observe and record vaginal blood loss. **E**
• Disposable pants in position	To secure the position of the sanitary towel. **E**
• A urinary catheter is in position and draining urine.	To ensure that urine is draining freely and to accurately monitor urinary output. **E**
2 Observe any blood loss and/or other discharge from the vagina.	To monitor for haemorrhage, shock and other post-operative complications. **E**
3 Ensure routine post-operative observations are performed until the patient is stable. Continue to monitor temperature, blood pressure and pulse throughout treatment at least 2–4 hourly.	To ensure early detection of possible complications. **E**
4 Administer prescribed analgesia, antiemetics and antidiarrhoeal agents.	For the patient's comfort and reduction of symptoms that may impact on the safe delivery of treatment using radiation sources. **E**

5 Encourage oral fluid intake as soon as the patient is allowed to drink. Encourage a fluid intake of 50–100% a day over and above the patient's normal intake.	To ensure adequate hydration. To reduce the risk of urinary tract infection (Beetz 2003, **R1a**).
6 A low-residue diet may be taken. Liaise with dietitian regarding suitable supplements.	To prevent the stimulation of a bowel action. **E**
7 The patient must remain in bed in a recumbent or semi-recumbent position while the applicators or implants are in place.	To prevent the applicators becoming dislodged or changing their position in relation to the adjacent internal organs. **E**
8 Log rolling the patient from side to side is permitted.	To promote comfort and relieve the skin of prolonged pressure on any one area, thus reducing pressure sores to at-risk tissue. **E**

217

Procedure guideline 5.10 Sealed source therapy: low dose rate Selectron treatment

Pre-procedure

Action	Rationale
1 Ensure written consent has been obtained, checking the patient is prepared to go ahead with the procedure.	To ensure consent has been obtained. To ensure the patient fully understands and agrees to the treatment planned and is offered the opportunity to ask any questions or mention any concerns they may still have (Faithfull and Wells 2003, **E**).
2 Ensure thorough nursing assessment of the patient has been undertaken by nursing staff.	To ensure the patient is suitable and will comply with treatment restrictions (Gosselin and Waring 2001, **E**).
3 Ensure full pre-operative medical assessment has been undertaken including baseline blood tests (FBC, clotting, U&E and LFT), ECG and chest X-ray.	To ensure the patient is fit for treatment. **E**
4 Administer antidiarrhoeal drugs the night before treatment. The patient should be monitored and if necessary treatment provided for radiation-induced enteritis.	To prevent bowel action during treatment which may then dislodge applicators during treatment. **E**

Procedure

5 Nurse the patient on a pressure-relieving mattress or with a foam wedge under her buttocks or a pillow under her knees to alter position.	To promote comfort and to relieve backache because rolling is not encouraged and in some areas is not permitted. **E**
6 Ensure the plastic transfer tubes are supported securely in the bed bracket, leaving slight slack.	To enable the patient to change position slightly without putting traction on the applicators. **E**
7 Limit the frequency and duration of interruptions to treatment. Visitors are discouraged unless the patient is markedly distressed.	To prevent unnecessary prolongation of treatment time. **E**
8 Check the patient's physical and psychological condition 2-hourly:	
• Temperature, pulse and vaginal loss.	To monitor for haemorrhage, shock or other post-operative complications. **E**
• Contents of catheter drainage bag.	To ensure urine is draining freely. **E**
• Assist the patient to adjust her position.	To promote comfort and relieve prolonged pressure on any one area. To maintain skin integrity and prevent friction. **E**
9 Check position of applicators. Marking the position of the applicators on the patient's legs can assist in the checking of their position.	To ensure no movement of the applicators has occurred. **E**
10 Administer prescribed analgesia, antiemetics, antidiarrhoeal and sedative agents as appropriate, observing and evaluating effect.	To promote the patient's comfort and well-being. **E**
11 Encourage fluid intake as soon as the patient is able to drink.	To ensure adequate hydration and reduce the risk of urinary tract infection and dehydration (Beetz 2003, **R1a**).
12 Encourage a light, low-residue diet to be taken, appropriate for consuming easily in a lying down position.	To maintain nutritional needs whilst reducing stimulation of a bowel action. **E**

Post-procedure

13 Perform accurate documentation.	To ensure accurate record keeping (NMC 2015, **C**).

Procedure guideline 5.11   Sealed source therapy: Selectron applicator removal

Essential equipment
- Gloves
- Plastic apron/gown
- Clinical waste bag
- Clean sanitary pad
- Gauze
- Catheter removal pack including syringe to remove water from catheter, large collecting tray for applicators and Central Sterile Supplies Department (CSSD) bag for returning applicators and rubber caps for ends of applicators
- Prescription chart
- Pre-removal medications
- Entonox and mask

Pre-procedure

Action	Rationale
1 Explain and discuss the procedure with the patient.	To ensure that the patient understands the procedure and gives her valid consent (Faithfull and Wells 2003, **E**).
2 Check treatment has been terminated by: • Ensuring the appropriate channel lights are green.	The applicators should be removed only on completion of treatment. **E**
• Ensuring the time display on the Selectron unit reads zero for the appropriate channels. • Ensuring the print-out indicates that treatment has stopped for those channels.	To ensure that the treatment completed corresponds with the patient. This is essential when delivering treatment via the same machine to two patients at the same time. **E**
3 Check that the closed-circuit television camera is not focused on the patient.	To ensure privacy and dignity. **E**

Procedure

Action	Rationale
4 Ensure any pre-removal drugs have been administered.	To allow analgesic and/or sedative medications time to be effective. **E**
5 Assist the patient into a comfortable position with her knees apart.	To allow access to the applicators. **E**
6 Uncouple the plastic transfer tubes by rotating the black coupling anticlockwise in the direction of the arrow and very carefully storing the tubes on the plastic supporting mantle attached to the Selectron unit.	To prevent the plastic catheter becoming damaged or kinked. **E**
7 Place rubber caps on the ends of the applicators.	To ensure no fluid or debris is allowed to enter the applicator tubes. **E**
8 Commence administration of Entonox (see Chapter 3) at least 2 minutes before removal of the applicators if patient has consented to that.	To allow the effect of the gas to become maximal. **E**
9 Prepare the equipment and put on non-sterile gloves.	This procedure is clinically clean and not aseptic (Rossoff et al. 1993, **R1b**).
10 Remove the vulval dressing pads and any sutures and vaginal packing.	These must be removed before the applicators can be eased out. **E**
11 Dismantle the applicators by loosening the screws holding them together.	To promote ease of removal. **E**
12 Remove the uterine tube first, ensuring it is taken out complete with its small white flange, and then remove the remaining applicators and the ovoids.	To prevent the flange being left in the patient's vagina. **E**
Check all parts of the equipment used in the procedure are accounted for.	To ensure no equipment or packing has been left in the patient. **E**
13 Remove the catheter after the balloon has been deflated, provide vulval care and ensure the patient has a clean sanitary pad and a fresh sheet under her.	To promote cleanliness and patient comfort. Observe for any bleeding post applicator removal. **E** To identify any changes to the vulva or surrounding skin areas. **E**
Educate the patient to inform the team when she has passed urine after the catheter has been removed.	To ensure that there is no urinary retention post catheter removal. **E**

14 The patient can then be assisted into a comfortable position. Instruct the patient to inform the nurse when she requires assistance with personal hygiene as she adjusts to an upright position.	To reassure the patient that the procedure has been completed, that she is no longer receiving radiation treatment and can resume normal activities. **E**

Post-procedure

15 Applicators are then placed into CSSD return bags and returned to CSSD for cleaning in accordance with local policies.	To ensure correct sterilization and/or disposal. **E**

Problem-solving table 5.1 Prevention and resolution (Procedure guidelines 5.10 and 5.11)

Problem	Cause	Prevention	Action
Patient removes the applicators herself.	Possible causes can be post-anaesthetic, infection and/or isolation issues.	Clear explanation to the patient about the problems of removing the applicators.	Check the room for any sources that may have escaped, using a contamination monitor; sources that have escaped should be placed in lead pots using long-handled forceps and the physics department notified. Remove applicators completely if partially removed as per instructions above. In the confused patient, this is a two-nurse procedure.
Applicator is partially dislodged.	Patient may have moved too much or too vigorously.	Explanation to patient about amount of movement allowed.	Interrupt treatment and inform physicist and radiotherapist; the applicator may have to be removed as in Procedure guideline 5.11.
Alarm sounding at nurse station.	Treatment has been interrupted and inadvertently left off.	Check all settings when leaving the patient.	Check the patient is not requiring any nursing intervention and then check the patient is unattended; if unattended, recommence treatment.
Sources are not transferred to the applicators.	Incorrect coupling or loose connection.	Check all connections.	Check print-out to identify which channel is at fault; tighten appropriate coupling device. If not resolved, contact physics department.
Alarm activated at remote control unit.	Failure in the system.	Check Selectron is kept maintained.	Check the error code on the print-out with the Selectron user's manual. Rectify as indicated in the manual or seek technical assistance from the physics department.
Pellets stuck in the applicator or transfer tubing.	A damaged or kinked catheter tubing.	Check the catheter tubing prior to use.	A risk assessment to be completed regarding the likelihood of this occurrence (HSE 2003a). Inform the patient of the problem and contact physics department and the medical team.

Post-procedural considerations

Ongoing care

Discharge of patient
Patients are usually discharged on the day of completion of brachytherapy. All patients must void after removal of applicators and vaginal packing.

Patients can sometimes be unsteady on their feet after prolonged bedrest and may require assistance. They should be informed that normal bowel actions may not return for a day or so; advice on managing diarrhoea or constipation should be given. Light spotting or discharge from the vagina is normal and should be discussed with patients to prevent any unnecessary concerns once at home. If patients experience pain or any more marked bleeding, hospital staff should be contacted immediately. Symptoms of urinary tract infection such as dysuria and/or elevated temperature should also be reported and a plan of care established prior to discharge. Contact numbers should be provided on who to call if any issues arise post discharge.

Complications
Early complications include pain, post-treatment fatigue, increased bowel activity, urinary urgency or frequency, dysuria, nocturia, vaginal discharge and perineal irritation (Faithfull and Wells 2003). Severe reactions, although uncommon, can include severe or prolonged proctitis in patients with pre-existing bowel disease and late complications, including bowel and bladder complications, vaginal dryness, vaginal narrowing, vaginal stenosis, dyspareunia, premenopausal symptoms and early menopause (Chen et al. 2004, Jefferies et al. 2007, Lancaster 2004).

The vaginal canal is included in the radiation field, therefore side-effects from treatment can be significant on the delicate tissue in the vagina. All patients need to be aware of possible complications associated with the treatment causing alteration to the elasticity and lubrication within the vagina, changes in sensation, vaginal stenosis and tissue fibrosis. It is therefore important, as stated earlier, for this patient population to be supported by a clinical nurse specialist to provide supportive care and intervention strategies that have the potential to reduce some of the short- and long-term toxicities associated with this treatment (Jefferies et al. 2007, Muscari Lin et al. 1999, White and Faithful 2006, White et al. 2004).

Possible interventions
- Women who are sexually active should be advised to continue intimate relations as tolerated with the use of analgesia as required.

- A provision for assessing discomfort and/or pain.
- Provide adequate and appropriate analgesia.
- Allow for radiation reactions to resolve, providing specific information on using vaginal dilators and personal hygiene care (Jefferies et al. 2007).
- The lifelong use of vaginal dilators (Jefferies et al. 2007).
- The use of water-soluble lubricants to help alleviate the dry mucosa (Muscari Lin et al. 1999).
- Short courses of localized hormone therapy to increase natural lubrication (Blake et al. 1998).

A review of 107 patients who had received radiotherapy found that advice from healthcare professionals was valuable in managing complications of treatment (Gami et al. 2003). Syed et al. (2002) completed a 20-year evaluation of the long-term survival and safety of interstitial and intracavity brachytherapy in the treatment of carcinoma of the cervix and found a reasonable chance of cure with acceptable morbidity. Teruya et al. (2002) found that all patients included in a retrospective review of HDR micro-Selectron brachytherapy reported vaginal mucosal changes but few complaints regarding sexual functioning.

However, this specific cancer treatment can cause persistent changes to the vagina, resulting in considerable distress by compromising sexual activity (Bergmark et al. 1999). Patients need to be reassured that many women regain their capacity for sexual activity and enjoyment. Extra support in the form of counselling or psychosexual counselling may help this patient population if difficult issues arise. Follow-up strategies focusing on specific areas such as self-esteem, body image and sexuality can provide a mechanism to identify these specific issues over the longer term (Farrell 2002).

Male partners of women with cancer reported difficulty in knowing how to behave and how to communicate with their partners (Lalos et al. 1995). Almost all male partners were given the news of the diagnosis exclusively by their ill partner, which provoked feelings of anger and bitterness (Lalos 1997). Coping improved if the men were integrated in the patient's care from the time the diagnosis of cancer was made (Lalos et al. 1995). See Chapter 8 for further information about responding to female sexual concerns related to cancer treatment.

Sealed source iodine-125 seeds used in prostate malignancies

Post-procedural considerations

Ongoing care

Seeds are implanted permanently into the tissue and the patient must agree to stay in hospital until the physics team states that the radioactivity is at a legally permissible level for discharge. The urine should be checked with the contamination monitor to ensure that the sources have not been expelled in the urine. If no radioactivity is found, the urine may be disposed of in the usual way.

The morning after implant, a CT scan is performed to check the number of seeds inserted and then the urinary catheter is removed. Once the patient has voided normally they may be discharged. Prophylactic antibiotics are prescribed to prevent infections for 5 days after the implant. Anti-inflammatory medication will also be prescribed to prevent discomfort and swelling.

In the event of accidental or sudden death within 1 year of the iodine seed implant, burial rather than cremation should be performed. It is also advised that burial should take place up to 3 years after implant. If cremation is planned during the 1–3 years post implant, the crematorium would first have to be told to contact the hospital for advice.

Education of patient

Advise the patient to observe for haematoma under the scrotum and give advice on reporting to the medical team. In the first weeks after the implant, the patient may experience dysuria or frequency. They should be advised to drink at least 2 litres of fluid a day and that any haematuria should resolve quickly. It should also be explained that some patients may experience soft stools or some diarrhoea or mucus in the faeces and that generally most of these symptoms disappear within a few days to a week.

The radioactive iodine seeds implanted into the prostate have a very limited range of radiation. This radiation is not harmful to the patient or their family at home and patients can be discharged when clinically stable. However, advice should be given regarding avoiding close contact with small children and pregnant women for the first few months after treatment.

Sexual intercourse is possible after treatment but advise the patient to wait for a few weeks after the procedure. If sexual intercourse is planned in the first 2 months after the procedure, patients should use a condom, in case of the rare occurrence when a radioactive seed may be expelled during ejaculation. For the first few occasions, the colour of the ejaculation fluid may be discoloured, ranging from a light red to black.

For the first few weeks after treatment, it may be possible that one or more radioactive seeds may be expelled during urination. For this reason, patients should be advised to sit down when using the toilet, rather than use a urinal. Any seeds that are expelled will then be flushed away. Patients must be informed not to touch any loose seeds with their hands but if necessary to use a spoon or a pair of forceps. All other social contact and activities can be resumed, including travelling.

Complications

Although rare, severe treatment-related side-effects cannot be totally excluded.

- There is a small risk of incontinence (less than 2%).
- *Erectile dysfunction:* occurs in 40–50% of men under the age of 60 and is more common in older men. Its frequency depends on the level of erectile function before treatment. Treatment is available for those men who develop difficulties.
- *Reduced volume of ejaculate:* the prostate is responsible for semen production and radiation treatments cause the relevant glands in the prostate to stop production.
- *Proctitis:* persistent inflammation of the rectum leading to increased urge to open bowels and the passing of mucus. This occurs rarely (in less than 1% of patients).

Intraoral sealed sources

Pre-procedural considerations

All patients receiving this treatment will have a dental assessment by an oral surgeon and any issues around dental caries, mouth infections and possible dental extractions will be addressed prior to the treatment because of the possible alteration of blood supply being impaired by treatment.

The patient is usually admitted 24 hours before the implant, during which time the nature of the procedure and the implications of having a radioactive source should be explained to them. The patient is nursed in a single controlled room away from other patients as per radiation protection guidance to keep exposure to staff and other patients and visitors as low as reasonably possible (ALARP). Only staff and visitors authorized to enter the controlled area should go into the room, and written arrangements for entering the room should be contained within the local rules displayed at the door of the room.

Procedure guideline 5.12   Sealed source therapy: insertion of sealed radioactive sources into the oral cavity

Essential equipment
- Lead pot
- Long-handled forceps
- Hand-held radiation monitor
- Shielding

- Disposable gloves
- Overshoes
- Plastic apron and/or gown

Pre-procedure

Action	Rationale
1 Before treatment begins, ensure the room is set up appropriately. This includes placing a lead pot and long-handled forceps in the room to hold any dislodged sources.	To reduce unnecessary time spent in the room once the patient returns from theatre (Hart 2006, **E**).
2 Switch on a controlled area radiation warning light outside the room and check it is working correctly.	To warn staff, visitors and other patients of the radiation risk and to ensure only trained personnel enter the room (Hart 2006, **E**).
3 Place a radiation warning notice outside the patient's room.	To ensure only authorized personnel enter the room. **E**

Procedure

Action	Rationale
4 A yellow radiation hazard board should accompany the patient back from theatre. This must remain at the bottom of the bed or outside the cubicle until the source is removed.	To alert everybody that the patient has a radioactive source. **E**
5 Place lead shields in position at the door. All staff entering the room should work behind the lead shield when in close contact with the patient.	To reduce radiation exposure of staff in close contact with the patient (Hart 2006, **E**).
6 When transferring patients from theatre to ward, the nurse and porter should remain at the head and foot of the bed and at least 120 cm from the centre of the bed in the event of any delay in the transfer.	To minimize the risk of exposure to radiation. **E**
7 Nursing staff must calculate the time allowed with the patient in any 24-hour period. This time should be written on the yellow warning notice on the bed or cubicle door.	To minimize exposure to radiation (Hart 2006, **E**).
8 A contamination monitor should be available on the ward.	To monitor radioactivity if a dislodged source is suspected, for example in the bedlinen (Hart 2006, **E**).
9 Although one nurse should be responsible for planning the nursing care of the patient, the time spent with the patient should be shared between all suitably trained nurses and all time spent in performing nursing procedures must be kept to a minimum. Only those staff whose presence is necessary should spend time with the patient.	To minimize the risk of overexposure to radiation (Hart 2006, **E**).
10 Every nurse must wear a radiation badge above the level of the lead shield.	To record the extent of exposure to radiation (Ionising Radiations Regulations 1999, **C**).
11 All bedlinen and waste materials removed from the patient area should be monitored before being removed from the ward.	To prevent loss of an accidentally dislodged source (Hart 2006, **E**).
12 If a source becomes dislodged, use the long-handled forceps to put the source into a lead pot. Care should be taken not to damage the source. It must never be handled directly with the fingers.	To minimize the dose of radiation received (Hart 2006, **E**).
13 Visitors must seek permission each time they wish to enter the room. Visitors must remain at least 120 cm away from the patient. Visitors must always sit behind one of the bed shields. The visit should not last longer than the time shown on the warning notice. No children or pregnant women are allowed to visit.	To minimize the risk of overexposure to radiation (DH 2000, **E**).
14 When the patient needs to visit another department, for example X-ray, the following must be ensured.	In order that medical care can continue to be provided while the patient is receiving radioactive sealed source therapy. **E**
• That the receiving department is aware of the hazard of exposure to radioactivity.	To allow the appointment to be made when the department is quiet, thus ensuring waiting time is kept to a minimum and to minimize exposure to others (Ionising Radiations Regulations 1999, **C**).

(continued)

Procedure guideline 5.12 Sealed source therapy: insertion of sealed radioactive sources into the oral cavity *(continued)*

Action	Rationale
• One porter and a nurse should accompany a patient in a wheelchair; two porters and a nurse should accompany a patient on a trolley. In the event of any delays, the nurse and porters should remain at the head and foot of the bed and at least 120 cm from the centre of the bed.	To minimize the risk of exposure of staff to radiation. **E**
• A radiation warning hazard sign should accompany the patient.	To warn all staff that the patient has a radioactive source *in situ* (Ionising Radiations Regulations 1999, **C**).
• Unless the patient is likely to be in the department for a long time, the nurse and porter should stay with the patient.	To ensure time, distance, shielding and segregation restrictions are maintained. **E**
• If the source becomes dislodged during transfer, the porter must ring the switchboard, who will send out an emergency call to the physics department. The nurse must ensure the area around the patient is kept clear of other patients, staff and visitors.	To minimize the risk of exposure to radiation. **E**
• A member of staff from the ward should take a lead pot, forceps and a monitor to the nurse who will place the source in the lead pot and monitor the area to ensure it is free of radioactivity.	To contain the radioactive source and minimize the risk of exposure (Hart 2006, **E**).
• The radiation protection adviser and supervisor should be informed of the incident.	To evaluate the incident, and to prevent it recurring (DH 2000, **C**).
15 *In the event of a cardiac arrest*, an Ambu-bag or similar device must be used, and the physics department must be informed immediately.	To minimize exposure. **E**
16 *In the event of a fire*, the fire policy must be followed. Following evacuation, the appropriate distance between the radioactive patient and other staff should be maintained; help should be sought from the physics department.	To minimize exposure. **E**
17 *In the event of a patient's death:* *Either:* *Removable sources*: the radiation sources should be removed by the radiotherapist. Inform the physics department.	Remove radioactivity to allow Last Offices to be undertaken as normal. **E**
Or: *Non-removable sources*: inform the physics department immediately. The body should be placed in a body bag.	In order for the physics department staff to begin making the necessary arrangements for removal of the body to the mortuary. Arrangements would include: segregated refrigerator, warning notices and use of body bag to contain sources if they became dislodged. **E**
Transfer of the body should be arranged by the physics department.	The physics staff will supervise the transfer of the body. **E**
18 *In the event of bleeding*: in order to stem bleeding in the vicinity of the implant, apply pressure using at least four thickness dressing pads. The padding should only be compressed for 15 minutes by any single person.	To minimize exposure. **E**
19 In the event of a confused or agitated patient, premature removal of sources may be required.	To prevent overexposure to radiation of the nurses attending the patient, as well as to prevent the patient removing or dislodging sources. **E**
20 Only staff who have received training and have been authorized may enter a controlled area. A list of suitably trained staff should be kept by the domestic and catering managers and by the ward's local radiation protection supervisor. A domestic or catering supervisor should undertake tasks if the ward-based employee is not trained.	To keep all radiation exposure as low as can be reasonably achieved (Ionising Radiations Regulations 1999, **C**).
21 Domestic and catering staff should not remove items such as cleaning equipment and crockery until they have been monitored by a nurse and deemed safe.	To prevent sources being removed from the room before it is safe to do so (Hart 2006, **E**).

Post-procedural considerations

Ongoing care

Mouth care
The patient may have difficulty in swallowing due to soreness and oedema and may be at risk of localized mouth infection (Ionising Radiations Regulations 1999) so frequent mouth care using a sterile saline solution as a mouthwash is important. Any rinsed solution should be collected in a disposable bowl to check for a dislodged source. Nurses should ensure that the patient has paper tissues and a bowl, crushed ice to suck and/or soluble aspirin as a mouthwash. Corticosteroids may also be prescribed to help reduce oedema.

A soft, puréed or liquid diet, avoiding spicy and/or hot foods, must be provided to maintain nutritional levels and reduce the complexity of eating when implants are present and further exacerbation of local reactions or soreness from the implants. This will also reduce the risk of the patient biting into the source or their tongue. Carbonated water can also alleviate dryness caused by the treatment.

Writing equipment must be provided for the patient to reduce the need for oral communication. Talking can increase soreness and pain, and potentially alter the distribution of the sources. The sources should be checked at regular intervals, for example at the beginning of each shift, to ensure they have not become dislodged. The patient should be confined to their room and only leave when necessary, for example to visit the X-ray department. This is to minimize the risk of radiation exposure to other people on the ward.

Discharge of the patient
The patient is usually discharged the day after the removal of the implant; they should be warned about the painful local reaction that they may experience from cell breakdown and cell death induced by the radiation. In order to minimize the risk of infection or soreness, the patient should be taught oral hygiene care and to observe the mouth for any infection (Hoskin and Coyle 2005, UKOMiC 2015).

Websites

Ionising Radiations Regulations 1999 (SI 3232)
www.legislation.hmso.gov.uk/si/si1999/19993232.htm

Ionising Radiation (Medical Exposure) Regulations 2000 (SI 1059)
www.legislation.hmso.gov.uk/si/si2000/20001059.htm

UK Oral Mucositis in Cancer Group (UKOMiC)
www.ukomic.co.uk

References

Agrawal, P.P., Singhal, S.S., Neema, J.P., et al. (2005) The role of interstitial brachytherapy using template in locally advanced gynecological malignancies. *Gynecologic Oncology*, 99(1), 169–175.

Anglesio, S., Calamia, E., Fiandra, C., et al. (2005) Prostate brachytherapy with iodine-125 seeds: radiation protection issues. *Tumori*, 91(4), 335–338.

Beetz, R. (2003) Mild dehydration: a risk factor for urinary tract infection? *European Journal of Clinical Nutrition*, 57(Suppl 2), S52–S58.

Bergmark, K., Avall-Lundqvist, E., Dickman, P.W., Henningsohn, L. & Steineck, G. (1999) Vaginal changes and sexuality in women with a history of cervical cancer. *New England Journal of Medicine*, 340(18), 1383–1389.

Blake, P.R., Lambert, H.E. & Crawford, R. (1998) *Gynaecological Oncology: A Guide to Clinical Management*. Oxford: Oxford University Press.

Blank, L.E., Gonzalez Gonzalez, D., de Reijke, T., et al. (2000) Brachytherapy with transperineal [125]-iodine seeds for localized prostate cancer. *Radiotherapy and Oncology*, 57(3), 307–313.

Bomford, C.K (2002a) Radiation protection. In: Bomford, C.K. & Kunkler, I.K. (eds) *Walters and Miller Textbook of Radiotherapy*, 6th edn. Edinburgh: Churchill Livingstone, pp. 69–88.

Bomford, C.K. (2002b) Brachytherapy. In: Bomford, C.K. & Kunkler, I.K. (eds) *Walters and Miller Textbook of Radiotherapy*, 6th edn. Edinburgh: Churchill Livingstone, pp. 225–244.

Brophy, P., Schmus, C. & Balistreri, L. (2004) Meeting the nursing challenge in treating children with 131 I-mIBG. *Journal of Paediatric Oncology Nursing*, 21(1), 9–15.

Budrukkar, A.N., Shrivastava, S.K., Jalali, R., et al. (2001) Transperineal low-dose rate iridium-192 interstitial brachytherapy in cervical carcinoma stage IIB. *Strahlentherapie und Onkologie*, 177(10), 517–524.

Chen, S.W., Liang, J.A., Yang, S.N., et al. (2004) Radiation injury to intestine following hysterectomy and adjuvant radiotherapy for cervical cancer. *Gynecologic Oncology*, 95(1), 208–214.

Cormack, J., Towson, J.E.C. & Flower, M.A. (1998) Radiation protection and dosimetry in clinical practice. In: Murray, I.P.C. & Ell, P.J. (eds) *Nuclear Medicine in Clinical Diagnosis and Treatment*, 2nd edn. Edinburgh: Churchill Livingstone, pp. 1651–1677.

Darby, S. (1999) Radiation risks. *BMJ*, 319 (7216), 1019–1020.

DH (2000) *Ionising Radiation (Medical Exposure) Regulations No. 1059*. London: HMSO.

DH (2016) Regulatory controls for radiation protection in the UK. Available at: https://www.gov.uk/guidance/regulatory-controls-for-radiation-protection-in-the-uk (Accessed: 1/5/2018)

Dougherty, L. & Lister, S. (eds) (2011) *The Royal Marsden Manual of Clinical Nursing Procedures: Professional Edition*. 8th edn. Oxford: Wiley-Blackwell.

Faithfull, S. & Wells, M. (2003) *Supportive Care in Radiotherapy*. Edinburgh: Churchill Livingstone.

Faithfull, S. & White, I. (2008) Delivering sensitive healthcare information challenging the taboo of women's sexual health after pelvic radiotherapy. *Patient Education and Counseling*, 71(2), 228–233.

Farrell, E. (2002) Premature menopause. 'I feel like an alien'. *Australian Family Physician*, 31(5), 419 421.

Fitch, M.I. & McGrath, P.N. (2003) The needs of family members of patients receiving radioactive iodine. *Canadian Oncology Nursing Journal*, 13(4), 220–231.

Fung, A.Y. (2002) The Syed temporary interstitial iridium gynaecological implant: an inverse planning system. *Physics in Medicine and Biology*, 47(16), N203–N208.

Gami, B., Harrington, K., Blake, P., et al. (2003) How patients manage gastrointestinal symptoms after pelvic radiotherapy. *Alimentary Pharmacology and Therapeutics*, 18(10), 987–994.

Gosselin, T.K. & Waring, J.S. (2001) Nursing management of patients receiving brachytherapy for gynaecologic malignancies. *Clinical Journal of Oncology Nursing*, 5(2), 59–63.

Grabenbauer, G.G., Rodel, C., Brunner, T., et al. (2001) Interstitial brachytherapy with Ir-192 low-dose-rate in the treatment of primary and recurrent cancer of the oral cavity and oropharynx. Review of 318 patients treated between 1985 and 1997. *Strahlentherapie und Onkologie*, 177(7), 338–344.

Hart, S. (2006) Ionising radiation: promoting safety for patients, visitors and staff. *Nursing Standard*, 20(47), 47–57.

Health Protection Agency (HPA) (2006) *Administration of Radioactive Substances Advisory Committee, Guidance Notes*. London: Health Protection Agency.

Health Protection Agency (HPA) (2010) www.hpa.org.uk/radiation.

Hoskin, P. & Coyle, C. (2005) *Radiotherapy in Practice: Brachytherapy*. Oxford: Oxford University Press.

HSE (2003a) *Five Steps to Risk Assessment*. Norwich: Health and Safety Executive Books.

HSE (2003b) *Safe Working and the Prevention of Infection in Clinical Laboratories and Similar Facilities*. Norwich: Health and Safety Executive Books.

Institute of Physics and Engineering in Medicine/Royal College of Nursing (IPEM/RCN) (2002) Procedures involving radiation. In: *Ionising*

223

Radiation Safety. A Handbook for Nurses. York: York Publishing, pp. 17–32.

International Commission on Radiological Protection (ICRP) (2004) Release of patients after therapy with unsealed radionuclide. *Annals of the ICRP*, 34(20), v–vi and 1–79.

International Commission on Radiological Protection (ICRP) (2005) Radiation safety aspects of brachytherapy for prostate cancer using permanently implanted sources. ICRP Publication 98. *Annals of the ICRP*, 35(3), iii–vi and 3–50.

Ionising Radiations Regulations (IRR) (1999) London: HMSO.

Ionising Radiation (Medical Exposure) Regulations (IRMER) (2000). Available at: https://www.gov.uk/government/publications/the-ionising-radiation-medical-exposure-regulations-2000 (Accessed: 3/4/2018)

Jefferies, H., Hoy, S., McCahill R. & Crichton, A. (2007) The development of Best Practice guidelines for the use of vaginal dilators following pelvic radiotherapy. *Nursing Times*, 103(30), 28–29.

Jones, B., Pryce, P., Blake, P. & Dale, R. (1999) High dose brachytherapy practice for the treatment of gynaecological cancers in the UK. *British Journal of Radiology*, 72(856), 371–377.

Karakoyun-Celik, O., Norris, C. Jr., Tishler, R., et al. (2005) Definitive radiotherapy with interstitial implant boost for squamous cell carcinoma of the tongue base. *Head and Neck*, 27(5), 353–361.

Kucera, H., Mock, U., Knocke, T., et al. (2001) Radiotherapy alone for invasive vaginal cancer: outcome with intracavitary high dose rate brachytherapy versus conventional low dose rate brachytherapy. *Acta Obstetrica et Gynecologica Scandinavica*, 80(4), 355–360.

Kuipers, T., Hoekstra, C., van't Riet, A., et al. (2001) HDR brachytherapy applied to cervical carcinoma with moderate lateral expansion: modified principles of treatment. *Radiotherapy and Oncology*, 58(1), 25–30.

Lalos, A. (1997) The impact of diagnosis on cervical and endometrial cancer patients and their spouses. *European Journal of Gynaecological Oncology*, 18(6), 513–519.

Lalos, A., Jacobsson, L., Lalos, O. & Stendahl, U. (1995) Experiences of the male partner in cervical and endometrial cancer – a prospective interview study. *Journal of Psychosomatic Obstetrics and Gynecology*, 16(3), 153–165.

Lancaster, L. (2004) Preventing vaginal stenosis after brachytherapy for gynaecological cancer: an overview of Australian practices. *European Journal of Oncology Nursing*, 8(1), 30–39.

Lapeyre, M., Bollet, M., Racadot, S., et al. (2004) Postoperative brachytherapy alone and combined postoperative radiotherapy and brachytherapy boost for squamous cell carcinoma of the oral cavity, with positive or close margins. *Head and Neck*, 26(3), 216–223.

Leborgne, F., Leborgne, J.H., Zubizarreta, E. & Mezzera, J. (2002) Cesium-137 needle brachytherapy boosts after external beam irradiation for locally advanced carcinoma of the tongue and floor of the mouth. *Brachytherapy*, 1(3), 126–130.

Leung, P.M. & Nikolic, M. (1998) Disposal of therapeutic 131-I waste using a multiple holding tank system. *Health Physics*, 75(3), 315–321.

Montgomery, C., Lydon, A. & Lloyd, K. (1999) Psychological distress among cancer patients and informed consent. *Journal of Psychosomatic Research*, 46(3), 241–245.

Muscari Lin, E., Aikin, J.L. & Good, B.C. (1999) Premature menopause after cancer treatment. *Cancer Practice*, 7(3), 114–121.

Nag, S., Yacoub, S., Copeland, L.J. & Fowler, J.M. (2002) Interstitial brachytherapy for salvage treatment of vaginal recurrences in previously unirradiated endometrial cancer patients. *International Journal of Radiation Oncology, Biology, Physics*, 54(4), 1153–1159.

NICE (2005) Low dose rate brachytherapy for localised prostate cancer [IPG132]. London: National Institute for Health and Clinical Excellence. Available at: www.nice.org.uk/IPG132 (Accessed: 3/4/2018)

NMC (2009) *Record Keeping: Guidance for Nurses and Midwives*. London: Nursing & Midwifery Council.

NMC (2010) *Standards for Medicines Management*. London: Nursing & Midwifery Council.

Nutting, C., Horlock, N., A'Hern, R., et al. (2006) Manually afterloaded 192Ir low-dose rate brachytherapy after subtotal excision and flap reconstruction of recurrent cervical lymphadenopathy from head and neck cancer. *Radiotherapy and Oncology*, 80(1), 39–42.

O'Dwyer, H.M., Lyon, S., Fotheringham, T. & Lee, M. (2003) Informed consent for interventional radiology procedures: a survey detailing current European practice. *Cardiovascular and Interventional Radiology*, 26(5), 428–433.

Pearson, D., Rogers, A.T. & Moss, E. (2001) A generic approach to risk assessment for the Ionising Radiation Regulations 1999. *British Journal of Radiology*, 74(877), 62–68.

Petereit, D.G., Sarkaria, J.N. & Chappell, R.J. (1998) Perioperative morbidity and mortality of high-dose-rate gynecologic brachytherapy. *International Journal of Radiation Oncology, Biology, Physics*, 42(5), 1025–1031.

Picano, E. (2004) Informed consent and communication of risk from radiological and nuclear medicine examination: how to escape from a communication inferno. *BMJ*, 329(7470), 849–851.

Public Health England (PHE) (2014) Guidance Radiation: products and services. Available at: https://www.gov.uk/guidance/radiation-products-and-services. (Accessed 18/6/18)

RIDDOR (1995) *The Reporting of Injuries, Diseases and Dangerous Occurrences Regulations*. London: HMSO.

Rossoff, L.J., Lam, S., Hilton, E., Borenstein, M. & Isenberg, H.D. (1993) Is the use of boxed gloves in an intensive care unit safe? *American Journal of Medicine*, 94(6), 602–607.

Skalla, K.A., Bakitas, M., Furstenberg, C.T., Ahles, T. & Henderson, J.V. (2004) Patients' need for information about cancer therapy. *Oncology Nursing Forum*, 31(2), 313–319.

Stajduhar, K.I., Neithercut, J., Chu, E., et al. (2000) Thyroid cancer patients' experience of receiving iodine-131 therapy. *Oncology Nursing Forum*, 27(8), 1213–1218.

Stock, R.G., Stone, N., Lo, Y., et al. (2000) Postimplant dosimetry for 125I prostate implants: definitions and factors affecting outcome. *International Journal of Radiation, Oncology, Biology, Physics*, 48(3), 899–906.

Syed, A.M., Puthawala, A.A., Abdelaziz, N.N., et al. (2002) Long-term results of low-dose-rate interstitial-intracavitary brachytherapy in the treatment of carcinoma of the cervix. *International Journal of Radiation Oncology, Biology, Physics*, 54(1), 67–78.

Takacsi-Nagy, Z., Oberna, F., Polgar, C., et al. (2001) The importance of interstitial radiotherapy in the treatment of the base of tongue tumors: a retrospective analysis. *Neoplasma*, 48(1), 76–81.

Tan, L.T., Russell, S. & Burgess, L. (2004) Acute toxicity of chemo-radiotherapy for cervical cancer: the Addenbrooke's experience. *Clinical Oncology*, 16(4), 255–260.

Teruya, Y., Sakumoto, K., Moromizato, H., et al. (2002) High-dose intracavitary brachytherapy for carcinoma in situ of the vagina occurring after hysterectomy: a rational prescription of radiation dose. *American Journal of Obstetrics and Gynecology*, 187(2), 360–364.

Tessa, M., Rotta, P., Ragona, R., et al. (2005) Concomitant chemotherapy and external radiotherapy plus brachytherapy for locally advanced esophageal cancer: results of a retrospective multicenter study. *Tumori*, 91(5), 406–414.

Thompson, M.A. (2001) Radiation safety precautions in the management of the hospitalized 131-I therapy patient. *Nuclear Medicine Technology*, 29(2), 61–66.

UK Oral Mucositis in Cancer Group (UKOMiC) (2015) Oral mucositis guidelines. Available at: http://ukomic.co.uk (Accessed: 1/5/2018)

Ung, Y.C., Yu, E., Falkson, C., Haynes, A.E., Stys-Norman, D. & Evans, W.K. (2006) The role of high-dose-rate brachytherapy in the palliation of symptoms in patients with non-small-cell lung cancer: a systematic review. *Brachytherapy*, 5(3), 189–202.

Velji, K. & Fitch, M. (2001) The experience of women receiving brachytherapy for gynecologic cancer. *Oncology Nursing Forum*, 28(4), 743–751.

Vialard-Miguel, J., Mazere, J., Mora, S., et al. (2005) [I131 in blood samples: management in the laboratory.] *Annales de Biologie Clinique (Paris)*, 63(5), 561–565.

Wadsley, J.C., Patel, M., Tomlins, C., et al. (2003) Iridium-192 implantation for T1 and T2a carcinoma of the tongue and floor of mouth: retrospective study of the results of treatment at the Royal Berkshire Hospital. *British Journal of Radiology*, 76, 414–417.

Wallace, K., Fleshner, N., Jewett, M., Basiuk, J. & Crook, J. (2006) Impact of a multi-disciplinary patient education session on accrual to a difficult clinical trial: the Toronto experience with the surgical prostatectomy versus interstitial radiation intervention trial. *Journal of Clinical Oncology*, 24(25), 4158–4162.

224

White, I., Faithfull, S. & Nicholls, P. (2004) *UK Survey of Current Practice in Vaginal Dilatation Associated with Pelvic Radiotherapy*. European Institute of Health and Medical Sciences (internal document), p. 13.

White, I.D. & Faithfull, S. (2006) Vaginal dilation associated with pelvic radiotherapy: a UK survey of current practice. *International Journal of Gynecological Cancer*, 16, 1140–1146.

Williams, C.E. & Woodward, A.F. (2005) Management of the hapless patient after radioiodine ablation therapy. Are we being too strict? *Nuclear Medicine Communications*, 26(10), 925–928.

Wong, F.C., Tung, S.Y., Leung, T.W., et al. (2003) Treatment results of high-dose-rate remote afterloading brachytherapy for cervical cancer and retrospective comparison of two regimens. *International Journal of Radiation, Oncology, Biology, Physics*, 55(5), 1254–1264.

Wust, P., von Borczyskowski, D., Henkel, T., et al. (2004) Clinical and physical determinants for toxicity of 125-I seed brachytherapy. *Radiotherapy and Oncology*, 73(1), 39–48.

Zelefsky, M.J. (2006) Quality of life of patients after permanent prostate brachytherapy in relation to dosimetry. *Urologic Oncology*, 24(4), 377–378.

Chapter 6
Wound management

Procedure guidelines

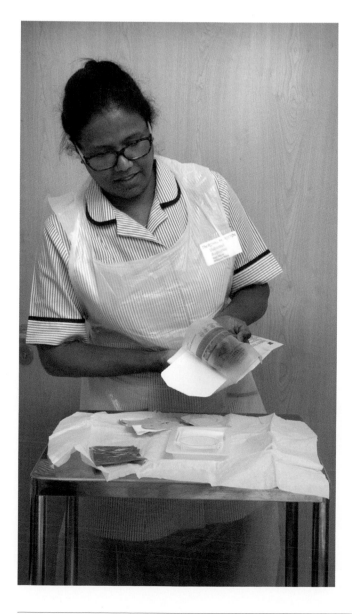

The Royal Marsden Manual of Cancer Nursing Procedures. Edited by Sara Lister and Lisa Dougherty, with Assistant Editor Louise McNamara.
© 2019 The Royal Marsden NHS Foundation Trust. Published 2019 by John Wiley & Sons, Ltd.

Overview

The aim of this chapter is to provide an overview of the management of oncological wounds; fungating malignant wounds, skin problems, wounds associated with graft-versus-host disease (GvHD) and radiotherapy wounds.

Malignant fungating wounds

Definition

A malignant fungating wound is the result of a cancerous mass that infiltrates through the skin epithelium and surrounding lymph and blood vessels (Pearson and Mortimer 2004). These wounds can develop anywhere on the body and can present as either an ulcerating crater or a 'fungating' wound with raised nodules similar in appearance to a cauliflower, or a combination of both, with maceration and inflammation of the surrounding skin (Benbow 2009a). A malignant fungating wound can grow rapidly, cause considerable damage to the skin (Alexander 2009a) and rarely heals (Bird 2000). Malignant fungating wounds can also be known as fungating wounds, cutaneous malignancies or tumour necrosis (Benbow 2009a).

Anatomy and physiology

Malignant fungating wounds are diagnosed based on a histological assessment. A malignant wound can develop from:

- a primary skin tumour such as a malignant melanoma or a squamous cell carcinoma
- an underlying tumour that invades through the surrounding skin structures, such as a breast cancer
- metastases that have spread along tissue planes, capillaries or lymph vessels from a distant primary tumour (Naylor 2002a).

Malignant fungating wounds are the result of a cancerous process in which the cells infiltrate and damage the local blood and lymph vessels, which then disrupts the normal flow of blood and lymph, leading to a loss of vascularity and resulting in tissue necrosis (Benbow 2009a) (Figure 6.1).

Tumour necrosis and ulceration tend to develop in the centre of the mass as this area is furthest from the surrounding blood supply. Tumours need a blood supply to grow and spread; growth occurs at the periphery of the tumour where the blood supply is rich due to surrounding healthy tissue. The central area of the tumour becomes ischaemic and then necrotizes and ulcerates.

When local invasion of the skin occurs, the initial presentation may be as patches or plaques, which may be inflamed, indurated and hot; the colour can range from deep red to brown/black (Seaman 2006). Lesions can initially present as demarcated nodules, ranging from a few millimetres to several centimetres in size. The areas may be tender to touch, although they are generally painless on initial presentation. The skin may be fixed to underlying tissue with a *peau d'orange* appearance (swollen pitted skin, resembling orange peel); the skin can then break and ulcerate as the tumour damages further tissues (Wilson 2005). When the lesions extend above the skin surface they may then develop into fungating or ulcerative areas, or a combination of both (Naylor 2001).

Fungating lesions develop through a proliferative process and often have a 'cauliflower' appearance (Figure 6.2).

An ulcerating lesion has a crater-like appearance (Naylor 2002a), which is undergoing a destructive process through cancer infiltration of the skin and subcutaneous tissues (Alexander 2009a) and may have a distinctive 'lip' around the edge (Moody and Grocott 1993) (Figure 6.3).

The presentation of a malignant wound bed can vary from pale pink to very friable, necrotic or a combination of all three. Malignant lesions are often friable and may bleed easily. The bleeding may occur due to the erosion of local blood vessels or tissue necrosis (Lloyd 2008), or because of impaired platelet function within the tumour (Haisfield-Wolfe and Rund 1997). The surrounding skin may be fragile, erythematous and tender to touch, with maceration from exudate. As the lesions extend they will produce necrotic areas due to poor vascularization. The necrotic tissue provides an ideal environment for aerobic and anaerobic bacteria to multiply, leading to localized infection with a subsequent increase in exudate and malodour (Benbow 2005). The level of pain experienced by the patient will be dependent on factors such as the depth of tissue invasion, damage to surrounding skin, nerve involvement, location of the wound and the patient's previous experience with pain (Naylor 2001).

Related theory

Malignant fungating wounds are associated with advanced cancer and often appear in the last 6 months of life, although they can develop earlier and the patient could have them for a prolonged period (Naylor 2002a). There is often an absence of pain in the early stages of the tumour developing, which can result in a delay in the patient presenting with the problem and consequently lead to a delay in treatment (Benbow 2005). There are occasions when patients present for help when their wounds are advanced. It is

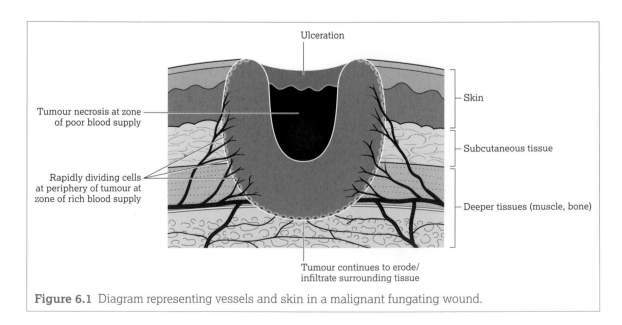

Figure 6.1 Diagram representing vessels and skin in a malignant fungating wound.

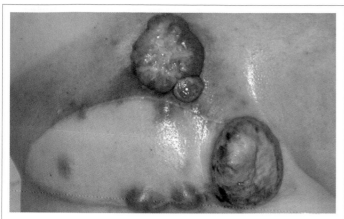

Figure 6.2 Fungating malignant wound from recurrent breast cancer – chest wall resurfaced with flap reconstruction. Recurrent nodules arising around and infiltrating the flap. *Source:* Naylor (2005). Reproduced with permission.

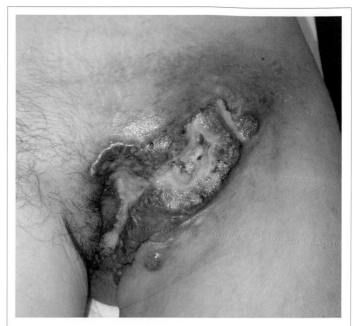

Figure 6.3 Deep ulcerating fungating malignant wound caused by untreated squamous cell carcinoma of the vulva. *Source:* Naylor (2005). Reproduced with permission.

thought that this may be through fear of the cancer diagnosis or embarrassment (Lund-Neilson et al. 2011).

The wounds often present as malodorous, necrotic and exuding areas which have a devastating effect on a patient's quality of life. Patients have often already endured a long, distressing treatment journey and the wounds then act as a constant physical reminder that their disease is both progressive and incurable (Naylor 2002a). Living with a fungating wound can have a profound impact on a patient's physical, psychological and social well-being and on their family and friends.

Healing of these wounds is rarely a realistic aim unless there is a good response to treatment, such as radiotherapy or chemotherapy, or the wound can be surgically excised. Recent developments such as electrochemotherapy may slow progression in a carefully selected group of patients (NICE 2015a). When palliative management of the wound is required, the concentration should be on addressing distressing and uncomfortable symptoms to minimize the impact of the wound on the patient, promoting comfort and enhancing their quality of life (Grocott 2007).

There are several case studies and articles with anecdotal evidence on the management of malignant wounds. However there is a dearth of formal research in this area. The wounds are often managed on a trial and error basis. This is contrary to good clinical governance which requires practice to be evidence based (Lloyd 2008). There are no formal recordings and exact statistics known for malignant wounds, and the statistics that are available have often been collected without consistent inclusion criteria (Alexander 2009a).

It is estimated that malignant fungating wounds occur in approximately 5% of patients with cancer and 10% of patients with metastatic cancer (Seaman 2006). They often occur in patients over 70 years of age (Dowsett 2002) and some may be due to neglect and late presentation. The most common presentation of malignant wounds is seen in breast tumours metastasizing in the breast or chest wall (62%) (McDonald and Lesage 2006). Lung and gastrointestinal tumours and melanomas account for most remaining fungating wounds, although they can develop from any other type of malignancy, including head and neck, ovary, genitourinary or from an unknown primary (Seaman 2006). They have also been found in unusual areas such as the nailbed, scrotum, eyelid and ear (Moore 2002).

Malignant wounds in the perineal or abdominal regions can lead to sinuses or fistulae with internal cavities, such as the bladder, vagina and bowel, which then increase problems of malodour and exudate as body substances such as faecal fluid may leak through the wound (Dowsett 2002). Wounds in the head and neck can result in distortion of the face, infiltration of the buccal cavity, which may lead to dribbling of saliva, and a wound exit point around the chin area (Grocott 2007).

Marjolin's ulcer

A Marjolin's ulcer is an aggressive malignant tumour that creates an ulcer in a chronic wound or scar tissue. It has a high rate of local recurrence and metastatic spread (Choi et al. 2013). Marjolin's ulcers most commonly occur in burn scars, although they can develop in chronic pressure ulcers, venous stasis ulcers or skin graft donor sites (Malheiro et al. 2001). The exact cause is not known, however there is general agreement that the lack of blood supply and chronic inflammation and immunity in the scar tissue form a 'cancerous environment'. The delicate, dry epithelium can be repeatedly damaged by slight injuries, movement over joints, flexion or prolonged itching. The regeneration of epithelium over this area is inferior and the persistent requirement for the marginal epithelium to regenerate and repair can eventually lead to neoplastic changes. The signs and symptoms of a Marjolin's ulcer can often be mistaken for infection, leading to a delay in diagnosis. The ulcers can present as indolent, flat, chronic ulcers, increasing in circumference and depth, with indurated and elevated margins and a granular base; there is often an increase in volume and consistency of exudate and malodour (Malheiro et al. 2001) (Figure 6.4). Biopsy confirmation is required to diagnose a Marjolin's ulcer to initiate prompt treatment to reduce the risk of metastatic spread. Treatment is by wide excision followed by chemotherapy or radiotherapy (Choi et al. 2013).

A high index of suspicion is required to diagnose Marjolin's ulcer so diagnosis is often delayed. Any wound that is not showing evidence of healing should be biopsied to rule out Marjolin's ulcer.

Principles of care

Psychosocial support for patients who present with a fungating tumour

There are many goals in caring for a patient with a fungating tumour; psychological support features heavily. In this, one

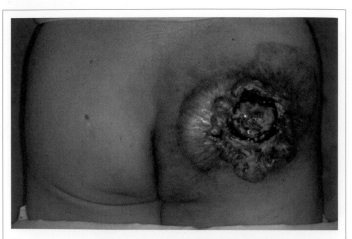

Figure 6.4 Marjolin's ulcer on a buttock arising in an area of previous skin graft or burn scar. *Source:* Choi et al. (2013). Reproduced with permission of The Korean Society of Reconstructive and Plastic Surgeons.

of the main aspects is controlling symptoms, which in turn may improve the patient's quality of life and psychosocial well-being.

There are many challenges to a patient presenting with a tumour of this type and an empathetic nurse–patient relationship is paramount in providing support. Patients often feel socially rejected and distressed, so allowing expression of fears and concerns is important. Studies have shown that living with a fungating wound causes distress, thus inducing feelings of worthlessness, embarrassment, fear of the stigma associated with cancer and a constant reminder of its presence (Piggin and Jones 2009).

For many patients there is a loss of sense of self when they are living with a tumour and they may feel unable to face the world on a day to day basis. Many female patients have highlighted a loss of femininity. The inability to wear a bra because of the tumour and dressing affects the ability to choose clothes of a feminine nature (Reynolds and Gethin 2015). Sensitivity, understanding and emotional intelligence shown by the nurse can greatly improve the patient's feelings and self-image. Knowing that someone understands what they are going through can often help.

Providing holistic and supportive care can often give the patient the opportunity to live as full a life as possible, within the limitations of their disease.

Choice of an appropriate dressing can be challenging for a nurse when caring for a patient presenting with a fungating tumour, yet this can affect how the patient reflects upon themselves. A nurse needs confidence in her communication skills and ability when being involved in a patient's care. Managing the odour can be part of the task, as this can affect the patient in many ways. Social relationship was found to have suffered as a direct result of malodour (Gibson and Green 2013). This breakdown in a patient's ability to be confident socially may also have financial implications for them or their families.

The continuous improvement of nursing knowledge is important as it reflects in a nurse's evidence-based practice. A passion for this area of nursing is not enough; there is a professional, personal and collective responsibility to continue to enhance knowledge and understanding in light of new strategies as well as applying proven strategies to patient care (Benbow 2009b).

The nurse may also be involved in giving support to the family or loved ones of a patient presenting with a fungating tumour. This often involves assessing if there are any gaps in care and assessing how he or she can offer practical assistance or help. Caring for a loved one with a malignant fungating tumour causes psychological distress (Probst et al. 2012).

Support offered by the nurse to the patient and family can help them on their constant course of adjustment that living with and learning how to manage a fungating tumour brings.

Wound assessment

Assessment and evaluation of a wound are discussed in *The Royal Marsden Manual of Clinical Nursing Procedures, Ninth Edition*: Chapter 15 Wound Management (2015).

Fungating wounds are unique and will have a range of different appearances, symptoms and problems that can be very difficult to treat and require individual, patient-specific management plans (Benbow 2005). Assessment is difficult due to the uniqueness and complexity of the wounds and how quickly they may change (Schulz et al. 2009). It is important that health professionals use sound clinical assessment skills, understand the dressing products that they use and are aware of the functions and limitations of a dressing. The management of wounds through dressings can have a significant impact on all areas of a patient's quality of life (Watret 2011).

An accurate holistic assessment is an extremely important aspect of a patient's care. The assessment should be ongoing and involve the patient's physical, nutritional intake, psychological, spiritual and cultural needs and social state as well as specific wound factors. It is important that the patient is encouraged to carry out a self-assessment that includes how they are coping with the wound, their overall coping strategies and ability to self-care, together with the impact the wound is having on their quality of life and their family. The patient should be involved in the management planning and implementation process to enable the development of a patient-centred treatment plan that considers the perspectives of the patient and of the healthcare practitioner (Alexander 2009a).

Wound assessment tools

Literature identifies that palliative care tools are most effective when they are simple to follow, complete and encompass the wide range of needs of the patient and their families (Schulz et al. 2009). Patient self-assessment is the optimum method of symptom reporting. However, if a patient is very unwell and communication is difficult then this is not realistic. It is then that accurate assessment is extremely important (Naylor 2002a).

The European Oncology Nursing Society (EONS 2015) looked at a range of assessment tools that can be used for patients with malignant fungating wounds. The tools help to structure individualized care in an area that is not often encountered by healthcare professionals (Table 6.1).

Figure 6.5 shows the wound assessment chart used at the Royal Marsden.

Pre-procedural considerations

Dressing changes should be scheduled where possible at times when the patient feels at their best. Pain medication should be offered at least 30 minutes prior to changing the dressing and it should have reached its maximum effectiveness prior to commencing the procedure (Rogers 2015). The dressing should be changed in a well-ventilated room, and consideration should be given to relaxation, comfortable position and music or complementary therapies where appropriate. If the patient experiences any discomfort during the dressing change the procedure should be stopped, further analgesia given if required, the patient given a break and the procedure not resumed until the patient has consented (Rogers 2015).

For further information please see Dougherty and Lister (2015) *The Royal Marsden Manual of Clinical Nursing Procedures, Ninth Edition*: Chapter 15 Wound Management.

Table 6.1 Some assessment tools for fungating wounds

Assessment tool	Description	Advantages/disadvantages
The TELER System (Grocott et al. 2011)	Covers all aspects of wound management and the psychosocial impact of wounds: discomfort from skin conditions, exudate, leakage and intrusion of dressings Designed to be completed by patients, carers and healthcare professionals	Enables the perspectives of patient and healthcare professionals to be considered when developing treatment plan (Alexander 2009a) Includes long-term goals negotiated with patient Available in digital format Identifies what patient finds the most challenging aspects of wound to influence choice of product management (Watret 2011)
The Wound and Symptoms Self-assessment chart (WoSSac) (Naylor 2002a)	Quantitative tool developed to enable patients to rate the symptoms and impact the wound has on them and their wider environment. Completed by patient or their carer, uses visual analogue scale and Likert scale when measuring the severity of the wound-related symptoms and impact on the patient	Tool has pre-determined set of criteria which may not reflect individual needs of the patient; further discussion would be required for comprehensive assessment (Alexander 2009a) Enables a patient to rate the most significant area they feel is the most challenging, considering the severity of symptoms and impact on their quality of life (Watret 2011).
Malignant fungating wound assessment tool (Schulz et al. 2009)	Completed by health professionals. Covers general information about the patient, wound and symptoms	Open-ended questions to enable assessment of patients' perceptions

Source: Adapted from EONS (2015).

Procedure guideline 6.1   Assessing a malignant fungating wound

Essential equipment
- Sterile dressing pack containing gallipots or an indented plastic tray, low-linting swabs, disposable forceps, gloves, sterile field, disposable bag and disposable plastic apron
- Fluids for cleaning and/or irrigation
- Hypoallergenic tape
- Appropriate dressing
- Appropriate hand hygiene preparation

- The nature of the dressing will determine any other material; special features of a dressing should be referred to in the patient's nursing care plan
- Detergent wipe
- Total traceability system for surgical instruments and patient record form, if required

Optional equipment
- Sterile scissors

Pre-procedure

Action	Rationale
1 Explain and discuss the procedure with the patient and check analgesia requirements.	To ensure that the patient understands the procedure and gives his or her valid consent, and to reduce anxiety (NMC 2017). **C**
2 Wash hands with soap and water; put on a disposable plastic apron.	Hands must be cleaned before touching a patient and prior to a procedure to prevent cross-infection and reduce the risk of healthcare-associated infection (WHO 2009). **C** Clothing may become contaminated with pathogenic micro-organisms, blood/body fluids (Loveday et al. 2014). **C**
3 Clean trolley with a detergent wipe.	To provide a clean working surface and reduce the risk of the environment providing a reservoir for cross-infection (Guizhen 2016). **C**
4 Place all the equipment required for the procedure on the bottom shelf of the clean dressing trolley. Check integrity and use-by dates of all equipment (i.e. packs are undamaged, intact and dry).	To maintain the top shelf as a clean working surface. To ensure sterility of equipment prior to use (Fraise and Bradley 2009, **E**).
5 Screen the bed area and provide privacy. Position the patient comfortably so that the area to be dealt with is easily accessible without exposing the patient unduly.	Maintain the patient's dignity and comfort (NMC 2017, **C**).
6 Take the trolley to the treatment room or patient's bedside; minimize the movement of bedding and screens as much as possible prior to dressing change.	To allow any airborne organisms to settle before the sterile field and the wound is exposed, to minimize airborne contamination (Bache et al. 2015). **C**

(continued)

Procedure guideline 6.1   Assessing a malignant fungating wound *(continued)*

Procedure

7	Clean hands with a bactericidal alcohol handrub.	To reduce the risk of wound infection and cross-contamination (WHO 2009). **C**
8	Open the outer cover of the sterile dressing pack and slide the contents onto the top shelf of the trolley.	To ensure that only sterile products are used (Fraise and Bradley 2009, **C**).
9	Open the sterile field using only the corners of the paper.	So that areas of potential contamination are kept to a minimum. **E**
10	Loosen the dressing tape (if necessary). If contamination on outer dressings, gloves should be worn.	To make it easier to remove the dressing. **E** For personal protection (Loveday et al. 2014, **C**).
11	Clean hands with a bactericidal alcohol handrub.	Hands may become contaminated by handling outer packets and dressings (WHO 2009). **C**
12	Using the plastic bag in the pack, arrange the sterile field. Pour cleaning solution into gallipots or an indented plastic tray.	The time the wound is exposed should be kept to a minimum to reduce the risk of contamination. To prevent contamination of the environment. To minimize risk of contamination of cleaning solution. **C**
13	Remove dressing by placing a hand in the plastic bag, lifting the dressing off and inverting the plastic bag so that the dressing is now inside the bag. Thereafter use this as the 'dirty' bag. Use gloves if there is difficulty removing dressing.	To reduce the risk of cross-infection. To prevent contamination of the environment (Fraise and Bradley 2009, **C**).
14	Attach the bag with the dressing to the side of the trolley below the top shelf on the side next to the patient.	To avoid taking soiled dressings across the sterile area. Contaminated material should be disposed of below the level of the sterile field. **C**
15	Assess wound healing (see Table 15.1 in *The Royal Marsden Manual of Clinical Nursing Procedures, Ninth Edition*)	To evaluate wound care (Dealey 2005, **E**; Hampton and Collins 2004, **E**; Hess 2005, **E**).

Treatment options

Initial diagnosis and evaluation

Managing the wound is vital but will not cure or control the disease. Fungating cancers are as heterogeneous as any presenting cancer and the treatment of the underlying disease should follow the same systematic process of diagnosis and treatment planning. It is no longer the case that the management of a fungating lesion equates to symptom control and wound care alone, although these are vital components.

Malignant fungating lesions may present in the presence or absence of metastatic disease and it is this criterion that determines treatment intent. The presence of metastatic disease (American Joint Committee on Cancer 2010) signifies that treatment is no longer able to eradicate disease. Long-term control is still a valid and realistic goal, however, with combinations of appropriate treatment.

The successful management of a fungating malignant wound requires comprehensive, accurate diagnosis and pretreatment assessment. It demands the involvement and coordination of the complete multidisciplinary team (MDT) from the outset.

Evaluation should include a full history of the symptoms and clinical examination to assess the extent of skin and local muscle involvement. It may be appropriate to biopsy the tumour to give information about nuclear grade and hormone receptor status to decide the most appropriate treatment. Staging scans may be required to ensure there is no distant disease. MDT discussion will confirm treatment intent, whether it be curative or palliative control.

The presence of metastatic disease will affect the treatment plan as the accepted approach is to employ less intensive treatments when the aim is not cure. It should be remembered that cancer in secondary sites, such as with breast cancers, can be controlled for significant periods. As such, treatments that improve the symptoms of a fungating malignant wound will offer more benefit proportionately.

Fungating tumours may be locally advanced because they are aggressive in nature. The patient may reliably describe only a short history of symptoms. It is to be hoped that such tumours will respond to chemotherapy to downsize them. An alternative scenario may be that of a patient who has been aware of changes for a significant time, sometimes even years, but has not sought help for a variety of reasons. Such a history indicates a slow progression. However, a treatment-naïve tumour may respond to systemic treatments.

Surgical considerations

Surgical approaches and the development of reconstructive techniques have increased the surgical remit and ability to remove larger tumours while maintaining good aesthetic results or reproduce increasingly natural-appearing reconstructions following operations such as a mastectomy. The role of the surgeon at diagnosis is to confirm whether surgery should be the primary treatment of choice for a fungating cancer. Seminal work published in the 1940s argued that the presence of certain characteristics, common to fungating lesions, absolutely contraindicated surgery as the primary treatment. Haagensen and Stout (1942) cited these, in relation to breast cancers, to be extensive local skin oedema, skin ulceration, fixation to the chest wall, fixed involved axillary nodes and satellite skin nodules. These remain accepted standards today. Rather, surgery should be employed as the definitive treatment following medical therapies.

In the presence of metastatic disease, the role of surgery to improve local control and palliate symptoms is unclear. Surgery

THE ROYAL MARSDEN WOUND ASSESSMENT CHART
Complete one chart for each wound

Patient name:						
Hospital number:						
Date of assessment (weekly)						
Wound dimensions						
Max length (cm)						
Max width (cm)						
Max depth (cm)						
Wound bed – approximate % cover (enter %)						
Necrotic (BLACK)						
Slough (YELLOW)						
Granulating (RED)						
Epithelializing (PINK)						
Skin around wound						
Intact						
Healthy						
Fragile						
Dry						
Scaly						
Erythema						
Maceration						
Oedema						
Eczema						
Skin nodules						
Skin stripping						
Dressing allergy						
Tape allergy						
Other (please state)						
Exudate level						
None						
Low						
Moderate						
High						
Amount increasing						
Amount decreasing						
Odour (see over for rating scale)						
None						
Slight						
Moderate						
Strong						
Bleeding						
None						
Slight						
Moderate						
Heavy						
At dressing change						
Pain from wound (see over for rating scale)						
Level (0–10)						
Continuous						
At specific times (specify)						
Wound infection suspected						
Swab taken (Y/N)						
Swab result						
Treatment						
Assessment review date						
Initials of assessor						

Figure 6.5 Wound assessment chart. *Source:* Dougherty and Lister (2015).

(continued)

Location (mark diagram):	Visual Analogue Scale (VAS) for Patient's Rating of Pain.

Right   Left   Left   Right

Visual Analogue Scale:

0 — 1 — 2 — 3 — 4 — 5 — 6 — 7 — 8 — 9 — 10
No pain   Worst pain imaginable

Rating Scale for Odour	
Score	Assessment
None	No odour evident, even when at the patient's bedside with the dressing removed.
Slight	Wound odour is evident at close proximity to the patient when the dressing is removed.
Moderate	Wound odour is evident upon entering the room (1.5 to 3 metres from patient) with the dressing removed.
Strong	Wound odour is evident upon entering the room (1.5 to 3 metres from patient) with the dressing intact.

Diagram of wound if appropriate (or attach tracing/photograph):

Date: _____	Date: _____
Date: _____	Date: _____
Date: _____	Date: _____

Notes on use
Use one chart per wound.
Complete a wound assessment at least once a week.
Measure the wound at its widest points using a clean ruler, use a sterile wound swab or blunt probe to measure wound depth.
For the 'skin around wound' assessment more than one box may be ticked.
Odour and pain should be assessed using the scales at the top of page 2.
Following the assessment a wound management care plan should be written and updated if necessary after each reassessment.

Figure 6.5 *continued*

in the breast cancer setting may often be extensive and may include plastics and thoracic teams to clear and resurface the area. Benefits may only be small. However, they may be of great importance to the patient living with a fungating lesion. Overall survival is unlikely to be affected.

Medical approaches

Neo-adjuvant chemotherapy
Where treatment intent is curative and surgery is planned following medical treatment, full immunohistochemistry of the tumour enables medical oncologists to plan intervention with appropriate drugs and drug combinations. This will include standard chemotherapy, often in combination with newer targeted drugs. The success of the human epidermal growth factor receptor (HER2) monoclonal antibody trastuzumab is well documented and has led to further development of other anti-HER2 agents such as pertuzumab and lapatinib, which are showing promise and increasing the rate at which medical oncology teams are seeing complete pathological responses to treatment. Other targeted therapies of note currently include everolimus and bevacizumab. Such evidence is obtained from trials in the

neo-adjuvant setting for all breast cancers and it is an extrapolation that the same responses can be expected with fungating lesions. Treatment response should be monitored both clinically and radiologically.

Neo-adjuvant or primary endocrine therapy

The use of endocrine therapy alone in a frailer patient can be effective in downsizing and treating a locally advanced tumour. Often response is slower and the neo-adjuvant phase may be longer. Endocrine therapies can also be used in conjunction with the targeted drugs described previously. Discussion regarding when and whether to intervene with surgery should be ongoing and include the patient.

Radiotherapy

Radiotherapy is a local treatment given to reduce the risk of locoregional recurrence. This is of paramount importance with a fungating lesion as the chance of such recurrence is higher due to involvement of lymphatics, skin and often muscle. The radiotherapy treatment destroys malignant cells and can reduce the size of the wound, alleviating symptoms such as exudate, bleeding and pain. Initially there can be a deterioration in the appearance of the wound as malignant cells die and skin reactions occur (Winnipeg Regional Health Authority [WRHA] 2014). Standard radiotherapy policies should be employed if the patient is being treated with curative intent. Research is not unequivocal and the question as to whether it should be accepted practice is unanswered. As the drive to personalize treatment continues this will be an important area of discussion.

Those fungating lesions that are deemed suitable for palliation only may well be improved and controlled by radiotherapy, which will improve a patient's quality of life. Unlike the use of surgery at this point it may be less demanding and more tolerable to the patient.

Electrochemotherapy

Electrochemotherapy is aimed at the treatment and palliation of primary skin cancers and melanomas, and cutaneous and subcutaneous metastases of areas of non-skin origin. It combines the administration of a cytotoxic chemotherapeutic agent, such as bleomycin or cisplatin, with electrical pulses applied to the tumour, which enhances the permeability of the tumour cells and leads to cellular uptake of the drug (Marty et al. 2006). There is increasing evidence for the effectiveness of electrochemotherapy in reducing tumour volume and in managing symptoms such as bleeding and exudate. It appears to be effective with minimal and transient side-effects. The treatment can be given in a single session in an outpatient setting, which is convenient and cost-effective, and patients can be retreated if the tumour recurs (Grocott et al. 2013).

Principles of the management of dressings for a malignant fungating wound

Dressing selection

The evidence to support the choice of dressings for managing malignant wounds is often poor and heavily biased. New products need to be carefully and objectively evaluated and compared to a gold standard. Unfortunately, this evidence is often lacking and nurses are often required to be innovative and resourceful in their choice of dressings. The products for successfully managing malignant wounds are limited, and the sizes and configurations required for such wounds are not available. Management may include the use of a wide range of dressings together with stoma bags and continence products.

It is important when choosing a dressing regimen to discuss it with the patient to see what is important to them. What is most appropriate for the wound may not be what is best for the patient (Clark 2002). It is often a major challenge to dress wounds in an inconspicuous way that protects a patient's dignity and is socially acceptable to them. Bulky dressings should be avoided when possible, dressings that are skin toned may be more acceptable for a patient, and clothing should be used creatively to cover the affected area (Rogers 2015).

Malignant wounds are often dressed with two or more layers. The primary layer should be non-adherent, not cause trauma on removal and allow the passage of moisture to the secondary layer. Following assessment of the wound it may be possible to leave the primary contact layer *in situ* for several days and change the outer dressing when required, which is more acceptable to the patient and also more cost-effective (Benbow 2015). The secondary or subsequent layers should be highly absorbent, not bulky and as aesthetically acceptable as possible to the patient (McManus 2007). Ideally the dressings should be capable of being left in place for longer periods of time, reducing the discomfort and inconvenience for the patient of dressing changes (Alexander 2009c).

When considering a dressing for a malignant wound the ideal dressing must fulfil the following functions:

- minimize the odour associated with a malignant wound
- allow gaseous exchange
- protect the wound from contamination
- allow removal of the dressing without pain or skin stripping
- be acceptable to the patient
- be highly absorbent (for heavily exuding wounds)
- be cost-effective
- require minimal replacement or disturbance
- be appropriate to the wound in terms of debridement activity and haemostatic properties (Thomas 2009).

Local wound management

Symptom management and local wound management are the foci of care for a patient with a malignant fungating wound. TIME wound bed preparation (TIME/WBP) principles comprise four components underpinning the wound bed preparation (European Wound Management Association 2004).

1 **T**issue management.
2 **I**nflammation/infection control.
3 **M**oisture balance.
4 **E**pithelial advancement.

These principles can be applied in palliative wound care (Grocott 2007) as autolytic debridement and moisture management can enhance quality of life. Effectively controlling symptoms can increase independence and help patients regain a measure of control over their lives (Grocott 2007).

Each patient responds individually to having such a wound, the consequences of which impinge on physical, psychological, social, sexual as well as spiritual well-being. The highest level of nursing expertise is required. Informing patients can lead them to understand their signs and symptoms and enable them to report accurately and live more positively with their wound (Lo et al. 2008).

Whilst the appearance and presenting symptoms of malignant fungating wounds are unique, the most common symptoms associated with fungating wounds are heavy exudates, malodour, bleeding, pain and pruritus (Grocott 2007, Hampton 2008, Lund-Neilson et al. 2005).

Exudate

When skin integrity is broken through the development of a wound, the body initiates an inflammatory response where mediators such as histamines make capillaries more permeable and facilitate the movement of electrolytes, nutrients and proteins, growth factors, matrix metalloproteinases, platelets and micro-organisms, producing additional fluid in the wound and forming the basis of an exudate (Barrett et al. 2012). Exudate is required in wound healing to provide nutrients to the wound bed, aid autolytic debridement and facilitate the process of epithelialization to allow the cells to move across the wound bed.

Malignant fungating wounds have the propensity to produce high amounts of exudate, which can be as much as one litre per day (EONS 2015). The high level of exudate is the result of abnormal capillary permeability within the wound which can be caused by disordered blood vessels within the tumour (Naylor 2002b), autolysis of necrotic tissue by bacterial proteases and the inflammatory process associated with infections (EONS 2015).

Effective clinical management of highly exuding wounds is essential for patients to reduce malodour, reduce the risk of leakage onto clothing and bedding, as well as increase their comfort and confidence (Grocott 2007). If patients experience leakage through their dressings it can lead to embarrassment, anxiety and feelings of being unclean which have the potential to lead to depression and social isolation with an overall negative impact on their quality of life. Failure to control wound exudate also results in an increased frequency of nursing interventions and an overall increase in the expenditure on wound management products and resources (Dowsett 2015).

Assessment of exudate

A description of exudate, including the appearance and amount, should be recorded at each dressing change. Healthcare professionals should understand the implications for the presence and appearance of exudate. A change in exudate should initiate a change in the wound management plan for the patient. Assessment of the level of the exudate has traditionally been in terms of 'low', 'moderate' and 'high' or +,++,+++, which can be very subjective (Tickle 2015).

Table 6.2 indicates the significance of the colour and Table 6.3 the significance of the consistency of wound exudate and what the nurse should take into consideration when assessing the patient.

Management of exudate

Table 6.4 sets out appropriate ways to manage exuding malignant fungating wounds.

Table 6.2 Significance of the colour of exudate

Characteristic	Possible cause
Clear, amber	Serous exudate, often considered 'normal', but may be associated with infection by fibrinolysin-producing bacteria such as *Staphylococcus aureus*; may also be due to fluid from a urinary or lymphatic fistula
Cloudy, milky or creamy	May indicate the presence of fibrin strands (fibrinous exudate – a response to inflammation) or infection (purulent exudate containing white blood cells and bacteria)
Pink or red	Due to the presence of red blood cells and indicating capillary damage (sanguineous or haemorrhagic exudate)
Green	May be indicative of bacterial infection, e.g. *Pseudomonas aeruginosa*
Yellow or brown	May be due to the presence of wound slough or material from an enteric or urinary fistula
Grey or blue	May be related to the use of silver-containing dressings

Source: World Union of Wound Healing Societies (WUWHS 2007). Reproduced with permission of WUWHS.

Table 6.3 Significance of exudate consistency

Characteristic	Possible cause
High viscosity (thick, sometimes sticky)	High protein content due to: – infection – inflammatory process Necrotic material Enteric fistula Residue from some types of dressings or topical preparations
Low viscosity (thin, 'runny')	Low protein content due to: – venous or congestive cardiac disease – malnutrition Urinary, lymphatic or joint space fistula Bacterial growth or infection Necrotic tissue Sinus/enteric or urinary fistula

Source: World Union of Wound Healing Societies (WUWHS 2007). Reproduced with permission of WUWHS.

Topical negative pressure

Topical negative pressure takes the fluid away from the wound by applying negative pressure. The system is not advocated for use in malignant wounds due to the potential for increasing cell activity; however, it may be appropriate to consider using a negative pressure pump as an alternative to conventional dressings in end of life care. Negative pressure may improve a patient's quality of life by managing three of the most challenging symptoms associated with dressing changes, namely exudate, odour and pain (Riot et al. 2015).

Periwound skin

If moisture becomes trapped under a dressing and the skin is in contact with the moisture for an extended time the epidermal cells can become waterlogged and prone to excoriation and stripping of the skin, potentially leading to an increase in the wound size. Exudate in chronic wounds appears to be more corrosive than in acute wounds and can lead to more damage to surrounding skin. It is possible to frame a wound using thin hydrocolloid dressings or semi-permeable films, which can help to protect the skin and can also be effective in anchoring the secondary dressings in place. A protective, non-alcohol based skin barrier such as Cavilon can be used prior to dressing application to protect the skin from damage due to excessive exudate (Benbow 2015) and can be beneficial in assisting adhesive dressings to form a good seal. Ideally the protective barrier should be used prior to any skin damage as pain and skin damage can impair the adherence of a dressing. Trauma to the skin can also be reduced by using atraumatic dressings, elastic vests and netting or tubular bandages to hold dressings in place (Draper 2005).

Malodour

The malodour from a malignant wound is often the most distressing symptom for a patient (Benbow 2009a) and can have a profound impact on their quality of life. Malodour can cause nausea, vomiting and involuntary gagging (Lund-Neilson et al. 2011) leading to a reduction in appetite and weight loss, with subsequent poor nutrition at a time when good nutrition is of high importance to their condition. A referral to the dietician service may be of benefit to the patient (Wilson 2005). Malodour can cause feelings of embarrassment and repulsion and lead to social isolation and depression. This is at a time when the support of family and friends is crucial for patients to cope with the physical and psychological impact of their progressive disease.

Malodour can be caused by necrotic and poorly vascularized tissue, the presence of bacteria, high levels of exudate (Gethin 2010) or stagnant exudate in the dressing. The type of tissue

Table 6.4 Dressings and equipment for the management of wound exudate

Amount	Dressings	
Lightly exuding wounds	Hydrogels/ hydrocolloids/absorbent vapour-permeable adhesive dressings	Contain exudate and maintain moist environment – minimize risk of pain/trauma/ bleeding at dressing change (Naylor 2002b)
Moderate– heavy exudate	Alginates/alginate plus (e.g. Sorbsan/Kaltostat)	When in contact with exudate forms a gel, which maintains a high humidity in the wound, they reduce the occurrence of exudate macerating surrounding skin
	Hydrofibre (e.g. Aquacel)	Hydrofibres have a different method of action to an alginate in that they absorb and retain fluid in the dressing
	Foam dressings (e.g. Allevyn/Mepilex)	Absorb exudate into the matrix of the dressing. Some can transmit the water vapour through the surface of the dressing so that it can evaporate into the air (Adderley 2010). Foams should not be covered with occlusive film or similar as their function will be affected
	High-absorbency dressings (e.g. Eclypse)	Some incorporate a gelling technology within the dressing similar to that used in disposable nappies. They are able to retain much higher levels of exudate within the dressing. They can reduce the number of dressing changes required. However, they can become heavy when saturated and cause the dressing to sag
Wounds with sinus/fistula	Wound manager bag systems	Can be beneficial in containing odour and keeping the exudate away from the surrounding skin. Particularly beneficial if there is a fistula or a deep open wound producing copious amounts of exudate (Adderley 2010)

present in the wound is often the cause of malodour: devitalized and necrotic tissue can be an ideal environment for anaerobic and aerobic bacteria which can produce volatile agents. Anaerobic bacteria such as Clostridium and aerobic bacteria such as Proteus, Klebsiella and Pseudomonas are the organisms most frequently isolated in malignant wounds (Thomas et al. 1998).

It is difficult to quantify and describe odour because a person's perception is very subjective (Benbow 2005) and this makes assessment of the wound and effectiveness of the dressings difficult. This could contribute to the reason for a lack of empirical research into the management of malodour in wounds and the effectiveness of dressings to control odour (Gethin et al. 2014).

Management of malodour
When changing dressings, ensure that the room is well ventilated and that the dressings are disposed of quickly and appropriately following removal (Wilson 2005). Finding a dressing large enough to contain leakage is often a challenge. The frequency of the dressing changes may need to be increased to reduce the odour. The dressings may quickly become saturated with wound exudate, blood and pieces of necrotic tissue and increase the malodour when left in place (Schiech 2002). Dressings appropriate for the management of malodour in malignant fungating wounds are listed in Table 6.5.

Wound cleansing
Wound cleansing is extremely important in the management of malignant wounds to remove surface contaminants, microorganisms and excess exudate and loosen debris. However, cleansing is not appropriate for all wounds; if the aim of the management of the wound is to keep the area dry, it may be contraindicated (Jones 2012). Stagnant exudate within the wound or dressing can lead to an increase in malodour (Collier 1994).

If appropriate, patients with malignant wounds can remove their dressing and shower the open wound with warm water. This can be beneficial psychologically for the patient and help them to feel clean and refreshed (Fairbairn 1994). NICE guidelines (2015b) recommend that when a clean technique is required, warm tap or shower water is the preferred choice. If a sterile technique is required in circumstances such as a patient being immunocompromised, exposed bone within the wound or prior to taking a microbiology swab, sterile 0.9% sterile saline should be used, preferably warmed to body temperature prior to use.

The use of antiseptic solutions is not recommended by NICE (2015b) because they may be detrimental to the healing of wounds

and toxic to tissues (Sibbald et al. 2000). Body fluids also quickly inactivate the solution (Naylor 2002b). If there is a biofilm present in the wound the use of sodium chloride and tap water may be ineffective as biofilms may be resistant to irrigation and antibiotics (Jones 2012). The use of a wound irrigation solution or gel which contains polyhexamethylene biguanide such as Prontosan was found to be effective in eliminating biofilms in an evaluation by Horrocks (2006). The study showed a significant improvement in wounds over a 3-week period and a reduction in the level of exudate.

A study by Bale et al. (2004), looking at the efficacy of metronidazole gel on malignant wounds, interestingly found that 76% of patients in the placebo arm reported an elimination in malodour. This was attributed to the fact that while the patients were on the study their wounds were thoroughly cleaned and their dressings changed on a regular basis. These findings support the need for regular cleansing and redressing of wounds to be carried out according to the requirements of the wound and the severity of the symptoms (Draper 2005).

Debridement
The management of malodour in a wound requires the odour to be contained and the cause to be treated. Debridement of devitalized tissue may be appropriate to reduce the concentration of the bacteria. The method of debridement should be based on the assessment of the wound, and guided by treatment goals and patient preference (Gethin 2011). Care should be taken with debridement as the wounds are often friable and tend to bleed; surgical or sharp debridement is therefore often contraindicated (Grocott 2007). It is also suggested that surgical debridement may 'seed' the malignant cells (Hampton 2004). Autolytic or enzymatic debridement is usually the preferred method (EONS 2015). However, consideration should be given to the impact on the patient of any form of debridement that may increase the exudate level while the necrotic tissue is liquefying.

Metronidazole
If an infection is suspected a wound swab should be taken and microbiology results obtained for a specific antibiotic to be prescribed.

There are several anecdotal reports affirming the effectiveness of metronidazole and the relief that is expressed by patients within a few days (Alexander 2009d). Metronidazole is a synthetic drug which prevents the replication of bacteria by binding to their DNA, thereby reducing the bacterial burden in a wound (Draper 2005).

NICE guidelines (2015b) recommend oral metronidazole for deep tissue infections which are causing odour, with a dosage

Table 6.5 Dressings and agents for the management of wound malodour

Dressing/agent	Description	Application	Comments
Charcoal, e.g. Clinisorb/Carboflex/Carbonet	Effective for reducing malodour Absorbs small molecules and bacterial spores, making it a powerful deodorizer (Williams 2000) Available as either carbon only or incorporated with an additional dressing such as an alginate or an antimicrobial	If used on dry wounds, apply over a non-adherent dressing Consult specific manufacturer's guidance	Conflicting studies as to effectiveness of carbon when wet Studies by Hampton (2003) and Morris (2008) showed Clinisorb could be used as a primary dressing without affecting malodour-controlling properties Draper (2005) found carbon dressings most effective when kept dry and applied as a sealed unit, not always possible with fragile skin Lee et al. (2006) found that fibres may break away from dressings and they were not effective when wet. Only absorb odour, do not act on source
Silver dressings, e.g. Aquacel Ag/Acticoat	Silver is an inert metal which becomes active when it interacts with wound exudate. Ionic silver is released into the wound bed. Silver ions bind to and denature bacterial DNA and RNA, inhibiting replication (Hampton 2008)	Consult specific manufacturer's guidelines Specific silver dressings such as Acticoat require activation with water prior to application	There is limited research in the use of silver dressings in malignant wounds but observation in clinical practice has shown that they can be effective in odour control (Hampton 2008). When there is an infection present, the reduction of bacteria should lead to reduction in odour and symptoms of infection Expensive and should only be used when requirement for antimicrobial dressing is confirmed (Alexander 2009d)
Manuka honey, e.g. Activon	Manuka honey has levels of hydrogen peroxide which have a destructive effect on bacteria. Bacteria are metabolized by honey's glucose to produce lactic acid instead of the amino acids that produce malodorous ammonia, amines and sulphur compounds (White 2005) Available as an ointment, impregnated gauze or alginate dressing	Medical grade honey should be replaced or refreshed if exudate is very high or it stops being effective Contraindications: • Patients with known allergy to bee venom • Blood sugar levels should be monitored in patients with diabetes Patients may experience a 'stinging/burning' sensation on initial application – remove dressing if patient not able to tolerate	Can reduce bacterial load, combat odour, assist with debridement and have an anti-inflammatory action, whilst thought to be harmless to healthy tissue (Booth 2004). Antimicrobial and debridement actions beneficial in management of malodour as they assist in removing slough and bacteria, often the cause of the odour Not suitable for highly exuding wounds
Iodine: • Cadexomer iodine: e.g. Iodoflex/Iodosorb • Povidone-iodine: Inadine	Cadexomer iodine is an antimicrobial agent that can be used to reduce malodour in malignant wounds (Hampton 2008, Seaman 2006) Iodine penetrates micro-organisms and attacks key protein groups, nucleotides and fatty acids, which kills the bacteria (Angel et al. 2008)	Consult specific manufacturer's guidance for application Available as impregnated knitted viscose, gel sheets or paste Contraindications: dry necrotic tissue or patients with known sensitivity. Do not use with children, pregnant or lactating patients/thyroid or renal impairment	Care should be taken when considering use of iodine in friable wounds as it has a tendency to cause wounds to bleed more easily (Hampton 2008) Cadexomer iodine formats are slow release and are activated on exposure to exudate. They are able to absorb high levels of exudate, forming a gel and reducing the wound bioburden
Larvae	Larval secretions liquefy necrotic and non-viable tissue Proteinaceous material is then ingested by the larvae (BioMonde 2016)	Maggots are sealed in a finely woven polyester net pouch. Check the wound daily and change secondary dressings. Larvae can remain on the wound for 4 days prior to changing (BioMonde 2016)	There is conflicting evidence on the use of larvae therapy in the management of malignant wounds. It is thought by some authors that larvae therapy may increase the incidence of bleeding in friable tissue (Alexander 2009d). Jones et al. (1998) and Sealby (2004) described the successful use of larvae therapy in the management of malignant wounds

Dressing/agent	Description	Application	Comments
Essential oils, aromatherapy candles, room deodorizers or fragrances	Pleasant and familiar smells can increase the production of endorphins, aiding relaxation (James 2009)	Essential oils can be vaporized in the room or drops applied to the dressing Care should be taken as strong scents may induce nausea	Mercier and Knevitt (2005) chose an essential oil that was only present during dressing changes. The oil was vaporized in the room before and after the dressing change. If odour was detectable when the dressing was in place, a few drops were applied to the dressing. Eucalyptus, tea tree and lemon myrtle were found to be the most promising scents in the trial Oils have been blended into creams and applied directly to a wound; however the safety of this practice cannot be recommended without discussion with a pharmacist and must only be used by healthcare professionals with the relevant skills and knowledge (Gethin 2011)
External odour absorbers, i.e. cat litter/activated charcoal	Can be placed under the patient's bed	The use of such methods should be discussed with patients and their families and friends to avoid causing distress or offence (EONS 2015)	The use of cat litter or charcoal in an open tray under the bed, which may assist in absorbing odour, has been written in anecdotal evidence There are also reports of an open dish of shaving foam or coffee beans being used to successfully manage wound odour

239

of 400 mg three times daily for 5–7 days. If a partial response is seen, consider continuing the drug for a further 7 days. However, patients may experience side-effects such as nausea and neuropathy and the reduction of odour may only be effective for a few days (Grocott 2000). The effect may be reduced if the blood supply to the wound is compromised (EONS 2015).

The use of topical metronidazole may avoid the effects associated with the oral drug. It is traditionally thought to be effective against anaerobic bacteria; however, Thomas et al. (1998) reported that it is also effective against aerobes. There can be limited effect when the wounds are extensive and penetration of the deep tissue to reach the anaerobic bacteria is not possible (Grocott 2000). It has also been questioned how therapeutic levels can be maintained when the drug is diluted with exudate in highly exuding wounds and can be absorbed in the dressings (Grocott 2000).

Topical metronidazole 0.75% gel can be applied directly onto the wound and can be more effective than oral metronidazole when excess necrotic tissue is present (NICE 2015b). The gel should be applied liberally to the ulcer once or twice daily for 7 days. If there is a partial response, consider continuing for a further 7 days (NICE 2015b). The contents of metronidazole capsules have also been sprinkled directly onto wounds; however, this may act as an irritant on the wound bed. The practice is unregulated and has only been documented through anecdotal evidence (EONS 2015).

Metronidazole gel can be used alone or with systemic therapy to manage malodorous wounds. The gel may also expedite debridement within the wound, through the facilitation of autolysis of the necrotic tissue and slough (Gethin 2011).

Dressings and agents for the management of wound malodour are summarized in Table 6.5.

Bleeding
Tumour-induced angiogenesis and coagulopathy can result in thin-walled blood vessels that bleed easily and have reduced coagulation (Lotti et al. 1998). As a tumour progresses, blood vessels may be eroded from the tumour or from the surrounding necrotic tissue, which can increase the risk of episodes of spontaneous bleeding or bleeding from trauma when a dressing is removed (Lloyd 2008).

The overall health conditions of the patient can increase the risk of bleeding, such as abnormal platelet function and vitamin K deficiency (Woo and Sibbald 2010). Systemic coagulopathy from existing co-morbidities can exacerbate the fragility of a malignant wound (Alexander 2009b).

The bleeding can be small or a significant bleed which is hard to control and may potentially necessitate the patient's admission to hospital. This can be extremely frightening for the patient and their family and can also be challenging and cause anxiety and apprehension for nursing staff managing their dressings (Lloyd 2008). A patient may be anxious and frightened about even the slightest leakage of blood from a wound (Lund-Neilson et al. 2005).

The tumour may erode through a major vessel, which can result in a catastrophic fatal bleed. It is rare for a fatal haemorrhage to occur; however, it is most likely in head and neck tumours adjacent to the carotid artery or tumours in the groin adjacent to the femoral artery (EONS 2015). This can be extremely distressing for everyone involved. If it is thought to be a possibility, preparation should be made in advance. If possible a strategic plan should be developed with the patient and family, using dark sheets and having dark towels available (Watson and Hughes 2015). Medication to sedate the patient, such as subcutaneous benzodiazepine, should be available and prescribed in advance (EONS 2015).

Management of bleeding wounds
Much of the literature on the management of bleeding in malignant wounds is prescriptive with minimal empirical evidence on interventions (Alexander 2009c).

- Consider antibiotics if signs or symptoms of infection are present – infected wounds are more prone to bleeding.
- The patient's bloods should be monitored to ensure they are not becoming anaemic due to bleeding from the wound (Benbow 2005).
- Consider the appropriateness of radiotherapy, chemotherapy, cauterization or embolization (Yorkshire Palliative Medicine Clinical Guidelines Group 2009), electrochemotherapy (Gehl and Geertsen 2006) or surgery, depending on the palliative care goals for the patient (Seaman 2006).
- If dressings are adherent to the wound, gently soak them off and review the dressing regimen to include non-adherent dressings.
- If required, wounds should be gently irrigated with warmed normal saline as opposed to swabbing to avoid further trauma.
- If bleeding occurs the initial intervention should be to apply direct pressure to the area for 10–15 minutes (Watson and Hughes 2015).

Dressings appropriate for the management of bleeding wounds are listed in Table 6.6.

Table 6.6 Dressings and agents for the management of bleeding wounds

Dressing/agent	Description	Application	Comments
Non-adherent/soft silicone dressings or moist wound products, e.g. NA Ultra/Mepitel	Specifically designed to be non-traumatic and enable pain-free removal from the wound	Apply with secondary dressing If silicone dressing used can be left *in situ* and secondary dressing changed – refer to specific manufacturer's guidelines	To reduce the risk of trauma to the wound and subsequent bleeding, a non-adherent dressing should be used that maintains a moist surface between the dressing and the wound (EONS 2015)
Alginate dressing, e.g. Kaltostat/Sorbsan (for mild–moderate bleed)	Some alginate dressings have haemostatic properties; however, they are not licensed as haemostatic dressings The calcium ions within the dressings are released into the wound, activating platelets and leading to haemostasis (Yorkshire Palliative Medicine Clinical Guidelines Group 2009)	Available as flat non-woven pad, ribbon for packing narrow wounds or sinuses and rope for packing cavities Requires a secondary dressing Forms a gel when in contact with wound exudate Contraindications: dry/low exuding wounds, or hard necrotic tissue	Alginates can adhere to the wound between dressing changes and then cause further trauma and bleeding on removal. A silicone non-adherent dressing may be placed directly onto the wound bed and left undisturbed and the secondary dressings changed as required (Watret 2011)
Silver nitrate sticks (for mild–moderate bleed)	Works by coagulating proteins, leading to tissue necrosis and eschar formation, which leads to thrombus formation and haemostasis (Glick et al. 2013)	Apply to specific small bleeding points within a wound Can cause permanent skin pigmentation Surrounding skin should be protected prior to use	Small bleeding points can be managed with silver nitrate sticks (Seaman 2006) Creates a thin eschar that sloughs off within several days
Sucralfate paste (for mild–moderate bleed)	For a slow capillary ooze	Sucralfate paste (1–2 g sucralfate crushed with a water-soluble gel) can be applied to the bleeding point 1–2 times a day (Yorkshire Palliative Medicine Clinical Guidelines Group 2009)	
Haemostatic surgical dressings, e.g. Surgicel (for moderate–heavy bleed)	Absorbable haemostat composed of oxidized cellulose polymer, absorbable knitted fabric that is flexible and adheres to bleeding surfaces (Keshavarzi et al. 2013)		For heavier bleeding, haemostatic surgical dressings (e.g. Surgicel) can provide rapid capillary haemostasis. They can be left in place on the wound and covered with a secondary dressing (Naylor 2002b)
Topical adrenaline (for moderate–heavy bleed)	Adrenaline is a vasoconstrictor that makes capillaries smaller, limiting blood flow to the wound	Topical adrenaline (1:1000, 1 mg in 1 mL) in the form of a gauze soak should be applied with pressure for 10 minutes (EONS 2015)	There can be rebound bleeding when the effect of the adrenaline has worn off (Yorkshire Palliative Medicine Clinical Guidelines Group 2009) The use of vasoconstriction methods may lead to tissue ischaemia and necrosis (Watret 2011) and is advocated only for use under medical supervision (Naylor 2002a). This can be difficult as most fungating wounds are managed in the community
Topical tranexamic acid (for moderate–heavy bleed)	Tranexamic acid is an antifibrinolytic that stops the conversion of plasminogen to plasma, preventing the degradation of fibrin and the breakdown of clots (Noble and Chitnis 2013)	Tranexamic acid 500 mg in 5 mL soaked into gauze can be used as an alternative and applied with pressure for 10 minutes	Topical tranexamic acid is thought to have a lower incidence of developing thrombotic complications than oral route (Emara et al. 2014)
Oral fibrinolytic antagonists, e.g. tranexamic acid (for moderate–heavy bleed)		See specific medication guidance for dosage	Oral fibrinolytic antagonists such as tranexamic acid can be given to stop bleeding and prevent further bleeding (Yorkshire Palliative Medicine Clinical Guidelines Group 2009)

Pain

This section will concentrate on the management of acute non-cyclic and acute cyclic pain particularly relating to malignant fungating wounds.

Patients consistently report pain as having a major impact on their quality of life and as one of the worst parts of living with a chronic wound (Price et al. 2008). It is recognized that pain is not only physical; it can also affect the psychological, social and spiritual well-being of a patient and can limit their physical activities and social contact and contribute to an increase in anxiety and depression (Wounds International 2012).

Patients may experience the following types of physical pain with malignant fungating wounds:

- non-cyclic acute pain – occurs when a procedure such as sharp debridement is being carried out
- cyclic acute pain – occurs on a regular basis and can be related to wound care, such as cleansing or dressing removal (procedural pain), or to movement and activity (incident pain) (Naylor 2005)
- chronic pain – consistent pain that is not related to the actual management of the wound (World Union of Wound Healing Societies 2004).

The physical sensation of pain in malignant wounds can be due to several different factors such as: pressure from the tumour on other body structures; damage to nerve endings from the tumour; exposure of nerve endings; recurrent infections; impaired lymphatic and capillary drainage; trauma from wound care procedures and inappropriate dressings (Alexander 2009b, Naylor 2005).

A study conducted by Woo (2008) found that 80% of patients experienced persistent pain between their dressing procedures. Szor and Bourguignon (1999) found that 87.5% of the patients they studied reported pain at dressing change; Sibbald et al. (2006) identified that pain is often at its worst during removal of the dressing.

A full and accurate assessment of the pain a patient is experiencing and the impact it has on their quality of life is crucial in understanding the correct management required. A valid and reliable assessment tool, such as a visual analogue scale, should be used to provide an accurate assessment of the type, frequency and duration of pain to identify aggravating and relieving factors and to allow implementation of an appropriate management plan. This should be an ongoing process so that the effectiveness of the analgesia can be monitored and adjusted as required to ensure that the patient is offered the maximum relief for any wound-related pain (Day 2013).

A compassionate caring approach by the healthcare professional, and providing patients with an explanation of what to expect through dressing changes and details of the strategies in place to minimize their pain can help to reduce a patient's fear and anxiety. Increased levels of stress and anxiety have been shown to lower a patient's tolerance to pain, and a cycle can develop where pain, stress and anxiety worsen the patient's experience of pain (Woo 2008). Anticipatory pain is a significant problem. If there is a high level of anxiety a patient will anticipate more pain and can consequently experience more intense pain (Woo 2008). If there is inadequate pain management at the first dressing change that a patient experiences, it can have an impact on future management and the patient may lose confidence in the team managing their care (Latarjet 2002).

Patients should be encouraged to participate in their own care, where appropriate, by removing their dressings themselves, giving them some control and autonomy (Day 2013). They should be aware that they can request regular breaks during the dressing change if required and be encouraged to express when they are in discomfort.

Management of pain

Dressing changes should be kept to a minimum to avoid distress to the patient and trauma to the wound.

The inappropriate use of dressings can cause or increase pain for patients. Care should be taken when removing any dressings and the manufacturer's instructions should be consulted to avoid trauma, for example film dressings should be lifted at the edge then stretched up and away from the wound. A medical adhesive remover should be considered when removal of the dressing is painful or traumatic to the skin. Traditional dressings such as gauze and paraffin tulle should be avoided as they have the tendency to dry out and adhere to wounds and can become incorporated into tissues when the granulation tissue grows through the mesh pores. Soaking to remove these dressings is rarely effective (Naylor 2001). Products with an overall layer of adherence, such as hydrocolloids, foams and films, should be used with caution as they can be painful on removal (Hollinworth and Collier 2000). Honey dressings can cause a stinging or burning sensation for patients. This could potentially be due to the acidity level or the osmotic pull that they exert. See Table 6.7 for appropriate dressings and agents to manage wound pain.

Table 6.7 Dressings and agents to manage wound pain

Dressing/agent	Description	Application	Comments
Soft silicone dressing/ non-adherent dressings, e.g. Mepitel	Soft silicone dressings reduce pain at dressing changes as they do not adhere to the wound surface. There is therefore no trauma, pain or stripping of skin on removal (Benbow 2009a)	Soft silicone dressings may be left *in situ* and secondary dressings changed as required	The use of soft silicone dressings together with appropriate analgesia has been shown to lead to a dramatic improvement in a patient's pain levels and emotional state (Naylor 2001)
Alginate dressings, i.e. Sorbsan/ Kaltostat	Alginate dressings transform to a gel when in contact with wound exudate. This provides a moist environment and facilitates pain-free removal of dressings	Alginate dressings should not be applied to wounds with low levels of exudate as they dry out, adhere to the wound and cause trauma on removal	Moist wound healing is advocated in malignant fungating wounds to provide an environment where exposed nerve endings are bathed in fluid, preventing stimulation of the nerve receptors through dehydration and minimizing pain levels (White 2008)

(continued)

Table 6.7 Dressings and agents to manage wound pain (*continued*)

Dressing/agent	Description	Application	Comments
Skin protector/ barrier film, e.g. Cavilon	Liquid barrier film that dries quickly to form a breathable, transparent coating on the skin. Designed to protect intact, damaged or at risk skin from exudate and adhesive trauma (3M 2016)	Consult manufacturer's guidelines for application	Patients can develop contact and allergic dermatitis in the periwound area from corrosive exudate and dressing materials, leading to erythema, oedema and blistering around the wound edges Macerated periwound skin can cause high levels of background pain. The application of a skin barrier film can prevent trauma to periwound skin
Topical opioids	Topical opioids can provide effective relief for up to 24 hours following application (Ashfield 2005) and can significantly improve the patient's comfort in between dressing changes	When using topical opioids, several factors should be taken into consideration such as the wound aetiology and size, the monitoring of the patient and their previous experience of treatment, the dose concentration and formulation (Graham et al. 2013) Treatment is usually a mixture of morphine and hydrogel, with a dosage of 1 mg morphine per 1 g of hydrogel (Naylor 2005)	The use of topical opioids is thought to be safe due to the low doses used and the minimal systemic absorption of topically applied opioids (EONS 2015) It is thought that topical opioids can relieve inflammatory pain without causing systemic side-effects Metronidazole can be used as a carrier for the opioid to combine pain and odour control (Grocott 2000)
Topical anaesthetics, e.g. lidocaine	Topical anaesthetic works by causing temporary numbness to the area of skin	Topical preparations may be suitable for use prior to a painful procedure under medical guidance Use with caution due to potential increased absorption (Maier 2012)	Can reduce pain during wound manipulation and it is thought that patient anxiety may be reduced as they are aware that an anaesthetic is being applied (Sibbald et al. 2006)
Entonox	Entonox is a gas mixture of 50% nitrous oxide and 50% oxygen used to manage procedural pain	Appropriate training is required for healthcare professionals prior to the administration of Entonox	It can be used for rapid short-lasting pain relief such as dressing changes with no lasting side-effects (Hollinworth and Collier 2000)
Transcutaneous nerve stimulation (TENS)	Produces effect by stimulating the large diameter nerve fibres that carry the signals to the spinal cord and then inhibit the transmission of pain signals (James 2009)	Someone with expertise in the area should apply the TENS machine as the electrodes should be applied to receptor sites in areas of intact skin (Grocott 2007)	
Complementary therapies, e.g. relaxation, distraction or visualization	Visualization and imagery focus a patient's attention away from painful stimuli by creating images. Visualization is consciously selected images, and imagery is spontaneously occurring images from the unconscious (Van Fleet 2000) Distraction draws attention away from pain using an actual physical stimulus such as conversation, music or television Aromatherapy – pleasant familiar smells can increase the production of endorphins		The use of relaxation and massage can help to reduce tension and anxiety, improving pain tolerance by breaking the cycle of anxiety and pain (Naylor 2001) Aromatherapy can create a relaxing atmosphere and help with wound odour. A combination of techniques can be used to provide optimal care for a patient, such as breathing techniques, relaxation and music during dressing changes (Naylor 2001)
Acupuncture, acupressure and hypnosis	Acupuncture – needle inserted into the median that runs through the area of pain to interrupt it (James 2009) Acupressure – exact mechanism unknown; believed it allows endogenous opioids to be released into the body and improves local circulation (James 2009) Hypnosis – induced state of consciousness where patient loses power of voluntary action and is responsive to suggestion or direction	All administered by appropriate skilled healthcare professionals	Hypnosis – thought to alter thoughts and feelings, behaviour or psychological states. Can help alleviate sensory or effective components of a pain experience (James 2009)

Table 6.8 Dressings and agents for the management of pruritus

Dressing/agent	Description	Application	Comments
Tricyclic antidepressants and paroxetine			Pruritus from malignant wounds generally does not respond to antihistamines
			Tricyclic antidepressants and paroxetine can be beneficial, although their use may be limited due to their toxicity (Zylicz et al. 1998)
Bedlinen and clothing			Garments and bedlinen that reduce pruritus in conditions such as eczema may be beneficial for patients with malignant fungating wounds (EONS 2015)
Hydrogel sheets, e.g. Novogel	Hydrogel sheets keep the skin well hydrated and can have a cooling effect (EONS 2015)	The dressing should be covered with a semi-permeable film to prevent the dehydration of the dressing. If the wound is exuding, cover with a dry dressing and secure in place (Naylor et al. 2001)	Dressings such as Novogel have a cooling effect which is enhanced if cooled in a non-food refrigerator prior to use
Menthol in aqueous cream	Pre-prepared lotion such Levomenthol cream	Can be applied to an itchy area 1–2 times a day. This should be applied to surrounding skin and not directly onto an open wound	Menthol in aqueous cream can have a cooling effect and the cream does not dry on the skin as calamine lotion would
TENS (transcutaneous electrical nerve stimulation)	TENS machines stimulate the nerves that carry non-painful messages to the brain which then overrides the pain messages and can also be beneficial in the treatment of pruritus (Grocott 2007)	Someone with expertise in the area should apply the TENS machine as the electrodes should be applied to receptor sites in areas of intact skin	

Appropriate treatment should be provided for any signs of infection. An increase, unexpected pain or change in the nature of the pain could indicate that there is an infection present in the wound (Gardner et al. 2001). There may be an increase in pain from a high bacterial load which can occur prior to any signs of an infection being observed.

To reduce discomfort wounds should be irrigated or showered with an appropriate temperature solution and not swabbed unnecessarily (EONS 2015). (See Dougherty and Lister [2015] *The Royal Marsden Manual of Clinical Nursing Procedures, Ninth Edition*: Chapter 15 Wound Management.)

Analgesia should be given at least 30–60 minutes prior to dressing changes to allow for maximum effect and can be systemic, local or topical (Lloyd-Jones 2008).

Pruritus

Pruritus can be one of the most troublesome symptoms of advanced cancer and may be so severe that patients scratch their skin until it bleeds (Alexander 2009b). Itching can often be disabling and is difficult to treat as the active tumour is often the cause of the itch. A patient's quality of life can be impaired with the resulting anxiety, depression and loss of sleep (Upton et al. 2013). The itching can be intense and is often described as creeping by patients. It can be caused by the stretching of the skin over the active tumour which irritates the nerve endings at the dermo-epidermal border, leading to a biochemical reaction (Zylicz et al. 1998). See Table 6.8 for appropriate dressings and agents for the management of pruritus.

Procedure guideline 6.2 Dressing a malignant fungating wound (continued from Procedure guideline 6.1)

After the nurse has assessed the wound and decided on the clinical management plan as outlined previously, the malignant fungating wound is redressed. In practice, this is a continuation of Procedure guideline 6.1. Please refer to this for the pre-procedure steps.

Procedure

Action	Rationale
16 Clean hands and put on sterile gloves.	To reduce the risk of cross-contamination of micro-organisms to staff and patients. Aseptic technique required to prevent hospital-acquired infection when the body's natural defence mechanisms are compromised by an open wound (Loveday et al. 2014). **C**
	Gloves provide greater sensitivity than forceps and are less likely to traumatize the wound or the patient's skin. **E**

(continued)

Procedure guideline 6.2 Dressing a malignant fungating wound *(continued)*

17 If necessary, gently irrigate the wound with 0.9% sodium chloride warmed to body temperature, unless another solution is indicated (warm saline solution in tap water).	To reduce the possibility of physical and chemical trauma to granulation and epithelial tissue (Hess 2005). **C** When wound temperature drops below body temperature cellular activity decreases, slowing the healing process (Naylor et al. 2001, **E**).
18 Apply skin barrier if required (see periwound skin, Table 6.5)	To protect skin from damage due to excessive exudate (Benbow 2009a, **E**).
19 Apply the dressing that is most suitable for the wound using the criteria for dressings (see section for relevant symptom).	To promote healing and/or reduce symptoms. **E**
20 Secure dressing in place with atraumatic tape/netting or tubular bandage.	To reduce the risk of trauma to surrounding tissue (Davis et al. 2015, **E**).
21 Make sure the patient is comfortable and the dressing is secure.	A dressing may slip or feel uncomfortable as the patient changes position. **E**
Post-procedure	
22 Dispose of waste in orange plastic clinical waste bags and sharps into a sharps bin. Remove gloves and wash hands.	To prevent environmental contamination and sharps injury. Orange is the recognized colour for clinical waste (DOH 2013, **C**).
23 Ensure the patient is comfortable and draw back the curtains.	To promote well-being and maintain dignity and comfort. **E**
24 Clean hands with bactericidal alcohol rub. Wipe trolley with detergent wipe and return to storage.	To prevent the risk of cross-contamination from previous episode of care (Fraise and Bradley 2009). **C**
25 Record assessment in relevant documentation at the end of the procedure.	To maintain an accurate record of wound-healing progress (NMC 2015, **C**). See Figure 6.5.

Post-procedural considerations

Ongoing care

Dressings need to be changed when 'strike-through' occurs; that is, the dressing becomes soiled and damp at the surface or edge or leakage of wound exudate occurs (see individual dressing packs for instructions to guide practice). The medical team may take the dressing down to view the wound and the nurse should be present to monitor this and reapply an appropriate dressing. Record any changes and/or instructions in the patient's notes or wound care plan (NMC 2015). Included in the notes should be the amount and appearance of exudate, any signs of inflammation, infection or odour, and appearance of the wound bed. The condition of the periwound skin should be recorded as should any pain at dressing change. The management plan for the next dressing change should be amended accordingly.

Complications

Malnutrition and dehydration

Patients with a malignant fungating wound often have additional nutritional requirements that may be due to the loss of protein through wound exudate, often combined with a poor appetite due to nausea from their disease process or the odour from their wound (EONS 2015).

The patients have a high metabolic demand and may require regular meals and snacks during the day and consideration to be given to nutritional supplements. Exudate from malignant fungating wounds can be up to one litre per day which puts an increased demand on the patient for proteins and additional fluid intake to reduce the risk of dehydration (EONS 2015).

A nutritional specialist or dietician should be involved in the care of the patient for a comprehensive nutritional assessment. For further nutritional information please refer to Chapter 8.

Graft-versus-host disease wounds

Definition

A wide variety of haematological malignancies are treated with haematopoietic stem cell transplantation (Hymes et al. 2006). Transplantation is the use of donor peripheral stem cells, cord blood stem cells or bone marrow to reconstitute the immune system following myeloablative chemotherapy/radiotherapy with the aim to eradicate disease and extend survival (Fiuza-Luces et al. 2016). For further haematological procedures, see Chapter 2. Graft-versus-host disease (GvHD) is the immunological interaction between the donor cells and host (patient) tissue and is a serious complication of transplantation (Rodgers et al. 2013). GvHD develops in up to 50% of all transplant recipients (Pavletic and Fowler 2012), commonly affects the skin, liver, gastrointestinal tract and lungs, and causes skin rashes, diarrhoea, deranged liver function and permanent pulmonary damage. GvHD can be divided into two categories: acute (aGvHD) and chronic (cGvHD). Historically, acute is defined as any time within 100 days post transplant, and chronic any time after; however, more recently it has been acknowledged that there are overlaps and it is the clinical features that determine GvHD as acute or chronic and not the time from transplant (Jagasia et al. 2015).

Skin GvHD

The skin is one of the organs most commonly affected by both aGvHD and cGvHD (Rodgers et al. 2013) with the skin integrity being damaged and the result of loss of skin function (Dignan et al. 2012). Severe or chronic GvHD is associated with skin ulcers, reduced skin integrity and poor wound healing (Jagasia et al. 2015).

Anatomy and physiology

It is important to understand the pathophysiology of GvHD when diagnosing and treating skin GvHD. Ferrara (2007) describes the process of GvHD in three stages:

1 The first is a conditioning regimen that causes tissue damage in the host.

2 The second is the activation of T cells against the host and clonal expansion.

3 The third is the release of inflammatory cells and cytokines that cause further tissue damage.

Scheinfeld (2016) describes acute skin GvHD as:

- scattered erythematous macules and papules (a red rash that can either be flat or slightly raised)
- a rash that covers a greater total body surface area as its severity increases
- in its most severe forms, erythroderma and bullae (an intensely red and widespread rash that has larger raised areas containing serous fluid).

The clinical features of chronic GvHD include (Jagasia et al. 2015):

- pigmentation changes
- lichen planus like rash (shiny pinkish purple papules with varying configuration and distribution)
- superficial sclerotic features (localized smooth or shiny skin, leather like)
- deep sclerotic features (smooth, waxy, thickened or tightened skin caused by deep and diffuse sclerosis causing limitation of joint mobility)
- lichen sclerosus like lesions (purple, grey-white moveable papules or plaques, shiny appearance with cigarette paper like texture).

Making the correct diagnosis of skin GvHD is essential but complicated by the fact that other skin reactions such as drug reactions and infections can have a similar appearance; response to treatment and a skin biopsy are often the most reliable tools to make a diagnosis (Scheinfeld 2016).

Related theory

Diagnosing and treating skin GvHD early is essential to minimize the risk of developing wounds. However, there are also contributing factors related to GvHD that put patients at a high risk for wounds:

- Immunosuppressive drugs such as cyclosporine are given as preventative medication for GvHD but increase the risk of infections (Hausermann et al. 2008).
- Immunosuppression and/or steroids are given systemically as the first-line treatment for both aGvHD and cGvHD and increase the risk of infection (Rodgers et al. 2013).
- Patients with GvHD are at an increased risk of bacterial, viral and fungal infections (Rodgers et al. 2013).
- The use of less toxic conditioning regimens prior to transplant has enabled stem cell transplant to be a treatment option for the older patient with potentially lower performance status (Pavletic and Fowler 2012). The risk of developing GvHD alongside other co-morbidities will increase their risk of infection.
- Long-term use of steroids in the treatment of cGvHD has been proven to cause skin thinning and striae and slow the healing process (Dignan et al. 2012).
- Acute skin GvHD is often associated with gastrointestinal and liver GvHD and chronic skin GvHD, and is also associated with oral GvHD. Gastrointestinal and oral GvHD affects nutrition and can lead to anorexia (Fiuza-Luces et al. 2016), which will leave the patient vulnerable to wounds and poor healing.
- In cGvHD, where there are sclerodermoid changes, joint contractures and limitations in joint movement are common. These cause immobility and are a risk factor for development of wounds (Scheinfeld 2016).
- Bullae are a serious complication as they can break down into ulcers that are slow to heal and at risk of infection (Hymes et al. 2006).

- The psychological impact of both aGvHD and cGvHD, especially if they overlap severely, affects quality of life, motivation and self-care (Fiuza-Luces et al. 2016, Fraser et al. 2006), increasing the risk of developing a wound.
- Recipients of donor stem cell transplants have a higher risk of secondary cancer and are therefore at a higher risk of developing a skin malignancy (Hymes et al. 2006).

Principles of care

Patients with GvHD should be treated by a team experienced in recognizing and managing transplant-related complications. A referral to a dermatologist and tissue viability clinical nurse specialist (with experience in transplant dermatology) for patients with moderate or severe GvHD with all growing, non-healing wounds should be made within 2 weeks (Dignan et al. 2012).

Treatment of xerosis (abnormally dry skin) is with an emollient such as Diprobase; treatment of pruritus and erythema is with emollients such as Diprobase and a topical corticosteroid. These are topical treatments: hydrocortisone 1% is low potency and can be used over the hands and face; betamethasone (Betnovate) is medium potency; and clobetasol (Dermovate) is high potency. If clobetasol is considered as a treatment choice, a referral to a dermatologist should also be made. If there is no response to topical treatment, systemic treatment with corticosteroids such as prednisolone and methylprednisolone is then advised. Application of Diprobase and other emollients should be 2–3 times a day to maintain skin integrity. It is recommended that steroid cream should be generously applied once a day for maximum effect as opposed to sparingly 2–3 times a day.

Second-line treatment for skin GvHD is extracorporeal photopheresis (ECP), an immunotherapy that involves collecting the patient's leukocytes and exposing them to ultraviolet light. This causes apoptosis of the treated cells and a reduction in GvHD (Klassen 2010). Referral to a specialized consultant dermatologist who offers this type of treatment should be made if the patient is non-responsive or refractory to first-line treatment.

Management with the multidisciplinary team is essential. Physiotherapy can help relieve the symptoms of sclerodermoid disease and dermatopathic strictures. Occupational therapy can offer advice on complementary therapies for management of symptoms; however, use of essential oils should only be recommended by a qualified practitioner who has knowledge of GvHD. Slow wound healing in this cohort of patients is associated with not only immunosuppressive medications but also poor diet, therefore inclusion of the dietician is essential to monitor nutritional intake.

Prevention of a wound is the best treatment. Patients at risk of or known to have GvHD should be closely monitored, with early referral to the appropriate specialist. Management of a wound caused by GvHD would not differ from that of a normal wound (as described previously) but there must be a collaborative approach to the management of the wound that involves haematologists, dermatologists and wound specialists.

Skin care following radiotherapy

Radiotherapy is a common cancer treatment given to over 50% of cancer patients (Delaney et al. 2006). Radiotherapy can be given as a high-dose treatment with curative intent or, usually at lower doses, may be used to provide palliation of cancer symptoms (see Chapter 5 for further information). A skin reaction from radiotherapy is one of the most common side-effects of treatment and can cause considerable distress to the patient and compromise delivery of the planned dose (Schnur et al. 2011). However, severe skin reactions are only observed with higher doses and longer fractionations (number of treatments). Radiation used for palliation should never provoke a skin reaction beyond a brisk erythema.

Anatomy and physiology

Radiation impairs stem cell division within the basal layer of the epidermis, disrupting or sometimes halting the normal process of skin regeneration (Archambeau et al. 1995). Skin damage occurs when the rate of repopulation of the basal layer cannot match the rate of cell destruction caused by the treatment. Radiotherapy-induced skin damage is usually noted around 10–14 days from the start of treatment. There are a number of stages of acute radiotherapy skin reactions:

Erythema is the first stage of an acute radiotherapy reaction caused by exposure of the skin to ionizing radiation. Erythema is characterized by reddening of Caucasian skin or darkening of more pigmented skin types. The change is caused by dilation of superficial capillaries as an inflammatory response to basal cell damage (McQuestion 2011). Erythematous skin can feel hot and itchy.

Continued exposure to radiation can promote increased mitotic activity, leading to a thickening of the stratum corneum. The reaction is exacerbated by a reduction in sweat and sebum production. At this point the reaction is described as *dry desquamation* and is characterized by itchy, blotchy and flaky skin. Deepening

of the pigmentation will continue due to stimulation of melanocytes, and epilation may start due to hair follicle damage.

The next stage of skin reaction seen in some patients is *moist desquamation*. This occurs when the basal layer produces insufficient cells to replace those lost, resulting in the epidermis becoming denuded and the dermis exposed. The skin will become inflamed with areas of blistering or ulceration. At this point there is a risk of infection. There is usually associated pain requiring pain medication. The reaction can be distressing and uncomfortable with an exudate of serum causing added discomfort.

The final stage of the acute skin reaction is *necrosis*, tissue death, and should rarely occur using modern radiotherapy techniques.

The severity of the skin reaction can increase for up to 2 weeks following completion of the course of radiotherapy. After this peak reaction, the skin will start to repair although it may take between 4 and 10+weeks for full healing to take place if the skin reaction has been severe.

A formal grading tool, the Radiation Therapy Oncology Group (RTOG) schema, grades radiation skin reactions, based on the appearance of the skin (see Table 6.9).

Table 6.9 RTOG radiation skin reaction scores

Assessment/observation	Effect on skin	Intervention
RTOG 0 No visible change to skin		Gently wash skin with warm water and pat skin dry. Continue with regular skin care products including soaps and moisturizers. Moisturizing creams provide symptomatic relief. (Avoid moisturizers containing sodium lauryl sulphate) Assess weekly
RTOG 1 Faint or dull erythema. Mild tightness of skin and itching may occur		Increase application of moisturizing cream as required for comfort. Consider prophylactic use of Cavilon No Sting barrier spray, Mepitel film or Mepilex Lite to reduce friction. Hydrogel sheets can soothe hot or irritated skin unless there is skin breakdown. Antihistamines or 1% corticosteroids can be considered for pruritus; use sparingly Assess weekly
RTOG 2a Bright erythema/dry desquamation. Sore, itchy and tight skin		Increase application of moisturizing cream as required for comfort. Polymem can be used for dry desquamation. Dampen for better skin contact. It contains a cleansing agent and maintains a moist healing environment. Continue with RTOG 1 interventions Assess daily
RTOG 2b Patchy moist desquamation. Yellow/pale green exudate. Soreness with oedema		Continue using moisturizing cream on unbroken skin. Refer to radiotherapy nurse for specialist advice and wound dressing. Saline soaks can be used to remove slough and are soothing. Amorphous hydrogels are particularly useful behind ears, in skin folds or on perineum. Cavilon No Sting Barrier spray acts as a second skin which prevents infection and reduces pain. Mepitel and Polymem as before Assess daily
RTOG 3 Confluent moist desquamation. Yellow/pale green exudate. Soreness with oedema		Stop moisturizing cream on broken skin. Continue with RTOG 2b interventions. Refer to radiotherapy nurse for specialist advice and wound dressing Assess daily
RTOG 4 Ulceration, bleeding, necrosis (rarely seen)		Seek specialist advice from tissue viability team. Debride any eschar/slough

Sources: Intervention data adapted from *The Royal Marsden Handbook* (2016). Other text and images from The Princess Royal Radiotherapy Review Team (2011). Reproduced with permission of Ellen Trueman. RN. Former Senior Sister. Princess Royal Radiotherapy Review Team, Bexley Wing, St James's Institute of Oncology, Leeds Teaching Hospitals NHS Trust. [Table created by Punita Shah, Practice Facilitator Radiotherapy Pre-treatment, from information contained in *The Royal Marsden Handbook* (2016), Radiotherapy Side Effects; text and images adapted from The Princess Royal Radiotherapy Review Team (2011), Managing Radiotherapy Induced Skin Reactions; A Toolkit for Health Professionals]

Related theory

The degree of skin reaction depends on intrinsic (patient-related) and extrinsic (treatment-related) factors (NHSQIS 2010). These factors should be considered when determining the risk of a patient developing a more severe radiotherapy-induced skin reaction (see Table 6.10).

Radiosensitizing chemotherapy drugs used concomitantly will increase all side-effects, including the skin reaction to radiotherapy. Monoclonal antibody treatment that targets the epidermal growth factor receptors is known to produce an acne-like rash which varies in severity (Saltz et al. 2004) but particularly affects treatment fields in head and neck areas (Bernier et al. 2008).

Evidence-based approaches

A baseline assessment should note the condition of the skin at commencement of treatment and highlight any specific risk factors (see Table 6.10).

The identification of patients with a higher risk of developing a severe skin reaction is important: the patient can be advised of the expected skin reaction and it may also allow prophylactic measures to be started. Consideration should be given to the educational needs of the patient and their family or carers and their ability to adhere to skin care advice (Maher 2005).

Historically, skincare advice for patients has been derived from clinical experience (Bernier et al. 2008, Kedge 2009, NHSQIS 2010). The Society and College of Radiologists' (SCoR) Radiotherapy Skincare Guidelines (Harris et al. 2012) were developed following an extensive review of the evidence collected from research. Much of the advice recommended in the new guidelines has remained unchanged from that which has always been given; for example, there is consensus that patients should avoid heat or ice packs and should be gentle with skin care. However, there have been a couple of noteworthy changes to traditional opinion.

- There is insufficient evidence to advise patients to avoid deodorants, unless the skin is broken.
- It is suggested that patients can continue with their regular skin care products, soaps and moisturizers, although now it is advised that the moisturizer should not include sodium lauryl sulphate (SLS) as it can lead to skin thinning and loss of moisture (Tsang and Guy 2010).

There are, unfortunately, omissions from the guidelines and if patients ask for advice it should be given following the general principles of reduced friction and gentle care.

A specific area where there is no advice in the new guidelines is regarding the use of perming or chemical straightening of hair during radiotherapy to the head. The need for gentle care suggests that strong chemicals should not be applied in the area, either during treatment or for several weeks following its completion. Locally, patients have been told to avoid colouring, perming or chemical straightening of their hair until the skin over the head shows no residual sign of treatment. It is important to stress to the patient that recommended skin or hair care is only applicable in the area receiving radiation.

Table 6.11 summarizes skincare advice from a variety of sources including the SCoR and advice given by radiotherapy departments nationally. The advice is also consistent with that given by internet sources such as Macmillan Cancer Support and Cancer Research.

Principles of care

Therapy radiographers will usually be responsible for daily assessment of the treated skin and will provide the patient with skin care information. Patients with advancing skin reactions should be referred to appropriate nursing support or specialist radiographers in line with local practice. Each patient should be treated on a case-by-case basis if they progress to moist desquamation as they

Table 6.10 Factors that increase the risk of skin reaction severity

Risk factor	Rationale
Intrinsic factors	
Increasing age	The ageing process affects the epidermal cell cycle, leading to extended healing times. Peripheral vasculature is compromised with age, leading to delayed healing
Ethnic origin	There is some evidence that patients with darker skin suffer more severe skin reactions (Ryan et al. 2007).
Poor nutritional status	Adequate nutritional status provides optimum tissue repair; undernourished patients have increased likelihood of impaired repair mechanisms
Obesity	Increases the likelihood of skin folds and friction. Adipose tissue heals slowly
Skin and connective tissue disorders, e.g. bacterial or fungal skin infection or underlying skin conditions such as eczema, psoriasis, lichen sclerosus	Many skin and connective tissue disorders can compromise normal skin repair
Smoking and alcohol	Decreased capillary blood flow and oxygen levels lead to increased skin reactions and impaired healing
Co-morbidities, e.g. diabetes, HIV-related disease	Certain conditions may compromise repair mechanisms due to impaired capillary blood flow or may lead to increased likelihood of wound complications
Genetic predisposition	Increasingly believed to influence skin sensitivity and repair mechanisms
Extrinsic factors	
Dose fractionation	High total dose/high dose per fraction
Bolus/build-up, electrons or superficial X-rays	Often used to bring the dose closer to the skin surface
Concurrent chemotherapy or monoclonal antibodies	Many concurrent pharmaceutical drugs are radiosensitizers (increase the effect of radiation)
Unmodified/less sophisticated treatment techniques	May lead to inhomogeneous doses to the skin
Entry/exit sites and techniques treating through skin folds or moist areas subject to friction	Friction is known to exacerbate radiotherapy skin reactions. Folds of skin and adipose tissue act as build-up for the underlying skin

will require specialist wound care which will vary according to the site and severity of the reaction (Bernier et al. 2008).

The principles of wound healing should be understood by those practitioners who assist the patient with managing an advanced skin reaction. The suggested management of different stages of skin reaction is summarized in Box 6.1.

247

Dealey, C. (2005) *The Care of Wounds: A Guide for Nurses*. Oxford: Blackwell Science.

Delaney, G., Jacob, S., Featherstone, C. & Barton, M. (2006) The role of radiotherapy in cancer treatment: estimating optimal utilization from a review of evidence-based clinical guidelines. *Cancer*, 107(3), 660.

Department of Health (DOH) (2013) Environment and sustainability Health Technical Memorandum 07-01: Safe management of health-care waste. Available at: https://www.gov.uk/government/uploads/system/uploads/attachment_data/file/167976/HTM_07-01_Final.pdf (Accessed: 5/3/2018)

Dignan, F.L., Scarisbrick, J.J., Cornish, J., et al.: Haemato-Oncology Task Force of the British Force of the British Committee for Standards in Haematology: British Society for the Blood and Marrow Transplantation (2012) Organ-specific management and supportive care in chronic graft-versus-host disease. *British Journal of Haematology*, 158(1), 62–78.

Dormand, E.L., Banwel, P. & Goodacre, T. (2005) Radiotherapy and wound healing. *International Wound Journal*, 2(2), 112–127.

Dougherty, L. and Lister, S. (2015) *The Royal Marsden Manual of Clinical Nursing Procedures*, Professional Edition, 9th. Oxford: John Wiley & Sons.

Dowsett, C. (2002) Malignant fungating wounds: assessment and management. *British Journal of Community Nursing*, 7(8), 394–400.

Dowsett, C. (2015) Breaking the cycle of hard-to-heal-wounds: balancing the cost of care. *Wounds International*, 6(2), 17–21.

Draper, C. (2005) The management of malodour and exudate in fungating wounds. *British Journal of Nursing*, 14(11), S4–S8.

Emara, W.M., Moez, K.K. & Elkhouly, A.H. (2014) Topical versus intravenous tranexamic acid as a blood conservation intervention for reduction of post-operative bleeding in hemiarthroplasty. *Anesthesia Essays and Researches*, 8(1), 48–53.

European Oncology Nursing Society (EONS) (2015) *Recommendations for the Care of Patients with Malignant Fungating Wounds*. Available at: http://www.cancernurse.eu/documents/EONSMalignantFungatingWounds.pdf (Accessed: 5/3/2018)

European Wound Management Association (2004) *Wound bed preparation in practice. Position document*. Available at: http://www.woundsinternational.com/media/issues/87/files/content_49.pdf (Accessed: 5/3/2018)

Fairbairn, K. (1994) A challenge that requires further research: management of fungating breast lesions. *Professional Nurse*, 9(4), 272–277.

Ferrara, J.L. (2007) Novel strategies for the treatment and diagnosis of graft-versus-host disease. *Best Practice Research Clinical Haematology*, 20(1), 91–97.

Fiuza-Luces, C., Simpson, R. J., Ramirez, M., Lucia, A. & Berger, N.A. (2016) Physical function and quality of life in patients with chronic GvHD: a summary of preclinical and clinical studies and a call for exercise intervention trials in patients. *Bone Marrow Transplantation*, 51, 13–26.

Fraise, A.P. & Bradley, T. (eds) (2009) *Ayliffe's Control of Healthcare-Associated Infection: A Practical Handbook*, 5th edn. London: Taylor & Francis.

Fraser, C. J., Bhatia, S., Ness, K., et al. (2006) Impact of chronic graft-versus-host disease on the health status of hematopoietic cell transplantation survivors: a report from the Bone Marrow Transplant Survivor Study. *Blood*, 108(8), 2867–2873.

Gardner, S.E., Frantz, R.A. & Doebbeling, B.N. (2001) The validity of the clinical signs and symptoms used to identify localized chronic wound infection. *Wound Repair and Regeneration*, 9(3), 178–186.

Gehl, J. & Geertsen, P.F. (2006) Palliation of haemorrhaging and ulcerated cutaneous tumours using electrochemotherapy. *European Journal of Cancer Supplements*, 4(11), 35–37.

Gethin, G. (2010) Managing wound malodour in palliative care. *Wounds UK*, Palliative Wound Care Supplement, 12–15.

Gethin, G. (2011) Management of malodour in palliative wound care. *British Journal of Community Nursing*, Supplement 1, S28–S36.

Gethin, G., Grocott, P., Probst, S. & Clarke, E. (2014) Current practice in the management of wound odour: an international survey. *International Journal of Nursing Studies*, 51, 865–874.

Gibson, S. & Green, J. (2013) Review of patients experiences with fungating wounds and associated quality of life. *Journal of Wound Care*, 22(5), 265–275.

Glick, J.B., Kaur, R.R. & Siegel, D. (2013) Achieving hemostasis in dermatology – Part II: Topical hemostatic agents. *Indian Dermatology Online Journal*, 4(3), 172–176. Available at: www.ncbi.nlm.nih.gov/pmc/articles/PMC3752468 (Accessed: 5/3/2018)

Graham, T., Grocott, P., Probst, S., Wanklyn, S., Dawson, J. & Gethin, G. (2013) How are topical opioids used to manage painful cutaneous lesions in palliative care? A critical review. *Pain*, 154, 1920–1928.

Grocott, P. (2000) The palliative management of fungating wounds. *Journal of Wound Care*, 9(1), 4–9.

Grocott, P. (2007) Care of patients with fungating malignant wounds. *Nursing Standard*, 21(24), 57–62.

Grocott, P., Blackwell, R., Pillay, E. & Young, R. (2011) Digital TELER: clinical note-making and patient outcome measures. *Wounds International*, 2(3), 13–16.

Grocott, P., Gethin, G. & Probst, S. (2013) Malignant wound management in advanced illness: new insights. *Current Opinions in Supportive Palliative Care*, 7(1), 101–105.

Guizhen, S. (2016) A collaborative approach to reduce healthcare-associated infections. *British Journal of Nursing*, 25(11), 582–586.

Haagensen, C.D. & Stout, A.P. (1942) Carcinoma of the breast – part I; results of treatment. *Annals of Surgery*, 116, 801–815.

Haisfield-Wolfe, M.E. & Rund, C. (1997) Malignant cutaneous wounds: a management protocol. *Ostomy Wound Management*, 43(1), 56–60, 62, 64–66.

Hampton, S. (2003) Reducing malodour in wounds: a dressing evaluation. *British Journal of Community Nursing*, 17(4), 28–33.

Hampton, S. (2004) Managing symptoms of fungating wounds. *Journal of Community Nursing*, 18(10), 22–26.

Hampton, S. (2008) Malodorous fungating wounds: how dressings alleviate symptoms. *British Journal of Community Nursing*, 13(6), S31–S36.

Hampton, S. & Collins, F. (2004) *Tissue Viability: The Prevention, Treatment, and Management of Wounds*. London: Whurr Publishers.

Harris, R., Probst, H., Beardmore, C., et al. (2012) Radiotherapy skin care: a survey of practice in the UK. *Radiography*, 18(1), 21–27.

Hausermann, P., Walter, R.B., Halter, J., et al. (2008) Cutaneous graft-versus-host disease: a guide for the dermatologist. *Dermatology*, 216, 287–304.

Herst, P. (2014) Protecting the radiation damaged skin from friction: a mini review. *Journal of Medical Radiation Sciences*, 61(2), 119–125.

Hess, C. (2005) *Wound Care*. Philadelphia: Lippincott Williams & Wilkins.

Hollinworth, H. & Collier, M. (2000) Nurses views about pain and trauma at dressing changes: results of a national survey. *Journal of Wound Care*, 9(8), 369–373.

Horrocks, A. (2006) Prontosan wound irrigation and gel: management of chronic wounds. *British Journal of Nursing*, 15(22), 1222–1228.

Hymes, S.R., Turner, M.L., Champlin, R.C. & Couriel, D.R. (2006) Cutaneous manifestations of chronic graft-versus-host disease. *Biology of Blood and Marrow Transplantation*, 12, 1101–1113.

Jagasia, M.H., Greinix, H.T., Arora, M., et al. (2015) National Institutes of Health Consensus Development Project on Criteria for Clinical Trials in Chronic Graft-versus-Host Disease: I. The 2014 Diagnosis and Staging Working Group Report. *Biology of Blood and Marrow Transplantation*, 21, 389–401.

James, S. (2009) Non-pharmacological methods of pain control. Wounds UK. Available at: www.wounds-uk.com/media/WUK/Books/trauma2-Chap_9_r.pdf (Accessed: 5/3/2018)

Jones, M. (2012) Wound cleansing: is it necessary, or just a ritual? *Nursing and Residential Care*, 14(8), 396–399.

Jones, M., Andrews, A. & Thomas, S. (1998) A case history describing the use of sterile larvae (maggots) in malignant wounds. Worldwide wounds. Available at: http://www.worldwidewounds.com/1998/february/Larvae-Case-Study-Malignant-Wounds/Larvae-Case-Study-Malignant-Wounds.html (Accessed: 5/3/2018)

Kedge, E.M. (2009) A systematic review to investigate the effectiveness and acceptability of interventions for moist desquamation in radiotherapy patients. *Radiography*, 15(3), 247–257.

Keshavarzi, S., MacDougall, M., Lulic, D., Kasasbeh, A. & Levy, M. (2013) Clinical experience with the surgical family of absorbable hemostats (oxidized regenerated cellulose) in neurosurgical applications: a review. *Wounds*, 25(6), 160–167.

Klassen, J. (2010) The role of photopheresis in the treatment of graft-versus-host disease. *Current Oncology*, 17(2), 55–58.

Latarjet, J. (2002) The management of pain associated with dressing changes in patients with burns. http://www.worldwidewounds.com/2002/november/Latarjet/Burn-Pain-At-Dressing-Changes.html (Accessed: 5/3/2018)

Lee, G., Anand, S.C., Rajendran, S. & Walker, I. (2006) Overview of current practice and future trends in the evaluation of dressings for malodorous wounds. *Journal of Wound Care*, 15(18), 344–346.

Lloyd, H. (2008) Management of bleeding and malodour in fungating wounds. *Journal of Community Nursing*, 22(8/9), 28–32.

Lloyd-Jones, M. (2008) Treatment of superficial wounds and management of associated pain. *Primary Health Care*, 18(4), 41–46.

Lo, S., Hu, W., Hayter, M., Chang, S., Hsu, M. & Wu, L. (2008) Experiences of living with a malignant fungating wound: a qualitative study. *Journal of Clinical Nursing*, 17(20), 2699–2708.

Lotti, T., Rodofili, C., Benci, M. & Menchin, G. (1998) Wound-healing problems associated with cancers. *Journal of Wound Care*, 7(2), 81–84.

Loveday, H.P., Wilson, J.A., Pratta, R.J., et al. (2014) Epic 3: National evidence-based guidelines for preventing healthcare associated infection in NHS Hospitals in England. *Journal of Hospital Infection*, 86(S1), S1–S70. Available at: https://www.his.org.uk/files/3113/8693/4808/epic3_National_Evidence-Based_Guidelines_for_Preventing_HCAI_in_NHSE.pdf (Accessed: 5/3/2018)

Lund-Neilson, B., Muller, K. & Adamsen, L. (2005) Malignant fungating wounds in women with breast cancer: feminine and sexual perspectives. *Journal of Clinical Nursing*, 14, 56–64.

Lund-Neilson, B., Midguard, J., Roth, M. Gottrup, F. & Adamsen, L. (2011) An avalanche of ignoring: a qualitative study of health care avoidance in women with malignant breast cancers. *Cancer Nursing*, 34(4), 277–285.

Maher, K.E. (2005) Radiation therapy: toxicities and management. In: Yarbro, C.H., Frogge, M.H. & Goodman, M. (eds) *Cancer Nursing: Principles and Practice*, 6th edn. Sudbury, MA: Jones and Bartlett, pp. 283–314.

Maier, M. (2012) Treatment of painful cutaneous wounds. Practical Pain Management. Available at: http://www.practicalpainmanagement.com/pain/other/treatment-painful-cutaneous-wounds (Accessed: 5/3/2018)

Malheiro, E., Pinto, A., Choupina, M., Barroso, L., Reis, J. & Amarante, J. (2001) Marjolin ulcer of the scalp: case report and literature review. *Annals of Burns and Fire Disasters* 14(1). Available at: http://www.medbc.com/annals/review/vol_14/num_1/text/vol14n1p39.htm (Accessed: 5/3/2018).

Marty, M., Sersa, G. & Garbay, J.R. (2006) Electrochemotherapy: an easy, highly effective and safe treatment of cutaneous and subcutaneous metastases: results of ESOPE (European Standard Operating Procedures of Electrochemotherapy). *European Journal of Cancer Supplements*, 4(11), 3–13.

McDonald, A. & Lesage, P. (2006). Palliative management of pressure ulcers and malignant wounds in patients with advanced illness. *Journal of Palliative Medicine*, 9(2), 285–295.

McManus, J. (2007) Principles of skin and wound care: the palliative approach. *End of Life Care*, 1(1), 8–19.

McQuestion, M. (2006) Evidence-based skin care management in radiation therapy. *Seminars in Oncology Nursing*, 22(3), 163–173.

McQuestion, M. (2011) Evidence-based skin care management in radiation therapy. *Seminars in Oncology Nursing*, 27(2), e1–e17: clinical update.

Mercier, D. & Knevitt, A. (2005) Using topical aromatherapy for the management of fungating wounds in a palliative care unit. *Journal of Wound Care*, 14(10), 497–501.

Moody, M. & Grocott, P. (1993) Let us extend our knowledge base: assessment and management of fungating wounds. *Professional Nurse*, 8(9), 58–79.

Moore, S. (2002) Cutaneous metastatic breast cancer. *Clinical Journal of Oncology Nursing*, 6(5), 255–260.

Morris, C. (2008) Wound odour: principles of management and the use of clinisorb. *British Journal of Nursing*, Tissue Viability Supplement, 17(6).

Naylor, W. (2001) Assessment and management of pain in fungating wounds. *British Journal of Nursing*, 10 (suppl22), 833–836.

Naylor, W. (2002a) Part 1: Symptom control in the management of fungating wounds. http://www.worldwidewounds.com/2002/march/Naylor/Symptom-Control-Fungating-Wounds.html (Accessed: 5/3/2018)

Naylor, W. (2002b) Malignant wounds: aetiology and principles of management. *Nursing Standard*, 16(52), 45–53.

Naylor, W. (2005) Guidelines for wound management in palliative care. Available at: https://www.nzwcs.org.nz/images/publications/wound-managementguidelines-text.pdf (Accessed: 5/3/2018)

Naylor, W., Laverty, D. & Mallett, J. (2001) *The Royal Marsden Hospital Handbook of Wound Management in Cancer Care*. Oxford: Blackwell Science.

NHSQIS (2010) Best Practice Statement: Skincare of Patients Receiving Radiotherapy. NHS Quality Improvement Scotland. Available at: http://www.healthcareimprovementscotland.org/previous_resources/best_practice_statement/radiotherapy_skincare.aspx (Accessed: 24/4/2018)

NICE (2015a) Electrochemotherapy for metastases in the skin from tumours of non-skin origin and melanoma. Available at: www.nice.org.uk/guidance/ipg446 (Accessed: 24/4/2018)

NICE (2015b) Palliative care – malignant skin ulcer. Available at: https://cks.nice.org.uk/palliative-care-malignant-skin-ulcer (Accessed: 5/3/2018)

NMC (2015) Record keeping guidance. Available at: https://www.nmc.org.uk/standards/code/record-keeping/ (Accessed: 5/3/2018)

NMC (2017) Principles of consent: guidance for nursing staff. Available at: https://www.rcn.org.uk/professional-development/publications/pub-006047 (Accessed: 24/4/2018)

Noble, S. & Chitnis, J. (2013) Case report: use of tranexamic acid to stop localised bleeding. *Emergency Medical Journal*, 30, 509–510.

Pavletic, S.Z. & Fowler, D.H. (2012) Are we making progress in GVHD prophylaxis and treatment? *Hematology*, 2012, 251–264.

Pearson, I. & Mortimer, P.S. (2004) Skin problems in palliative medicine. In: Doyle, D., Hanks, G., Cherny, N. & Calman, K. (eds) *Oxford Textbook of Palliative Medicine*. Oxford: Oxford University Press, pp. 618–627.

Piggin, C. & Jones, V. (2009) Malignant fungating wounds: an analysis of the lived experience. *Journal of Wound Care*, 18(2), 57–64.

Price, P.E., Fagervik-Morton, H. & Mudge, E.J. (2008) Dressing-related pain in patients with chronic wounds: an international patient perspective. *Internal Wound Journal*, 5, 159–171.

Probst, S., Arber, A., Trojan, A. & Faithfull, S. (2012) Caring for a loved one with a malignant fungating tumour. *Support Cancer Care*, 20, 3065–3070.

Reynolds, H. & Gethin, G. (2015) The psychosocial effects of malignant fungating wounds. *EMWA Journal*, 15(2), 29–32.

Riot, S., DeBonnecaze, G., Garrido, I., Ferron, G., Grolleau, J. & Chaput, B. (2015) Is the use of negative pressure wound therapy for a malignant wound legitimate in a palliative context? 'The concept of NPWT ad vitam': a case series. *Palliative Medicine*, 29(5), 470–473.

Ristic B (2004) Radiation recall dermatitis. *International Journal of Dermatology*, 43(9), 627–631.

Rodgers, C.J., Burge, S., Scarisbrick, J. & Peniket, A. (2013) More than skin deep? Emerging therapies for chronic cutaneous GVHD. *Bone Marrow Transplantation*, 48, 323–337.

Rogers, G. (2015) Palliative wound care: Part 2. *Wound Care Advisor*, 4(2), 30–38.

Roy, I., Fortin, A. & Larochelle, M. (2001) The impact of skin washing with water and soap during breast irradiation: a randomized study. *Radiotherapy and Oncology*, 58(3), 333–339.

Ryan, J.L., Bole, C., Hickok, J.T., et al. (2007) Post-treatment skin reactions reported by cancer patients differ by race, not by treatment or expectations. *British Journal of Cancer*, 97(1), 14–21.

Saltz, L.B., Meropol, N.J., Loehrer, P.J., Sr., et al. (2004) Phase II trial of cetuximab in patients with refractory colorectal cancer that expresses the epidermal growth factor receptor. *Journal of Clinical Oncology*, 22(7), 1201–1208.

Scheinfeld, N.S. (2016) Dermatologic manifestations of graft versus host disease. Available at: http://emedicine.medscape.com/article/1050580-overview (Accessed: 5/3/2018)

Schiech, L. (2002) Malignant cutaneous wounds. *Clinical Journal of Oncology Nursing*, 6(5), 1–5.

Schnur, J.B., Ouellette, S.C., DiLorenzo, T.A., Green, S. & Montgomery, G. (2011) A qualitative analysis of acute skin toxicity among breast cancer radiotherapy patients. *Psychooncology*, 20(3), 260–268.

Schulz, V., Kozell, K., Biondo, P.D., et al. (2009) The malignant wound assessment tool: a validation study using a Delphi approach. *Palliative Medicine*, 23(3), 266–273.

Sealby, N. (2004) The use of maggot therapy in the treatment of a malignant foot wound. *British Journal of Community Nursing*, 9(3), S16–S19.

Seaman, S. (2006) Management of malignant fungating wounds in advanced cancer. *Seminars in Oncology Nursing*, 22(3), 185–193.

Sibbald, R., Williamson, G.D., Orsted, H., et al. (2000) Preparing the wound bed – debridement, bacterial balance, and moisture balance. *Ostomy/Wound Management*, 46(11), 14–35.

Sibbald, R., Katchky, A. & Queen, D. (2006) Medical management of chronic wound pain. *Wounds UK*, 2(4), 74–89.

Szor, J.K. & Bourguignon, C. (1999) Description of pressure ulcer pain at rest and at dressing change. *Journal of Wound Ostomy & Continence Nursing*, 26(3), 115–120.

Thomas, S. (2009) *Formulary of Wound Management Products*, 10th edn. Liphook: Euromed Communications.

Thomas, S., Fisher, B., Fram, P. & Waring, M. (1998) Odour absorbing dressings: a comparative laboratory study. World Wide Wounds. Available at: http://www.worldwidewounds.com/1998/march/Odour-Absorbing-Dressings/odour-absorbing-dressings.html (Accessed: 5/3/2018)

Tickle, J. (2015) Wound exudate: a survey of current understanding and clinical competency. *British Journal of Nursing*, 24(20), S38–S43.

Tsang, M. & Guy, R.H. (2010) Effect of Aqueous cream BP on human stratum corneum in vivo. *British Journal of Dermatology*, 163, 954–958.

Upton, D., Richardson, C., Andrews, A. & Rippon, M. (2013) Wound pruritus: prevalence, aetiology and treatment. *Journal of Wound Care*, 22 (9), 501–508.

Van Fleet, S. (2000) Relaxation and imagery for symptom management: improving patient assessment and individualising treatment. *Oncology Nursing Forum*, 27(3), 501–510.

Watret, L. (2011) Management of a fungating wound. *Journal of Community Nursing*, 25(2), 31–36.

Watson, H. & Hughes, A. (2015) Symptom Management Guidelines: Care of Malignant Wounds. BC Cancer Agency. Available at: http://www.bccancer.bc.ca/nursing-site/Documents/10.%20Malignant%20Wounds.pdf (Accessed: 24/4/2018)

Westbury, C., Hines, F., Hawkes, E., Ashley, S., & Brada, M. (2000) Advice on hair and scalp care during cranial radiotherapy: a prospective randomized trial. *Radiotherapy and Oncology*, 54(2), 109–116.

White, R.J. (2005) The benefits of honey in wound management. *Nursing Standard*, 20(10), 57–64.

White, R.J. (2008) Pain assessment and management in patients with chronic wounds. *Nursing Standard*, 22(32), 62–68.

Williams, C. (2000) Clinisorb activated charcoal dressing for odour control. *British Journal of Nursing*, 9(15), 1016–1019.

Wilson, V. (2005) Assessment and management of fungating wounds: a review. *British Journal of Community Nursing*, 10, 828–834.

Winnipeg Regional Health Authority (WRHA) (2014) Malignant fungating wounds. Available at: http://www.wrha.mb.ca/extranet/eipt/files/EIPT-013-007.pdf (Accessed: 5/3/2018)

Woo, K.Y. (2008) Meeting the challenges of wound associated pain: anticipatory pain, anxiety, stress and wound healing. *Ostomy Wound Management*, 54(49), 10–12.

Woo, K.Y. & Sibbald, R.G. (2010) Local wound care for malignant and palliative wounds. *Advances in Skin & Wound Care*, 23, 417–428.

World Health Organization (WHO) (2009) WHO Guidelines on Hand Hygiene in Health Care. Available at: http://apps.who.int/iris/bitstream/10665/44102/1/9789241597906_eng.pdf (Accessed: 5/3/2018)

World Union of Wound Healing Societies (WUWHS) (2004) Principles of best practice. A WUWHS initiative: minimising pain at wound dressing-related procedures. A consensus document. http://www.woundsinternational.com/consensus-documents/view/minimising-pain-at-wound-dressing-related-procedures-a-consensus-document (Accessed: 5/3/2018)

World Union of Wound Healing Societies (WUWHS) (2007) Principles of best practice: wound exudate and the role of dressings: a consensus document. Available at: http://www.woundsinternational.com/media/issues/82/files/content_42.pdf (Accessed: 5/3/2018)

Wounds International (2012) International consensus. Optimising wellbeing in people living with a wound. Available at: http://www.woundsinternational.com/consensus-documents/view/international-consensus-optimising-wellbeing-in-people-living-with-a-wound (Accessed: 5/3/2018)

Yorkshire Palliative Medicine Clinical Guidelines Group (2009) Guidelines on the management of bleeding for palliative care patients with cancer – summary. Available at: www.palliativedrugs.com/download/090331_Summary_bleeding_guidelines.pdf (Accessed: 5/3/2018)

Zylicz, Z., Smits, C. & Krajnik, M. (1998) Paroxetine for pruritus in advanced cancer pain. *Journal of Pain Symptom Management*, 16(2), 121–124.

Chapter 7

Acute oncology

Procedure guidelines

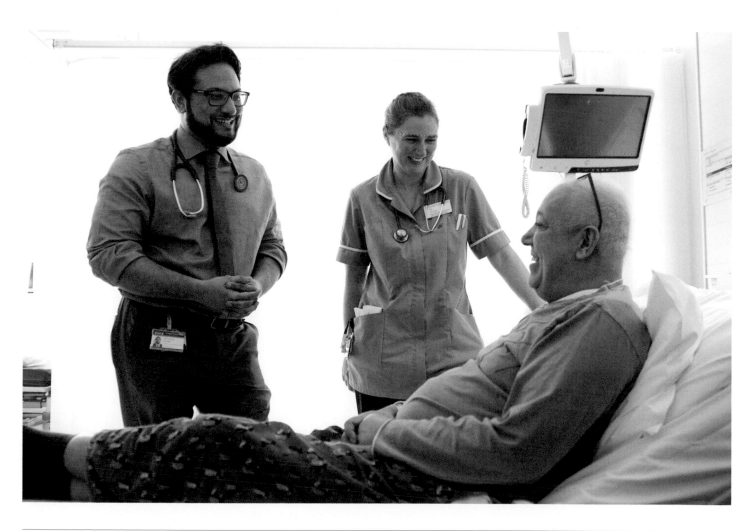

Overview

Acute oncology is an area of cancer care that deals with oncological emergencies. These can occur either because of the cancer itself or from its treatments (Watson et al. 2006). It has been shown that early diagnosis and treatment in any acute deterioration are necessary to prevent major morbidity or mortality.

Cancer is the second leading cause of death across most of the Western world (McCurdy and Shanholtz 2012). People with cancer may present at some point in their cancer journey with a cancer-related emergency; this may even be their initial presentation. They may also present via many routes, not just through the accident and emergency department (A&E) (DH 2011, National Cancer Intelligence Network 2010, Putt and Jones 2014). The literature now suggests that slightly less than 50% of cancer patients will die from their cancer, accentuating the need for optimal symptom management and recognition of any acute deterioration that may be reversible (Hjermstad et al. 2016).

Inpatient care accounts for 50% of all cancer expenditure, and inpatient cancer care accounts for 12% of all acute inpatient bed stays (National Audit Office 2010). Emergency admissions for cancer rose by 30% from 1997 to 2007 (Mort et al. 2008). It is estimated that an average hospital will have five cancer patients admitted to A&E every day (Mort et al. 2008, National Chemotherapy Advisory Group [NCAG] 2009). Acute oncology cancer nursing is about recognizing these patients and their symptoms and instituting appropriate care and management in conjunction with the whole team. Aggressive management may be appropriate even in advanced disease if the toxicity is reversible. However these decisions should be made on an individual basis and as far as possible with information regarding the patient's treatment plan, prognosis and wishes.

Most oncological emergencies can be classified as metabolic, haematological, structural (as seen in Table 7.1), or side-effects from chemotherapy agents (Higdon and Higdon 2006). Some

Table 7.1 Examples of oncological emergencies, cancer of origin, signs and symptoms

Oncological emergency	Cancer or treatment causes	Common presenting symptoms	Rare presenting symptoms
Neutropenic sepsis	All cancers where the disease or treatment causes bone marrow suppression	• Temperature >38°C (101°F) • Temperature >37.5°C and feeling generally unwell and associated coryzal symptoms • Coryzal symptoms (cough, runny nose, etc.) • Absolute neutrophil count less than 500/mm^3 (0.5×10^9/L)	• Rash • Mouth ulcers and feeling unwell
Metastatic spinal cord compression (MSCC)	Lung, breast, prostate, multiple myeloma, renal, lymphoma	• Back pain – increased by straining or laying flat • Limb weakness • Difficulty walking • Sensory loss • Altered bowel or bladder sensation or incontinence • Neurological signs	• Nocturnal spinal pain • Crush fracture • Impotence • Saddle anaesthesia
Hypercalcaemia of malignant origin	Lung (particularly squamous cell), breast, kidney, myeloma, leukaemias	• Nausea • Vomiting • Constipation • Fatigue • Weakness • Cardiac arrhythmias • Polydipsia • Polyuria • Cognitive dysfunction • Incidental	• Depression • Pancreatitis • Renal calculi
Superior vena cava obstruction (SVCO)	Lung (particularly squamous origin), mediastinal metastases, lymphoma (particularly non-Hodgkin), central venous access devices	• Facial oedema • Superficial venous dilatation (neck and upper thorax) • Dyspnoea • Headache • Dizziness • Nasal congestion • Hoarseness • Cough • Stridor • Alteration of consciousness	
Tumour lysis syndrome (TLS)	Any advanced cancer, beginning of antineoplastic treatment (particularly for lymphomas, leukaemias, metastatic germ cell)	Signs of: • Hyperuricaemia • Hyperkalaemia – cardiac arrhythmias • Hyperphosphataemia – muscle cramps, tetany • Hypocalcaemia – memory loss, confusion, muscle cramps • Acute kidney injury	

Oncological emergency	Cancer or treatment causes	Common presenting symptoms	Rare presenting symptoms
Acute kidney injury (AKI)	Any cancer or its treatment (particularly nephrotoxic drugs)	• Dehydration • Oliguria • Sepsis • Swelling in legs, ankles, and around the eyes • Fatigue or tiredness • Shortness of breath • Confusion • Nausea	• Chest pain or pressure • Seizures or coma in severe cases

Source: Adapted from Cassidy et al. (2015), Higdon and Higdon (2006), McCurdy and Shanholtz (2012).

oncological emergencies are insidious and may take months to develop, whereas others can manifest in hours and are potentially life threatening (Higdon and Higdon 2006). If patients with potentially serious symptoms do not present in a timely manner, optimum management might not be possible. The National Confidential Enquiry into Patient Outcome and Death audit into deaths within 30 days of receiving systemic anticancer therapy (Mort et al. 2008) confirmed that substantial numbers of patients did not recognize toxic effects or seek advice appropriately or did not want to bother health professionals. Therefore, before any cancer treatment, including supportive therapies, is delivered, patients and carers must be educated about the optimum management of potentially life-threatening effects and their role in recognizing and reporting side-effects. An assessment at every clinical meeting of the symptoms being experienced by the patient is essential, along with reiteration of the information.

In many areas across the UK cancer patients have access to 24-hour patient advice lines. The UK has led the way in the development of these services, with the UK Oncology Nursing Society (UKONS) establishing a validated telephone triage tool (Figure 7.1) and toxicity grading guide (Figure 7.2).

These tools provide nurses with a framework for improving patient safety and empowering them to make the correct patient management decision (UKONS 2016). The initial assessment undertaken at telephone triage provides evidence either that the patient requires further assessment or supports the nurse to provide advice, avoiding unnecessary admissions or visits to emergency settings. Optimal management of oncological emergencies requires the nurse to:

• promptly recognize signs of deterioration in the patient
• have a good knowledge of the clinical symptoms of the more common acute oncology presentations
• understand cancer's natural history and have an appreciation of the purpose of the treatment
• be aware of the side-effects of the main treatment modalities
• prioritize patients and their management and know when to escalate.

When caring for a cancer patient who presents as or becomes acutely unwell there are some simple questions to ask that will aid clinical reasoning:

1 Is there a previous diagnosis of malignancy?
2 Are symptoms due to tumour or complications of treatment?
3 What treatment is the patient having (or has had)?
4 How quickly are symptoms progressing?
5 What is the interval between treatment and onset of symptoms?
6 Should treatment be directed at treating the malignancy or the complication?
7 What are the patient's other existing medical conditions?

The oncological emergencies described in this chapter have been ordered according to the Higdon and Higdon (2006) classification:

• Haematological:
  – central venous access device complications
  – major artery vessel rupture
  – superior vena cava obstruction.
• Metabolic:
  – hypercalcaemia of malignancy
  – hypomagnesaemia.
• Side-effects from chemotherapy agents:
  – diarrhoea
  – nausea and vomiting
  – neutropenic sepsis
  – pneumonitis.
• Structural:
  – ascites (malignant)
  – bowel obstruction (malignant)
  – metastatic spinal cord compression
  – pericardial effusion (malignant)
  – raised intracranial pressure due to malignant disease.

Haematological emergencies

Central venous access device complications

Definition
A central venous access device (CVAD) is a catheter that is inserted into the central venous system (Dougherty and Lister 2015, RCN 2016) with the tip placed within the:

• superior vena cava (SVC)
• inferior vena cava (IVC)
• right atrium (RA).

CVADs allow medications to be delivered directly into larger veins, are less likely to clot, and can be left in for long periods. They are small, flexible tubes placed in large veins for people in whom frequent access to the bloodstream is required. The most common uses of CVADs and their advantages are shown in Table 7.2.

There are several risks and complications related to CVADs, of which the most common will be discussed in this section. For further information regarding the insertion, care, use or management of vascular access devices, including extravasation of systemic anticancer therapy (SACT), please refer to Chapter 4.

The most common complications associated with CVADs are thrombosis, infection and extravasation (Dougherty 2006, Kayley 2008, RCN 2016). The patient should be told to report signs of redness and tracking at the exit site, along the skin tunnel or up the arm, any oozing at the exit site and fevers or rigors.

255

ONCOLOGY/HAEMATOLOGY ADVICE LINE
TRIAGE TOOL, VERSION 2 (NOVEMBER 2016)

UKONS Oncology Nursing Society

All Green = self care advice | 1 Amber = review within 24 hours | 2 or more amber = escalate to red | Red = attend for assessment as soon as possible

Patients may present with problems other than those listed below, these would be captured as "other" on the log sheet checklist. Practitioners are advised to refer to the NCI-CTCAE common toxicity criteria V4.03 to assess the severity of the problem and/or seek further clinical advice regarding management.

CAUTION! Please note patients who are receiving or have received **IMMUNOTHERAPY** may present with treatment related problems at anytime during treatment or up to 12 months afterwards. If you are unsure about the patient's regimen, be cautious and follow triage symptom assessment.

Toxicity/Symptom	0	1	2	3	4
Fever - receiving or has received Systemic Anti Cancer Treatment (SACT) within the last 6-8 weeks or immunocompromised.	None.	**ALERT** - patients who have taken analgesia or steroids or who may be dehydrated or who may not present with an abnormal temperature but may still have an infection and be at risk of sepsis - if in doubt do a count. **Advise URGENT A&E for medical assessment- 999** **NB if infusional SACT in place arrange for disconnection.**			
Chest pain STOP oral and intravenous Systemic Anti Cancer Treatment until reviewed by oncology or haematology team.	None.				
Dyspnoea/shortness of breath Is this a new symptom? How long for? Is it getting worse? Do you have a cough? How long for? Is it productive? If yes, what colour is your phlegm/spit? Is there any chest pain or tightness? - if yes refer to chest pain Consider: SVCO / Anaemia / Pulmonary embolism / Pneumonitis / Infection.	None or no change from normal.	New onset shortness of breath with moderate exertion.			
Performance Status Has there been a recent change in performance status?	No change to pre-treatment normal - or fully active, able to carry on all pre-disease performance without restriction.	Restricted in physically strenuous activity but ambulatory and able to carry out work of a light or sedentary nature, such as light housework or office work.	Ambulatory and capable of all self care but unable to carry out any work activities. Up and about more than 50% of waking hours.		
Diarrhoea How many days has this occurred for? How many times in a 24 hour period? Is there any abdominal pain or discomfort? Is there any blood or mucus in the stool? Has the patient taken any antidiarrhoeal medication? Is there any change in urine output? Is the patient drinking and eating normally? Consider: Infection / Colitis / Constipation. N.B. Patients receiving immunotherapy or Capecitabine should be managed according to the drug specific pathway and assessment arranged as required.	None or no change from normal.	Increase of up to 3 bowel movements a day over pre-treatment normal or mild increase in ostomy output. Drink more fluids Obtain stool sample. Commence regimen specific antidiarrhoeal.	Increase of up to 4-6 episodes a day or moderate increase in ostomy output or nocturnal movement or moderate cramping. Drink plenty of fluids Obtain stool sample. Commence regimen specific antidiarrhoeal. If diarrhoea persists after taking regimen specific antidiarrhoeal escalate to red. If patient is or has been on immunotherapy escalate to red →		
Constipation How long since bowels opened? What is normal? Is there any abdominal pain and/or vomiting? Has the patient taken any medication? Assess the patients urinary output and colour.	None or no change from normal.	Mild - no bowel movement for 24 hours over pre-treatment normal. Dietary advice, increase fluid intake, review supportive medications.	Moderate - no bowel movement for 48 hours over pre-treatment normal. If associated with pain / vomiting move to red. Review fluid and dietary intake. Recommend a laxative.		
Urinary Disorder Are you passing urine normally? Is this a new problem or is this normal for you? Is there any change in the urine colour? Is there any blood in the urine? Is there any incontinence, frequency or urgency? Are you passing your normal amount? Are you drinking normally, are you thirsty? Consider: Infection	None or no change from normal.	Mild symptoms. Minimal increase in frequency, urgency, dysuria nocturia. Slight reduction in output. Drink more fluids. Obtain urine sample for analysis.	Moderate symptoms. Moderate increase in frequency, urgency, dysuria nocturia. Moderate reduction in output. Drink more fluids. Obtain urine sample for analysis.		
Fever NOT receiving Systemic Anti Cancer Treatment (SACT) and NOT at risk of immunosuppression.		Normal.	<36.0°c or >37.5°c - 38.0°c		
Infection Has the patient taken their temperature? If so when? What is it? - if pyrexial see fever toxicity. Are there any specific symptoms, such as: • pain, burning / stinging or difficulty passing urine? • cough, any sputum, if so what colour? • any shivering, chills or shaking episodes?	None.	Localised signs of infection otherwise generally well.	* If on active SACT treatment follow neutropenic sepsis pathway. * If not on active treatment arrange urgent local review.		

Figure 7.1 UKONS telephone triage tool. *Source:* UKONS (2016). Reproduced with permission of UKONS.

	None / no change	Grade 1	Grade 2	Grade 3	Grade 4
Nausea How many days? What is the patient's oral intake? Is the patient taking antiemetics as prescribed? Assess patient's urinary output and colour.	None.	Able to eat/drink reasonable intake. Review anti emetics according to local policy	Able to eat/drink but intake is significantly decreased. Review anti emetics according to local policy.		
Vomiting How many days? How many episodes? What is the patient's oral intake? Is there any constipation or diarrhoea? - if yes see specific toxicity. Assess patient's urinary output and colour.	None.	1-2 episodes in 24 Hours. Review anti emetics according to local policy.	3-5 episodes in 24 hours. Review anti emetics according to local policy.		
Oral / stomatitis How many days? Are there any mouth ulcers? Is there evidence of infection? Are they able to eat and drink? Assess patient's urinary output and colour.	None.	Painless ulcers and/or erythema, mild soreness but able to eat and drink normally. Use mouthwash as directed.	Painful ulcers and/or erythema, mild soreness but able to eat and drink normally. Continue with mouthwash as directed, drink plenty of fluids. Use painkillers either as a tablet or mouthwash.		
Anorexia What is appetite like? Has this recently changed? Any recent weight loss?	None or no change from normal.	Loss of appetite without alteration in eating habits. Dietary advice.	Oral intake altered without significant weight loss or malnutrition. Dietary advice.		
Pain Is it a new problem? Where is it? How long have you had it? Have you taken any pain killers? Is there any swelling or redness? If pain associated with swelling or redness consider **thrombosis or cellulitis**. Back pain consider **metastatic spinal cord compression (MSCC)**.	None or no change from normal.	Mild pain not interfering with daily activities. Advise appropriate analgesia.	Moderate pain interfering with daily activities. Advise appropriate analgesia.		
Neurosensory / motor When did the problem start? Is it continuous? Is it getting worse? Is it affecting mobility/function? Any perineal or buttock numbness (Saddle paresthesia)? Any constipation? Any urinary or faecal incontinence? Any visual disturbances? Is there any pain? If yes refer to specific problem / symptom. **Consider** - Metastatic spinal cord compression, cerebral metastases or cerebral event.	None or no change from normal.	Mild paresthesia, subjective weakness. No loss of function. Contact the advice line immediately if deterioration.			
Confusion/cognitive disturbance Is this a new symptom? How long have you had this symptom? Is it getting worse? Is it constant? Any recent change in medication?	None or no change from normal.	Mild disorientation not interfering with activities of daily living. Slight decrease in level of alertness.		999 - Urgent assessment in A&E.	999 - Urgent assessment in A&E.
Fatigue Is this a new problem? Is it getting worse? How many days? Any other associated symptoms? Do you feel exhausted?	None or no change from normal.	Increased fatigue but not affecting normal level of activity. Rest accompanied with intermittent mild activity / exercise.	Moderate or interfering with some normal activities.	Severe or loss of ability to perform some activities.	
Rash Where is it? Is it localised or generalised? How long have you had it? Is it getting worse? Is it itchy? Are you feeling generally unwell? Any signs of infection, such as pus, pyrexia Moderate = 10-30% of the body surface area (BSA) Severe = greater than 30% of the body surface area (BSA) NB Haematology, follow local guidelines.	None or no change from normal.	Rash covering <10% BSA with or without symptoms, such as pruritus, burning, tightness.			
Bleeding Is it a new problem? Is it continuous? What amount? Where from? Are you taking anticoagulants? NB Haematology, follow local guidelines.	None or no change from normal.	Mild, self limited controlled by conservative measures. Consider arranging a full blood count.	999 - Urgent assessment in A&E.	999 - Urgent assessment in A&E.	
Bruising Is it a new problem? Is it localised or generalised? Is there any trauma involved?	None or no change from normal.	Localised - single bruise in only one area.			
Ocular/eye problems Is this a new problem? Any associated pain? Any visual disturbance? Any discharge/sticky eyes?	None or no change from normal.	Mild symptoms not interfering with function.			
Palmar Plantar syndrome If on active oral SACT therapies follow drug specific pathways. Drug may need to be suspended and medical review arranged.	None.	Mild numbness, tingling, swelling of hands and/or feet, with or without pain or redness. Rest hands and feet, use emollient cream.	Painful redness and/or swelling of hands and/or feet. Follow drug specific pathway - may require dose reduction or treatment deferral. Advise painkillers.	Moist desquamation, ulceration, blistering and severe pain. Follow drug specific pathway - arrange urgent appointment for review by specialist team within 24 hours. May require dose reduction or treatment deferral. Advise painkillers.	
Extravasation Any problems after administration of treatment? When did the problem start? Is the problem around or along the injection site? Has the patient got a central line in place? Describe the problem.	None.	Non Vesicant. Review the next day.	Arrange urgent review.		

SoR   WE ARE MACMILLAN. CANCER SUPPORT

Figure 7.1 Continued

TO RE-ORDER THIS FORM, EMAIL STUDIO@TELFORDREPRO.CO.UK FORM REF: T.L.S.1

HOSPITAL NAME / DEPT:	UKONS 24 HOUR TRIAGE LOG SHEET (V2 2016)

Patient Details

Name:

Hospital no...................................

DOB...

Tel no...

Patient History

Diagnosis:

Male ☐   Female ☐

Consultant.................................

Has the caller contacted the advice line previously Yes ☐   No ☐

Enquiry Details

Date................... Time.................

Who is calling?

....

Contact no.................................

Drop in Yes ☐   No ☐

Reason for call
(in patients own words)

Is the patient on active treatment? SACT ☐ Immunotherapy ☐ Radiotherapy ☐ Other ☐ Supportive ☐ No ☐

State regimen..   Are they part of a clinical trial Yes ☐   No ☐

When did the patient last receive treatment?   1-7 days ☐   8-14 days ☐   15-28 days ☐   Over 4 weeks ☐

What is the patient's temperature? ☐ °C (Please note that hypothermia is a significant indicator of sepsis)

Has the patient taken any anti-pyretic medication in the previous 4-6 hours Yes ☐   No ☐

Does the patient have a central line? Yes ☐   No ☐   Infusional pump in situ Yes ☐   No ☐

CAUTION! Please note patients who are receiving or have received **IMMUNOTHERAPY** may present with treatment related problems at anytime during treatment or up to 12 months afterwards. If you are unsure about the patient's regimen, be cautious and follow triage symptom assessment.

Advise	24 hour follow up	Assess
Remember: two ambers equal red!		
Fever - on SACT		
Chest Pain		
Dyspnoea/shortness of breath		
Performance Status		
Diarrhoea		
Constipation		
Urinary disorder		
Fever		
Infection		
Nausea		
Vomiting		
Oral/stomatitis		
Anorexia		
Pain		
Neurosensory/motor		
Confusion/cognitive disturbance		
Fatigue		
Rash		
Bleeding		
Bruising		
Ocular/eye problems		
Palmar Plantar syndrome		
Extravasation		
Other, please state:		

Significant medical history

Current medication

Action Taken

Attending for assessment, receiving team contacted Yes ☐   No ☐

© P.Jones et al/UKONS

Triage practitioner

Signature.. Print... Designation.................................. Date / /

Follow Up Action Taken:

Consultants team contacted Yes ☐   No ☐   Date / /

Signature................................. Print...................................... Designation.............................. Date / / Time:

Figure 7.2 UKONS toxicity grading guide. *Source:* UKONS (2016). Reproduced with permission of UKONS.

Table 7.2 Central venous access devices: most common uses and advantages

Common uses	Advantages
Administration of medications: antibiotics, chemotherapy drugs, other intravenous drugs	Avoids problems that result over time from administering highly irritant medications through small veins with peripheral devices such as irritation of the vein and thrombosed veins
Administration of fluids and nutritional compounds	High rates can be given over a short period
Transfusion of blood products	
Multiple blood tests for diagnostic testing	Avoids inflammation and scarring from multiple needlesticks
	Increases comfort and reduces anxiety of possible multiple venous access

Thrombosis (catheter related)

Definition

A thrombosis is a clot of blood that can be present at the tip of a catheter or can surround the catheter, for example a thrombosis in the upper arm caused by the presence of a peripherally inserted central catheter (PICC). An SVC thrombus occurs when a catheter chronically rubs against the wall of the SVC, provoking a thrombosis at the site, and is often associated with a fibrin sheath. A fibrin sheath is defined as a heterogeneous matrix of cells and debris that have formed around catheters (Hacker et al. 2012). Three factors are required for a thrombosis to develop. These are known as Virchow's triad:

1 stasis
2 endothelial damage
3 a hypercoagulable state, caused by the following conditions: diabetes, malnutrition, dehydration, pregnancy, osteomyelitis, smoking, chronic renal failure, cirrhosis, cancer, obesity, sickle cell disease, surgery, congestive heart failure, oestrogen therapies (Gorski et al. 2010, Qinming 2012, Wilkes 2011).

Related theory

The association between venous thromboembolism (VTE) and cancer has been evaluated in recent years with increasing interest (Timp et al. 2013). Patients with cancer are at four- to seven-fold higher risk for VTE than patients without cancer, and about 15% of patients with cancer suffer an episode of VTE (Agnelli and Verso 2011, Baskin et al. 2012). The overall incidence can be 1–5% (Qinming 2012), with rates in PICCs of 4–5% (Aw et al. 2012, Lobo et al. 2009).

On the other hand, approximately 20% of patients presenting with VTE have an active cancer. Patients with VTE and cancer are hospitalized more frequently than VTE patients without cancer, are sicker and are more prone to suffer side-effects related to anticoagulant treatment. Patients with cancer have more frequently bilateral deep vein thrombosis (DVT) of the lower limbs and venous thrombosis in unusual sites (Timp et al. 2013).

When a patient has a CVAD in situ, this increases the risk of a thrombosis related to suboptimal tip position, with the risk decreasing with the use of the subclavian approach, small-bore catheters, the basilic rather than the cephalic vein and secure fixation (Bodenham and Simcock 2009). VTE may initially present as persistent withdrawal occlusion or resistance to flushing (Bodenham and Simcock 2009). Symptoms can be very acute or vague. The patient will usually complain of pain in the area such as the arm or neck, oedema of neck, chest and upper extremity, periorbital oedema, facial tenderness, tachycardia, shortness of breath and sometimes a cough, signs of a collateral circulation over the chest area, jugular venous distension and discolouration of the limb (Bodenham and Simcock 2009, Qinming 2012).

Thrombosis can be prevented by correct placement of the tip in the SVC, IVC or RA (Bodenham and Simcock 2009), monitoring of catheter function and flushing with pulsatile positive pressure (Mayo 2000). The use of prophylactic anticoagulants such as low-dose warfarin has been shown to be of no apparent benefit (Agnelli and Verso 2011, Couban et al. 2005, Debourdeau et al. 2013, Young et al. 2005). Full anticoagulation may be necessary if the patient has had previous thromboembolic events (Bishop 2009). Therefore, it should be stressed to the patient that any of the following signs or symptoms should be reported immediately: breathlessness and pain and/or swelling over the shoulder, across the chest and into the neck and arm. Early reporting may enable effective treatment and avoid removal of the device (Bishop 2009). There is, however, a lack of consensus around the management in cancer patients and heterogeneity in clinical practice worldwide (Debourdeau et al. 2013).

Diagnosis of a thrombus

If a thrombus is suspected it is important to rule out any obvious mechanical obstruction (e.g. a kink in the catheter tubing, a suture that is too tight, a clamp inadvertently left closed, a catheter tip blocked by the blood vessel wall, or malposition of the subcutaneous port needle) by carefully inspecting the CVAD and repositioning the patient (Baskin et al. 2012, Mason et al. 2014). Repositioning manoeuvres include raising the ipsilateral arm, having the patient sit or stand, or rolling the patient onto one side.

If these are all negative and a thrombus is suspected, venography or ultrasound can help evaluate the venous system (Baskin et al. 2012). Venography is the current gold standard but is not often performed because it is invasive and requires the patient to be exposed to intravenous contrast and radiation. Ultrasonography is often used as it is non-invasive, readily available and accurate (Sajid et al. 2007). In paediatrics, venography remains the most reliable diagnostic tool, however Doppler ultrasonography has been found to be a less invasive alternative (Gupta et al. 2007).

Management of a thrombus

The management of a CVAD thrombus depends on whether the patient needs the device to remain in situ for ongoing treatment (see Figure 7.3).

Patients who no longer need a CVAD

For patients who have developed a thrombus but no longer need a CVAD or in whom it is no longer functioning, removal of the catheter after 3–5 days of anticoagulation therapy is recommended (Kearon et al. 2008). However, some believe that the CVAD can be removed once a patient has been appropriately anticoagulated, as documented by an appropriate partial thromboplastin time (if unfractionated heparin is used) or anti-Xa level (if low

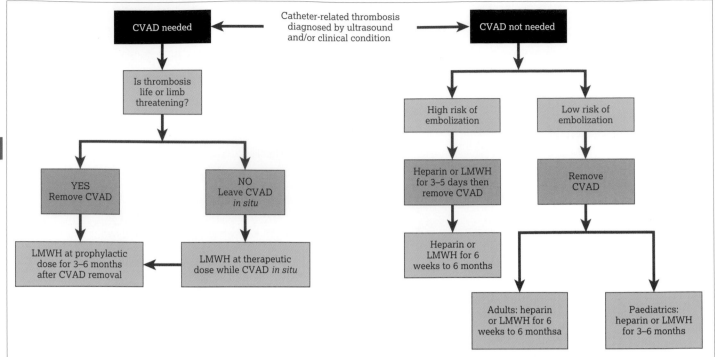

Figure 7.3 Algorithm for managing central venous access device (CVAD) related thrombosis. LMWH, low molecular weight heparin.

molecular weight heparin is used) (Baskin et al. 2012). In adults, an adequate anti-Xa level has not been associated with improved clinical outcomes with low molecular weight heparin, and some clinicians do not advocate routine monitoring of the anti-Xa level in uncomplicated patients (Debourdeau et al. 2013). In paediatrics, the response to low molecular weight heparin is less predictable and most clinicians advocate measurement of anti-Xa levels until therapeutic and then periodically to ensure that they remain within a therapeutic range (Monagle et al. 2012). The length of time a patient should be anticoagulated following removal of the CVAD is controversial. Although some physicians advocate anticoagulation for 3 months after the CVAD has been removed, others may shorten the course depending on the patient and the severity of the clot (Debourdeau et al. 2013, Monagle et al. 2012).

Patients who continue to need a CVAD

If the CVAD is required and is functional, well-positioned and not infected, the catheter can be left in place and anticoagulation therapy initiated (Debourdeau et al. 2013). If the thrombosis threatens life or limb or anticoagulation is contraindicated, the CVAD will probably require removal regardless of the patient's need for continued central venous access (Baskin et al. 2012).

For patients who retain their catheter, current recommendations include initial anticoagulation for several days with unfractionated heparin or low molecular weight heparin, followed by at least 3 months of anticoagulation with a vitamin K antagonist or low molecular weight heparin (Agnelli and Verso 2011, Debourdeau et al. 2013, Kearon et al. 2008). Low molecular weight heparin is preferred for cancer patients because it more effectively prevents recurrent thrombosis, and because warfarin interferes with some chemotherapy regimens and is more difficult to adjust when thrombocytopenia occurs (Gorski et al. 2010). Thrombolytic treatment for an upper extremity DVT is not recommended for initial therapy of a catheter-related thrombus (CRT). Additionally, if the catheter remains in place once the course of full-dose anticoagulation is complete, continued anticoagulation therapy at a prophylactic dose until the catheter is removed is recommended (Kearon et al. 2008, Monagle et al. 2012).

However, some paediatric patients require an indwelling catheter for a long period secondary to their treatment regimens and long-term anticoagulation prophylaxis may be difficult to continue. Therefore, physicians sometimes individualize the duration of anticoagulation for documented CRT based on the size and location of the clot, perceived length of time the patient has had the thrombosis, persistence of risk factors such as continued use of thrombophilic medications such as glucocorticoids and L-asparaginase, and the time span for which the catheter is required (Monagle et al. 2012).

Sepsis

Infection is one of the most common complications associated with a central venous catheter (Dougherty 2006). The catheter provides the ideal opportunity for micro-organisms to either track along the outside of the catheter or be administered via the hub internally into the central venous system. Infections can occur locally on the skin at the insertion site, in the skin tunnel/port pocket or systemically (Wilkes 2011). Signs of infection at the insertion site include erythema, oedema, tracking along the length of the catheter, tenderness at the site, exudate such as pus and offensive smell (Wilkes 2011).

Septicaemia is a systemic infection which is usually characterized by pyrexia, flushing, sweating and rigors (rigors occur particularly when the catheter is flushed) (Wilkes 2011). Prevention consists of the use of good aseptic non-touch technique and evidence-based guidelines, for example the central venous catheter (CVC) care bundle (DH 2010, Loveday et al. 2014, Wilkes 2011), as well as the use of catheters with antiseptic properties, for example those that are impregnated, bonded or coated with antibiotics or chlorhexidine or the addition of chlorhexidine in an impregnated patch or integrated into a gel dressing (DH 2007, Wilkes 2011). If the patient develops symptoms of an infection, site swabs should be taken along with blood cultures (from the device and peripheral veins). The needle should be removed from a port if there is a skin infection and the port should not be reaccessed until the infection has cleared (Wilkes 2011). Depending on the clinical condition of the patient, the CVAD may be removed and/or intravenous antibiotics may be commenced (Gorski et al. 2010).

Major artery rupture

Definition
Carotid artery rupture (CAR) is an acute major bleed with major cardiovascular manifestations, whose origin is the carotid artery in the neck (Upile et al. 2005). The term 'sentinel' or 'herald' bleed is defined as prodromal bleeding occurring 24–48 hours before the rupture of an artery that resolves either spontaneously or with packaging or pressure (Harris and Noble 2009). Carotid artery blowout is a rupture of the carotid artery or branches caused by the tumour mass compromising the vascular axis or by chemoradiation therapy (Casey 1988, Peguero et al. 2015).

Anatomy and physiology
The common carotid arteries arise from the aorta on the left and from the brachiocephalic artery on the right, and they supply almost all the blood to the head and neck. They run upwards on either side of the trachea and divide at the level of the hyoid bone into the internal and external carotids. It is at this bifurcation that there is an area of increased risk of damage due to the thinness of the arterial wall (Casey 1988, Shumrick 1983). There are three distinct layers to an artery: the outermost layer (adventitia) protects the artery and is nourished by the vasa vasorum which provides 80% of the nutrition to the arterial wall (Schiech 2000). When this essential nourishment is interrupted, destruction of the arterial wall occurs over 6–10 days (Lesage 1986).

Related theory
Studies show that CAR can occur in 3–4% of all patients who have undergone head and neck surgery (Koch 2009, Lesage 1986, Morrissey et al. 1997). However, in advanced disease CAR can account for over 11.6% of head and neck cancer deaths (Shedd and Shedd 1980). Haemorrhage may occur either externally from the neck, internally from within the oropharynx or directly into the airway or tracheostomy. Hypovolaemic shock is often the cause of death (Kane 1983), however asphyxiation from blood may also be a contributory factor. CAR can be dramatic and some preparation for the event is essential (Feber 2000, Gagnon et al. 1998, Kane 1983). This event needs immediate action and can be traumatic for all those involved.

There are several risk factors such as previous surgery, radiotherapy, post-operative healing problems, pharyngocutaneous fistula, fungating tumour invading the artery and some pre-existing medical conditions (Frawley and Begley 2005).

- *Previous surgery.* Any patient who has undergone head and neck surgery to sites local to the carotid artery is a potential candidate for a major bleed (Casey 1988, Cohen and Rad 2004). Life-threatening haemorrhage is a well-recognized complication following a radical neck dissection (Rodriguez et al. 2001). A radical neck dissection removes the sternomastoid muscle and internal jugular vein and often involves sacrifice of the accessory nerve. This is done to rid the neck of lymph nodes that may contain metastatic tumour cells. Skin flaps in the neck are raised to expose the deep cervical fascia. The fascia is also dissected from the internal jugular vein, vagus nerve and carotid artery. Surgical interventions of this nature increase the risk of CAR occurring, especially if the adventitial arterial wall is exposed and removed due to tumour infiltration, and if there are subsequent wound healing complications, infection (Nieto et al. 1980) and previous irradiation to the area (Cohen and Rad 2004). Please note if the patient has had surgery, it is crucial that their resuscitation status is clarified.

- *Radiotherapy.* Previous neck irradiation is the most common factor leading to CAR (Kane 1983, Rodriguez et al. 2001). Almost 100% of CARs occur within an irradiated field, especially if the treatment is delivered within 2 months of surgery (Nieto et al. 1980). Irradiation has been associated with a sevenfold increase in the risk of CAR in patients with head and neck cancer (Cohen and Rad 2004).

- *Post-operative healing problems.* Impaired wound healing can occur following surgery to the neck such as a radical neck dissection (Feber 2000). Deficits in circulation, oxygen and nutrients can all affect wound healing. If wound breakdown occurs this can have disastrous consequences. The carotid artery can be exposed and flap necrosis can occur, allowing the invasion of bacteria and leading to possible sepsis and desiccation of the adventitia (Cohen and Rad 2004, Lesage 1986, Nieto et al. 1980).

- *Pharyngocutaneous fistula.* Pharyngocutaneous fistula can occur as a result of wound breakdown following surgery and is recognized as an important causative factor in CAR (Feber 2000, Nieto et al. 1980). The fistula results in the adventitia being bathed in saliva, which is bacteria laden and damaging to the outer lining of the arterial wall (Casey 1988, Nieto et al. 1980).

- *Fungating tumour invading the artery.* Direct infiltration by the tumour can result in destruction of the arterial wall. A fungating wound will contain necrosis and often infected tissue, which only exacerbates the vulnerability of the arterial wall (Upile et al. 2005).

- *Systemic factors.* Pre-existing medical conditions may also increase the risk of CAR. These are: diabetes mellitus and immune deficiencies (Johangten 1998), generalized atherosclerosis (Nieto et al. 1980, Schiech 2000) and malnutrition (Okamura et al. 2002). Age of 50 years and over and/or weight loss of 10–15% are also predisposing factors to CAR (Casey 1988, Schiech 2000).

The management and care of the patient with an advanced malignancy in the head and neck demand much from the healthcare professionals involved. A CAR or carotid 'blowout' remains one of the most feared complications of head and neck cancer and its treatment (Cohen and Rad 2004, Lovel 2000). The goal of care in the event of a patient with a CAR is to ensure death with dignity, providing a calm, reassuring and caring atmosphere, to minimize the distress, anxiety and fear felt by the patient and family and often the professionals involved (Frawley and Begley 2006, Grahn et al. 2008).

Signs and symptoms
There are several signs and symptoms that should prepare the nurse for an imminent major bleed. It must be remembered, however, that there may be no warning at all in some cases and an assessment of risk factors must always be taken into consideration.

- 'Sentinel' or 'herald' bleeds can present as minor bleeding from a wound, flap site, tracheostomy, or the mouth (Forbes 1997, Lovel 2000). As the process of erosion is gradual, impending rupture of the artery may be recognized by sentinel bleeding (Macmillan and Struthers 1987). Even seemingly trivial bleeding may herald a CAR (Fortunato and Ridge 1995).
- Pulsations from the artery or tracheostomy or flap site (Casey 1988, Kane 1983).
- Sternal or high epigastric pain several hours before rupture (Anon. 1995).
- 'Ballooning' of an artery (Casey 1988, Luo et al. 2003, Schiech 2000).

There may be other indicators that a patient is at high risk of a CAR, specifically, direct observation by the surgeon that the tumour is infiltrating the arterial wall at the time of surgery. There may also be indications through scanning of the head and neck area, for example with MRI scans. The multidisciplinary

261

head and neck cancer meeting can be the ideal forum to identify those patients who are at risk (Frawley and Begley 2005, 2006, Grahn et al. 2008).

Pre-procedural considerations

Preparing the patient

When to warn a patient and family that CAR might occur is difficult to judge. It must be remembered that, although patients and families have a 'right to know', there is also a corresponding 'right not to know' and that they should have the option of choosing how much information they want to be given. It is suggested that two healthcare professionals should be present when talking to the family and have discussed prior to the meeting exactly what might be said to the patient and relatives. An open and honest approach is the best way of helping the patient and family (Bildstein and Blendowski 1997, Feber 2000, Forbes 1997, Johantgen 1998). For the patient and family who are unprepared, this will be a horrifying experience and the shock of the death can contribute to complex bereavement issues (Cherny et al. 2015, Dickenson and Johnson 1993).

Many patients and families will have contemplated how the death will occur and in most cases haemorrhage may already be an unexpressed fear (Feber 2000). Contemplating the truth and knowing what to expect, what to do and how distress can be relieved can be helpful to the patient and family (Kane 1983). It may also help the patient and family to know that in the event of a massive carotid rupture there should be little pain and that death is usually very quick (Cohen and Rad 2004). The information should ensure that patients/relatives are aware that no resuscitation will take place and this should be clearly documented in the patient's medical and nursing notes. Decide with the family if they wish to stay with the patient in the event of a CAR and be respectful of their wishes. It is important to stress to the patient/relatives that they may change their minds at any time and opt for care at home or in the hospice setting if available. Explain to the family that they will be offered a follow-up meeting to discuss the event, allowing them a chance to debrief. The family should be offered the support of the hospital relative support co-ordinator.

It is important that all the multiprofessional team are prepared; at handover the patient who is at risk of a CAR and their resuscitation status should be highlighted. Where possible the patient should be nursed in a single room to avoid shock and distress to other patients and relatives, and the equipment required in the event of a rupture must be available (see Procedure guideline 7.1) (Feber 2000). CAR happens quickly and equipment must be to hand in order to minimize the distress, anxiety and fear felt by the patient and family and often professionals involved (Frawley and Begley 2006, Grahn et al. 2008, Schiech 2000).

Pharmacological support

The pharmacological management of major life-threatening bleeding should involve the use of an appropriate sedative drug (e.g. midazolam) (Lovel 2000). In most cases an injection of 10 mg of midazolam will adequately sedate the patient. However, some patients may require further, larger doses of midazolam, for example patients on long-term benzodiazepine therapy (Roodenburg and Davies 2005). The subcutaneous route should be used in patients without intravenous access, although the intravenous route should be used in patients with intravenous access. The onset of action for intravenous midazolam is 2–3 minutes, whereas the onset of action for subcutaneous midazolam is 5–10 minutes (Twycross et al. 2014). The only indication for the use of opioids in this situation is the concurrent presence of pain.

Superior vena cava obstruction

Definition

Superior vena cava obstruction (SVCO) is caused by compression or invasion of the superior vena cava (SVC) by thrombus, lymph nodes or tumour in the region of the right main bronchus (Watson et al. 2006). The gradual compression of the SVC leads to oedema and retrograde flow (Beeson 2014).

Anatomy and physiology

The SVC is a thin-walled vessel approximately 4–6 cm in length and 1.5–2 cm wide in adults. It extends from the confluence of the brachiocephalic veins and terminates in the superior right atrium and is confined by the chest wall and surrounding structures (Watson et al. 2006, Wilson et al. 2007). A mediastinal mass, for example, impinging on the SVC can easily obstruct the blood flow; after a short period (1–2 weeks) this results in high venous pressure and upstream vessel engorgement. This in turn promotes collateral vein dilatation to reduce the pressure (McCurdy and Shanholtz 2012).

Related theory

SVCO was first described in 1757 due to obstruction from syphilitic aortitis (McCurdy and Shanholtz 2012). Lung cancer is the most common malignant cause (90%), although lymphoma, metastatic mediastinal tumours and indwelling catheters (including pacemaker leads) can also cause superior vena cava syndrome (Beeson 2014, Cohen et al. 2008, McCurdy and Shanholtz 2012). Patients with SVC syndrome usually have advanced disease,

---

Procedure guideline 7.1 Carotid artery rupture (CAR)

Essential equipment
- A selection of needles and syringes
- Non-sterile gloves
- Plastic apron
- Green/blue towels or other dark-coloured disposable towels
- Goggles
- Syringes for cuff inflation on a tracheostomy tube (10 mL non-Luer lock)

Medicinal products
- Sedation must be kept in a locked cupboard/room

Pre-procedure

Action	Rationale
1 Ensure that the patient and family are aware of the risk of CAR.	It may help the patient and family to know that, in the event of a massive carotid rupture, there should be little pain and that death is usually very quick (Cohen and Rad 2004, **E**; Kane 1983, **E**).

Procedure

Procedure	Rationale
2 Stay with the patient. Calmly call for assistance from other staff members and press the emergency call bell for assistance to aid with patient and family care and to administer any medication. Avoid panic.	To minimize the distress, anxiety and fear felt by the patient and family and often the professionals involved (Frawley and Begley 2006, **E**; Grahn et al. 2008, **E**).
3 Talk gently and calmly to the patient and hold their hand. Try to keep them in the same place if possible. Remember that being calm will greatly reassure the relatives.	To minimize the distress, anxiety and fear felt by the patient and family and often the professionals involved (Frawley and Begley 2006, **E**; Grahn et al. 2008, **E**).
4 Apply towels to the bleeding site and absorb the bleeding if possible.	Applying pressure to the area will reduce the aggressive nature of the bleed and allow time for sedation to work (Upile et al. 2005, **E**).
5 Apply gentle suctioning to mouth and trachea as necessary.	To reduce the discomfort to the patient and the family due to the sound the suctioning can make (Schiech 2000, **E**).
6 Prepare and administer sedation (i.e. midazolam) by appropriate route.	The onset of action for intravenous midazolam is 2–3 minutes, whereas the onset of action for subcutaneous midazolam is 5–10 minutes (Twycross et al. 2014, **E**).
7 If the patient has a cuffed tracheostomy tube *in situ*, inflate the cuff.	Cuff inflation prevents soiling of the lower airway with blood (Upile et al. 2005, **E**).
8 Contact the patient's medical team for advice and assistance.	This can be a chaotic situation and additional support, especially if a clear plan is not in place, will be required (Fawley and Begley 2006, **E**; Harris and Noble 2009, **E**).
9 Be aware of family presence and needs. Be respectful of the decision by the family whether they wish to stay with the patient. Ensure support is given to family and friends at this time.	For the patient and family who are unprepared, this will be a horrifying experience and the shock of the death can contribute to complex bereavement issues (Cherny et al. 2015, **E**; Dickenson and Johnson 1993, **E**).

Post-procedure

Post-procedure	Rationale
10 Relatives and friends should be offered a follow-up meeting to discuss the event, allowing a chance to debrief. They should also be offered bereavement counselling as appropriate.	For the patient and family who are unprepared, this will be a horrifying experience and the shock of the death can contribute to complex bereavement issues (Cherny et al. 2015, **E**; Dickenson and Johnson 1993, **E**).
11 All staff should be offered support, not just those immediately involved but all in the vicinity of the incident, i.e. domestic colleagues, ward receptionist, junior nurses and doctors. Other visitors may also be debriefed.	This can be a traumatic experience for those involved and staff who know the patient (Frawley and Begley 2006, **E**).

and less than 10% survive more than 30 months after treatment (Beeson 2014).

Diagnosis

Understanding the regional anatomy will enable the cancer nurse to appreciate the clinical manifestations of SVC syndrome (Cohen et al. 2008). SVC syndrome presents with symptoms related to engorgement of the upper extremities, upper thorax and head as the venous drainage is obstructed. The extent of the obstruction and therefore degree of SVC compromise will determine the clinical presentation (Higdon and Higdon 2006).

Symptoms can be as mild as slight facial and upper extremity oedema or as extreme as intracranial swelling, seizures, haemodynamic instability and tracheal obstruction (Higdon and Higdon 2006). The patient may report that their symptoms are worse in the morning and when lying flat or bending forward. Along with these symptoms there may also be venous hypertension, headaches, visual changes, dizziness, cough, engorged conjunctivae, periorbital oedema, non-pulsatile dilated neck veins and dilated collateral veins in the chest and arms.

Baseline observations are the start of diagnosis and must include respiratory rate and oxygen saturations. If the patient is breathless then cannulation and bloods, from the opposite side to the SVCO or CVAD if present (venous lactate, full blood count [FBC], urea and electrolytes [U&Es]), will help determine the level of physiological distress of the patient (Manzi et al. 2012). Although SVC syndrome is a clinical diagnosis, plain radiography, computed tomography (CT) and venography are used for confirmation of the cause (Higdon and Higdon 2006). CT scan may differentiate between extrinsic compression and intravascular thrombosis, but on occasion a venogram may be necessary, particularly if an intravascular stent is being considered (Walji et al. 2008).

Management

Management of SVCO includes symptomatic relief and treatment of the complications and underlying clinical condition (McCurdy and Shanholtz 2012).

In a patient who presents in advanced acute SVCO the following actions are recommended:

- Sit the patient upright and give 60% oxygen via a facemask.
- Maintain calmness. This will help to reduce anxiety and thus improve the efficacy of breathing in the patient. Low-dose subcutaneous midazolam may be required.
- Ensure that blood pressure is not monitored on the right arm as this may increase pressure on the SVCO. The use of a manual cuff may be required if the electronic monitor upper limit cannot be reset.

- Give any medication as soon as it is prescribed, explaining to the patient the rationale for its use. Clear communication will help reduce the patient and their family's anxiety.
  - Dexamethasone 16mg PO/IV.
  - Furosemide 40mg PO/IV.
- If the SVCO is due to a thrombus along the outside of the CVAD, initial management is removal of the device. It is recommended that the patient has an ultrasound to ascertain the size and location of the thrombosis and then is commenced on anticoagulant therapy (see Figure 7.3). If the catheter is to be removed, this should be done 72 hours after commencing anticoagulants (Pittiruti 2015). If a patient has a thrombosis but the catheter lumen is still patent, it can be used for IV therapy. The exception to this would be if the thrombosis were occluding the tip of the catheter. This can be distressing for the patient if they are needle phobic or have remaining cycles of chemotherapy. Working with the clinician is essential to ensure that the rationale is simply explained to the patient.
- Recommended treatments include chemotherapy and radiation to reduce the tumour that is causing the obstruction (Beeson 2014, McCurdy and Shanholtz 2012). However, treatment with intravenous stents is becoming increasingly common (Beeson 2014). In cases of compression, dilation and stenting of the SVC may be performed; in some cases a bypass of the SVC may be indicated (Cohen et al. 2008). Percutaneous stent placement in cases of SVC syndrome in malignancy is a simple, safe and effective technique to rapidly relieve SVC syndrome. Alleviation of severe compressive symptoms using tracheal and SVC stents in a patient with advanced lung carcinoma has been reported (McCurdy and Shanholtz 2012).

Metabolic emergencies

Hypercalcaemia of malignancy

Definition

Hypercalcaemia is a common biochemical abnormality in the blood that can be potentially life-threatening (Grandjean and McMullen 2010). It is defined as a serum calcium concentration (following adjustment) of 2.65 mmol/L or higher on two occasions and can also be classified according to severity (Clinical Knowledge Summaries [CKS] 2014a). Hypercalcaemia can be caused by malignancy, hyperparathyroidism, medications or underlying medical conditions. The initial signs and symptoms can be quite vague but it can also present as dehydration, cardiac arrhythmias or coma. Severe hypercalcaemia is an emergency and requires prompt management to prevent life-threatening complications to the kidneys, heart and brain (CKS 2014a). The nurse's understanding of the pathophysiology, signs and symptoms of hypercalcaemia enables effective diagnosis and holistic management of the patient with complex health needs (Walker 2015).

Anatomy and physiology

Calcium is predominantly found in the bone and calcified cartilage but is also present in the intracellular and extracellular fluids. Calcium is required for muscle and cell contraction, neurotransmission and bone formation (Walker 2015). Calcium levels in the blood (serum calcium) are kept in the normal reference range by parathyroid hormone (PTH), 1,25-dihydroxy vitamin D_3 (calcitriol) and calcitonin (Grandjean and McMullen 2010). PTH and calcitriol physiologically regulate calcium homeostasis, with calcitonin playing a lesser role (Sargent and Smith 2010). These regulators are known to help in the prevention of hypocalcaemia, but are less effective in hypercalcaemia (Sargent and Smith 2010). For hypercalcaemia to develop, normal calcium regulation in which bone is continuously resorbed (removed) by osteoclasts and replaced with new bone created by osteoblasts must be overwhelmed by an excess of PTH, calcitriol or a huge calcium

load (Green 2016). Cancer cells release proteins and cytokines that stimulate osteoclasts and enhance bone resorption, causing calcium to be released into the blood and increasing levels of calcium (Sargent and Smith 2010).

Related theory

Eighty per cent of cases of hypercalcaemia are caused by primary hyperparathyroidism and cancer, in particular those of breast, lung and multiple myeloma, with or without bone metastases. In the other 20%, bone metastases cause lysis and release of skeletal calcium. It is important to recognize that drugs such as thiazide diuretics, vitamin D and antacids with calcium co-prescribed can also be a factor as these drugs are commonly used in cancer care. About 20–30% of all people with cancer develop hypercalcaemia at some point during their illness (Joshi et al. 2009). For most people with malignancy-associated hypercalcaemia, an underlying cause has already been identified (Bushinsky and Monk 1998, Clines 2011, Twycross et al. 2009). When hypercalcaemia occurs, it is usually a sign of advanced cancer with a median survival of 3–4 months (Seccareccia 2010).

Symptoms

The symptoms of hypercalcaemia are often non-specific, and patients who suffer chronically can often be asymptomatic (Minisola et al. 2015). The extent of the symptoms relates to the severity and rate of onset. Symptoms can be grouped together according to the system affected (see Table 7.3).

Diagnosis

The only way to confirm the diagnosis is a venous blood sample to measure both serum calcium and albumin concentrations (Minisola et al. 2015). Patients who present with symptoms or have severe hypercalcaemia based on blood results should commence treatment immediately and investigation of the underlying cause should be delayed until the life-threatening situation is under control (Pettifer and Grant 2013). Unless the patient is symptomatic or the classification is severe, the patient can be treated as an outpatient (CKS 2014a, Legrand 2011, Pettifer and Grant 2013).

For people with unexplained, asymptomatic mild (2.65–3.0mmol/L) or moderate hypercalcaemia (3.01–3.4mmol/L), there may be more than one cause. Review the medical and family history, clinical features and drug treatments, looking for an underlying cause. Referral to the appropriate specialist, depending on the suspected cause or causes, is recommended (CKS 2014a, Minisola et al. 2015). The healthcare professional may also organize the following additional investigations to provide further information as to the cause:

- Chest X-ray (to exclude lung cancer or metastases, sarcoidosis or tuberculosis).
- Renal function and serum electrolytes, including magnesium and phosphate (to assess for chronic kidney disease).
- FBC (to diagnose or exclude anaemia of chronic disease).
- Erythrocyte sedimentation rate (ESR) or C-reactive protein (CRP) (may be increased in cancer or other inflammatory or granulomatous conditions).
- Serum and urine protein electrophoresis, including testing for urinary Bence Jones protein (to exclude myeloma).
- Liver function tests (LFTs) (to exclude liver metastases or chronic liver failure; also alkaline phosphatase may be increased in primary hyperparathyroidism, Paget's disease with immobilization, myeloma or bone metastases).
- Thyroid function tests (to exclude thyrotoxicosis).
- Serum cortisol (morning sample, at 8–9 am if Addison's disease [a rare cause of hypercalcaemia] is suspected).
- Urinalysis for urine protein (if chronic kidney disease is suspected).

In patients with a known malignancy the main cause is likely to be their cancer but this must not exclude testing for primary

Table 7.3 Symptoms of acute and chronic hypercalcaemia according to anatomical system

System	Acute hypercalcaemia	Chronic hypercalcaemia
General	Flushing, itching, keratitis, conjunctivitis, fatigue, weight loss	Fatigue, corneal calcification
Cardiovascular	Hypertension, prolonged PR interval, widened QRS complex, shortened QT interval, bundle branch block, bradycardia, arrhythmias, syncope, cardiac arrest	Prolonged PR interval, widened QRS complex, shortened QT interval, bundle branch block, bradycardia, arrhythmias, hypertension, valvular heart disease, vascular calcification
Renal	Thirst, polydipsia; dehydration (due to nephrogenic diabetes insipidus); polyuria; nocturia; frequent urination; renal failure from obstructive uropathy, nephrolithiasis, nephrocalcinosis or pre-renal causes	Renal impairment (nephrocalcinosis), renal colic (nephrolithiasis), chronic renal failure, renal osteodystrophy
Neurological	Tiredness, obtundation, lethargy, confusion, delirium, somnolence, stupor, coma, hypotonia, hyporeflexia, paresis	Impaired concentration and memory loss, dementia, sleep disturbance, decreased concentration
Psychiatric	Depression, anxiety, hallucination, psychosis	Irritability, depression, anxiety
Gastrointestinal	Anorexia, nausea, vomiting, abdominal pain, dyspepsia, constipation, pancreatitis, peptic ulcer	Anorexia, dyspepsia, weight loss, constipation, pancreatitis, peptic ulcer
Skeletal and muscle	Bone pain, muscle weakness	Bone pain, muscle weakness, myalgias, osteoporosis, osteopenia, fragility fractures, osteitis fibrosa cystica, bone cysts, brown tumours of long bones, chondrocalcinosis, joint calcification
Haematological	Anaemia	Anaemia
Ocular	—	Band keratopathy (cornea)

Source: Adapted from CKS (2014a), Minisola et al. (2015), Pettifer and Grant (2013).

265

hyperparathyroidism. If hypercalcaemia is detected, a blood sample for PTH levels is required as primary hyperparathyroidism may co-exist with malignancy.

Assessment and management

Nursing management of hypercalcaemia relies on having a high index of suspicion in any patient known to have predisposing pathology, such as breast cancer, or known chronic hypercalcaemia (Walker 2015). Due to the nature of hypercalcaemia, patients present often with vague symptoms, therefore initial nursing assessment is essential to highlight hypercalcaemia as a potential differential diagnosis. If the patient has a known malignancy, then the treatment is the same but be mindful that although this is the likely cause for the hypercalcaemia there may be an additional cause (Twycross et al. 2009). Consider the patient's underlying cancer and whether it is appropriate to treat the hypercalcaemia (Seccareccia 2010). Table 7.4 provides initial nursing actions when hypercalcaemia is suspected.

Hypercalcaemia can cause acute kidney injury (AKI) via the concurrent effects of a hypovolaemic state and vasoconstrictive effects of calcium (Carroll and Schade 2003). It is important that the cancer nurse is aware of this risk as many cases of AKI can be prevented by following the four Ms (Table 7.5). Management of AKI should be based on local policies; an example can be found in NICE (2013) clinical guideline 169.

In adults, AKI is diagnosed using any of the following criteria (NICE 2013):

- a rise in serum creatinine of 26 µmol/L or greater within 48 hours
- a 50% or greater rise in serum creatinine known or presumed to have occurred within the past 7 days
- a fall in urine output to less than 0.5 mL/kg/hour for more than 6 hours.

To support management, the nurse should ensure that the patient's volume status (including pulse, blood pressure, peripheral perfusion and jugular venous pressure), renal function and serum potassium level (to exclude hyperkalaemia) have been assessed (CKS 2014b, NICE 2013). Management of AKI in hypercalcaemia is linked directly to reducing the serum calcium level through rehydration and bisphosphonates (Moyses-Neto et al. 2006). Bisphosphonates (pamidronate or zoledronic acid) are classified as first-line therapy for malignant hypercalcaemia (CKS 2014a, Mallik et al. 2016, McCurdy and Shanholtz 2012). Bisphosphonates bind to hydroxyapatite and inhibit osteoclastic reabsorption and bone crystal dissolution (Higdon and Higdon 2006, McCurdy and Shanholtz 2012). The effects of these are expected to be seen 2–4 days after administration, supporting the use of this treatment in the palliative setting (Mallik et al. 2016).

The key to management is avoiding hypovolaemia by maintaining haemodynamic stability to ensure adequate renal perfusion (Rahman et al. 2012). If fluid resuscitation is required, isotonic solutions (e.g. 250 mL 0.9% sodium chloride in increments) are preferred over hyperoncotic solutions (e.g. dextrans, hydroxyethyl starch, albumin) (NICE 2013). If the patient has persistent hypotension they may require vasopressors; the critical care outreach team should be involved at this point (Prowle et al. 2011). Attention to electrolyte imbalances (e.g. hyperkalaemia, hyperphosphataemia, hypermagnesaemia, hyponatraemia, hypernatraemia, metabolic acidosis) is important. This is particularly important in AKI due to hypercalcaemia as these parameters may already be altered (CKS 2014b).

The use of diuretics is not recommended in hypercalcaemia and should only be used in AKI in the management of volume overload (NICE 2013, Rahman et al. 2012). It should also be noted that diuretics do not improve morbidity, mortality or renal outcomes, and should not be used to prevent or

Table 7.4 Initial actions on suspicion of hypercalcaemia

Action	Rationale
Regular observations: blood pressure (BP), pulse (P), respiratory rate (RR), oxygen saturation (Sats), temperature, National Early Warning Score (NEWS), AVPU ('alert, voice, pain, unresponsive' – record of conscious status)	Ensures close monitoring for signs of deterioration, enabling prompt action (Clinical Knowledge Summaries [CKS] 2014a)
Take bloods (outlined above) if not already done, ensuring that corrected calcium, potassium, magnesium and phosphorus is selected. Avoid prolonged tourniquet application	Provide diagnostic information Potassium, magnesium and phosphorus also likely to be deranged (McCurdy and Shanholtz 2012) Prolonged tourniquet application can increase the corrected calcium result (CKS 2014a)
Ensure electrocardiogram (ECG) is taken and reviewed for possible prolonged or shortened QT interval, widened QRS complex, or bundle branch block	In severe hypercalcaemia the electrical functioning of the heart can be affected (McCurdy and Shanholtz 2012)
Cannulate the patient and administer IV fluids (1000 mL sodium chloride 0.9%) in preparation	Promotes renal excretion of calcium and protects kidneys (Dark and Razak 2014)
Monitor urine output – risk of acute kidney injury (AKI) or cardiac overload	Hypercalcaemia can cause renal impairment and calculi (McCurdy and Shanholtz 2012) Speed of administration and amount of fluids can cause cardiac overload in frail patients (Seccareccia 2010)
Administer bisphosphonates as prescribed	In severe hypercalcaemia they cause inhibition of osteoclast activity and may have an effect on osteoblasts by allowing them to work more effectively thus reducing levels of circulating calcium (Dark and Razak 2014, Seccareccia 2010)
Encourage the patient to mobilize if symptomatically able	Helps the body to reabsorb the calcium (CKS 2014a, Walker 2015)
Ensure serum calcium and other electrolytes are monitored regularly (at least 1 week post bisphosphonate)	Hypercalcaemia will usually return within 4–6 weeks of initial treatment if the underlying cause is not treated (Seccareccia 2010)
Ensure loop diuretics have been stopped	Loop diuretics are not recommended as they can inhibit calcium reabsorption by the bone (Bower and Cox 2004)

Table 7.5 The four Ms to monitor if a patient is at risk of acute kidney injury (AKI)

Action	Rationale
Monitor the patient: use NEWS, regular blood tests, fluid charts and urine volumes	A change in observations and subsequent increase in NEWS will alert to a potential deterioration in condition and trigger a response (NICE 2007b)
Maintain circulation: hydration, resuscitation and oxygenation	Ensuring that the patient is adequately perfused and oxygenated and has a patent airway will reduce risk of kidney injury or general deterioration (NICE 2013). Vigorous fluid administration (normal saline) is aimed at reversing renal ischaemia and diluting nephrotoxins (Prowle et al. 2011)
Minimize kidney insults: review nephrotoxic medications and the use of contrast media and treat infections	Reduce the stress placed on the kidneys and prevent further damage (Rahman et al. 2012)
Manage the acute illness: dehydration, sepsis, heart and liver failure. Untreated, all of these can contribute to AKI	AKI is a medical emergency and is associated with a high incidence of mortality (up to 80%) (Rahman et al. 2012)

treat AKI in the absence of volume overload (Lewington and Kanagasundaram 2011).

Medications that potentially affect renal function by direct toxicity or by haemodynamic mechanisms should be discontinued; for example, metformin (Glucophage) should not be given to patients with diabetes mellitus who develop AKI (Lewington and Kanagasundaram 2011). The dosages of essential medications should be adjusted for the lower level of kidney function. This includes supportive therapies (e.g. antibiotics, maintenance of adequate nutrition, mechanical ventilation, glycaemic control, anaemia management) which should be pursued based on standard management practices.

If the person is asymptomatic with mild or moderate hypercalcaemia (adjusted serum calcium 3.40 mmol/L or less), repeat the blood test a week later to exclude rapidly increasing hypercalcaemia suggestive of cancer (CKS 2014a). Ensure that the patient is given clear information regarding signs and symptoms along with advice to drink six to eight glasses of water a day to prevent nephrolithiasis, provided there are no contraindications such as renal impairment or heart failure, and to maintain a normal diet

(Clines 2011, Walker 2015). The literature suggests that restriction of dietary calcium and vitamin D can lead to malnutrition (CKS 2014b).

For all patients ensure that they avoid any drugs or vitamin supplements containing calcium and encourage mobilization as this aids the reabsorption of calcium (CKS 2014a). Calcium levels should be checked within 2 weeks after initial treatment as it is noted that calcium levels can begin rising within 4 weeks of treatment (Seccareccia 2010). It is known that cancer-associated hypercalcaemia is more likely to become symptomatic at lower serum calcium levels and that the serum calcium increases more rapidly (Clines 2011, Ralston et al. 1990).

Hypomagnesaemia

Definition
Hypomagnesaemia is defined as serum magnesium of less than 0.75 mmol/L; normal values of serum magnesium are between 0.75 and 1.5 mmol/L (Efstratiadis et al. 2006).

Related theory
Magnesium is the second in abundance intracellular ion and is known to have a significant role in the cardiovascular system, arterial tension, central nervous system, skeletal muscles and pregnancy (Efstratiadis et al. 2006, Martin et al. 2009). Hypomagnesaemia is a life-threatening condition as it affects nearly every organ of the body but it is usually picked up through routine testing when the patient is being assessed for other reasons. Therefore, most patients are asymptomatic as levels are only mildly depressed (>0.5 mmol/L). Due to the underlying pathophysiology of hypomagnesaemia it is common for patients to have associated hypokalaemia (occurring in 40–60% of cases), partly due to underlying disorders that cause magnesium and potassium losses, including diuretic therapy, chemotherapy and diarrhoea (Fulop 2016). It is important to acknowledge that in many chemotherapy regimens diuretic therapy is standard, therefore monitoring of magnesium is imperative and, if patients present at risk of dehydration or oedema, review of their magnesium level should be included (Martin et al. 2009).

Assessment
As most cases of hypomagnesaemia are identified through routine blood tests, most patients are asymptomatic on presentation. Hypomagnesaemia is also commonly found in association with hypocalcaemia, hypokalaemia and hyponatraemia, therefore these must be investigated through the addition of these tests within the blood profile. In any patient who presents with an acute deterioration of their condition with unknown or unclear cause the standard assessment should be carried out as stated in the introduction of this chapter. Review of the patient's history, including cancer treatment, will guide further investigations such as inclusion of magnesium in the bloods and undertaking an ECG to look for arrhythmias (Box 7.1).

Management
Management of hypomagnesaemia is dependent on grade (Table 7.6) however patients with recurrent low magnesium should be encouraged to have a diet rich in sources of magnesium such as green vegetables (spinach), beans and peas, nuts and seeds, and whole, unrefined grains and seafood (Guerrera et al. 2009).

Box 7.1 Symptoms arising once serum magnesium levels fall below 0.5 mmol/L

Neuromuscular
- Muscular weakness
- Cramping
- Tremors
- Seizure
- Paraesthesias
- Tetany
- Positive Chvostek sign (metacarpal hyperflexion) and Trousseau sign (facial nerve hypersensitivity)
- Vertical and horizontal nystagmus
- Ataxia
- Depression
- Hyperactive deep tendon reflexes
- Altered mental state (in severe cases)

Cardiac
- Tachycardia
- Palpitations
- Non-specific T-wave changes – U waves
- Prolonged QT and QU interval
- Repolarization alternans
- Premature ventricular contractions – monomorphic ventricular tachycardia
- Torsades de pointes
- Ventricular fibrillation
- Enhanced digitalis toxicity

Metabolic
- Hypokalaemia
- Hypocalcaemia

Table 7.6 Grading and management of hypomagnesaemia

Grade (UKONS classification)	Serum magnesium	Management
1 (Green)	<0.5 mmol/L	If patient is asymptomatic consider oral Mg replacement and advise a Mg-rich diet
		If patient is symptomatic review other electrolytes and treat as per grade 3 or 4 (red)
2 (Amber)	<0.5–0.4 mmo/L	Consider oral replacement and advise a Mg-rich diet.
		Recheck bloods in 24–48 hours
		Correct any other electrolyte imbalance as necessary
		If patient is symptomatic review other electrolytes and treat as per grade 3 or 4 (red)
3 (Red)	<0.4–0.3 mmol/L	Administer IV Mg 10–20 mmol diluted in 0.9% sodium chloride over 3–6 hours
		Correct any other electrolyte imbalance as necessary
4 (Red) Life threatening	<0.3 mmol/L	Admit for slow IV Mg
		If arrhythmias on ECG then admit to ICU for bolus IV Mg

Source: UKONS (2018). Reproduced with permission of UKONS. Adapted from Martin et al. (2009), Pfennig and Slovis (2014).

Side-effects from chemotherapy agents

Diarrhoea (chemotherapy and radiotherapy induced)

Definition

Diarrhoea is defined as the passage of three or more loose or liquid stools per day (or more frequent passage than is normal for the individual). Frequent passing of formed stools is not diarrhoea, neither is the passing of loose stools (World Health Organization [WHO] 2013). In cancer patients it must be acknowledged that the accepted 'normal' has been changed due to the disease or surgical management, therefore diarrhoea is defined as an abnormal increase in stool frequency (four to six times or more per day over the baseline) and stool liquidity, with or without nocturnal bowel movements or moderate abdominal cramping (Muehlbauer et al. 2009, Stein et al. 2010).

Diarrhoea has been described as one of the most distressing symptoms affecting medical oncology patients due to its impact on their nutritional status (Tong et al. 2009). It may lead to dehydration, electrolyte imbalance, renal insufficiency, immune dysfunction and, in extreme cases, possibly even death (Cherny 2008). The psychological effects of diarrhoea include anxiety, depression, social isolation, low self-esteem and caregiver strain (Viele 2003).

Anatomy and physiology

The gastrointestinal (GI) tract starts at the buccal cavity of the mouth and ends at the anus. It is usually divided into the upper GI tract, which consists of the mouth, pharynx, oesophagus and stomach, and the lower GI tract which encompasses the small and large intestines. It is a muscular tube, approximately 9 metres in length, and is controlled by the autonomic nervous system (McGrath 2005). The three primary functions of the GI tract are the ingestion of food and water, the digestion of food and absorption of nutrients and the expulsion of waste matter. These primary functions occur in conjunction with the accessory digestive organs which include the salivary glands, pancreas, liver and gallbladder (Nightingale 2015). As food is taken into the mouth the salivary glands switch into action, and as it continues through the GI tract, enzymes found in the stomach, small intestine, pancreas and liver continue the process. It is this secretion of fluids that helps maintain the function of the tract (Tortora and Derrickson 2014).

Diarrhoea induced by cancer treatment is a multifactorial process in which acute damage to the intestinal mucosa (including loss of intestinal epithelium, superficial necrosis and inflammation of the bowel wall) causes an imbalance between absorption and secretion in the small bowel (Gibson and Stringer 2009, Keefe 2007, Keefe et al. 2000). This is a simplistic explanation as the underlying pathophysiology is related to each particular mode of treatment and beyond the remit of this chapter.

Related theory

The GI tract is lined with epithelial cells that are rapidly dividing which, when affected by cancer treatment, especially radiotherapy and anticancer drugs, leads to an array of symptoms (Stein et al. 2010).

With the development of new anticancer treatment modalities, such as ipilimumab, it is important to recognize that the management of treatment-induced diarrhoea requires different approaches dependent on the underlying cause. Diarrhoea can result from chemotherapy-induced cellular damage, which reduces absorption from the gastrointestinal (GI) tract and increases the secretion of electrolytes into the stool. Severe diarrhoea can cause hyponatraemia, which can lead to seizures and coma, and severe hypokalaemia which can impair cardiac function (Grenon and Chan 2009).

Anticancer drugs

Diarrhoea induced by anticancer drugs is common and can cause morbidity and mortality: grade 3–4 serious adverse events are reported with a frequency of 5–47% in randomized clinical trials (Andreyev et al. 2014). As a result treatment is frequently compromised as diarrhoea can sometimes lead to hospital admission and can be life threatening. Clinical trials have reported death due to fluorouracil-induced diarrhoea in 1–5% of patients (Tveit et al. 2012). Chemotherapy-induced diarrhoea remains an important complication and the risk of death is increased when the patient is also neutropenic (Andreyev et al. 2014). Chemotherapeutic agents frequently associated with diarrhoea are listed in Table 7.7 although this is not exhaustive and the toxic effects depend on the schedule and dose of the drug.

Working within the acute cancer care setting, an understanding of the main treatments used helps the nurse to predict the likely cause of the patient's symptoms. The following information provides examples of how practical knowledge of GI side-effects of anticancer treatment can assist the cancer nurse to better support patients through treatment and recognize side-effects early.

Fluorouracil

Fluorouracil is frequently used to treat GI tract cancers. If given as a bolus injection, the drug causes more myelosuppression and stomatitis, whereas infused fluorouracil is more frequently associated with grade 3–4 diarrhoea. The severity of the diarrhoea is increased by the addition of folinic acid (leucovorin) which is not a chemotherapy drug but is often given as part of anticancer treatment to reduce the side-effects of drugs such as high-dose methotrexate. However, when used with fluorouracil, it is found to increase the effectiveness of fluorouracil (Andreyev et al. 2014).

Clinical factors predictive for fluorouracil-induced diarrhoea include being female, increasing age (although the threshold is not known), normal body mass index, white ethnic origin and diabetes mellitus (McCollum et al. 2002, Meyerhardt et al. 2004).

Prodrugs of fluorouracil, such as capecitabine, produce similar effects (Malet-Martino and Martino 2002).

Plant alkaloids

Irinotecan is associated with dose-limiting diarrhoea when given either as a 30-minute bolus every 3 weeks or as a continuous infusion over 7 days (Masi et al. 2004). Acknowledging the patient's past medical history is also important as those with Gilbert's syndrome, characterized by decreased bilirubin glucuronidation, have an increased risk of severe diarrhoea (Andreyev et al. 2014).

Monoclonal antibodies

Diarrhoea is one of the most common adverse events recorded following treatment with *tyrosine kinase inhibitors* (TKIs) (Keefe and Anthony 2008). In patients treated with TKIs, diarrhoea is second only to rash as the most common adverse event, affecting up to 50% of patients, although these symptoms have been suggested to predict tumour response (Bowen 2013). Diarrhoea grade 3 or higher occurs in up to 28% of patients taking TKIs (Gibson et al. 2013).

In contrast to TKIs, up to 66% of patients prescribed *vascular endothelial growth factor (VEGF) inhibitors* (e.g. pazopanib, sunitinib, sorafenib) develop diarrhoea (Bowen 2013).

Diarrhoea might start as early as 2–3 days after initiation of *epidermal growth factor receptor (EGFR) inhibitor therapy*. With most monoclonal antibodies, the severity of diarrhoea is dose dependent and can be modulated by a decrease in total dose. Third-generation EGFR inhibitors that irreversibly block EGFR, such as afatinib, are associated with dose-limiting diarrhoea (Yang et al. 2013).

Agents that interfere with crucial regulatory biological molecules are increasingly being used to induce tumour regression. An example is *ipilimumab*, a fully human monoclonal antibody to CTLA-4 that prolongs the time to progression in patients with

Table 7.7 Categories of chemotherapy-induced gastrointestinal tract injuries

Gastrointestinal injury	Drug classification	Drug
Panenteritis, enterocolitis, mucositis	Antimetabolites	Cytosine arabinoside, methotrexate
		Fluoropyrimidines: fluorouracil, capecitabine, tegafur–uracil
		Multitargeted folinic acid antagonists: pemetrexed, raltitrexed, gemcitabine
	Plant alkaloids	Vinca alkaloids: vincristine, vinorelbine
		Epipodophyllotoxins: etoposide
		Taxanes: paclitaxel, docetaxel
		Topoisomerase I inhibitors: irinotecan
	Cytotoxic antibiotics	Anthracyclines: doxorubicin, daunorubicin, idarubicin, aclarubicin, dactinomycin with prednisone
	Alkylating agents	Cyclophosphamide, cisplatin, carboplatin, oxaliplatin, nedaplatin
Abdominal pain	Antimetabolites	Gemcitabine
Autoimmune colitis	Monoclonal antibodies	Ipilimumab
Ischaemic colitis	Monoclonal antibodies	Antibodies against vascular endothelial growth factor (VEGF): bevacizumab
	Plant alkaloids	Taxanes: docetaxel, paclitaxel
Gastrointestinal leucocytoclastic vasculitis	Miscellaneous	Sirolimus

Source: Adapted from Andreyev et al. (2014). Reproduced with permission of Elsevier.

269

melanoma and ovarian, prostate and renal-cell cancers. Immune-mediated side-effects include severe diarrhoea; this is associated with perforation in less than 1% of patients and with death in 5%. Treatment is mainly supportive, although in severe cases high-dose corticosteroids should be started early. If steroids fail, the use of anti-tumour necrosis factor (TNF) drugs such as infliximab that block the action of TNF and so reduce inflammation has been advocated (Pagès et al. 2013).

Radiotherapy
Although radiotherapy is discussed in detail in Chapter 5, it is important to highlight this treatment modality here because diarrhoea is a common adverse event. The severity of acute GI symptoms during pelvic radiation depends partly on the dose given and volume of bowel treated; other risk factors include diabetes, inflammatory bowel disease, collagen vascular disease, HIV, old age, smoking and low body mass index (Fuccio et al. 2012). Acute intestinal side-effects of radiation begin at approximately 10–20 Gy and peak between weeks 3 and 5 of treatment (Faithfull 2006). Acute diarrhoea is an independent prognostic factor of

outcome during treatment for colorectal cancer, but more severe acute effects are also associated with long-term consequences of treatment (Bowen 2013).

Evidence-based approaches
Diarrhoea can have an effect on performance status and the ability of the patient to perform daily activities. Patients may become housebound because of embarrassment, fatigue, dehydration, abdominal, rectal and perianal pain, excoriation or discomfort, and the fear of needing to defaecate suddenly (Andreyev et al. 2014). This can result in social isolation, time off work, relationship difficulties and psychological distress; some individuals doubt their ability to complete treatment (Elting et al. 2008). If patients do not present in a timely manner with potentially serious symptoms, optimum management might not be possible.

Assessment
The seriousness of diarrhoea is frequently defined using the common terminology criteria for adverse events (CTCAE; US Department of Health and Human Services 2010) (Table 7.8).

Table 7.8 Common Terminology Criteria for Adverse Events grades of diarrhoea and UKONS triage grading

Grade	Symptoms
Grade 1	Increase to two to three bowel movements per day additional to number before treatment or mild increase in stoma output
Grade 2	Increase to four to six bowel movements per day additional to number before treatment, moderate increase in stoma output, as well as moderate cramping or nocturnal stools
Grade 3	Increase of seven to nine bowel movements per day additional to number before treatment, incontinence, or severe increase in stoma output, as well as severe cramping or nocturnal stools, that interfere with activities of daily living
Grade 4	Increase to more than ten bowel movements per day additional to number before treatment, grossly bloody diarrhoea, need for parenteral support, or a combination of these features

Source: UKONS (2018). Reproduced with permission of UKONS.

The most important decision is whether the patient can be managed as an outpatient or needs admission for fluid resuscitation; this depends on the risk of adverse outcomes. Patients with grade 1–2 diarrhoea without worrying clinical features and test results can usually be managed at home. Those with grade 3–4 diarrhoea generally need immediate admission unless clinical review suggests the patient is well hydrated, has not yet had any antidiarrhoeal medication, and can be reviewed daily (Andreyev et al. 2014). Several features should alert clinicians to the fact that diarrhoea is clinically worrying, including abdominal cramps not relieved by loperamide, an inability to eat, increasing fatigue, increasing weakness, chest pain, nausea not controlled by antiemetics, vomiting, dehydration accompanied by reduced urine output, fever (temperature higher than 38.5°C), gastrointestinal bleeding and previous admission for diarrhoea.

If an acute oncology helpline is available, the patient should be encouraged to telephone for advice after starting antidiarrhoeal medication to confirm the severity and whether face-to-face assessment is required.

Guidance in the UK on the management of GI side-effects of cancer therapies emphasizes three crucial factors:

- whether the patient is being woken from sleep to defaecate
- whether there is any steatorrhoea
- whether there is urgency of defaecation or any faecal incontinence.

Other important factors to consider are:

- the degree of fatigue
- changes in medication
- changes in diet
- other chemotherapy-induced toxic effects
- whether the patient is presenting with overflow diarrhoea.

Fatigue
The intensity of fatigue correlates with the severity of diarrhoea at 3 weeks (Alhberg et al. 2005). Fatigue can also be associated with a significant decrease in albumin concentrations in serum ($p < 0.001$) (Jakobsson et al. 2010).

Changes in medication
Recent changes to medication (within the previous 10–14 days) should be taken into account, as the introduction of proton pump inhibitors, non-steroidal anti-inflammatory drugs, laxatives, or antibiotics can increase the likelihood of diarrhoea.

Changes in diet
When assessing diet, it should be established whether patients are eating very little or excessive amounts of fibre. Foods containing lactose might trigger diarrhoea and should be suspected, especially if the diarrhoea is accompanied by marked bloating. Other causes to consider are excessive alcohol intake and an inability to eat and drink normally.

Other chemotherapy-related toxic effects
These include nausea, vomiting, or both, odynophagia, mouth ulceration and red hands or feet.

Overflow diarrhoea
If the patient has loss of appetite, abdominal pain, bloating and increased frequency of soft or loose stool rather than profuse watery diarrhoea, overflow diarrhoea should be suspected.

When treatment-induced diarrhoea is suspected, initial assessment follows the same pattern as the UKONS tool but with the following specific considerations (Andreyev et al. 2014, Muehlbauer et al. 2009):

1 Identify: is the patient at risk of immunosuppression (chemotherapy or radiotherapy within the last 6 weeks, bone marrow transplant or disease-related immunosuppression) as there may also be an underlying sepsis (± neutropenia)?

2 Obtain baseline observations: temperature, pulse, blood pressure, respiration rate, oxygen saturations and early warning score (EWS). If the patient is tachycardic or dehydrated or if sepsis is suspected, fluid resuscitation should be started and 4 mg loperamide given before investigations are performed.

3 Initial investigations: FBC, U&Es, LFTs, CRP, lactate (if sepsis is suspected), stool sample (sent for microscopy, culture and sensitivity [MC&S], faecal pathogens and *Clostridium difficile* toxin [CDT]).

4 History of presenting complaint:
- What chemotherapy is the patient on and when was the last treatment?
  - Are any of these drugs commonly associated with chemotherapy-induced diarrhoea (CID)?
- Is the patient receiving any radiotherapy and to which area – when was their last treatment?
- How often do their bowels usually move?
  - If the patient has not already done so, ask them to commence a stool chart.
- How many stools a day are they currently passing above their normal?
  - If the patient has a stoma – how often does their stoma work usually and how many times more currently?
- Are the stools/stoma output formed, loose or watery?
  - Associated with any faecal incontinence and/or nocturnal movements?
  - Any blood noted in the stool or toilet paper after wiping themselves?
- Are there any associated symptoms?
  - Abdominal cramping – is this associated with a bowel movement?
  - Nausea or vomiting – if they have vomited, what colour and amount was it?
  - Passing urine as usual – any change in colour or smell?
- Are they able to eat and drink as usual?
- Is it interfering with their activities of daily living?
- Do they have any other chemotherapy-associated symptoms – mouth ulcers, etc?
- Any recent antibiotic use?
- Current medications – laxatives or antisickness or antidiarrhoeal medications within the last 24 hours?

Pharmacological support
Patients can be encouraged to self-medicate but should keep a record of their drug use. How much to take, how often, and when in relation to meals patients can take antidiarrhoeal medication must be made clear if patients are to keep medications at home (Andreyev et al. 2014). For CID it is important to determine if the patient is currently taking any oral chemotherapy; if they are, they should be advised to stop taking it and commence oral loperamide (UKONS 2018). Importantly, if the first dose of loperamide does not work, patients should be informed that it is likely that they have not taken enough. After starting loperamide, patients need to know when they must contact their chemotherapy unit and when they can delay contact; generally, patients should make contact if taking eight 2 mg tablets in 24 hours has had no effect as they may need intravenous fluids and other treatments (Andreyev et al. 2014). A starting dose of 4 mg followed by 2 mg every 2 h after an episode of diarrhoea is often recommended. If the patient can still eat, however, this treatment might be more effective if taken 30 minutes before food (Benson et al. 2004, Nightingale et al. 1992, Remington et al. 1982).

Loperamide can be discontinued when the patient has been diarrhoea free for 12 hours (Benson et al. 2004). If mild to moderate diarrhoea persists for more than 24 hours, high-dose loperamide may be given and oral antibiotics should be initiated as prophylaxis against infection (Benson et al. 2004, Cherny 2008). If mild to moderate CID persists for more than 48 hours while the patient is on high-dose loperamide, loperamide should be discontinued and a second-line antidiarrhoeal agent should be started, such as octreotide (starting at 100–150 µg subcutaneously [SC]) (Benson et al. 2004, Muehlbauer et al. 2009).

Complicated cases of CID require aggressive treatment involving hospitalization and intravenous fluids (Cherny 2008). Higher doses of loperamide have not been shown to be effective for grade 3–4 CID, and a change to octreotide 100–150 µg (SC or intravenous [IV]) with a dose escalation up to 500 µg until diarrhoea is controlled should be considered (Benson et al. 2004, Muehlbauer et al. 2009). Patients can become dehydrated because of diarrhoea with or without vomiting but the physiological requirements must be established before and reviewed regularly after replacement of fluids is started (Andreyev et al. 2014). Patients with severe CID can lose up to 4–6 L of diarrhoea per day, putting them at risk of becoming severely hypovolaemic, which can make exclusion or differentiation from sepsis difficult (they might coincide). If hypovolaemia is uncertain, the response to a 500 mL bolus (250 mL in patients with a history of cardiac failure) of a balanced crystalloid (0.9% sodium chloride is preferred if potassium concentrations are higher than 5.5 mmol/L or if oliguric AKI is possible) should be assessed to see if blood plasma volume increases (Benson et al. 2004). In severely ill patients who are hypotensive, tachycardic and potentially septic and have high lactate concentrations, an initial fluid bolus of 20 mL/kg should be given (Rivers et al. 2001). Consensus guidelines (Figure 7.4) have been produced to support evidence-based practice in this growing problem.

Non-pharmacological support

The initial treatment for mild to moderate diarrhoea includes non-pharmacological interventions. Dietary modifications such as eliminating all lactose-containing products, alcohol and high-osmolar dietary supplements may help decrease CID. Sorbitol-containing products, such as sugar-free gum and confectionery, should be eliminated as they can cause diarrhoea (Muehlbauer et al. 2009). Any medications or foods that may enhance the diarrhoea should be discontinued. The patient should be instructed to document stool frequency and promptly report symptoms of fever or dizziness upon standing (Benson et al. 2004, Cherny 2008). Other non-pharmacological interventions include hydrating with 8–10 glasses of clear liquids per day and eating small frequent meals (Benson et al. 2004). Oral rehydration with fluids that contain water, sugar and salt will help prevent hyponatraemia and hypokalaemia; such fluids are sports drinks, broth, gelatine and decaffeinated, decarbonated soft drinks (Benson et al. 2004, Richardson and Dobish 2007).

Autoimmune colitis (enterocolitis) requires different management to other forms of treatment-induced diarrhoea. This is due to the mode of action of the monoclonal antibodies that work using the body's immune response such as ipilimumab. The severity of side-effects is directly correlated to the treatment dose (Fecher et al. 2013). Therefore, ascertaining the patient's current treatment modality (specifically the drug) is imperative in being able to manage the type of treatment-induced diarrhoea. For the purposes of this section the drug ipilimumab will be used as this is most commonly used in practice. Ipilimumab-related diarrhoea of any grade is reported in approximately 30–35% of patients, and grade 3–5 diarrhoea or enterocolitis in 5–8% (Hodi et al. 2010). Mild, intermittent changes in bowel movements are commonly

seen with this drug, therefore all diarrhoea is suspect and most likely related to the drug.

As with all treatment-induced diarrhoea, patient education will ensure that diarrhoea is reported and managed promptly. It can be self-limited; however, ipilimumab-related diarrhoea is not typical of the drug-induced or idiopathic diarrhoea seen with other cancer therapies. It often presents around the second dose of therapy, but its timing of onset can vary and is not predictable. Symptoms can progress rapidly to potentially life-threatening status if untreated (Fecher et al. 2013). If a diagnosis of ipilimumab-induced colitis is established, treatment should be initiated with oral or IV steroids, depending on the grade of diarrhoea. Once an intervention is initiated, reassessment within 24 hours in the hospital or by telephone is necessary. Frequent re-evaluation is recommended as symptoms and course can change rapidly and response to interventions cannot be assumed. Referral to a gastroenterologist for flexible sigmoidoscopy or colonoscopy should be considered for persistent grade 2 diarrhoea or any grade 3–4 diarrhoea.

Patients presenting with grade 3–4 diarrhoea may need hospital admission for work-up, monitoring, IV hydration, bowel rest (nil by mouth) and high-dose IV steroids. For patients with refractory symptoms despite maximal medical support and treatment with high-dose steroids for approximately 5 days, a single dose of infliximab 5 mg/kg has demonstrated rapid resolution of symptoms and durable efficacy and should be considered (Johnston et al. 2009). Infliximab may also be considered for persistent grade 2 symptoms that do not resolve despite treatment with steroids. Infliximab can be repeated, but should not be used if there is concern for perforation or sepsis. The immune-related adverse event (irAE) gastrointestinal management algorithm (Figure 7.5) sets out what steps should be taken in the management of ipilimumab-induced gastrointestinal toxicities.

Education

Education of patients and their carers about the risks associated with, and management of, CID is the foundation for optimum treatment of toxic effects. Ensuring that the patient and their carer are aware of the rationale for adequate and, if necessary, repeated assessment, appropriate use of loperamide, and fluid resuscitation requirements is the second crucial step to incorporating the patient in their care and ongoing management.

Personal cleanliness is a fundamental value in society and of particular importance in preventing infection and reducing the risk of pressure ulcers. See Chapters 8 and 15 of the *The Royal Marsden Manual of Clinical Nursing Procedures, Ninth Edition* for further detail.

Nausea and vomiting

Definition

Nausea and vomiting are often referred to as a single symptom but are separate physiological conditions (Glare et al. 2011, Heskeeth 2008):

- *Nausea* is defined as an unpleasant feeling of the need to vomit and is often accompanied by autonomic symptoms such as pallor, cold sweat, salivation and tachycardia (Heskeeth 2008).
- *Vomiting* (emesis) is defined as the forceful expulsion of gastric contents through the mouth (Twycross and Black 1998).
- *Retching* is defined as the gastric and oesophageal movements of vomiting without the expulsion of vomit (Twycross and Black 1998). It may occur in isolation without discharge of gastric contents from the mouth and is often referred to as 'dry heaves'.
- *Chemotherapy-induced nausea and vomiting* (CINV) is one of the most common side-effects of chemotherapy; however,

271

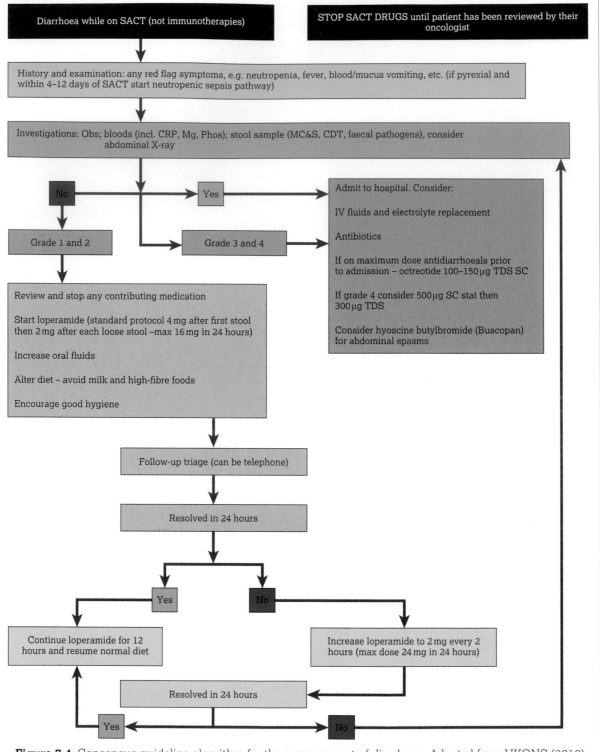

Figure 7.4 Consensus guideline algorithm for the management of diarrhoea. Adapted from UKONS (2018) and Kornblau et al. (2000).
CDT, *Clostridium difficile* toxin; CRP, C-reactive protein; MC&S, microscopy, culture and sensitivity; SACT, systemic anticancer therapy; SC, subcutaneous(ly); TDS, three times a day.

persistent nausea and vomiting are now fairly rare with the use of the modern antiemetic drugs. CINV is often grouped into three phases, with two additional subclassifications (Molassiotis and Borjeson 2006, Nasir and Schwartzberg 2016):
– Acute: within 24 hours of receiving chemotherapy.
– Delayed: from 24 hours after chemotherapy. Seldom persists beyond 1 week.

– Anticipatory: occurs prior to any chemotherapy and is a learned response to previous treatments.
– Breakthrough: development of symptoms (nausea and vomiting) despite standard antiemetic therapy which require treatment with an additional pharmacological agent.
– Refractory: patients who have failed on both standard and rescue medication.

272

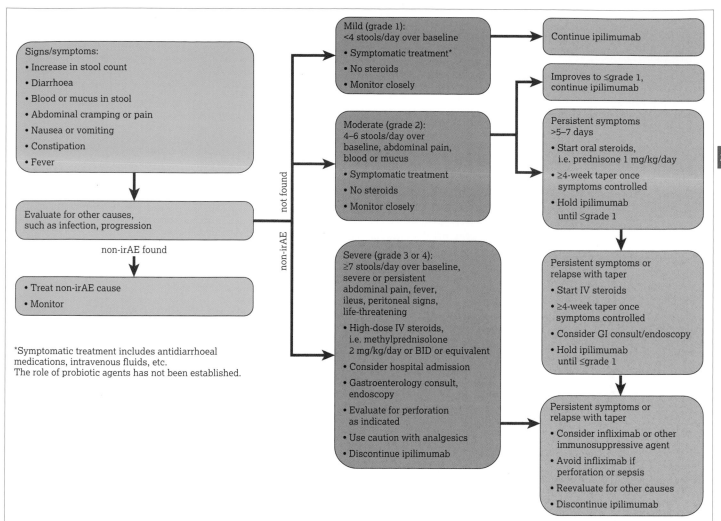

Figure 7.5 The immune-related adverse event (irAE) gastrointestinal management algorithm. *Source:* Fecher et al. (2013). Reproduced with permission of AlphaMed Press, permission conveyed through Copyright Clearance Center, Inc.

Anatomy and physiology

Several neural structures and a variety of neurotransmitters and receptors have been identified that relate to nausea and vomiting. Most of the relevant receptors are excitatory and induce nausea and vomiting when stimulated (Twycross and Black 1998). The afferent and efferent reflexes that result in nausea and vomiting are thought to be stimulated at brainstem level through the chemotherapy trigger zone and integrative trigger zone (Figure 7.6).

The chemoreceptor trigger zone (CTZ) is located in the floor of the fourth ventricle and is outside the blood–brain barrier (Pleuvry 2012). As it sits outside the blood–brain barrier it is exposed to various noxious agents such as toxins, biochemical products and drugs, borne in the blood and cerebrospinal fluid (O'Brien 2008). Neural pathways from the CTZ provide the main stimulus to the vomiting centre (Mannix 2002, Pleuvry 2012). The CTZ is stimulated by chemicals in cerebrospinal fluid and blood as well as vestibular and vagal afferents and contains receptors for dopamine (D2), serotonin (5-HT3), acetylcholine (ACH) and opioids (MU2).

The vomiting centre (VC) is situated in the medulla oblongata outside the blood–brain barrier and is thought to co-ordinate the vomiting process (Mannix 2002, Pleuvry 2012). The VC receives input from the CTZ, vestibular apparatus (the part of the internal ear concerned with balance), glossopharyngeal and splanchnic nerves, cerebral cortex, thalamus, hypothalamus and the vagus nerve through the stimulation of stretch of mechanoreceptors and activation of 5-HT3 receptors in the GI tract (Mannix 2002). These pathways then prompt the vomiting reflex, which stimulates peristalsis in the upper GI tract, the pylorus and oesophagus relax, and the intercostal muscles, diaphragm and abdominal wall contract culminating in the forced expulsion of the gastric contents through the mouth past a closed glottis (Nasir and Schwartzberg 2016).

Evidence-based approaches

Background

An estimated 60% of patients who receive chemotherapy as part of their treatment experience some degree of nausea and vomiting (Bender et al. 2002, Warr 2008). It is reported as one of the most dreaded side-effects and can have both a physical and psychological effect on the patient (Molassiotis and Borjeson 2006). Cancer itself or the many treatments used can cause nausea and vomiting (Table 7.9). It is therefore important to ascertain what treatment the patient is on in order to rule this out as a cause. Do not assume that nausea and vomiting are chemotherapy related. Many chemotherapies have no significant emetic potential, and chemotherapy will seldom cause nausea and vomiting more than 1 week after administration (London Cancer Alliance 2015).

274

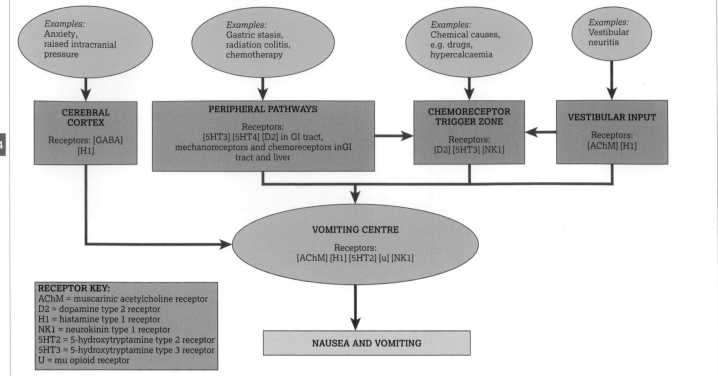

Figure 7.6 The emetogenic pathway. *Source:* Harris (2010). Reproduced with permission of Oxford University Press, permission conveyed through Copyright Clearance Center, Inc.

Within this section nausea and vomiting will be referred to as 'emesis' as this incorporates both symptoms along with retching. CINV will be discussed, however the assessment and management of emesis in the acutely unwell patient is the same. The pharmacological management will differ according to the cause.

Also, as part of the global assessment, the following risk factors can contribute to a greater experience of emesis for some patients (Molassiotis and Borjeson 2006):

- below the age of 40
- female
- susceptibility to nausea when eating food
- taste of the drug during administration
- low alcohol use
- history of labyrinthitis and vestibular disturbance
- susceptibility to motion sickness
- a desire to control the choice of antiemetic used.

Chemotherapy regimens can be classified according to their emetic potential and treatment recommended accordingly (National Comprehensive Cancer Network [NCCN] 2016). Several types of CINV exist (Janelsins et al. 2013). CINV can result in altered nutritional and performance status and poor quality of life, which may affect patients' ability and desire to receive additional treatment. Prevention or effective treatment of CINV is, therefore, an important aspect of successful therapy. Owing to the potential side-effects associated with antiemetic agents themselves (e.g. constipation, headaches), use of the lowest possible effective antiemetic dose is desirable. Antiemetic regimens should be chosen based on the emetogenic potential of the chemotherapy regimen as well as patient-specific risk factors (London Cancer Alliance 2015, Nasir and Schwartzberg 2016).

Assessment

When treatment-induced emesis is suspected, initial assessment follows as outlined in the introduction to this chapter but with the addition of the following specific questions:

History of presenting complaint

1 What chemotherapy is the patient on and when was the last treatment?
  a Are any of these drugs commonly associated with CINV?
2 Are they receiving any radiotherapy and to which area – when was their last treatment?
3 Frequency and nature of emesis?
  a Any blood noted in the vomit?
  b Does anything make it better or worse?
4 Any associated symptoms?
  a Is the emesis associated with any particular time of the day?
  b Any change in bowel movement?
    i Signs of constipation, diarrhoea or bowel obstruction?
  c Any evidence of reflux or gastritis?
  d Abdominal pain?
5 Are they able to eat and drink as usual?
  a How much fluid are they able to drink and what type?
6 Any signs of dehydration – decreased urine output, fever, thirst, dry mouth?
7 Current medications – are they taking any antiemetics and how are they taking them?
8 What is the extent of their disease – known brain, bone or liver metastases?

Identify

Is the patient at risk of immunosuppression (chemotherapy or radiotherapy within the last 6 weeks, bone marrow transplant or disease-related immunosuppression) as there may also be an underlying sepsis (±neutropenia)?

Obtain baseline observations

These should include temperature, pulse, blood pressure, respiration rate, oxygen saturations and the Early Warning Score. If the patient is showing signs of sepsis (see Neutropenic sepsis section), fluid resuscitation should be started before investigations are performed.

Initial investigations include FBC, U&Es, LFTs and bone profile. If sepsis is suspected add CRP, lactate and blood cultures.

Table 7.9 Potential causes of nausea and vomiting in cancer patients

System	Possible causes	
Gastrointestinal	• Intestinal obstruction • Gastric outlet obstruction • Constipation • Gastroparesis • Ileus • Gastritis/dyspepsia • Ascites	
Metabolic	• Hypercalcaemia • Renal failure • Electrolyte disturbance • Liver failure	
Toxic	• Chemotherapy • Radiotherapy • Infection	
Drugs	Gastrointestinal irritation	Non-steroidal anti-inflammatory drugs Iron supplements Antibiotics Tranexamic acid
	Gastric stasis	Opioids Tricyclic antidepressants Phenothiazines Anticholinergics
	Chemoreceptor trigger zone stimulation	Opioids Digoxin Anticonvulsants Antibiotics Imidazoles Cytotoxics
	5-HT3 receptor stimulation	Cytotoxics Selective serotonin reuptake inhibitors
Other	• Raised intracranial pressure, e.g. brain metastases • Vestibular problems • Pain • Cough • Pharyngeal irritation, e.g. *Candida* • Psychological – fear, anxiety	

Source: Adapted from Warr (2008)

Management

Pharmacological support

As previously stated, for many patients this is one of the worst side-effects; providing a calm and dignified environment will help to calm them. The causes of nausea and vomiting in cancer patients can be multifactorial, therefore careful assessment is essential to explore the cause and identify any reversible causes (Roila et al. 2016). The basic principles of managing emesis with medication (as outlined in Tables 7.10 and 7.11) are as follows (Warr 2008).

- Identify and treat underlying causes if possible.
- If possible, discontinue any drugs thought to be responsible for nausea and vomiting.
- Give antiemetics regularly.
- Consider route – give parenterally if the patient is likely to vomit or has poor absorption.
- Tailor antiemetic according to likely cause of nausea/vomiting and receptors involved.

- Maximize dose before switching.
- In a third of patients, there may be more than one cause of nausea/vomiting.
  - Any added antiemetic should have a different mode of action.
  - Use a broad-spectrum antiemetic.
  - Consider adding a second agent.
  - Consider a broad-spectrum antiemetic (e.g. levomepromazine) if CINV is multifactorial
- Use the non-oral route if vomiting prevents drug absorption (e.g. in bowel obstruction).

Non-pharmacological support

It is important to acknowledge the place of non-drug treatments (e.g. control of malodour, avoidance of large meals, avoidance of exposure to food smells that may precipitate nausea). It is key for the nurse to facilitate this. Some dietary considerations include:

- Eating foods cold or at room temperature as they often smell less strongly than hot foods.
- Avoiding fatty foods.

Table 7.10 Common causes of nausea and vomiting in cancer patients and treatment options

Cause	Treatment options
Anxiety	Lorazepam; antidepressants in the longer term: seek advice from the patient's GP or from the oncology team
Bowel obstruction	Levomepromazine or haloperidol or cyclizine
Chemotherapy	Treat according to emetogenic potential of drugs:
	Mild (level 1): domperidone or metoclopramide (do not use together)
	Moderate (level 2): levomepromazine (6.25 mg BD PO) or cyclizine or prochlorperazine (25 mg rectally). These agents replace metoclopramide/domperidone
	Severe (level 3): ondansetron (effective in acute – maximum use 3 days) or lorazepam (effective in anticipatory – 1 mg PO, IV or sublingual) or levomepromazine (SC infusion) or haloperidol (1–2 mg QDS PO or 1–3 mg TDS IV)
Constipation	Treat cause
Delayed gastric emptying	Metoclopramide
Drugs* (non-chemotherapy)	Stop drug if possible
	Haloperidol or levomepromazine
Gastric irritation	Treat cause (e.g. proton pump inhibitor)
	Metoclopramide if needed
Metabolic causes including hypercalcaemia	Treat cause
	Haloperidol or levomepromazine
Renal failure	Haloperidol or levomepromazine
Raised intracranial pressure	Treat cause
	Dexamethasone and cyclizine

*Common culprits include antibiotics, antidepressants, non-steroidal anti-inflammatory drugs and opiates. *Source:* LCA (2015). Reproduced with permission of London Cancer Alliance.
BD PO, twice a day *per os*, by mouth; IV, intravenous(ly); QDS, four times a day; SC, subcutaneous(ly); TDS, three times a day.

Table 7.11 Drugs used to control emesis and their classification. This list is not exhaustive; each trust may have local clinical guidelines

Putative site of action	Class	Example
Central nervous system		
Vomiting centre	Anticholinergic	Hyoscine hydrobromide
	Antihistamine	Cyclizine, dimenhydrinate
	5-HT2 antagonist	Phenothiazines
		Levomepromazine
Central nervous system	Neurokinin-1 antagonist	Aprepitant
Chemoreceptor trigger zone	Dopamine (D2) antagonist	Haloperidol, phenothiazines, metoclopramide, domperidone
	5-HT3 antagonist	Levomepromazine
		Granisetron, ondansetron, tropisetron
Cerebral cortex	Benzodiazepine	Lorazepam
	Cannabinoid	Nabilone
	Corticosteroid	Dexamethasone
Gastrointestinal tract		
Prokinetic	5-HT4 agonist	Metoclopramide
	Dopamine (D2) antagonist	Metoclopramide, domperidone levomepromazine
Antisecretory	Anticholinergic	Hyoscine butylbromide, glycopyrronium
	Somatostatin analogue	Octreotide
Vagal 5-HT3 receptor blockade	5-HT3 antagonist	Granisetron, ondansetron, tropisetron
Anti-inflammatory	Corticosteroid	Dexamethasone

Source: Adapted from Collis and Mather (2015), Twycross and Black (1998).

- Eating carbohydrates.
- Eating small, frequent meals.
- Avoiding foods that increase the patient's nausea.
- Educating family members who, in their desire to 'do the right thing', encourage the patient to eat more than they can comfortably manage.

It can be argued that the patient's favourite food should be avoided during episodes of nausea in case it provides a future stimulus for nausea and vomiting, so depriving the patient of a pleasurable experience.

Avoiding the sight and smell of food may reduce episodes of nausea. The inpatient should be protected from unpleasant odours, for example from bedside commodes, episodes of incontinence or malodorous wounds. Once the patient has finished eating, any remaining food should be quickly cleared away. Any used receptacles should be removed promptly after episodes of vomiting.

Other measures include the use of acupressure bands (see Chapter 4) and acupuncture (see Chapter 3) (Ezzo et al. 2005, Pan et al. 2000).

Education

Non-pharmacological interventions are based around educating the patient and their family in techniques that may help reduce the frequency and severity of symptoms, enhance the effect of antiemetics and increase the patient's sense of control.

Neutropenic sepsis

Definition

Neutropenic sepsis is defined as a temperature greater than 38°C with a neutrophil count of less than 0.5×10^9/L in a patient receiving systemic anticancer treatment (NICE 2012b).

Related theory

Patients with neutropenia are vulnerable to invasive infection, which can be rapidly overwhelming, causing septic shock and death (Clarke et al. 2013). It is acknowledged that neutropenic sepsis, as with all forms of sepsis, is a medical emergency. Early recognition combined with urgent administration of intravenous antibiotics is essential to ensuring a good patient outcome (Ford and Marshall 2014, NICE 2012b).

Despite this, neutropenic sepsis remains a major and one of the most common complications of cancer chemotherapy, with an associated mortality rate ranging from 2% to 21% (Ford and Marshall 2014, National Institute for Clinical Excellence [NICE] and the National Collaborating Centre for Cancer 2012). The condition contributes to 50% of deaths associated with leukaemia, lymphomas and solid tumours (Viscoli 1998). Younger patients and patients on corticosteroids are more likely to present with ill-defined symptoms and, despite baseline observations being abnormal, may look quite well (Mort et al. 2008). Bacterial infections are common in patients with febrile neutropenia, but fungal sources are increasingly prevalent (Ford and Marshall 2014). There is considerable variation in symptoms, which can include a temperature of 101°F (38.3°C) or more and an absolute neutrophil count (ANC) less than 500 per mm^3 (0.5×10^9/L) (Ford and Marshall 2014, Quint 2000). The defining presenting features of general sepsis are two or more of the following symptoms: fever (>38°C) or hypothermia (<36°C), tachypnoea (>21–24 breaths per minute), tachycardia (91–130 beats per minute [bpm]), hypotension (systolic BP<90mmHg or 40 below normal) or oliguria for 12–14 hours (NICE 2016). However, in many patients with neutropenia, particularly those taking corticosteroids, the systemic inflammatory response to infection is attenuated, meaning that the diagnostic criteria for sepsis might not be fulfilled and a clear focus of infection might not be found. For this reason, there must be a high index of suspicion for infection in all patients undergoing chemotherapy who become unwell, even in the absence of fever. The only evidence of neutropenic sepsis might be a general deterioration in condition, or non-specific signs such as confusion. The neutrophil count typically reaches its nadir approximately 5–7 days after administration of SACT, at which time patients are particularly susceptible to infection. Once sepsis is established a situation develops in which oxygen consumption at tissue level rises and cannot be met by the circulation, which will eventually show as tachycardia, hypotension, hypoxia and tachypnoea (Dellinger et al. 2008).

Investigations

Although it is important to undertake a thorough investigation into the presenting complaint with this oncological emergency, time is of the essence (NICE 2012b, 2016). The national recommendation for the initial management of sepsis (±neutropenia) is to give initial empiric therapy within 1 hour of presentation of the patient to a healthcare professional (Dellinger et al. 2008, NICE 2012b, 2016). Although blood cultures should be taken initially it must be appreciated that it will take 24–48 hours to get a result and treatment should start immediately. Specification of antibiotics can be done once results are available.

A high index of suspicion of neutropenic sepsis must be acted upon if a cancer patient presents feeling unwell, with or without a temperature, on active cancer treatment, or if they have received treatment in the last 6 weeks (Clinical Knowledge Summaries [CKS] 2015). A simple history of the presenting complaint will provide information regarding the speed of onset of symptoms along with any co-morbidities (Marrs 2006). Baseline observations (including EWS) plus initial blood work on presentation should include (Dellinger et al. 2008, NICE 2012b, 2016):

- Temperature – although fever is usually the alerting sign (37.5°C on more than two occasions or 38°C on one occasion), patients may also present with hypothermia or confusion.
- Pulse – manual as well as via a monitor as this will inform of the regularity, strength and contour.
- Oxygen saturations – confirmed on blood gas.
- Respiratory rate – this is the simplest observation to take and the one that will change most quickly in a deteriorating patient.
- Blood pressure – looking for signs of septic shock. It may be that the patient is hypertensive prior to becoming hypotensive.
- Conscious level – AVPU.
- IV access and blood tests:
  - Lactate (venous blood gas is appropriate at this point), FBC, coagulation screen, U&Es, LFTs (including albumin), glucose (also take a capillary blood glucose level), calcium, magnesium, CRP.
- Full septic screen:
  - Blood cultures – from peripheral vein and central venous access device (if *in situ*).
  - Urine dip and specimen.
  - Swab all skin breaks.
  - Stool if the patient has complained of loose motion in last 24 hours.
- Commence fluid balance monitoring.

Certain drugs may mask these signs, such as beta blockers which will reduce tachycardia allowing hypotension to develop more easily. Corticosteroids and NSAIDs (e.g. regular ibuprofen) may affect temperature regulation leading to a minimal rise in temperature that would otherwise be easy to ignore (de Naurois et al. 2010). If respiratory symptoms are present, chest radiography is recommended, although it may not detect an infiltrate until the patient's ANC has improved enough to enable an inflammatory response (Hughes et al. 2002). This, however, can wait until empiric antibiotics are given along with antipyrexials (if required).

Management

Suspected neutropenic sepsis should be treated as a medical emergency and empiric antibiotic therapy commenced immediately, prior to blood results (NICE 2012b). Local policy will guide the initial empirical management of sepsis which will normally include monotherapy using a broad-spectrum agent such as piperacillin with tazobactam (NICE 2012b). See Figure 7.7 for an example of a neutropenic sepsis management pathway.

278

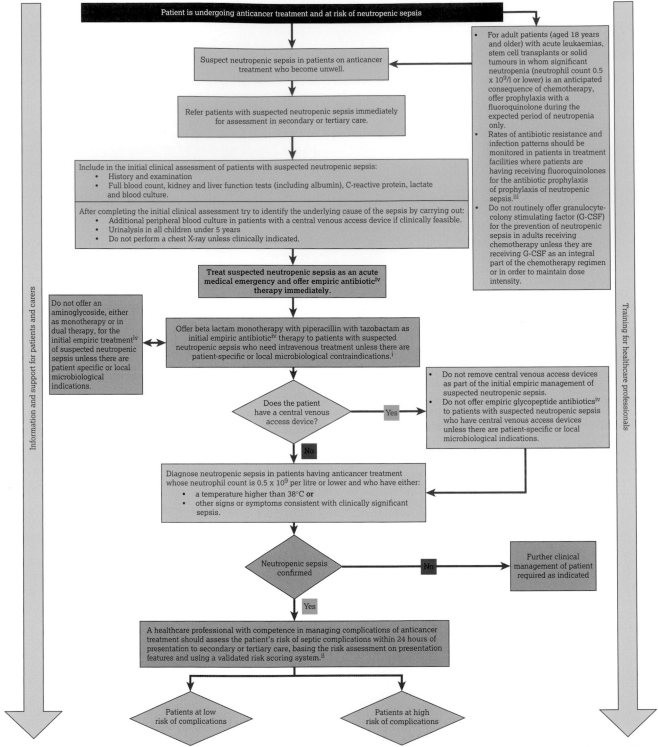

Patient is undergoing anticancer treatment and at risk of neutropenic sepsis

Suspect neutropenic sepsis in patients on anticancer treatment who become unwell.

Refer patients with suspected neutropenic sepsis immediately for assessment in secondary or tertiary care.

Include in the initial clinical assessment of patients with suspected neutropenic sepsis:
- History and examination
- Full blood count, kidney and liver function tests (including albumin), C-reactive protein, lactate and blood culture.

After completing the initial clinical assessment try to identify the underlying cause of the sepsis by carrying out:
- Additional peripheral blood culture in patients with a central venous access device if clinically feasible.
- Urinalysis in all children under 5 years
- Do not perform a chest X-ray unless clinically indicated.

Treat suspected neutropenic sepsis as an acute medical emergency and offer empiric antibiotic[iv] therapy immediately.

Do not offer an aminoglycoside, either as monotherapy or in dual therapy, for the initial empiric treatment[iv] of suspected neutropenic sepsis unless there are patient specific or local microbiological indications.

Offer beta lactam monotherapy with piperacillin with tazobactam as initial empiric antibiotic[iv] therapy to patients with suspected neutropenic sepsis who need intravenous treatment unless there are patient-specific or local microbiological contraindications.[i]

Does the patient have a central venous access device? — Yes →

Do not remove central venous access devices as part of the initial empiric management of suspected neutropenic sepsis.
Do not offer empiric glycopeptide antibiotics[iv] to patients with suspected neutropenic sepsis who have central venous access devices unless there are patient-specific or local microbiological indications.

No

Diagnose neutropenic sepsis in patients having anticancer treatment whose neutrophil count is 0.5×10^9 per litre or lower and who have either:
- a temperature higher than 38°C or
- other signs or symptoms consistent with clinically significant sepsis.

Neutropenic sepsis confirmed — No → Further clinical management of patient required as indicated

Yes

A healthcare professional with competence in managing complications of anticancer treatment should assess the patient's risk of septic complications within 24 hours of presentation to secondary or tertiary care, basing the risk assessment on presentation features and using a validated risk scoring system.[ii]

Patients at low risk of complications

Patients at high risk of complications

For adult patients (aged 18 years and older) with acute leukaemias, stem cell transplants or solid tumours in whom significant neutropenia (neutrophil count 0.5 x 10^9/l or lower) is an anticipated consequence of chemotherapy, offer prophylaxis with a fluoroquinolone during the expected period of neutropenia only.
Rates of antibiotic resistance and infection patterns should be monitored in patients in treatment facilities where patients are having receiving fluoroquinolones for the antibiotic prophylaxis of prophylaxis of neutropenic sepsis.[iii]
Do not routinely offer granulocyte-colony stimulating factor (G-CSF) for the prevention of neutropenic sepsis in adults receiving chemotherapy unless they are receiving G-CSF as an integral part of the chemotherapy regimen or in order to maintain dose intensity.

Information and support for patients and carers

Training for healthcare professionals

[i] At the time of publication (September 2012) piperacillin with tazobactam did not have a UK marketing authorization for use in children aged under 2 years. The prescriber should follow relevant professional guidance, taking full responsibility for the decision. The child's parent or carer should provide informed consent, which should be documented. See the GMC's Good practice in prescribing medicines – guidance for doctors and the prescribing advice provided by the Joint Standing Committee on Medicines (a joint committee of the Royal College of Paediatrics and Child Health and the Neonatal and Paediatric Pharmacists Group) for further information.
[ii] Example of risk scoring include The Multinational Association for Supportive Care risk index: a multinational scoring system for identifying low-risk febrile neutropenic cancer patients (Journal of Clinical Oncology 2000; 18: 3038-51) and the modified Alexander rule for children (aged under 18 (European Journal of Cancer 2009; 45: 2843-9)
[iii] For more information see the Department of Health's Updated guidance on the diagnosis and reporting of Clostridium difficile and guidance from the Health Protection Agency and the Department of Health on Clostridium difficile infection; how to deal with the problem.
[iv] An empiric antibiotic is given to a person before a specific microorganism or source of the potential infection is known. It is usually a broad-spectrum antibiotic and the treatment may change if the microorganism or source is confirmed.

Figure 7.7 The NICE neutropenic sepsis pathway (NICE 2012b). *Source:* Ford and Marshall (2014) Neutropenic sepsis: a potentially life-threatening complication of chemotherapy. *Clinical Medicine*, 14(5), 538–542. Reproduced with permission.

The role of the cancer nurse in this group of patients is to respond immediately when neutropenic sepsis is suspected and ensure that it is acknowledged as a medical emergency. Early recognition and treatment of sepsis is key to improving outcomes. In order to support the effective and efficient management of patients in suspected severe sepsis, six basic therapies (bundles) were developed based on best practice guidelines (NHS England 2013). The use of 'bundles' has been shown to simplify the complex processes of the care of patients with severe sepsis (NHS England 2013). A bundle is a selected set of elements of care that, when implemented as a group, have an effect on outcomes beyond implementing the individual elements alone (Surviving Sepsis 2015). One such bundle dealing with basic therapies, the 'sepsis six' (Table 7.12), has been shown to improve outcomes in septic patients. If the six factors are completed within the first hour following recognition of sepsis, the associated mortality has been reported to reduce by as much as 50% (Surviving Sepsis 2015).

Neutropenia has been found to be independently associated with a higher risk of AKI (urine output of less than 0.5 mg/kg/h for 6 hours) therefore close monitoring of the patient's haemodynamic status, including urine output, is essential (Reilly et al. 2016). Combined with the risk of hypotension in sepsis, fluid resuscitation may be required. If the patient's history includes oliguria or they present with hypotension, fluid resuscitation may be required. Treating hypotension through fluid resuscitation should be a central tenet in treating sepsis (Daniels 2011). Fluid resuscitation is as follows:

- Give 500 mL of 0.9% sodium chloride (NaCl) over 15 minutes. There is no evidence to suggest the use of a colloid is any more effective.
- Observe the patient and check vital signs at end of infusion and then every 15 minutes.
- If a satisfactory response has been achieved, give maintenance fluids to cover general anticipated fluid losses.
- Continue monitoring every 15 minutes for the first hour, then every 30 minutes for the second hour, and then hourly.

- If there is no response and jugular venous pressure (JVP) is not raised, repeat the fluid challenge.
- If a third fluid challenge is required, the clinical team and critical care outreach team should have been called.

NICE and the National Collaborating Centre for Cancer (2012) recommend that immediately following empiric IV antibiotic treatment the patient be risk assessed using a validated tool such as the Multinational Association for Supportive Care in Cancer (MASCC) scoring system for grading neutropenic sepsis. Table 7.13 shows how this has been adapted for use at The Royal Marsden to determine the risk of prolonged septic complications to guide ongoing management. If a patient is risk stratified as having low-grade neutropenia (a score of >21) outpatient management with oral antibiotics and robust follow-up with access to expert cancer triage in the ambulatory setting may be appropriate (Cooksley et al. 2015, NICE and the National Collaborating Centre for Cancer 2012). There is currently no consensus as to the period of monitoring low-risk patients should undergo prior to being discharged from hospital; this ranges from 24 to 48 hours (Freifeld et al. 2011). In high-risk patients (a score of <21) or where an organism has been isolated, treatment should be continued for 5 days (NICE 2012b).

In addition, effective written local policies are essential to ensure a rapid response whenever neutropenic sepsis is suspected. Some patients may present with neutropenic sepsis via the Emergency Department, and in this situation clear protocols must be in place to manage these patients appropriately.

Patient education
Successful management of neutropenic sepsis requires prompt recognition of, and reaction to, potential infection. Patient education to promptly recognize symptoms is vital, with clear written instructions on when and how to contact the appropriate service (de Naurois et al. 2010, Marrs 2006, Mort et al. 2008). Also essential is educating outpatient and emergency departments to suspect sepsis until proven otherwise in any patient who presents with ill-defined symptoms such as confusion or gastrointestinal

Table 7.12 Severe sepsis care bundle

Procedure	Rationale
Oxygen: start with high flow (15 L via non-rebreathe mask and titrate down) – target saturations >94%	Intended to restore the imbalance between oxygen supply and demand to the tissues
Fluid resuscitation: give boluses of 0.9% sodium chloride (500 mL) over 15 minutes Observe response and repeat as necessary until hypotension/organ dysfunction is improved (up to max 1.5–2 L then call senior doctor/ICU)	Intended to restore the imbalance between oxygen supply and demand to the tissues
Blood cultures: take at least two sets, including at least one from a fresh venepuncture • Culture any vascular access devices in situ >48 hours • Request other cultures/swabs/imaging as appropriate	Assists with identification of sepsis source, systemic and CVAD related (NICE and the National Collaborating Centre for Cancer 2012, Surviving Sepsis 2015)
IV antibiotics as per trust/local guidelines: ensure they are given immediately (within 1 hour of suspected neutropenic sepsis)	Decreases the risk of mortality and morbidity (NICE 2012b)
Arterial blood gas to measure lactate: a venous sample is OK if respiratory status is stable • Repeat lactate measurement after first-hour duties completed	A failure of lactate to improve with therapy is indicative of a poor outcome. Lactate clearance has been shown to correlate positively with survival
Take bloods for FBC, U&Es, clotting • Arrange transfusion if Hb<7	Enables assessment of patient condition and management (NHS England 2013, NICE 2012b)
Commence hourly fluid balance • Catheterize if necessary, checking platelet count first	Risk of AKI due to sepsis (Reilly et al. 2016) Increased risk of bleeding if platelet count <50×10^9/L

Source: Adapted from NHS England (2013).

Table 7.13 The metastatic spinal cord compression (MASCC) scoring system adapted for local use at The Royal Marsden for grading neutropenic sepsis risk

		Yes	No	Score*
Does the patient have a solid tumour or lymphoma (except Burkitt lymphoma)?		4	0	
Is the patient dehydrated or requiring IV fluids?		0	3	
Is the systolic BP<90mmHg?		0	5	
How sick is the patient?	No/mild symptoms	5	0	
	Moderate symptoms	3	0	
	Severe symptoms	0	0	
Is the patient aged<60 years?		2	0	
Does the patient have chronic obstructive pulmonary disease?		0	4	
Did the patient develop febrile neutropenia while an inpatient?		0	3	
Total MASCC score				

*Points attributable to burden of illness are not cumulative. The maximal theoretical score is therefore 26. A threshold of ≥21 points defines 'low risk'. *Source:* NICE (2012b).

upset and who has had SACT within 6 weeks of presentation (Ford and Marshall 2014, Mattison et al. 2016).

Nurses have been shown to have a significant impact on the outcome of patients with neutropenic sepsis through preventative interventions that monitor and educate the cancer patient population along with their healthcare colleagues from other departments (Marrs 2006, Mattison et al. 2016).

Pneumonitis

Definition

Pneumonitis is a general term that refers to inflammation of lung tissue. Technically, pneumonia is a type of pneumonitis because the infection causes inflammation, however pneumonitis is used when referring to other causes of lung inflammation. Pneumonitis can be caused by disease, infection, radiotherapy, allergies or irritation of the lung tissue by inhaled substances and SACT (National Cancer Institute 2016).

Anatomy and physiology

The primary function of the lungs is to provide gaseous interchange; therefore the lungs must be accessible to both the external and internal environments via inhalation and the circulation, respectively, leading to the evolutionary development of critical structural and physiological relationships between the air passages, respiratory parenchyma and vascular system (Notter et al. 2005). These relationships, together with the ease of access, make the lungs especially susceptible to a multitude of physical, chemical and biological stressors that appear to be able to disrupt the delicate functional balance of this system with relative ease. Depending on the source and severity, under many circumstances there is progression to a persistent, chronic pathology, which occurs through a complex cascade of processes beginning with the acute injury and followed by an associated innate inflammatory response, culminating in abnormal remodelling and tissue repair (Notter et al. 2005).

Related theory

Pneumonitis is the lung tissue's reaction to cancer treatment; it is deemed dose-limiting and thereby can compromise treatment and also lead to quality-of-life issues in survivors (Williams et al. 2010).

Radiation pneumonitis can occur within 6–12 weeks after thoracic radiotherapy and occurs in between 5% and 15% of patients (Oie et al. 2013, Williams et al. 2010). The risk of pneumonitis is related to the volume of normal lung irradiated and the dose of radiotherapy delivered (Libshitz 1993, McDonald et al. 1995). Therefore, it is most likely to occur with radical (potentially curative) treatments for lung and oesophageal cancer but can also occur following treatment for breast cancer and lymphoma (Williams et al. 2010). Symptoms usually arise within the first 90 days of radiotherapy treatment (acute effects of radiation) but can occur later than this during the development of lung fibrosis (McDonald et al. 1995). The chance of radiation pneumonitis is increased by the concomitant use of chemotherapy and is more likely to occur in patients with pre-existing lung disease such as chronic obstructive pulmonary disease.

SACT, including bleomycin, busulfan, cyclophosphamide, carmustine, the taxanes and methotrexate, can cause inflammation in the alveoli, filling them with white blood cells and fluids which can lead to the development of pneumonitis (Limper 2004, Matsuno 2012, Vander et al. 2004). Targeted therapies such as mammalian target of rapamycin (mTOR) and EGFR inhibitors along with immunotherapies (CTLA-4 or PD-1/PD-L1) are known to cause pneumonitis although the exact mechanism is unknown (Duran et al. 2014, Zhang et al. 2016). Discontinuation of the drugs with prednisolone treatment in severe cases will resolve the pneumonitis (Duran et al. 2014, Matsuno 2012).

Diagnosis

Clinical awareness and early identification of possible symptoms of pneumonitis in high-risk patients is essential to reduce interruptions, reduction in dose (if SACT), and treatment discontinuation and maintain quality of life and, ultimately, patient outcomes (Peterson 2013).

Pneumonitis must always be considered as a differential diagnosis in patients receiving radiotherapy to the thorax and SACT (including targeted therapies) with known respiratory side-effects (McDonald et al. 1995, Peterson 2013, Williams et al. 2010). The symptoms of pneumonitis can be vague in some patients or mimic those of their cancer itself. These include:

- shortness of breath on exercise
- chest pain
- cough
- low-grade fever.

In some cases there are no symptoms but the diagnosis is made on routine chest X-ray or high-resolution CT. If symptoms are present, a full set of observations should be taken including an arterial blood gas. This will help the clinician to evaluate the level of respiratory distress of the patient. When taking blood samples, inflammatory markers (ESR, CRP and FBC differentials) should be included to support diagnosis and rule out infective pneumonitis (Peterson 2013). A chest X-ray is a quick diagnostic test to obtain; if pneumonitis is present it may show as ground-glass

Table 7.14 Clinical management of pneumonitis induced by targeted therapy

Grade	Symptom	Management	Dose modification
1	Asymptomatic (radiographic findings only)	Initiate appropriate monitoring	No dose adjustment required
2	Symptomatic, not interfering with activities of daily living	Rule out infection. Consider treatment with corticosteroids (prednisolone 40 mg)	Consider interruption of therapy until symptoms improve to grade ≤ 1. Reinitiate at a lower dose. Discontinue treatment if failure to recover within 4 weeks
3	Symptomatic, interfering with activities of daily living; oxygen required	Rule out infection. Consider treatment with corticosteroids	Hold treatment until recovery to grade ≤ 1. Consider reinitiating at a lower dose. If toxicity recurs at grade 3, consider discontinuation
4	Life threatening	Ventilator support indicated	Discontinue treatment

Source: Adapted from Cancer Therapy Evaluation Program, Division of Cancer Treatment and Diagnosis, National Cancer Institute, National Institutes of Health (2010), Novartis (2012), Porta et al. (2011).

opacities with focal consolidation, predominantly in the lower lobes (Porta et al. 2011). Bronchoalveolar lavage may be required to rule out infections and evaluate lung inflammation (Porta et al. 2011).

Management

Pharmacological support
Treatment consists of corticosteroids such as prednisolone 40 mg daily until symptoms subside then slow reduction of the dose. The majority of patients recover with treatment but some may be left with pulmonary fibrosis that shows up on their chest X-ray; this will be permanent (McDonald et al. 1995, Oie et al. 2013). It is important to note that many patients receiving radiotherapy to the lung will have abnormal radiology subsequently and this does not necessarily indicate recurrent disease. The radiology should be interpreted in the context of clinical symptoms and by clinicians experienced in interpreting imaging post radiotherapy.

In targeted therapies the management is dependent on severity of the symptoms. An example is outlined in Table 7.14.

Structural

Ascites (malignant)

Definition
Ascites is a central oedema in which fluid accumulates in the peritoneal cavity (Witte and Witte 1983). Abdominal paracentesis is a technique used to drain a pathological collection of ascitic fluid from the abdomen (Campbell 2001). This technique is performed to help diagnose the cause of ascites (diagnostic paracentesis) or to relieve the discomfort associated with this condition (therapeutic paracentesis) (McGibbon et al. 2007).

Anatomy and physiology
The peritoneum is a semi-permeable serous membrane consisting of two separate layers: the parietal layer and the visceral layer. The parietal layer covers the abdominal and pelvic walls and the undersurface of the diaphragm. The visceral layer lines and supports the abdominal organs and the parietal peritoneum (Figure 7.8). The space between the parietal and visceral layers is known as the peritoneal cavity (Thibodeau and Patton 2010). The normal peritoneal cavity contains a small amount of free fluid – approximately 50 mL (McGibbon et al. 2007).

In a healthy individual, around 50–100 mL of fluid passes every hour from the peritoneal cavity into the lymphatic vessels and through the lymphatic vessels in the diaphragm due to changes in

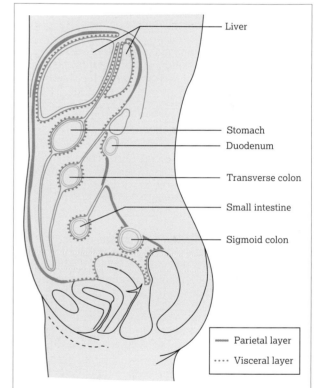

Figure 7.8 Peritoneum of female in lateral view. *Source:* Dougherty and Lister (2015). Reproduced with permission from John Wiley & Sons.

pressure as a result of breathing (Bronskill et al. 1977). The fluid is produced from the capillaries lining the peritoneal cavity and is drained by lymphatic vessels under the diaphragm. The fluid is collected by the right lymphatic duct which drains into the vena cava. The peritoneum forms the largest serous membrane in the body (Tortora and Derrickson 2014). However, in patients with malignant ascites, this balance of production and drainage is disrupted and ascitic fluid collects in the peritoneal cavity (Box 7.2).

Related theory
Ascites can be caused by non-malignant conditions such as cirrhosis of the liver, advanced congestive heart failure, chronic pericarditis and nephrotic syndrome (Hou and Sanyal 2009, Sargent 2006). In the absence of malignancy, liver disease is responsible

Box 7.2 Functions of the peritoneum

- The peritoneum is a serous membrane that enables the abdominal contents to glide over each other without friction.
- It forms a partial or complete cover for the abdominal organs.
- It forms ligaments and mesenteries that help to keep the organs in position.
- The mesenteries contain fat and act as a store for the body.
- The mesenteries can move to engulf areas of inflammation and this prevents the spread of infection.
- It has the power to absorb fluids and exchange electrolytes.

Source: Adapted from Thibodeau and Patton (2010), Tortora and Derrickson (2014).

for over 80% of cases of ascites (Royal College of Obstetricians and Gynaecologists 2014). Malignant conditions such as metastatic cancer of the ovary, stomach, colon or breast can also cause ascites. If a definitive diagnosis is needed to establish the cause, to aid staging and possible surgical intervention, then a peritoneal tap and analysis of fluid will be useful (Marincola and Schwartzentruber 2001).

It is not possible to distinguish between malignant and benign ascites by physical examination or radiographic techniques so invasive testing is necessary to differentiate the two types (Sangisetty and Miner 2012).

The pathogenesis of ascites differs depending on its primary related factors. Cirrhotic ascites is believed to be related to portal hypertension (Hou and Sanyal 2009, Lee and Grap 2008). The increased pressure occurs due to fibrosis and scarring of the liver from chronic liver disease, causing obstruction to venous flow (Whiteman and McCormick 2005). In the case of heart failure and constrictive pericarditis, the heart loses its ability to pump blood and this causes a back-up of blood and increases pressure in the portal venous system, leading to portal hypertension and ascites (Lee and Grap 2008).

The underlying physiological process causing malignant ascites is often multifactorial and is not as well understood as non-cancer-related ascites (Seike et al. 2007). It is thought to be caused by obstruction of lymphatic drainage preventing absorption of intra-abdominal fluid and protein, producing a high volume of fluid with a high protein content, hypoproteinaemia and occasionally portal hypertension secondary to hepatic cancer. This is thought to be the result of cytokines, mechanical obstruction and hormonal influence. Cytokines such as VEGF and vascular permeability factor regulate vascular permeability. The obstruction of lymphatic drainage by the disseminating malignant cells in the peritoneal cavity reduces absorption of peritoneal exudates (Seike et al. 2007). This reduction activates the renin–angiotensin–aldosterone system and leads to sodium retention, which then further exacerbates the ascites.

Ascites can be split into two main groups: exudates, which are high in protein, and transudates, which are low in protein (Runyon et al. 1988, Witte and Witte 1983). Exudates are more common and derive from a combination of increased permeability of capillaries and lymphatic obstruction, whereas transudates are likely to arise where liver metastases cause portal hypertension. Non-malignant ascites is more likely to produce a transudative ascites in which there is a marked increase in production of fluid and the lymphatic system reaches capacity with flow rates of 200 mL of ascites per hour (Bronskill et al. 1977). Ascites resulting from compression of the hepatic vein causing portal hypertension will also produce a transudative ascites. In malignancy that has spread to the peritoneal cavity, an exudative ascites is produced and lymphatic flow markedly decreases to levels as low as 15 mL per hour as the lymphatic vessels have become obstructed by tumour and cannot cope with the increased permeability of blood vessels, hence fluid accumulates.

Ascites is often accompanied by debilitating symptoms as large amounts of fluid collect in the peritoneal cavity, causing an increase in intra-abdominal pressure and resulting in pressure on internal structures. The fluid accumulation may occur over several weeks or rapidly over a few days (Lee and Grap 2008). Symptoms initially include vague abdominal discomfort, which can go on to affect the respiratory and gastrointestinal systems, depending on the amount of fluid present. Pressure on the diaphragm decreases the intrathoracic space and causes shortness of breath. Gastric pressure may cause anorexia, indigestion or hiatus hernia. Intestinal pressure may result in constipation, bowel obstruction or decreased bladder capacity (Royal College of Obstetricians and Gynecologists 2014). Patients also become increasingly fatigued, finding simple daily tasks difficult (Slusser 2014). Additionally, body image can be affected even when minimal distension is present.

Malignant ascites is most commonly seen in patients with a known diagnosis of ovarian or gastrointestinal cancer, but it can occur in any oncology patient (Ayantunde and Parsons 2007). Cytological confirmation of malignant cells is, however, difficult, with only a 50% chance of success (Fentiman 2002). In addition, more than 50% of patients with malignant ascites present with ascites at the initial diagnosis of their cancer (Ayantunde and Parsons 2007).

The onset and progression of malignant ascites is associated with deterioration in quality of life and a poor prognosis. Ascites is rarely an emergency but can be extremely uncomfortable for patients and it is not uncommon for over 8 litres of fluid to accumulate (Ayantunde and Parsons 2012). Ascites accumulates due to the presence of widespread peritoneal deposits, which leak fluid, and in some cases involvement of retroperitoneal nodes by disease may prevent drainage. Patients may complain of abdominal distension, pain, breathlessness, nausea and vomiting.

Abdominal paracentesis (drainage) will provide symptomatic relief in over 90% of cases, often very rapidly (Ayantunde and Parsons 2012). In a patient who has had no prior abdominal surgery, who is in significant pain and distress and who has a large volume of ascites, blind drainage is acceptable, however ultrasound marking is preferable. Paracentesis is effective in relieving the symptoms associated with malignant ascites but it requires repeated treatments, leads to frequent hospitalizations, depletes the patient of protein and electrolytes, and exposes the patient to a small but significant risk of peritonitis (Royal College of Obstetricians and Gynaecologists 2014).

Evidence-based approaches

Rationale

There is much debate about whether it is safe to drain large volumes of fluid rapidly from the abdomen. One concern is that profound hypotension may follow because of the sudden release of intra-abdominal pressure and consequent possible vasodilation (Lee et al. 2000). However, it is suggested that up to 5 litres of fluid may be safely drained over a few hours and it is not necessary to drain the abdomen until dry (Pericleous et al. 2016, Stephenson and Gilbert 2002). In cases of cirrhosis, however, Moore and Aithal (2006) suggest that all fluid should be drained to dryness in a single session as rapidly as possible over 1–4 hours, assisted by gentle mobilization of the cannula or turning the patient on their side if needed.

It is generally not necessary to have intravenous fluid or albumin replacement. However, patients with ascites who have large tumours, cirrhosis of the liver or renal impairment may require slower drainage of fluid and possible fluid replacement, depending on their clinical condition. Abdominal and peritoneal tumours can cause ascites to develop independently of the circulatory system and therefore hypotension is not usually seen as the ascites is drained.

A small study has shown that the success of blind paracentesis is directly related to the amount of fluid present (44% with 300 mL and 78% with 500 mL) (McGibbon et al. 2007). The literature suggests the use of ultrasound-guided paracentesis to confirm the presence of ascites and also to identify the best site to perform paracentesis, particularly when a small amount of fluid is present (McGibbon et al. 2007).

Indications
- To obtain a specimen of fluid for analysis for diagnostic purposes (diagnostic paracentesis).
- To relieve the symptoms associated with ascites, both physical and psychological (therapeutic paracentesis).
- To administer substances such as cytotoxic drugs (e.g. bleomycin, cisplatin) or other agents into the peritoneal cavity, to achieve regression of serosal deposits responsible for fluid formation (Hosttetter et al. 2005).

Contraindications
- *Relative contraindications:* pregnancy, severe bowel distension and previous extensive abdominal or pelvic surgery (McGibbon et al. 2007). When relative contraindications are present, paracentesis without the assistance of ultrasound (blind paracentesis) is not recommended (McGibbon et al. 2007).
- *Absolute contraindication:* clinically evident fibrinolysis or disseminated intravascular coagulation (McGibbon et al. 2007).

Preparatory investigations
The patient's clinical condition and purpose of the procedure must be taken into account when deciding what investigations are necessary but pre-procedure investigations usually include a blood screen and ultrasound examination. To keep intrusion to a minimum for palliative patients, fewer investigations may be performed. Blood is usually checked for FBC, U&Es, creatinine, LFTs, plasma proteins and coagulation screen (Rull 2013). In the case of a diagnostic paracentesis, the ascitic fluid should be analysed for cell count, bacterial culture, total protein and albumin (Hou and Sanyal 2009).

Methods of managing ascites
Interventions used to treat ascites range from an aggressive approach to a purely palliative approach. There have been few definitive studies that have evaluated the different approaches in the treatment of malignant ascites (Hosttetter et al. 2005). While paracentesis is effective, ascites recurs, requiring repeated procedures. This imposes a further burden on patients and their families (Mercadante et al. 2008). Methods for treating ascites may include the use of diuretics, paracentesis and a diet low in sodium, instillation of peritoneal agents or the insertion of long-term catheters (Ayantunde and Parsons 2012).

In terms of the use of drains, there is no consensus in the literature in relation to how long the drain should stay in place, whether the volume of fluid drained should be replaced intravenously, whether the drain should be clamped to regulate the drainage of fluid and whether any vital observations should be regularly recorded (Keen et al. 2010). However, many UK guidelines (London Cancer Alliance 2015) suggest that the ascites can be left to drain freely; clamping of the tube is not necessary unless the patient becomes hypotensive, in which case the drain is clamped for 20 minutes. The blood pressure should then be checked before further drainage.

In practice, most local guidelines suggest draining 1 litre, then clamping before checking the blood pressure. If the patient is not hypotensive (systolic < 90) then drainage can continue and this process should be repeated after every litre drained. There is no evidence that albumin support is beneficial and intravenous fluids are only used if the patient becomes hypotensive despite clamping the drain (Moore and Aithal 2006). The evidence suggests that drainage limited to 5–8 litres provides the greatest symptomatic relief and a reduction in potential complications. This evidence makes day case paracentesis a preferred option for many patients (Becker et al. 2006).

In chronic management, ascites frequently reaccumulates and drainage tends to provide ever-decreasing symptomatic benefit, but it is still worth performing. With recurrent drainage, there is an increasing risk that the ascites can become loculated, therefore a more permanent drain such as a PleurX™ may be appropriate (NICE 2018). Types of catheters are discussed further under 'Equipment'.

Common interventions in ascites include:

- *Paracentesis:* This is the most common way of managing ascites as it has an immediate effect in 90% of cases (Campbell 2001, Marincola and Schwartzentruber 2001).
- *Sodium-restricted diet.* The amount of fluid retained in the body depends on the balance between sodium ingested in the diet and sodium excreted in the urine. A reduced sodium intake of 2 g per day is considered a realistic goal (Sargent 2006).
- *Diuretics.* There is limited evidence supporting a role for diuretics such as spironolactone in malignant ascites, with only a handful of small case series reporting the outcomes after oral or intravenous therapy (Royal College of Obstetricians and Gynaecologists 2014). However, surveys of clinical practice suggest that diuretics are commonly used and are useful mainly in cirrhotic-type ascites. They may be used for malignant ascites together with a restriction of salt and fluid intake, and have been found to be effective in about one-third of patients (Hosttetter et al. 2005, Sangisetty and Miner 2012). Pockros et al. (1992) suggested that diuretic therapy was unlikely to mobilize ascitic fluid and that any weight loss was from loss of fluid outside of the peritoneal cavity and could lead to patients becoming dehydrated if not carefully supervised. Spironolactone is the diuretic of choice (Hou and Sanyal 2009). The most effective way of monitoring the fluid loss is by weighing the patient daily (Sargent 2006).
- *Instillation of intraperitoneal agents.* Cytotoxics, sclerosants and biological substances have been tried in an attempt to control the recurrence of ascites. To date, intraperitoneal agents have not been proven, unequivocally, to have a greater beneficial effect than the use of diuretics (Fentiman 2002).

It should however be noted that the literature available is mostly generated from studies in patients suffering from acute or chronic liver failure; this should be taken into account when managing patients with non-malignant ascites.

Anticipated patient outcomes
Nursing and medical care of patients with malignant abdominal ascites should be aimed at improving quality of life by relieving suffering caused by the symptoms (Cope 2005). Each patient should be carefully assessed with consideration of their individual circumstances, maintaining respect for their wish to have or not to have interventional treatment (Campbell 2001).

For many patients accumulation of ascitic fluid is a poor prognostic indicator and therefore the management is palliative (Ayantunde and Parsons 2012).

Legal and professional issues
Nurses should ensure that patients are educated about the nature of the procedure, what results can realistically be expected, and the risks and benefits. It is essential that the patient, family and carer are involved in the discussion so that an informed and joint decision may be made in order to achieve the best possible outcome.

Competencies
The procedure is performed by a doctor or a practitioner trained in paracentesis assisted by a nurse or healthcare professional throughout. There is no accredited pathway or course for learning

283

this clinical skill and specific training has to be negotiated and developed locally (Vaughan 2013).

Assessment

Clinical examination usually suffices; however, it is rare to be able to detect ascites unless there are at least 2–3 litres present. It is common practice to perform paracentesis under ultrasound control to identify the deepest pool of fluid and to ensure that there are no vital organs beneath the drainage site. A drainage catheter is usually placed following an ultrasound to mark an appropriate area into which it can be introduced. The catheter can be inserted at the same time as the scan or, more commonly, afterwards on the ward. The period between drainage and ultrasound can be a few hours, in which case the bowel may have moved, making bowel perforation an increased risk (Royal College of Obstetricians and Gynaecologists 2014). Abdominal X-ray is not useful in this setting unless it is needed to exclude small bowel obstruction (Sangisetty and Miner 2012).

Pre-procedural considerations

Equipment

Three types of long-term catheter are generally used:

- *Peritoneovenous shunt:* generally used in patients with a long-term prognosis. These shunts drain ascitic fluid into the superior vena cava and require general anaesthesia for insertion (Mamada et al. 2007, Seike et al. 2007).
- *PleurX™ drain:* a tunnelled catheter placed under ultrasound and fluoroscopic guidance. This device is associated with low rates of serious adverse clinical events, catheter failure, discomfort and electrolyte imbalance (Courtney et al. 2008). Additionally, it may allow patients to avoid spending added time in hospital for repeated paracentesis.
- *Peritoneal port-catheter:* similar to but larger than central venous access ports in order to make access easier and to decrease possible catheter occlusion (Ozkan et al. 2007). There are a very limited number of studies supporting its use.

Nurses should describe the equipment to be used during paracentesis to the patient. This may be more relevant when looking after a patient undergoing the procedure for the first time to whom the size of the catheter may be concerning.

Assessment and recording tools

A detailed and consistent nursing assessment is important when caring for patients requiring paracentesis. Nurses should pay attention to the cause of the ascites and the frequency with which the procedure is occurring. The involvement of the palliative care team may be indicated at this stage. In cases of ascites secondary to cirrhosis, nurses should pay special attention to unresolved issues surrounding alcohol abuse, offering support and information to the patient and family. As well as assessing the patient's psychological well-being, nurses must pay attention to the skin condition and pain levels.

In preparation for the paracentesis, the following investigations should take place to ensure patient safety: a full set of observations and baseline blood tests (FBC, U&Es and clotting). It is recommended that platelets are $>50\times10^9$/L and international normalized ratio (INR) 5 L/24 hours (NICE 2012d). However, an abnormal INR or thrombocytopenia is not a contraindication to paracentesis, and in most patients there is no need to transfuse fresh frozen plasma or platelets prior to the procedure (Runyon 1986). Of patients with ascites, 70% have an abnormal prothrombin time, but the actual risk of bleeding following paracentesis is very low (less than 1% of patients require transfusion). Exceptions are patients with clinically apparent disseminated intravascular coagulation or clinically apparent hyperfibrinolysis, who require treatment to decrease their risk of bleeding before undergoing paracentesis (McVay and Toy 1991). The patient's girth around the umbilicus should be measured and weight checked before the procedure; this should be clearly documented to allow for subsequent comparisons to be made. There is no need for the patient to fast prior to this procedure.

Pharmacological support

The healthcare professional performing the paracentesis must use a local anaesthetic (e.g. lidocaine 1%). The lidocaine is injected subcutaneously initially with a 25 G needle and subsequently with a 23 G needle until optimal pain control is achieved, not exceeding the maximum dose of 4.5 mg/kg (or 200 mg). Optimal pain control is achieved between 2 and 5 minutes after the drug is injected and it is important for the practitioner to assess the effectiveness of the local anaesthetic before the insertion of the catheter and drainage of ascites. Lorazepam at a dose of 1 mg can be of benefit prior to the procedure for patients who are anxious, due to its muscle relaxant and anxiolytic effects (Joint Formulary Committee 2018).

Non-pharmacological support

The nurse should enquire about the patient's fears and concerns regarding paracentesis. For some patients, music or relaxation, physical relaxation and visualization techniques are of great benefit so use of these approaches should be considered, if available (Misra 2016).

Procedure guideline 7.2 Abdominal paracentesis

Essential equipment

- Sterile abdominal paracentesis set containing scalpel blade and blade holder, swabs, towels, trocar and cannula (or other approved catheter and introducer), connector to attach to the cannula and guide fluid into the container (Figure 7.9)
- Sterile dressing pack
- Sterile specimen pots
- Local anaesthetic
- Needles and syringes
- Chlorhexidine 0.5% in 70% alcohol
- Adhesive dressing
- Large sterile drainage bag or container (with connector if appropriate to attach to cannula)
- Gate clamps
- Sterile gloves and apron
- Sharps bin

Optional equipment

- Weighing scales
- Tape measure

Pre-procedure

Action	Rationale
1 Explain and discuss the procedure with the patient.	To ensure that the patient is involved in the decision and understands the procedure, the agreed aim, the risks and benefits. Informed consent may then be obtained (Campbell 2001, **R5**; Cope 2011, **R5**; NMC 2015, **C**).

2	Ask the patient to empty their bladder prior to ultrasound (US) marking.	If the bladder is full there is a chance of it being punctured when the trocar is introduced (McGibbon et al. 2007, **E**). If the bladder is emptied post US marking it will alter the site of marking, making it inaccurate. **E**
3	Weigh the patient before the procedure and measure the girth and record.	To assess weight changes and fluid loss. **E**
4	Ensure privacy.	To maintain dignity (DH 2006, **C**).
5	Lie the patient supine in bed with the head raised 45–50 cm with a backrest.	Normally the pressure in the peritoneal cavity is no greater than atmospheric pressure, but when fluid is present pressure becomes greater than atmospheric pressure. This position will aid gravity in the removal of fluid and the fluid will drain of its own accord until the pressure is equalized. **E**
6	Using US, mark the area of greatest depth on the abdomen using a skin marker.	To indicate the site for the drain in order to reduce the risk of perforating vital organs, specifically bowel, if under the site of insertion (Royal College of Obstetricians and Gynaecologists 2014, **C**). A depth of >3.5 cm is recommended. **E**
7	Following the US marking and when it is safe to proceed, ensure that the patient has signed a consent form.	Informed consent may then be obtained (Campbell 2001, **R5**; Cope 2011, **E**; NMC 2015, **C**).

Procedure

8	Wash hands.	To minimize risk of contamination. **E**
9	Perform the procedure using an aseptic technique. Always perform the procedure in hospital with a second, appropriately trained, person.	To minimize risk of contamination. **E** To ensure patient safety at all times. **E**
10	Bring equipment to the bedside on a cleaned trolley. Remove the sterile abdominal paracentesis pack from its outer wrapping and open it on the trolley.	To minimize the risk of infection. **E** To facilitate access to the equipment. **E** To create a clean working area. **E**
11	Put on a disposable plastic apron and sterile gloves; open inner pack, arranging the contents as required.	To protect the professional and patient from the risks of cross-infection. **E**
12	Clean the skin thoroughly at the marked site for the paracentesis with an antiseptic solution, for example chlorhexidine 0.5% and alcohol solution, and allow to dry. Drape with sterile towels.	To reduce the risk of local and/or systemic infection. The peritoneal cavity is normally sterile (Fraise and Bradley 2009, **E**; Lee et al. 2000, **R5**). To prevent contamination (Loveday et al. 2014, **C**).
13	Draw up 10 mL of 1 or 2% lidocaine into a 10 mL syringe and attach a 25 G needle. Administer local anaesthetic to raise a small lidocaine skin wheal around the skin entry site. Switch to the longer 20 G needle, and administer 4–5 mL of lidocaine along the catheter insertion tract. Make sure to anaesthetize all the way down to the peritoneum. Alternate injection and intermittent aspiration down the tract until ascitic fluid is noticed in the syringe.	To minimize pain during the procedure (Runyon 2015, **E**). To have medications prepared for use. **E** To ensure that the catheter insertion tract is anaesthetized **E.** To note the length of the tract prior to reaching the peritoneum to assist with anticipated length of catheter to be inserted to reach the fluid within the peritoneum. **E**
14	Once the anaesthetic has taken effect, make an incision with the scalpel (approximately 5 mm length by 3 mm depth) into the skin of the abdomen (the position may have been marked previously in radiology following US). The incision should be long enough to aid entry of the trocar.	Allows for easier passage of the catheter. **E** To minimize pain during the procedure and thus maximize patient comfort and facilitate co-operation (Runyon 2015, **E**).
15	Depending on the type of catheter used, the trocar and cannula are inserted perpendicular to the skin via the incision either together or in succession. Slowly insert in increments of 5 mm. Upon entry into the peritoneal cavity, loss of resistance is felt and flashback of ascetic fluid is present.	To ensure correct insertion of the trocar and cannula. **E** Slow insertion reduces the risk of vascular entry or puncture of the small bowel. **E**
16	Once there is flashback of ascitic fluid, insert the trocar and cannula further. The depth of insertion is the depth of subcutaneous tissue plus a third of the depth of fluid as dictated by US measurements.	To ensure the cannula is in the correct position. **E**
17	Attach a sterile syringe to the end of the catheter and withdraw 3–10 mL of free-flowing ascites and then advance the cannula.	If the fluid return in the syringe is bubbling this may signal bowel perforation. To ascertain there is no bowel perforation and ensure the cannula is in free-flowing fluid. **E**

(continued)

Procedure guideline 7.2 Abdominal paracentesis *(continued)*

18 The trocar is removed and disposed of in a sharps container.	To reduce the risk of accidental needlestick injury (NHS Employers 2011, **C**).
19 Attach the closed drainage system to the cannula using a connector if appropriate. Apply an appropriate dry dressing to ensure the drain exit site is protected and the drain is taped firmly in position.	A sterile container with a non-return valve is necessary to maintain sterility. To reduce local and/or systemic infection. **E**
20 Collect ascitic fluid from the sterile drainage bag prior to it being hung by the bedside (20–100 mL as instructed by the patient's clinical team) and send for cytology, biochemistry (albumin, lactate dehydrogenase [LDH], protein) and microbiology. This can be taken directly from the tap on the drainage bag as this is sterile immediately post procedure.	If necessary, in order to diagnose the cause of ascites and for continued monitoring of fluid (Fentiman 2002, **E**; Hosttetter et al. 2005, **E**). Enables the clinician to ascertain if the ascites is exudate or transudate.
21 If the cannula is to remain in position, ensure that it is secured using a sterile dry dressing fixed in position by adhesive tape (e.g. Mefix) covering the entire dressing.	To prevent the cannula becoming dislodged and to prevent local trauma to the patient. **E**

Post-procedure

22 Dispose of the equipment and remove gloves and apron.	To reduce the risk of environmental contamination (Fraise and Bradley 2009, **E**).
23 Monitor the patient's blood pressure, pulse and respirations after each litre of fluid is drained.	To observe for signs of shock and/or infection. **E**
24 Observe the rate and nature of the drainage. Reduce the flow of fluid using the clamp available in the tube if the patient complains of light-headedness.	To ensure safe and unobstructed drainage. **E**
25 Monitor and record the drain output.	To ensure accurate recording of the amount of ascitic fluid drained. **E**
26 If draining < 200 mL per hour, encourage the patient to walk about to move ascitic fluid within the abdominal cavity.	To encourage fluid drainage (Runyon 2015, **E**).
27 When there is no further output remove the drain and apply a dry dressing.	To reduce the risk of infection (Fraise and Bradley 2009, **E**; Lee et al. 2000, **R5**).
28 Weigh the patient after the catheter is removed and record.	To assess weight changes and fluid loss. **E**
29 Measure the patient's girth around the umbilicus after the procedure and record.	This provides an indication of fluid shift and how much fluid has reaccumulated. **E**

286

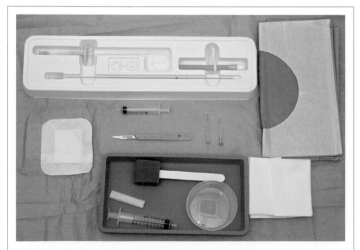

Figure 7.9 Example of sterile equipment tray for abdominal paracentesis. *Source:* Dougherty and Lister (2015). Reproduced with permission from John Wiley & Sons.

Problem-solving table 7.1 Prevention and resolution (Procedure guideline 7.2)

Problem	Cause	Prevention	Suggested action
Patient exhibits shock.	Major circulatory shift of fluid or sudden release of intra-abdominal pressure, vasodilation and subsequent lowering of blood pressure.	Monitor blood pressure and consider administration of intravenous fluid if volumes larger than 5 litres are expected to drain.	Clamp the drainage tube with a gate clamp to prevent further fluid loss. Record the patient's vital signs. Refer to the medical staff for immediate intervention.
Cessation of drainage of ascitic fluid.	Abdomen is empty of ascitic fluid.		Check the total output of ascitic fluid given on the patient's fluid balance chart.
			Ask the patient to move around to stimulate fluid movement within the peritoneal cavity.
			Measure the patient's girth; compare this measurement with the pre-abdominal paracentesis measurement. Suggest to medical staff that the cannula should be removed. Discontinue the drainage system.
	Patient's position is inhibiting drainage.	Teach the patient to avoid exerting pressure on the drainage tubing.	Change the patient's position, that is, move the patient upright or onto their side to encourage flow by gravity. Encourage the patient to mobilize.
	The ascitic fluid has congealed in the drainage system.	Keep the drainage bag on a stand and lower than the puncture site to facilitate drainage by gravity.	'Milk' the tubing. If this is unsuccessful, change the drainage system aseptically. Refer to the medical staff.
Cannula becomes dislodged.	Ineffective dressing or trauma at the puncture site.	Collaborate with medical staff about applying a suture or alternatively apply a secure dressing. The tube is taped to the skin further down to prevent pulling with movement at the puncture site.	Apply a secure dry dressing. Reassure the patient. Inform the medical staff. US may be required to confirm that the tube is in position.
Pain.	Pressure of ascites or position of drain.	Offer analgesia 30 minutes prior to procedure. Apply a dressing, allowing enough padding around the puncture site but avoiding drain movement within the abdomen.	Identify the cause. Anchor the drain securely to avoid pulling at the insertion site or movement within the abdomen. Assist the patient with repositioning. Administer an appropriate prescribed analgesic, monitor the patient's response and inform medical staff.

287

Post–procedural considerations

After paracentesis patients show relief of nausea, vomiting, dyspnoea and/or abdominal discomfort (Sangisetty and Miner 2012). Information should be given about post-procedure care of the puncture site and about the importance of diet and fluid intake to replace proteins and fluid lost in the ascitic fluid.

Complications

Complications of ascitic drains include pain, wound infection, leak from the puncture site, perforation, hypotension and secondary peritonitis (Duggal et al. 2006). In a study of 171 patients, major complications were seen in 1.6% and tended to be associated with a low platelet count ($<50\times10^9$/L) or alcoholic cirrhosis (De Gottardi et al. 2009).

Bowel obstruction (malignant)

Definition

It is important to differentiate between constipation and malignant bowel obstruction (MBO). Constipation is the irregular and infrequent or difficult evacuation of the bowels and can be associated with obstruction or diverticulitis and also hypercalcaemia or metastatic spinal cord compression (MSCC) (London Cancer Alliance 2015). A generic definition of both benign and malignant bowel obstruction is any mechanical or functional obstruction of the intestine that prevents physiological transit and digestion (Tuca et al. 2012). The diagnostic criteria of MBO are: (i) clinical evidence of bowel obstruction, (ii) obstruction distal to the Treitz ligament, (iii) the presence of primary intra-abdominal or extra-abdominal cancer with peritoneal involvement, and (iv) the absence of reasonable possibilities for a cure (Anthony et al. 2007).

Anatomy and physiology

Abdominal tumour growth may cause MBO by extrinsic intestinal compression, endoluminal obstruction, intramural infiltration or extensive mesenteric infiltration (Ripamonti et al. 2001). Intraluminal tumours may occlude the bowel lumen or provoke intussusception. Intramural infiltration through the mucosa may obstruct the lumen or impair peristaltic movements. Mesenteric and omental tumour involvement may angulate the bowel and provoke extramural bowel occlusion. Infiltration of the enteric or coeliac plexus may cause severe impairment in peristalsis and consequent obstruction due to dysmotility.

Fluid retention and intestinal gases proximal to the occlusive level produce a marked increase in endoluminal intestinal pressure. This abdominal distension favours the release of 5-HT3 by the intestinal enterochromaffin cells which, in turn, activates the enteric interneuronal system through its different mediators (substance P, nitric oxide, acetylcholine, somatostatin and vasoactive intestinal peptide). This stimulates the secretomotor neurones that are especially mediated by vasoactive intestinal peptide, which leads to splanchnic vasodilatation and hypersecretion of the cells of the intestinal crypts. The consequences of these phenomena are the appearance of intense intestinal oedema, an increase in the secretions retained, and endoluminal pressure, all of which are mechanisms that perpetuate the physiopathological process of MBO.

Related theory

MBO may appear at any time during the evolution of the patient's cancer but is more frequent in cases of advanced cancer (Ferguson et al. 2015, Tuca et al. 2012). MBO is estimated to occur in 2% of all patients with advanced malignancy but has a greater frequency in colorectal (10–28.4%) and ovarian (5.5–42%) malignancies (Tuca et al. 2012). Obstruction may originate in the small (61%) or large bowel (33%) or in both simultaneously (20%) (Ripamonti et al. 2001). Obstruction may be complete or partial and may appear as a sub-occlusive crisis or may involve one or multiple intestinal levels. Factors that may favour the appearance of MBO but are not directly dependent on abdominal tumour growth include paraneoplastic neuropathies, chronic constipation, intestinal dysfunction induced by opioids, inflammatory bowel disease, renal insufficiency, dehydration, mesenteric thrombosis, surgical adhesions, and radiogenic fibrosis (Ripamonti et al. 2008). In advanced and inoperable patients, multiple occlusive levels are presented in 80% of cases and peritoneal carcinomatosis is previously diagnosed in more than 65% of cases (Tuca et al. 2012). The prognosis of advanced oncological patients from the diagnosis of inoperable MBO is estimated at an average of 4 weeks (Tuca et al. 2012).

Diagnosis

MBO can present subacutely with the presence of colic pain, abdominal distension, nausea and vomiting which spontaneously cease (sub-occlusive crisis) (Tuca et al. 2012). The prevalence of symptoms in consolidated MBO is: nausea 100%, vomiting 87–100%, colic pain 72–80%, pain due to distension 56–90%, and the absence of stools or emission of gases in the previous 72 hours (85–93%) (Ripamonti et al. 2008). In upper MBO, the nausea is intense and presents early; vomiting is frequent, has an aqueous, mucous or biliary appearance and has little odour. Vomiting in lower obstruction usually occurs later, is dark, and has a strong odour (Tuca et al. 2012). Bacterial liquefaction of the retained intestinal content in the zone proximal to the obstruction confers the characteristic appearance and smell of faecaloid vomit (Ripamonti et al. 2001).

Patients with partial obstruction may present with liquid stools due to bacterial liquefaction of the digestive content and intestinal hypersecretion. The colic pain is due to giant peristaltic waves and spasms in the bowel with increased endoluminal pressure and no possibility of effective transit. Intestinal distension and tumoural infiltration of the abdominal structures are responsible for the continuous pain.

Assessment

The nurse can start the assessment of the patient suspected of MBO by undertaking a focused history, asking questions such as:

- What is their current cancer treatment?
- When did bowels last move (what consistency/colour/smell/ amount)?

- What is their normal bowel habit; medication history and any laxatives, change of medication, oral intake, nausea or vomiting (faecal smelling), abdominal swelling, discomfort or pain (Ferguson et al. 2015)?
- What the stool consistency was like prior to the loose stool (many patients will present with liquid or loose stools, before presuming diarrhoea, always ask as this could be overflow, but a stool sample should always be sent for MC&S (Tradounsky 2012)?

The patient should be cannulated and blood samples taken (FBC, U&Es, LFTs, calcium, magnesium, CRP); the results can be helpful in the evaluation of hydration or presentation with a metabolic disturbance (Tradounsky 2012). SACT should be stopped until clinical review and the diagnosis is confirmed as this may exacerbate symptoms and underlying pathophysiology (Ferguson et al. 2015).

The healthcare professional should undertake an abdominal assessment. If MBO is present, inspection of the abdomen will often show abdominal distension, but other important signs such as previous abdominal incisions and abdominal wall hernias must be noted for accurate diagnostic synthesis. Abdominal palpation may identify a specific tumour mass, or indeed a 'woody' abdomen secondary to diffuse malignant infiltration. Percussion of the abdomen is useful to differentiate the tympanic note of intestinal obstruction from the dull percussion note in cases where malignant ascites predominates as the cause of abdominal distension. In cases of true intestinal obstruction, hyperactive bowel sounds may be present, as may borborygmi. However, if a paralytic picture predominates, bowel sounds may be absent. This clinical sign is a useful discriminating factor when cross-sectional imaging is unavailable.

A digital rectal examination is essential as severe constipation can mimic, worsen or co-exist with symptoms of intestinal obstruction. A full rectum should be emptied by the use of local suppository or enema preparations before presuming a diagnosis of bowel obstruction. Stercoral perforation can and does occur in terminal disease, often due to the combination of long-term opiate medication and immobility, so obstructive symptoms, especially pain, should be treated seriously even when constipation is suspected (Ripamonti et al. 2001, 2008, Tuca et al. 2012). In patients with advanced cancer, MBO is also associated with anaemia (70%), hypoalbuminaemia (68%), alterations in hepatic enzymes (62%), dehydration and pre-renal renal dysfunction (44%), cachexia (22%), ascites (41%), palpable abdominal tumour masses (21%) and marked cognitive deterioration (23%) (Ferguson et al. 2015).

An abdominal X-ray is usually the initial radiological test requested; signs of MBO are distension of the intestinal loops, fluid retention and gases, with the presence of air–fluid levels in the zone proximal to the occlusion as well as a reduction in gas and stools in the segments distal to the obstruction. The presence of gas in the large bowel is usually a sign of subacute obstruction (Ferguson et al. 2015, Tuca et al. 2012).

Management

Management of MBO depends on the obstruction. A collaborative approach by surgeons and the oncologist and/or palliative care physician as well as an honest discourse between physicians and patients can offer an individualized and appropriate symptom management plan (Ferguson et al. 2015, Ripamonti et al. 2008).

The cancer nurse's role is to work with the patient to ensure advice and support is given regarding the symptoms and management of MBO. Additional support may be necessary for patients who are aware of the symptoms of MBO in the context of their disease (Tradounsky 2012). For patients who have not had a bowel movement for the last 48 hours (constipation), advice regarding diet and fluid intake along with a review of medication (stopping or changing constipating medication) and possible change of laxatives to include a softener and stimulant is appropriate. The patient must feel listened to and encouraged to report if symptoms worsen. For patients who have not had a bowel motion in the last 72 hours admission may be required to manage associated symptoms such as pain and nausea and vomiting. Reviewing medication, including laxatives, and dietary advice remains the same.

If the patient is considered to be in bowel obstruction (paralytic ileus) then admission is essential. Initially, efforts should be made to correct any biochemical imbalance that may be contributing to intestinal dysmotility, most commonly hypercalcaemia or hypokalaemia (Ferguson et al. 2015). Intravenous fluids, emesis control and pain management are essential, along with recognizing when surgical management may be an option and therefore keeping the patient nil by mouth until a decision has been made. Total parenteral nutrition (TPN) is often discussed in the context of managing MBO, however it is only recommended in MBO for those patients who are undergoing surgery to enable subsequent chemotherapy and have a post-operative survival likely to be more than 3 months (Shariat-Madar et al. 2014). Surgery is recommended as the primary treatment for selected patients with MBO, however patients known to have poor prognostic criteria for surgical intervention such as intra-abdominal carcinomatosis, poor performance status and massive ascites should be managed conservatively (Ripamonti et al. 2008). A number of treatment options are now available for patients unfit for surgery.

Conservative management consists of two mechanisms: obviating any precipitating factors, and decreasing the intraluminal pressure associated with MBO (Ferguson et al. 2015). Certain medications commonly used in advanced malignancy can worsen the obstructive picture, notably opioids and antispasmodic medications. A careful symptom exploration should be performed to ascertain if it is possible to stop or reduce these medications without precipitating symptomatic crises. Opioids can rarely be omitted, as acute pain also needs to be addressed, and have originally been commenced for ongoing significant pain. Conversion of background opioids to fentanyl can markedly reduce gastrointestinal dysmotility in appropriate cases (Ferguson et al. 2015). Active medical palliation in MBO focuses around the use of corticosteroids, antisecretory medications and antiemetics, with sufficient analgesia. Bowel rest is an aspect of medical management (Tuca et al. 2012). If the patient has nausea and vomiting, antisecretory drugs or/and antiemetics may be used. The insertion of a nasogastric Ryles tube may be necessary to aid stomach decompression and aid symptom control in severe nausea and vomiting but is only a temporary measure (Ripamonti et al. 2008). Somatostatin analogues (e.g. octreotide, from 300 to 600 µg per day) have been recommended, with good symptomatic outcomes reported; they reduce gastrointestinal secretions very rapidly and have a particularly important role in patients with high obstruction if hyoscine butylbromide fails (Ferguson et al. 2015).

The medical management of MBO will often take several days before there is a significant resolution of symptoms. Spontaneous resolution of MBO occurs in 36% (31–42%) of patients with inoperable MBO: 92% of those who settled spontaneously had done so by day 7, however 72% of those who settled spontaneously subsequently developed another episode of obstruction (Tuca et al. 2012).

Ongoing care

MBO is a frequent complication in advanced cancer patients, especially in those with abdominal tumours. Clinical management of MBO requires a specific and individualized approach that is based on disease prognosis and the objectives of care. Surgery should always be considered for patients in the initial stages of the disease with a preserved general status and a single level of occlusion. The priority of care for inoperable and consolidated MBO is to control symptoms and promote the maximum level of comfort possible. The spontaneous resolution of an inoperable obstructive process is observed in more than one-third of patients. Patients with consolidated MBO have a mean survival of no longer than 4–5 weeks.

Metastatic spinal cord compression

Definition

Metastatic spinal cord compression (MSCC) is the compression of the spinal cord or cauda equina, by direct pressure and/or vertebral collapse because of metastatic spread, that compromises the function of the spinal cord and may cause neurological deficit and paralysis (NICE 2014).

Anatomy and physiology

The spinal cord is about 45 cm in length and extends from the base of the brain, surrounded by the vertebrae, to the pelvis. Nerves situated within the spinal cord, called upper motor neurones, carry the messages between the brain and spinal nerves along the spinal tract. Spinal nerves are classified as lower motor neurones. Spinal nerves branch out from the spinal cord at each vertebral level to communicate with specific areas of the body (Harrison 2000).

MSCC is caused by the following (Loblaw et al. 2003):

- direct soft tissue extension from vertebral bony metastases
- tumour growth through intravertebral foramina (e.g. from retroperitoneal tumours or paravertebral lymphadenopathy)
- compression due to bony collapse
- intramedullary metastases (rare).

The damage to the spinal cord causes 'spinal shock' which is a temporary suppression of spinal cord activity caused by swelling at and below the level of the lesion in spinal cord injury. Within the confines of the vertebral canal, the oedematous cord is compressed against the surrounding bone. A complex series of physiological and biochemical reactions occur due to the resulting oedema and vascular damage. Circulation of blood and oxygen is disrupted; ischaemic tissue necrosis follows with an immediate cessation of conductivity within the spinal cord neurones. This can persist for 2–6 weeks (Harrison 2000).

Related theory

MSCC is one of the most serious and devastating complications of cancer. Unnecessary delays in diagnosis and treatment impact on patients' quality of life and prognosis. However, with prompt diagnosis and treatment many patients can retain good levels of function and independence. MSCC can occur in virtually all types of malignancy, but myeloma, lung, prostate and breast cancer are the most common (Bach et al. 1990).

Most MSCC cases occur in patients with a pre-existing cancer diagnosis; however, in around 20% of patients it is their first cancer presentation (Bucholtz 1999). A patient with a cancer diagnosis and confirmed vertebral metastases is at high risk of developing MSCC and it can have catastrophic consequences if diagnosis is delayed. It is important that these patients are educated about the risks of developing MSCC, how to identify the symptoms, what to do and who to contact.

It is reported that 30% of patients after diagnosis of MSCC may survive for 1 year (L'Esperance et al. 2012). Of patients that were ambulant on presentation 70% will retain function, but only 5% who presented paraplegic will regain some function (Loblaw et al. 2003). The predominant poor prognostic indicator with regards to regaining function is loss of sphincter function at presentation.

The true incidence of MSCC is unknown due to current restrictions in detection rate and coding systems in the UK (NICE 2014). Post mortem evidence indicates that it is present in 5–10% of patients with advanced cancer.

Classification

MSCC is classified as either stable or unstable.

- *Stable*. Spinal alignment is intact with no further risk of progression of neurological symptoms as the spine is still able to maintain and distribute weight appropriately.

289

- *Unstable.* Spinal fractures/lesions pose a risk of spinal cord injury and potentially irreversible neurological symptoms due to (potential) abnormal movement at the fracture site. Additionally, unstable MSCC can be further classified as complete or incomplete.
  - *Complete spinal cord injury.* The cord 'loses all descending neuronal control below the level of the lesion' (Lundy-Ekman 2007).
  - *Incomplete spinal cord injury.* 'The function of some ascending and/or descending fibres is preserved within the spinal cord' (Lundy-Ekman 2007).

Legal and professional issues

National guidance

MSCC can lead to serious disability, including permanent paralysis, and early death. *NICE Support for Commissioning Metastatic Spinal Cord Compression in Adults* (NICE 2014) covers adults who have or may develop MSCC because they have malignancy elsewhere in their body that has spread to their spine. Although it is not mandatory, healthcare professionals and commissioners are expected to fully refer to this guideline as well as consider the individual needs, informed choices and values of their patients and service users. NICE (2014) states that every cancer network should ensure that appropriate services are commissioned and in place for the efficient and effective diagnosis, treatment, rehabilitation and ongoing care of patients with MSCC. These services should include the establishment of an MSCC co-ordinator to provide 24-hour cover to guide and co-ordinate the care of patients with suspected MSCC.

Competencies

Patients should only be moved with adequate numbers of staff who have been fully trained in moving patients with spinal cord compression or injury, which should be covered within their trust's mandatory training.

Signs and symptoms

New back pain in patients with cancer suggests epidural spinal cord compression. Pain that worsens when the patient is lying down or with percussion of vertebral bodies is characteristic of this condition (Quint 2000). Late neurological signs such as incontinence and loss of sensory function are associated with permanent paraplegia (Newton 1999). The most common cause is extradural deposits due to the vertebral body extending into the anterior epidural space.

By recognizing symptoms that manifest early, such as back pain, a sensation of leg weakness or vague sensory changes, maximum functionality can be retained. Late signs such as profound weakness, a defined sensory level or sphincter disturbance are associated with a poor prognosis and the compression being less reversible.

Common symptoms include (NICE 2014):

- back pain and/or radicular pain nerve root symptoms resulting in pain or loss of sensation within a dermatome; patients may report:
  - pain in the middle of their spine
  - progressive or unremitting lower spinal pain
  - spinal pain aggravated by straining (for example at stool, or when coughing or sneezing)
  - localized spinal tenderness
  - nocturnal spinal pain preventing sleep
- limb weakness
- difficulty walking
- sensory loss
- cauda equina signs (saddle anaesthesia, bladder or bowel dysfunction)
- sexual dysfunction.

Investigations

Whole spine magnetic resonance imaging (MRI) is the investigation of choice; however, if MRI is absolutely contraindicated, spinal CT is an alternative (Levack et al. 2002). Imaging must be performed within 24 hours of presentation for any patient with spinal pain suggestive of spinal metastases and with neurological signs or symptoms suggestive of MSCC (NCAT 2011, NICE 2014). Imaging must be performed more urgently if there is clear neurological deficit or deterioration. In these situations, if out-of-hours MRI is not available, investigations must not be delayed. Instead, the patient should be transferred to the relevant regional MSCC treatment centre.

For patients with pain suggestive of spinal metastases but no neurological signs or symptoms, imaging should be performed as an outpatient within 1 week of presentation. An up-to-date CT of brain, chest, abdomen and pelvis must be considered as this assists surgical planning with regard to bone strength, structural integrity and ensuring that surgery is used appropriately (NICE 2014).

A full neurological assessment including per rectum examination and a respiratory assessment will be undertaken by the healthcare professional (NICE 2014). The nurse should undertake baseline observations (blood pressure, pulse, respiratory rate, temperature, oxygen saturations) as well as blood tests (FBC, U&Es, LFTs and bone profile).

Management

Patients with severe pain suggestive of spinal instability, or any neurological signs or symptoms suggestive of MSCC, should be nursed flat with neutral spine alignment (including 'log rolling' and use of a slipper bed pan) until bony and neurological stability are ensured (Levack et al. 2002). Healthcare professionals must assume that the spine is unstable until clearly documented in the medical notes. For cervical lesions, immobilization must be ensured with a hard collar.

If the patient is walking with minimal weakness or sensory change then there is a one in three chance of regaining leg strength, and initial management is:

- bedrest while the patient awaits clinical review
- an urgent MRI
- then oral or intravenous dexamethasone 16 mg (8 mg twice daily) with proton pump inhibitor cover to relieve peri-tumoural oedema (NICE 2014).
- a prescription of adequate analgesia that takes into account what the patient is currently taking.

All patients with radiologically confirmed MSCC must be discussed urgently with a consultant clinical oncologist, consultant neuro- or spinal surgeon and, where possible, the treating oncology consultant prior to definitive treatment decisions. Decisions regarding the role of surgery or radiotherapy should be made bearing in mind the cancer diagnosis, characteristics of the MSCC, functional level of the patient (neurological and performance status), overall disease status and likely prognosis. It may be appropriate to manage patients with MSCC palliatively, without surgery or radiotherapy; however, this decision should be made by a consultant oncologist, neurosurgeon or palliative medicine physician, usually following joint discussion. Although palliative radiotherapy is the main treatment modality, for a certain group of patients surgical decompression is appropriate (Rades et al. 2010).

MSCC co-ordinators must be contactable 24 hours a day for:

- rapid access to the MSCC pathway
- all urgent referrals
- review of patients with suspected MSCC.

If there is a neurological deficit, the patient must immediately be discussed with the local MSCC co-ordinator and managed as an emergency. Assessment and investigation must not be delayed due to lack of local out-of-hours services. If these are not available, the local MSCC co-ordinator must be contacted to arrange urgent transfer to the regional MSCC treatment centre (NICE 2014).

Initial nursing management is associated with maintaining spinal alignment and monitoring sensory and pain levels as well as baseline observations. Whilst waiting for a clear clinical management plan, the role of the nurse is to support the patient with analgesia, ensure that steroids are given and that the patient and their family understand the need to maintain bedrest, and supporting the patient with their activities in daily living (NICE 2014). The cancer nurse needs to understand the principles of moving and handling a patient with possible spinal instability to ensure that no further damage occurs. This is explored in greater detail later in this section.

Good nursing care remains the cornerstone of patient management. Throughout all of this the nurse must be able to recognize promptly the signs of the deteriorating patient with regards to back pain, leg weakness, sensory and functionality changes. This includes being able to prioritize patients and their management and know when to escalate and an awareness of the main side-effects of the treatment modalities being used. Patients with urinary retention should be catheterized. The hydration and nutritional status of patients should be assessed and appropriately managed. Measures should be instituted to reduce the risk of pressure sores and thromboembolic events. The pain status of the patient should be assessed and controlled with appropriate analgesia. Care should be taken that patients do not become constipated, and where necessary laxatives should be prescribed. Patients should be encouraged to mobilize as soon as spinal stability has been documented as this will aid their rehabilitation and reduce the risk of pressure sores, chest infections and thromboembolic events (Walji et al. 2008).

Evidence-based approaches

Rationale
When moving and turning the patient with confirmed or suspected spinal instability who is being nursed flat, log rolling must be used. This is a technique to maintain neutral spinal alignment. It is an essential method to enable the patient to use a slipper pan and to maintain pressure areas through regular turning every 2–3 hours (NICE 2014). Patients should only be moved with adequate numbers of staff who have been fully trained in moving patients with spinal cord compression or injury.

Indications
The pelvic twist for pressure care and a log roll with five people is indicated for patients with cervical and thoracic lesions T4 and above (Harrison 2000). A log roll with four people is indicated for thoracolumbar lesions (Harrison 2000).

Contraindications
The pelvic twist is contraindicated in the presence of thoracolumbar or pelvic injury/damage and pre-existing spinal deformity or rigidity, for example ankylosing spondylitis (Harrison 2000).

Principles of care
Further principles are dependent upon whether the patient has a stable or unstable spine.

Stable spine
Patients need to be assessed for adequate pain control prior to moving and positioning, and care should be taken to avoid excessive rotation of the spine when turning.

Unstable spine
For patients with an unstable spine or severe mechanical pain suggestive of spinal instability, specific instructions for moving must be followed until bony and neurological stability is radiologically confirmed (Harrison 2000, NICE 2014). This is to ensure spinal alignment and reduce the risk of further spinal damage and potential loss of function (Harrison 2000, NICE 2014).

This group of patients may require additional considerations to enable safe practice without compromising their clinical condition. These may include:

- Lateral surface transfer (for example moving from bed to trolley using a rigid lateral transfer board). Manual support of the patient's head and neck should be given for any flat surface

transfer (Harrison 2000). This ensures appropriate spinal alignment and patient comfort.
- Log rolling for personal and pressure care (Procedure guidelines 7.3, 7.4 and 7.5).

'Careful handling, positioning and turning can prevent secondary cord damage during transfer and movements for patients with spinal cord injury' (Harrison 2000). The procedure guidelines on how to position patients who are supine or side-lying, as well as the neurological patient with tonal problems, are all relevant to moving patients with MSCC. For further information please refer to Dougherty and Lister (2015) *The Royal Marsden Manual of Clinical Nursing Procedures, Ninth Edition*: Chapter 6 Moving and positioning.

Pre-procedural considerations
Prior to moving and handling a patient with MSCC, the nurse should determine whether the patient is able to assist with moving, positioning and transfers. This is dependent on:

- spinal stability
- pain
- level of lesion
- muscle power
- sensory impairment
- exercise tolerance
- patient confidence.

The nurse should not attempt to move a patient without fully appraising the clinical situation and reviewing the clinical notes.

Equipment

Spinal brace/cervical collar
When a patient has confirmed spinal instability, or is at risk of developing this because of vertebral injury or collapse, external spinal support will be required. This may be in the form of a spinal brace or collar. A properly fitted hard collar (Figure 7.10) must be used when there is suspicion of spinal instability (Harrison 2000, NICE 2014). This is available from surgical appliances and orthotics or some physiotherapy departments. Manufacturer's product details and care instructions are provided upon issue. Staff should be guided by medical advice and local policy.

Moving and handling aids
Patients may be able to assist with transfers using transfer boards, standing aids, mobility aids, frames, crutches and sticks.

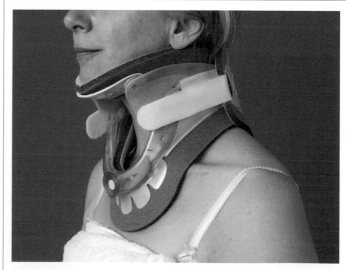

Figure 7.10 Hard collar *in situ. Source:* Dougherty and Lister (2015). Reproduced with permission from John Wiley & Sons.

If they are unable to assist, there are a variety of moving and handling aids, for example lateral patient transfer boards, hoists and standing hoists, which maintain the safety of both the patient and the carer (HSE 1992). For lesions affecting the cervical and thoracolumbar spine or where injuries make turning difficult, an electric turning bed can be used (Harrison 2000).

Assessment and recording tools

The focus of an initial neurological assessment is to establish the level of cord injury and act as a baseline against which future improvements or deterioration may be compared (Harrison 2000). Standard assessments, including pain, motor and sensory charts, should be used as a baseline and updated with any change in a patient's presentation. Assessments will depend on local policy and may include:

- American Spinal Injury Association (ASIA) Spinal Cord Injury Classification (ASIA 2002)
- ASIA Spinal Cord Injury Impairment Scale (ASIA 2002)
- Spinal Cord Independence Measure (SCIM III) (Catz and Itzkovich 2007, Catz et al. 2007, Itzkovich et al. 2007)
- pain assessment chart, for example visual analogue scale (Tiplady et al. 1998)
- manual handling risk assessment
- pressure ulcer assessment, refer to Dougherty and Lister (2015) *The Royal Marsden Manual of Clinical Nursing Procedures, Ninth Edition*: Chapter 15: Wound management.

Pharmacological support

As already discussed, pain is the primary indicator of MSCC in the first instance, but in relation to moving and handling it can also be suggestive of changes in neurology once gradual sitting and mobilization commences (NICE 2014). Implementation of a pain assessment chart can enable continuity of care, allowing accurate assessment and evaluation of all pharmacological needs such as non-steroidal anti-inflammatory drugs, opiates, bisphosphonates and epidural analgesia.

Non-pharmacological support

Nurses should always consider the use of complementary therapies during care planning for MSCC. The following techniques may be helpful to individual patients following appropriate assessment and have been incorporated into the protocols on management of MSCC by some acute oncology groups (Misra 2016).

Massage

Massage can decrease pain, anxiety, fear and depression. It can also increase comfort, circulation and self-esteem. It can promote sleep, stimulate the immune system and help to lower blood pressure. Perception of touch varies according to disease, medication and psychological state. Massage to the calf may be given for 2 minutes to patients not on anticoagulants, to help prevent deep vein thrombosis. For patients with peripheral neuropathies, gentle work on the soles of the feet can assist proprioception. Massage may also be given for patients who have constipation (Misra 2016).

Relaxation methods

These can decrease feelings of pain, tension, fear and anxiety and allow the patient to achieve relaxation and peace of mind. These methods may be used with visualization and guided imagery (Misra 2016).

Therapeutic touch

Therapeutic touch can provide comfort, support and relaxation and may be particularly helpful for patients with a rapid respiration rate due to anxiety. It should be considered when the use of massage is contraindicated (Misra 2016).

Procedure guideline 7.3 Log rolling for suspected/confirmed cervical spinal instability

See Figure 7.11

Essential equipment
- Pillows – minimum of four
- Collar or spinal brace
- A minimum of five people is needed to move a person with cervical spinal instability

Optional equipment
- Slipper pan
- Clean sheets
- Hygiene equipment
- Continence pads
- Pressure care

Pre-procedure

Action	Rationale
1 Explain and discuss the procedure with the patient.	To ensure that the patient understands the procedure and gives their valid consent (NMC 2015, **C**).
2 Wash hands thoroughly or use an alcohol-based handrub.	To reduce the risk of contamination and cross-infection (Fraise and Bradley 2009, **E**).
3 Ensure that the bed is at the optimum height for handlers. If two or more handlers are required, try to match handlers' heights as far as possible.	To minimize the risk of injury to the practitioner (Smith et al. 2011, **C**).
4 Ensure there are sufficient personnel available to assist with the procedure (minimum five for patients with cervical spinal instability).	Four staff to maintain spinal alignment and one to perform personal/pressure care check during the procedure (Harrison 2000, **C**).

Procedure

Action	Rationale
5 Assess the patient's motor and sensory function.	To provide a baseline to compare against after the procedure (Harrison 2000, **C**).
6 The lead practitioner stabilizes the patient's neck, supporting the patient's head.	To co-ordinate and lead log roll. **E** To take responsibility for providing instructions and ensuring all other practitioners are ready before commencing the manoeuvre (Harrison 2000, **C**).

7 Ideally, the lead practitioner's hands should offer support for the entire cervical curve from the base of the skull to C7.	To immobilize the patient's head. **E** To ensure spinal alignment is monitored throughout the procedure (Harrison 2000, **C**).
8 The second practitioner stands at the thorax and positions their hands over the patient's lower back and shoulder.	To ensure the lower spine remains aligned (Harrison 2000, **C**).
9 The third practitioner stands at the hip area and places one hand on the patient's lower back and the other under the patient's upper thigh.	To prevent movement at thoracolumbar site (Harrison 2000, **C**).
10 The fourth practitioner stands at the patient's lower leg and places one hand under knee and the other under ankle.	To ensure the lower spine remains aligned (Harrison 2000, **C**).
11 Ensure there is a fifth person standing on the opposite side of bed.	To position the equipment or take care of hygiene needs. **E** To assess upper back and occiput. This needs to be carried out once a day to check pressure areas (Harrison 2000, **C**).
12 The lead practitioner holding the head provides clear instructions to the team; for example, 'We will roll on three: One, two, three'.	To ensure a co-ordinated approach to the move. **E**
13 Each practitioner remains in place while the necessary action is performed.	To ensure a co-ordinated approach to the move. **E**
14 The person holding the head then provides clear instructions to return to supine.	To complete the move. **E**
15 In order to leave the patient in a lateral position: (a) All practitioners must stay in place until the practitioner holding the patient's head confirms neutral spine alignment.	To ensure the lower spine remains aligned (Harrison 2000, **C**). To ensure patient comfort. **E**
(b) Position the patient between 30 and 50° lateral tilt.	To ensure pressure care. **E** To prevent excessive pressure being exerted on lower trochanter (Harrison 2000, **C**).
(c) The fifth person places a pillow lengthwise behind the patient from shoulder to hip.	To ensure the lower spine remains aligned (Harrison 2000, **C**). To ensure patient comfort. **E**
(d) The fifth person places a pillow under the patient's upper thigh lengthwise from hip to foot.	To ensure the lower spine remains aligned (Harrison 2000, **C**). To ensure patient comfort. **E**
(e) The fifth person places a pillow between the patient's foot and end of the bed.	To ensure the lower spine remains aligned (Harrison 2000, **C**). To ensure patient comfort. **E**

Post-procedure

16 Reassess and record neurological symptoms.	To ensure clinical status is maintained (Harrison 2000, **C**).

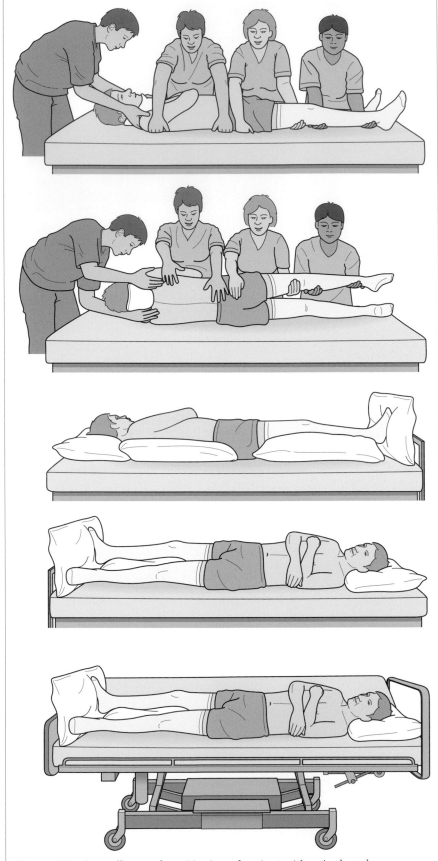

Figure 7.11 Log rolling and positioning of patient with spinal cord compression or injury. *Note:* In practice five people are needed for this manoeuvre. *Source:* Adapted from SIA (2000). Illustrations © Louise E Hunt and SIA. Reproduced from the Spinal Injuries Association (www.spinal.co.uk/) with permission.

Procedure guideline 7.4 Positioning for suspected/confirmed cervical spinal instability: pelvic twist to right

See Figure 7.12. This procedure is for cervical and upper thoracic spinal injuries only. It is contraindicated in the presence of thoracolumbar or pelvic trauma.

Essential equipment
- Collar or spinal brace
- Foam wedge or pillows

Optional equipment
- Equipment required for the purpose of the log roll, for example clean sheets, hygiene equipment, pads or pressure care

Pre-procedure

Action	Rationale
1 Explain and discuss the procedure with the patient.	To ensure that the patient understands the procedure and gives their valid consent (NMC 2015, **C**).
2 Wash hands thoroughly or use an alcohol-based handrub.	To reduce the risk of contamination and cross-infection (Fraise and Bradley 2009, **E**).
3 Ensure that the bed is at the optimum height for handlers. If two handlers are required, try to match handlers' heights as far as possible.	To minimize the risk of injury to the practitioner (Smith 2011, **C**).
4 Ensure there are three people available to assist with the procedure.	To ensure a co-ordinated approach to the move. **E**

Procedure

Action	Rationale
5 The lead practitioner stands at the head and places their hands firmly on the patient's shoulders.	To take responsibility for providing instructions and ensuring all other practitioners are ready before commencing the manoeuvre. **E** To prevent movement of unstable cervical spine. **E**
6 A second practitioner positions themselves on the left side of the bed to which the patient will be turned.	To ensure a co-ordinated approach to the move. **E**
7 The third practitioner assists the second practitioner to lift the patient's leg to allow them to place their left hand under the leg to the right hip and their right hand under the patient's lumbar region.	To prevent an angle of more than 30°. **E**
8 The patient's left hip is then upwardly rotated by the second practitioner.	The second practitioner's hands provide a barrier against friction during the turn. **E**
9 Both the lead and second practitioners maintain their position while the third practitioner places a folded pillow beneath the patient's left buttock above the sacrum. Place an additional pillow under the patient's upper buttock if required.	To prevent undue pressure risk to sacral/buttock region (Harrison 2000, **C**).
10 Place two pillows below the patient's left leg.	To support the left leg. **E**
11 Position a pillow at the foot end of the bed.	To minimize the risk of foot drop (Harrison 2000, **C**).

Post-procedure

Action	Rationale
12 In the event of a worsening of pain or neurological symptoms, reassessment by the medical team.	To ensure clinical status is maintained (Harrison 2000, **C**).

Procedure guideline 7.6   Early mobilization of the patient in bed

Essential equipment

• Collar/spinal brace for patients with unstable spine

Pre-procedure

Action	Rationale
1 Explain and discuss the procedure with the patient.	To ensure that the patient understands the procedure and gives their valid consent (NMC 2015, **C**).
2 Wash hands thoroughly or use an alcohol-based handrub.	To reduce the risk of contamination and cross-infection (Fraise and Bradley 2009, **E**).
3 Ensure that the bed is at the optimum height for patients or handlers. If two handlers are required, try to match handlers' heights as far as possible.	To minimize the risk of injury to the practitioner (Smith 2011, **C**).
4 Ensure there are sufficient personnel available to assist with the procedure (minimum of four for patients with thoracolumbar spinal instability).	Three staff to maintain spinal alignment and one to perform personal/pressure care check during the procedure (Harrison 2000, **C**).

Procedure

Action	Rationale
5 Assess stabilization of neurological symptoms.	To assess and evaluate clinical symptoms (NICE 2008, **C**).
6 Confirm mobilization status with medical staff.	To ascertain spinal stability to guide level of movement to reduce risk of further spinal damage (NICE 2008, **C**).
7 Ensure collar/brace is *in situ* for patients with unstable spine.	To ensure safety and stability (Harrison 2000, **C**; NICE 2008, **C**).
8 Assist the patient to move from supine to sitting at 60° in bed over 3–4 hours by gradually lifting the bed head.	To reduce the risk of orthostatic hypotension (NICE 2008, **C**).
9 Perform regular close monitoring of blood pressure and neurological symptoms.	To assess and evaluate clinical symptoms (NICE 2008, **C**).
10 On confirmation of stable symptoms, assist the patient to sit over the edge of the bed unsupported (see Dougherty and Lister [2015] *The Royal Marsden Manual of Clinical Nursing Procedures, Ninth Edition*: Chapter 6 Moving and positioning).	To ensure safe handling (CSP 2014, **C**; HSE 1992, **C**).
11 Closely monitor any changes in symptoms.	To assess and evaluate clinical symptoms (NICE 2008, **C**).
12 On confirmation of stable symptoms, proceed to standard principles of mobilization (see Dougherty and Lister [2015] *The Royal Marsden Manual of Clinical Nursing Procedures, Ninth Edition:* Procedure guideline 6.6: Moving from sitting to standing: assisting the patient) and follow risk assessment consideration. Refer to the general principles for moving patients with neurological impairment.	To ensure safe handling (CSP 2014, **C**; HSE 1992, **C**).

Problem-solving table 7.2 Prevention and resolution (Procedure guidelines 7.3, 7.4, 7.5 and 7.6)

Problem	Cause	Prevention	Action
1 **Autonomic dysreflexia (mass reflex):** • Severe hypertension (abrupt rise in blood pressure) – systolic blood pressure can easily exceed 200 mmHg.	Overstretching of bladder or rectum (urinary obstruction being the most common cause). Ingrown toenail or other painful stimuli. Fracture (#) below level of lesion. Pressure sore/burn/scald/sunburn. UTI/bladder spasm. Renal or bladder calculi. Visceral pain or trauma.	Closely monitor urinary drainage. Ensure effective bowel management regimen.	THIS IS A MEDICAL EMERGENCY: Identify or eliminate the most common (most lethal) cause of autonomic dysreflexia, which is non-drainage of urine.

299

Problem	Cause	Prevention	Action
• Bradycardia. • Pounding headache. • Flushed or blotchy appearance of skin above the level of lesion. • Profuse sweating above the level of lesion. • Pallor below the level of lesion. • Nasal congestion. • Non-drainage of urine.	DVT/PE. Severe anxiety/emotional distress (Harrison 2000, Lundy-Ekman 2007).		If this is not the cause, then proceed to investigate alternative causes according to the list given. Reassure the patient throughout because anxiety increases the problem. Remove the noxious stimulus, for example recatheterize immediately in the event of a blocked catheter. Do not attempt a bladder washout because there is no guarantee that the fluid will be returned. If possible, sit the patient up, or tilt the bed head up, to induce some element of postural hypotension. If symptoms remain unresolved after removal of noxious stimulus, or if the noxious stimulus cannot be identified, administer a proprietary chemical vasodilator, such as sublingual glyceryl trinitrate or captopril 25 mg, sublingually. (*Note*: Nifedipine capsules, which were previously recommended for use in treating or preventing autonomic dysreflexia, are being withdrawn as they have been implicated in episodes of severe hypotension.) Record blood pressure and give further reassurance. Monitor patient's condition. Refer to local spinal injuries unit for a specialist opinion/referral (Harrison 2000).
2 **Orthostatic hypotension**	Loss of sympathetic vasoconstriction. Loss of muscle-pumping action for blood return.	Antiembolic stockings. Careful assessment and monitoring during early mobilization/upright position changes.	Refer for medical review.
3 **Pain** Increased pain on movement to the extent that the patient perceives it as severe or does not reverse with rest.	Potential extension of spinal cord compression.	Ensure patients with unstable spine are moved appropriately.	Nurse the patient flat. Reassess spinal stability prior to further movement (NICE 2008).
4 **Respiratory function** Reduced respiratory function in patient with cervical level SCC.	Ineffective use of main respiratory muscles for effective ventilation for tetraplegic patients with lesions at C3 and above. Most patients with tetraplegia (paresis/paralysis of arms, trunk, lower limbs and pelvic organs) at C4 and below are able to make sufficient respiratory effort to avoid the need for mechanical ventilation. They will, however, require oxygen therapy (Harrison 2000).	Ensure effective GI clearance/management – constipation and impaction of the bowel are a common complication of SCI management. This may place undue pressure on the diaphragm and lessen breathing space for effective respiratory function (Harrison 2000). Closely monitor respiratory function during any procedure.	Ensure appropriate head/neck support as required – collar/cervicothoracic brace for unstable cervical spinal involvement during any moving and positioning but if patient's respiratory function decreases contact medical team urgently.

(continued)

Problem-solving table 7.2 Prevention and resolution *(continued)*

Problem	Cause	Prevention	Action
5 **Cardiac syncope** • Fainting with unconsciousness of any cardiac cause. • Second degree hypoxia following initial injury. • Second degree turning to left side.	A cervical collar applied too tightly may cause cardiac syncope (Harrison 2000). Sustained hypoxia increases vagal activity with a high risk of cardiac syncope (Harrison 2000). Turning the patient on to their left side for prolonged periods can increase vagal stimulation and may induce cardiac syncope. This problem is not usual during routine turning or twisting to the left side for pressure relief.	Ensure appropriate fit of cervical collar. Avoid turning the patient on to their left side for prolonged periods (e.g. during a back wash or sheet change). Turning the patient onto their right side does not have the same effect.	Check cervical collar is not too tight. Liaise with orthotist/PT. Administer high concentrations of oxygen and atropine (Harrison 2000). Measure dynamic trend of the patient's observations (Harrison 2000).

Post-procedural considerations

Ongoing care
Reassessment by the medical team will be necessary in the event of an increase in pain or neurological symptoms.

Anticipated patient outcomes
Many patients can retain good levels of function and independence with the appropriate care. The successful rehabilitation of a patient is often dependent on the action taken by the healthcare professional during the acute presentation. It is therefore essential that an early and accurate diagnosis is made and, if appropriate, treatment given to optimize neurological functioning. Timely referral to rehabilitation services is imperative for assessment, appropriate intervention and thorough discharge planning to enable smooth transition back into the community (NICE 2014).

Active rehabilitation may be postponed until the medical team has confirmed that the patient's spine is stable. However, there is a significant role for members of the rehabilitation team in the acute management of these patients in terms of:

- assessment of motor recovery
- minimizing further complications such as chest infections which may arise as a result of prolonged bedrest
- effective, co-ordinated discharge planning. The positioning and moving needs of these patients are often complex and so discharge planning may be lengthy and multifaceted, requiring ongoing support and rehabilitation in the community to optimize functional independence (Miller and Cooper 2010).

A referral to a physiotherapist is essential for patients with complex symptoms such as spinal instability, weakness and sensory impairment.

Documentation
Any changes in (neurological) presentation and/or function must be documented both prior to and following any procedure.

Complications
There are many potential long-term complications that may occur during or after moving and positioning MSCC patients. These are due to initial injury, the subsequent effects of changes in bowel and bladder functions and paralysis (complete loss of motor function) associated with their disease or injury through autonomic and peripheral nervous system dysfunction, and those associated with bedrest (Furlan et al. 2016, Kaplow and Iyere 2016).

Spinal shock
Following initial injury or lesion development, spinal shock can occur due to the loss of vasomotor tone throughout the paralyzed areas of the body. This is most pronounced in cases of tetraplegia. Patients present with hypotension, bradycardia and poikilothermia (having a body temperature that varies with the temperature of the surroundings). This is due to a temporary or permanent loss of reflexes and muscle tone and control potentially leading to a compromised cardiac output. The patient must be closely monitored throughout and following any procedure or transfer, as recommended by medical staff (Furlan et al. 2016).

Autonomic dysfunction
Following injury or lesion development, secondary effects occur due to autonomic dysfunction, a potential complication for all patients with complete spinal cord lesions above the level of T6 (see Problem-solving table 7.2) (Kaplow and Iyere 2016).

Autonomic dysreflexia
This is a mass reflex due to excessive activity of the sympathetic nervous system elicited by noxious stimuli below the level of the lesion. It is a medical emergency and, unresolved, it can cause fatal cerebral haemorrhage. Patients present with severe hypertension (abrupt rise in blood pressure), systolic blood pressure that can easily exceed 200 mmHg, bradycardia, 'pounding' headache, flushed or blotchy appearance of skin above the level of lesion, profuse sweating above the level of lesion, pallor below the level of lesion, nasal congestion and non-drainage of urine (Milligan et al. 2012).

Orthostatic hypotension
There is an extreme fall in blood pressure on assuming an upright position (systolic >20 mmHg, diastolic >10 mmHg). It is more common in tetraplegia than quadriplegia (Krassioukov et al. 2009, Lundy-Ekman 2007).

Poor thermoregulation
There is compensatory sweating above the level of lesion and loss of ability to shiver below the level of lesion. Patients should avoid exposure to excessive heat/cold temperatures; peripheral vasodilation means that the patient's core temperature can soon equal the environmental temperature through circulatory conduction poikilothermia. Ensure that the patient's body temperature is maintained at an appropriate level during all procedures, treatments, investigations and transfers. Active warming should be

undertaken cautiously for fear of causing skin damage (Harrison 2000).

Pressure care
There is a risk to skin integrity and the development of pressure sores due to a lack of movement, poor circulation and altered sensation (Kaplow and Iyere 2016).

Circulation
There is a risk of DVT due to the loss of vasomotor tone throughout the paralyzed areas of the body. Application of thigh-length thromboembolic deterrent (TED) stockings can replace some of the lost muscle resistance, as well as reducing the risk of DVT (Harrison 2000).

Pericardial effusion (malignant)

Definition
A pericardial effusion is the accumulation of fluid in the pericardial sac (Longmore et al. 2014).

Anatomy and physiology
The pericardium surrounds the heart and the great blood vessels and is composed of a thin visceral membrane, a fibrous parietal membrane, and the pericardial space between the membranes, which normally contains less than 50 mL of pericardial fluid (Braunwald 2012, Petrofsky 2014). Understanding the properties of the pericardium can help to predict changes within the heart under physiological stress. The pericardium plays a pivotal role in the distribution forces across the heart, playing a significant role in the physiological concept of ventricular interdependence whereby changes in pressure, volume and function in one ventricle influence the function of the other (Little and Freeman 2006, Strimel 2016).

The parietal membrane is composed primarily of collagen and elastin fibres, which give the membrane some elasticity (Braunwald 2012). As a result of this elasticity, the normal pericardium has a non-linear pressure–volume curve.

In non-altered function the right atrium and ventricle fill during inspiration; the pericardium limits the ability of the left-sided chambers to dilate. This contributes to the bowing of the atrial and ventricular septa to the left, which reduces left ventricular filling volumes and leads to a drop in cardiac output. Intrapericardial pressures rise, as occurs in the development of a pericardial effusion. Small pericardial fluid volume changes do not generally result in any change in pericardial pressure, but a large sudden increase in pericardial volume can cause a steep change in pericardial pressure, which can lead to a clinically significant fall in stroke volume leading to tamponade (Imazio and Adler 2013). With a slowly enlarging pericardial effusion, the pericardial membranes stretch to accommodate the growing fluid volume without any significant change in the pericardial pressure until the limit of pericardial membrane stretch is reached (Little and Freeman 2006, Strimel 2016).

Related theory
Malignant pericardial effusions are often undiagnosed in patients with cancer, and some patients with otherwise treatable cancer succumb to undiagnosed pericardial effusion (Rhodes and Manzullo 1997). Metastatic lung or breast cancer causes most effusions but they may also develop from malignant melanoma, leukaemia, lymphoma and where there has been radiation therapy to the chest wall (Higdon and Higdon 2006). Chemotherapies that can cause pericardial effusion include cyclophosphamide, cytarabine, dasatinib, doxorubicin and gemcitabine, along with other cardiotoxic agents (Svoboda 2010). Pericardial effusions, if left untreated, can cause cardiac tamponade which is a life-threatening oncological emergency. This situation occurs from an excess accumulation of fluid in the pericardial sac. This fluid causes an increase in pressure around the heart and a decrease in blood flow to the heart. The amount of fluid surrounding the heart varies and may range from 50 mL to 1 litre. As excess fluid accumulates it compresses the right ventricle which therefore is unable to fill resulting in a reduction in the amount of blood leaving the left side of the heart (Longmore et al. 2014). Severity is based on the amount of fluid and how rapidly it is accumulating.

Diagnosis
It is important to remember that pericardial effusions may not always be due to the cancer and to ensure that all causes are considered (Lestuzzi 2010). Clinical manifestations of pericardial effusion are highly dependent on the rate of accumulation of fluid in the pericardial sac. Rapid accumulation of pericardial fluid may cause elevated intrapericardial pressures with as little as 80 mL of fluid, while slowly progressing effusions can grow to 2 L without symptoms (Kim et al. 2010, Strimel 2016).

Clinical symptoms can include dyspnoea, orthopnoea, fatigue, heart palpitations, dizziness, pulsus paradoxus, tachycardia, distended neck veins with a raised JVP and narrow pulse pressure, and distant heart sounds may be present (Longmore et al. 2014, McCurdy and Shanholtz 2012, Odor and Bailey 2013). The most common sign of pericardial effusion is pulsus paradoxus (a fall of systolic blood pressure of >10 mmHg during the inspiratory phase along with a weakening of the pulse), occurring in about 30% of presentations of malignant pericardial effusion (Karam et al. 2001) and 77% of cases of acute tamponade (Karam et al. 2001). In cases caused by malignancy, exertional dyspnoea is the most common presenting symptom, observed in roughly 80% of presentations (Karam et al. 2001, Svoboda 2010).

The role of the cancer nurse is to identify an effusion before it progresses to cardiac tamponade (Flounders 2003, Magan 1992). Accurate and thorough ongoing assessment of cardiopulmonary and haemodynamic status is necessary to identify early abnormal changes. This should include strict monitoring of vital signs, including assessment for pulsus paradoxus, as well as assessment of level of consciousness, ECG tracings, respiratory status, and skin and temperature changes (Flounders 2003).

Accurate monitoring of intake and output is necessary, including assessment for oedema or oliguria and anuria, as well as measurement of abdominal girth to detect ascites (Schafer 1997). Dyspnoea is the most common sign of pericardial effusion in cancer patients. A chest X-ray is usually the first diagnostic test requested as this will show an enlarged cardiac silhouette and increase in transverse diameter (water bottle heart) (Karam et al. 2001, Peebles et al. 2011, Petrofsky 2014).

Echocardiography is the preferred diagnostic study and will enable the clinician to ascertain the impact on cardiac function as findings include low amplitude waveforms and electrical alternans due to swinging heart (Karam et al. 2001, Peebles et al. 2011, Petrofsky 2014). An ECG is useful to rule out acute pericarditis and will also aid the clinician to ascertain the impact of the perfusion on cardiac function (Troughton et al. 2010). Beck's triad of hypotension, increased JVP and decreased heart sounds is found mostly with a rapidly forming effusion and acute tamponade, but only infrequently in patients with chronic pericardial effusion (Karam et al. 2001, Odor and Bailey 2013, Strimel 2016). Ewart's sign (bronchial breathing at the left base) is present in large effusions due to compression of the left lower lobe and the patient may also demonstrate signs of cardiac tamponade (Longmore et al. 2014, Strimel 2016).

Management
The patient's prognosis from their underlying cancer along with their other co-morbidities should be taken into consideration when choosing the appropriate treatment of the pericardial effusion (Imazio and Adler 2013). Small asymptomatic effusions may be left alone, and stable patients without evidence of tamponade can be managed with careful monitoring, serial echo studies, avoidance of volume depletion, and therapy aimed at the underlying cause of the pericardial effusion (Odor and Bailey 2013,

301

Petrofsky 2014). By understanding the risk factors and goal of management which is the removal of fluid, restoration of hemodynamic functioning and prevention of fluid reaccumulation the nurse can provide emotional support and reassurance (Flounders 2003, Magan 1992).

Patients with evidence of tamponade who are hypovolaemic should be given volume resuscitation if systolic BP is below 100 mmHg (Odor and Bailey 2013). In tamponade there is a significant increase in the pericardial pressure, and the central venous pressure must be kept higher than the pericardial pressure in order for the heart to fill. If volume resuscitation results in haemodynamic improvement, such patients may be observed closely without urgent need for pericardiocentesis (Hoit 2011).

In patients with cancer and symptomatic cardiac tamponade with chamber collapse shown on echo, pericardiocentesis is indicated (Kim et al. 2010, Odor and Bailey 2013). Fluid samples should be analysed with cytology (Longmore et al. 2014, Petrofsky 2014). Systemic anticancer therapy in conjunction with pericardiocentesis has been found to be effective in reducing the recurrence of malignant effusions (Lestuzzi 2010, Strimel 2016). If the tumour is chemo-resistant or refractory to systemic treatment, pleurodesis may be considered as this may prevent the reaccumulation of fluid after the effusion is drained through promotion of the visceral and parietal pericardial layers (Lestuzzi 2010).

Raised intracranial pressure due to malignant disease

Definition
Intracranial pressure (ICP) is defined as the pressure of the cerebrospinal fluid in the subarachnoid space (the space between the skull and the brain) (Allan 2006). In healthy adults, ICP is maintained nearly constant between 0 mmHg and 15 mmHg (Woodrow 2006). A level of ICP higher than 15 mmHg is considered abnormal and is defined as raised ICP, or intracranial hypertension (Woodrow 2006).

A space-occupying lesion (SOL) is any abnormal tissue found on or in an organism, usually damaged by disease or trauma. A space-occupying lesion of the brain (CNS SOL) is usually due to malignancy but it can be caused by other pathology such as an abscess or a haematoma.

Anatomy and physiology
The central nervous system (CNS) consists of two parts: the brain and spinal cord. The brain consists of four lobes (frontal, temporal, parietal and occipital), the midbrain, pons, medulla oblongata and cerebellum. Each has individual and joint roles, and interconnects with the others via a complex system of pathways producing automatic and volitional movement and cognitive function. These connect with every part of the body via the peripheral nervous system, consisting of cranial and spinal nerves which carry motor (efferent) and sensory (afferent) fibres (refer to Dougherty and Lister (2015) *The Royal Marsden Manual of Clinical Nursing Procedures, Ninth Edition*: Chapter 11 Observations).

Many neurological complications caused either by primary brain cancer or secondary malignancy SOL result from a rise in ICP. This may result directly from the mechanical forces generated by the tumour mass or from cerebral oedema caused by altered capillary permeability. As the tumour infiltrates normal brain tissue, obstruction of venous drainage in the brain or obstruction of cerebrospinal fluid may contribute to elevation in ICP. Changes in blood supply due to the pressure caused by the growing tumour cause brain tissue necrosis. This and haemorrhage into the tumour may also elevate ICP (Behin et al. 2003). The skull can be viewed as a rigid box which the brain sits inside. Rapidly growing tumours cause the greatest dysfunction and it is when masses grow larger than 3 cm that they compress brain tissue, its blood supply and adjacent neuronal pathways (Lefebvre 2016).

The impaired arterial blood supply generally manifests as an acute loss of function and may be confused with primary cerebrovascular disorders. Seizures, as a manifestation of neurosensitivity changes, may be associated with compression due to SOL invasion thus impairing blood supply to the brain tissue. Some SOLs form cysts that can also suppress the surrounding brain parenchyma causing focal neurological disorders.

Related theory
CNS malignancy accounts for only 2% of all cancers but its aggressive nature and proximity to vital CNS structure makes it the fourth leading cause of cancer-related death in adults (Guilfoyle et al. 2011, Lefebvre 2016). In general, CNS tumours have a poor prognosis. Both their anatomical position and pathology play an important role in prognosis and decisions about appropriate investigation and treatment. Sometimes, the risks of obtaining tissue for histopathological assessment are considered clinically unacceptable, and the patient is managed on the basis of a diagnosis made on neuroradiological features. The anatomical location influences symptoms that include physical, cognitive and psychological components. For this reason, adults with CNS tumours pose a unique challenge to healthcare professionals; the patient may not be the best person to explain his or her symptoms, and cognitive dysfunction may greatly increase the need for psychological/psychiatric, social and physical support. In view of the poor survival of many patients, even with optimal treatment, an important aspect of improving outcome is maximizing quality of life (NICE 2007a).

Metastases in the brain occur in 20–40% of patients with other primary cancers. Brain metastases are usually associated with a poor prognosis. Adult-onset epilepsy is a common feature of brain tumours and may present as either focal or generalized seizures. It usually presents without other neurological symptoms or signs (NICE 2007a).

Diagnosis
Patients presenting with neurological deterioration require immediate assessment to determine the underlying cause (Lefebvre 2016). If the cause is a brain tumour (primary or metastatic), early identification allows measures to be initiated to control cerebral oedema and limit damage to CNS structures. As with any emergency situation, assessment of haemodynamic stability must be addressed first. If the patient is haemodynamically stable a comprehensive clinical history to identify the clinical signs and symptoms of CNS deterioration and exclude trauma, infection, drug or toxin exposure is the starting point (Lefebvre 2016). CNS symptoms and deterioration usually occur sequentially and will identify the urgency of the clinical situation. The chronology of symptoms should be acknowledged to assist rapid diagnosis. These can be generic such as headache (usually worse in the morning); nausea and vomiting; weakness; somnolence (radiotherapy-induced fatigue); seizures; but can also be dependent on the area of the brain affected and include (Dunn 2002, Lefebvre 2016, NICE 2007a):

- temporal lobe – dysphasia, contralateral homonymous hemianopia, amnesia
- frontal lobe – hemiparesis, personality change (irritability, lack of concentration, socially inappropriate behaviour), executive dysfunction
- parietal lobe – hemisensory loss, astereognosis (inability to recognize objects by touch alone), reduced two-point discrimination, papilloedema
- occipital lobe – contralateral visual field defects, palinopsia (seeing things again once the stimulus has left the field of vision)
- cerebellum – DASHING: dysdiadochokinesis, ataxia, slurred speech, hypotonia, intention tremor, nystagmus, gait abnormalities.

A full neurological examination, including fundoscopy to assess for papilloedema, is an essential aspect of the physical examination (Lefebvre 2016). The minimum documented neurological observations should include vital observations, level of consciousness, pupillary activity and limb movements (NICE 2007a). Vital observations include blood pressure, pulse, respiration, oxygen saturations and temperature monitoring (Pemberton and Waterhouse 2006). Blood glucose, ECG, FBC (including differentials) and electrolytes provide information regarding the acute nature of the situation and also information regarding possible reversible causes (Farrell and Dempsey 2013, Lefebvre 2016).

If the patient has hypertension with a widening pulse pressure, bradycardia and bradypnoea, they are demonstrating the signs of Cushing's triad. This is seen when increased ICP decreases the cerebral blood flow significantly and triggers an increased arterial pressure in order to overcome the increased ICP (Farrell and Dempsey 2013). This is a medical emergency and requires treatment to stabilize the ICP. If this does not occur, herniation of the brainstem and occlusion of the cerebral blood flow can occur with dire consequences (Farrell and Dempsey 2013).

An MRI scan is best for visualizing oedema, however it is acknowledged that this is not always available at initial presentation therefore CT scan is appropriate (Eberhart et al. 2001, NICE 2007a).

Management

Patients who present with no prior cancer diagnosis must be referred to the neurosurgeons for immediate review, and management will depend on the type of malignancy (Lefebvre 2016, NICE 2007a). This section will focus on the management of patients with known cancer who present with raised ICP. As noted this can be caused by the cancer or its treatment.

Surgical decompression or debulking of the tumour is effective in reducing intracranial pressure and preventing further oedema (Raslan and Bhardwaj 2007). Unifocal brain tumours are potentially curable with radiation therapy. Radiation itself causes an increase in brain oedema but is used once the patient is stabilized to treat the underlying cause of oedema (Becker and Baehring 2011). Chemotherapy is limited in use due to its inability to cross the blood–brain barrier (Becker and Baehring 2011).

Objective management in the emergency setting is to treat promptly to prevent further deterioration. If the patient's neurological condition is deteriorating rapidly, IV access, oxygen and airway management is primary treatment. Aggressive therapy is necessary to sustain or restore optimal neurological function (Rangel-Castillo et al. 2008). IV fluids should be limited unless the patient is hypotensive as they may worsen the situation (Lefebvre 2016). Sodium chloride 0.9% is the preferred fluid because dextrose can exacerbate cerebral oedema. If the patient has a fluctuating or depressed level of consciousness airway management should be considered, noting that coughing can increase ICP (Raslan and Bhardwaj 2007). Reversible causes of reduced conscious level such as hypoglycaemia or opioid toxicity should be reversed prior to commencing management of raised ICP (Lefebvre 2016).

Elevation of the patient's head (raising the head of the bed 30°) has been shown to decrease ICP due to the promotion of intracranial outflow (Hickey 2002, Mestecky 2007, Raslan and Bhardwaj 2007). Oxygenation of the patient should also be maximized through oxygen administration as guided by saturations which in turn reduces cerebral vasodilation and ICP (Raslan and Bhardwaj 2007, Sippell 2011).

Osmotic therapy aims to drive excess water from the brain tissue (Rangel-Castillo et al. 2008). Mannitol is recommended in acute deterioration at a dose of 0.25–1 g/kg IV as a 15–25% solution over 30–40 minutes with a maximum of 200 g/day (London Cancer Alliance 2015, Raslan and Bhardwaj 2007). The effects should be seen within 20–40 minutes post infusion but provide a temporary solution. Mannitol can worsen an intracranial bleed and should not be used unless this has been ruled out (Raslan and Bhardwaj 2007).

Use of glucocorticoids in raised ICP is indicated if the cause is due to infection, a brain tumour or its treatment (Fields 2014). The dose of dexamethasone is dependent on the severity of symptoms. In the event of serious neurological deficit such as paralysis or seizures (more than three in a week) an initial dose of dexamethasone 10 mg intravenously with proton pump inhibitor cover should be given and then converted to 4 mg every 6 hours for 5–7 days (Fields 2014, London Cancer Alliance 2015). The dose is tapered once neurological symptoms are controlled and reduced usually over a period of 2–3 weeks to avoid adrenal insufficiency. If symptoms occur during tapering then increasing the dose to its pre-symptom level is recommended followed by clinical review (Cross and Glantz 2003).

If patients have seizures, they should be placed on anticonvulsant therapy as per local guidelines (Dunn 2002, London Cancer Alliance 2015, NICE 2012a). Seizures cause an increase in cerebral metabolism thus increasing the risk of herniation due to a sudden rise in ICP, therefore prompt management and prophylaxis is imperative (Cross and Glantz 2003). Immediate discussion with the doctor is essential and additional support from the critical care outreach team may be required (Hickey 2002). The nurse should consider other pathologies as the cause of the seizure and exclude syncopal attacks, cardiac arrhythmias and transient ischaemic attacks. Reversible metabolic causes such as hypoglycaemia, hyponatraemia and hypoxia should be corrected and infective causes considered (Dunn 2002).

Bowel management is a simple but important aspect of raised ICP management. Constipation causes the patient to strain, therefore increasing intra-abdominal pressure and thus raising ICP. Monitoring bowel habits, understanding the causes of constipation and use of laxatives are an important yet often forgotten aspect of nursing care in this patient group (Hickey 2002).

References

Agnelli, G. & Verso, M. (2011) Management of venous thromboembolism in patients with cancer. *Journal of Thrombosis and Haemostasis*, 9(suppl 1), 316–324.

Ahlberg, K., Ekman, T. & Gaston-Johansson, F. (2005) The experience of fatigue, other symptoms and global quality of life during radiotherapy for uterine cancer. *International Journal of Nursing Studies*, 42, 377–386.

Allan, D. (2006) Disorders of the nervous system. In: Alexander, M.F., Fawcett, J.N. & Runciman, P.J. (eds) *Nursing Practice: Hospital and Home*, 3rd edn. Edinburgh: Churchill Livingstone, pp. 395–442.

Andreyev, J., Ross, P., Donnellan, C., et al. (2014) Guidance on the management of diarrhoea during cancer chemotherapy. *Lancet Oncology*, 15, e447–e460.

Anon. (1995) Practice guideline: carotid artery rupture. Society of Otorhinolarology and Head-Neck Nurses. *ORL-Head and Neck Nursing*, 13(4), 31.

Anthony, T., Baron, T., Mercandante, S., et al. (2007) Report of the clinical protocol committee: development of randomized trials for malignant bowel obstruction. *Journal of Pain and Symptom Management*, 34(1 Suppl), S49–S59.

ASIA (2002) *Impairment Scale*. Atlanta, GA: American Spinal Injury Association.

Aw, A., Carrier, M., Koczerginski, J., et al. (2012) Incidence and predictive factors of symptomatic thrombosis related to peripherally inserted central catheters in chemotherapy patients. *Thrombosis Research*, 130(3), 323–326.

Ayantunde, A.A. & Parsons, S.L. (2007) Pattern and prognostic factors in patients with malignant ascites: a retrospective study. *Annals of Oncology*, 18(5), 945–949.

Ayantunde, A.A. & Parsons, S.L. (2012) Predictors of poor prognosis in patients with malignant ascites: a prospective study. *Clinical Medicine and Diagnostics*, 2(2), 1–6.

Bach, F., Larsen, B.H., Rohde, K., et al. (1990) Metastatic spinal cord compression. Occurrence, symptoms, clinical presentations and prognosis in 398 patients with spinal cord compression. *Acta Neurochirurgica*, 107, 37–43.

Baskin, J.L., Reiss, U., Williams, J.A., et al. (2012) Thrombolytic therapy for central venous catheter occlusion. *Haematologica*, 97(5), 641–650.

Becker, G., Galandi, D. & Blum, H.E. (2006) Malignant ascites: systematic review and guideline for treatment. *European Journal of Cancer*, 42(5), 589–597.

Becker, K.P. & Baehring, J.M. (2011) Increased intracranial pressure. In: DeVita, V.T. Jr, Lawrence, T.S. & Rosenberg, S.A. *Cancer: Principles & Practice of Oncology*, 9th edn. Philadelphia: Wolters Kluwer Health/ Lippincott Williams & Wilkins, pp. 2130–2141.

Beeson, M.S. (2014) Superior Vena Cava Syndrome in Emergency Medicine. Available at: http://emedicine.medscape.com/article/760301-overview (Accessed: 6/4/2018)

Behin, A., Hoang-Xuan, K., Carpentier, A.F. & Delattre, J.Y. (2003) Primary brain tumours. *Lancet*, 361(9354), 323–332.

Bender, C.M., McDaniel, R.W., Murphy-Ende, K., et al. (2002) Chemotherapy-induced nausea and vomiting. *Clinical Journal of Oncology Nursing*, 6, 94–102.

Benson, A.B. 3rd, Ajani, J.A., Catalano, R.B., et al. (2004) Recommended guidelines for the treatment of cancer treatment-induced diarrhoea. *Journal of Clinical Oncology*, 22, 2918–2926.

Bildstein, C.A. & Blendowski, C. (1997) Head and neck malignancies. In: *Cancer Nursing Principles and Practice*, 4th edn. London: Jones and Bartlett.

Bishop, L. (2009) Aftercare and management of central access devices. In: Hamilton, H. & Bodenham, A. (eds) *Central Venous Catheters*. Oxford: John Wiley & Sons, pp. 221–237.

Bodenham, A.R. & Simcock, L. (2009) Complications of central venous access devices. In: Hamilton, H. & Bodenham, A. (eds) *Central Venous Catheters*. Oxford: John Wiley & Sons, pp. 175–205.

Bowen, J.M. (2013) Mechanisms of TKI-induced diarrhea in cancer patients. *Current Opinions in Support and Palliative Care*, 7, 162–167.

Bower, M. & Cox, S. (2004) Endocrine and metabolic complications of advanced cancer. In: Doyle, D., Hanks, G., Cherny, N.I. & Calman, K. (eds) *Oxford Textbook of Palliative Medicine*, 3rd edn. New York: Oxford University Press, pp. 688–690.

Braunwald, E. (2012) Pericardial disease. In: Longo, D. L., et al. (eds) *Harrison's Principles of Internal Medicine*, 18th edn, Vol. 1. New York: McGraw-Hill.

Bronskill, M.J., Bush, R.S. & Ege, G.N. (1977) A quantitative measurement of peritoneal drainage in malignant ascites. *Cancer*, 40(5), 2375–2380.

Bucholtz, J.D. (1999) Metastatic epidural spinal cord compression. *Seminars in Oncology Nursing*, 15(3), 150–159.

Bushinsky, D.A. & Monk, R.D. (1998) Calcium. *Lancet*. 352:306–311.

Campbell, C. (2001) Controlling malignant ascites. *European Journal of Palliative Care*, 8(5), 187–190.

Cancer Therapy Evaluation Program, Division of Cancer Treatment and Diagnosis, National Cancer Institute, National Institutes of Health (2010) Common terminology criteria for adverse events [Internet]. Version 3.0. Available from: https://ctep.cancer.gov/protocoldevelopment/electronic_applications/docs/ctcaev3.pdf (Accessed: 26/4/2018)

Carroll, M.F. & Schade, D.S. (2003) A practical approach to hypercalcaemia. *American Family Physician*, 67(9), 1959–1966.

Casey, D. (1988) Carotid "blow-out". *Nursing Standard*, 2(47), 30.

Cassidy, J., Bissett, D., Spence, R.A.J., Payne, M. & Morris-Stiff, G. (eds) (2015) *Oxford Handbook of Oncology*, 4th edn. Oxford: Oxford Medical Handbooks.

Catz, A. & Itzkovich, M. (2007) Spinal Cord Independence Measure: comprehensive ability rating scale for the spinal cord lesion patient. *Journal of Rehabilitation and Research Development*, 44(1), 65–68.

Catz, A., Itzkovich, M., Tesio, L., et al. (2007) A multicenter international study on the Spinal Cord Independence Measure, version III: Rasch psychometric validation. *Spinal Cord*, 45(4), 275–291.

Cherny, N. I. (2008). Evaluation and management of treatment-related diarrhoea in patients with advanced cancer: a review. *Journal of Pain and Symptom Management*, 36(4), 413–423.

Cherny N., Fallon M., Kaasa S., Portenoy R.K. & Currow D.C. (2015) *Oxford Textbook of Palliative Medicine*, 5th edn. Oxford: Oxford University Press.

Clarke, R.T., Jenyon, T., van Hamel Parsons, V. & King, A.J. (2013) Neutropenic sepsis: management and complications. *Clinical Medicine*, 13, 185–187.

Clines, G.A. (2011) Mechanisms and treatment of hypercalcemia of malignancy. *Current Opinions in Endocrinology and Diabetes Obesity*, 8, 339–346.

Clinical Knowledge Summaries (CKS) (2014a) Hypercalcaemia. Available at: http://cks.nice.org.uk/hypercalcaemia#!topicsummary (Accessed: 6/4/2018)

Clinical Knowledge Summaries (CKS) (2014b) Acute Kidney Injury. Available at: http://cks.nice.org.uk/acute-kidney-injury#!topicsummary (Accessed: 6/4/2018)

Clinical Knowledge Summaries (CKS) (2015) Neutropenic Sepsis. Available at: http://cks.nice.org.uk/neutropenic-sepsis#!topicsummary (Accessed: 6/4/2018)

Cohen, J. & Rad, I. (2004) Contemporary management of carotid blowout. *Current Opinion in Otolaryngology and Head and Neck Surgery*, 12, 110–115.

Cohen, R., Mena, D., Carbajal-Medoza, R., Matos, N. & Karki, N. (2008) Superior vena cava syndrome: a medical emergency? *International Journal of Angiology*, 17(1), 43–46.

Collis, E. & Mather, H. (2015) Nausea and vomiting in palliative care. *British Medical Journal*, 351, 6249.

Cooksley, T., Holland, M. & Klatersky, J. (2015) Ambulatory outpatient management of patients with low-risk neutropenia. *Acute Medicine*, 14(4), 178–181.

Cope, D. (2005) Malignant effusions and edema. In: Yarbro, C., Frogge, M. & Goodman, M. (eds) *Cancer Nursing Principles and Practice*, 6th edn. Sudbury, MA: Jones and Bartlett, pp. 826–840.

Cope, D. (2011) Malignant effusions. In: Yarbro, C.H., Wujcik, D. & Gobel, B.H. (eds) *Cancer Nursing Principles and Practice*, 7th edn. Sudbury, MA: Jones and Bartlett, pp. 863–879.

Couban, S., Goodyear, M., Burnell, M., et al. (2005) Randomized placebo-controlled study of low-dose warfarin for the prevention of central venous catheter-associated thrombosis in patients with cancer. *Journal of Clinical Oncology*, 23(18), 4063–4069.

Courtney, A., Nemcek, A.A. Jr, Rosenberg, S., Tutton, S., Darcy, M. & Gordon, G. (2008) Prospective evaluation of the PleurX catheter when used to treat recurrent ascites associated with malignancy. *Journal of Vascular Interventional Radiology*, 19(12), 1723–1731.

Cross, N. & Glantz, M. (2003) Neurological complications of cancer therapy. *Neurological Clinics of North America*, 21, 279–318.

CSP (2014) *Guidance in Manual Handling for Chartered Physiotherapists*, 4th edn. London: Chartered Society of Physiotherapy.

Daniels, R. (2011) Surviving the first hours in sepsis: getting the basics right (an intensivist's perspective). *Journal of Antimicrobial Chemotherapy*, (suppl 2), ii11–ii23.

Dark, C. & Razak, A. (2014) Oncology. In: Walker, B., Colledge, N., Ralston, S., et al. (eds) *Davidson's Principles & Practice of Medicine*, 22nd edn. Edinburgh: Churchill Livingstone, Elsevier, Chapter 11, p. 259.

De Gottardi, A., Thévenot, T., Spahr, L., et al. (2009) Risk of complications after abdominal paracentesis in cirrhotic patients: a prospective study. *Clinical Gastroenterology and Hepatology*, 7(8), 906–909.

de Naurois, J., Novitzky-Basso, I., Gill, M.J., Marti Marti, F., Cullen, M.H. & Roila, F. (2010) Management of febrile neutropenia: ESMO Clinical Practice Guidelines. *Annals of Oncology*, 21(Suppl 5), 252–256.

Debourdeau, P., Farge, D., Beckers, M., et al. (2013) International clinical practice guidelines for the treatment and prophylaxis of thrombosis associated with central venous catheters in patients with cancer. *Journal of Thrombosis and Haemostasis*, 11, 71–80.

Dellinger, R.P., Levy, M.M., Carlet, J.M., et al. (2008) Surviving Sepsis Campaign: international guidelines for management of severe sepsis and septic shock. *Critical Care Medicine*, 36, 296–327.

DH (2006) *Dignity in Care Public Survey. Older People and Disability Division*. London: Department of Health.

DH (2007) *Saving Lives: Reducing Infection, Delivering Clean and Safe Care. High Impact Intervention No 1(Central Venous Bundle) and No 2 (Peripheral IV Cannula Care Bundle)*. London: Department of Health.

DH (2010) *Clean Safe Care. High Impact Intervention. Central Venous Catheter Care Bundle and Peripheral IV Cannula Care Bundle*. London: Department of Health.

DH (2011) *Acute Oncology Measures Manual for Cancer Services: Acute Oncology – Including Metastatic Spinal Cord Compression Measures*. London: Department of Health.

Dickenson, D. & Johnson, M. (1993) *Death, Dying and Bereavement*. London: Sage Publications.

Dougherty, L. (2006) *Central Venous Access Devices: Care and Management*. Oxford: Blackwell.

Dougherty, L. & Lister, S. (Eds) (2015) *The Royal Marsden Manual of Clinical Nursing Procedures*, 9th edn. Oxford: Wiley-Blackwell.

Duggal, P., Farah, K.F., Anghel, G., et al. (2006) Safety of paracentesis in inpatients. *Clinical Nephrology*, 66(3), 171–176.

Dunn, L.T. (2002) Raised intracranial pressure. *Journal of Neurology, Neurosurgery & Psychiatry*, 73(suppl 1).

Duran, I., Goebell, P.J., Papazisis, K., et al. (2014) Drug-induced pneumonitis in cancer patients treated with mTOR inhibitors: management and insights into possible mechanisms. *Expert Opinion on Drug Safety*, 13(3), 361–372.

Eberhart, C., Morrison, A., Gyure, K., Frazier, J., Smialek, J.E. & Trancoso, J.C. (2001) Decreasing incidence of sudden death due to undiagnosed primary CNS tumours. *Archives of Pathology and Laboratory Medicine*, 125, 1024–1030.

Efstratiadis, G., Sarigianni, M. & Gougourekis, I. (2006) Hypomagnesemia and cardiovascular system. *Hippokratia*, 10(4), 147–152.

Elting, L.S., Keefe, D.M., Sonis, S.T., et al. and the Burden of Illness Head and Neck Writing Committee (2008) Patient-reported measurements of oral mucositis in head and neck cancer patients treated with radiotherapy with or without chemotherapy: demonstration of increased frequency, severity, resistance to palliation, and impact on quality of life. *Cancer*, 113, 2704–2713.

Ezzo, J., Vickers, A., Richardson, M.A., et al. (2005) Acupuncture-point stimulation for chemotherapy-induced nausea and vomiting. *Journal of Clinical Oncology*, 23(28), 7188–7198.

Faithfull, S. (2006) Radiotherapy. In: Kearny, N. & Richardson, A. (eds) *Nursing Patients with Cancer: Principles and Practice*. Edinburgh: Elsevier Churchill Livingstone.

Farrell, M. & Dempsey, J. (eds) (2013) *Smeltzer & Bare's Textbook of Medical-Surgical Nursing*, 3rd edn. Broadway: Lippincott, Williams & Wilkins.

Feber, T. (2000) *Head and Neck Oncology Nursing*. London: Whurr Publishers Ltd, Chapter 2.8, pp. 245–252.

Fecher, L.A., Agarwala, S.S., Hodi, F.S. & Weber, J.S. (2013) Ipilimumab and its toxicities: a multidisciplinary approach. *Oncologist*, 18(6), 733–743.

Fentiman, I. (2002) Serous effusions. In: Souhami, R.L., Tannock, I., Hohenbuerger, P. & Horiot, J.C. (eds) *Oxford Textbook of Oncology*, 2nd edn. Oxford: Oxford University Press, pp. 887–895.

Ferguson, H.J.M., Ferguson, C.I., Speakman, J. & Ismail, T. (2015) Management of intestinal obstruction in advanced malignancy. *Annals of Medicine and Surgery*, 4(3), 264–276.

Fields, M.M. (2014) Increased intracranial pressure. In: Yarbro, C.H., Wujicik, D. & Gobel, D.H. (eds) *Cancer Symptom Management*, 4th edn. Burlington MA: Jones and Bartlett, pp. 439–455.

Flounders, J.A. (2003) Cardiovascular emergencies: pleural effusion and cardiac tamponade. *Oncology Nurses Forum*, 20(2), E48–E55.

Forbes, K. (1997) Palliative care in patients with cancer of the head and neck. *Clinical Otolaryngology Allied Science*, 22(2), 117–122.

Ford, A. & Marshall, E. (2014) Neutropenic sepsis: a potentially life-threatening complication of chemotherapy. *Clinical Medicine*, 14(5), 538–542.

Fortunato, L. & Ridge, J.A. (1995) Surgical palliation of head and neck cancer. *Current Problems in Cancer*, 19(3), 153–165.

Fraise, A.P. & Bradley, T. (eds) (2009) *Ayliffe's Control of Healthcare-Associated Infection: A Practical Handbook*, 5th edn. London: Hodder Arnold.

Frawley, T. & Begley, C.M. (2005) Causes and prevention of carotid artery rupture. *British Journal of Nursing*, 14(22), 1198–1202.

Frawley, T. & Begley, C.M. (2006) Ethical issues in caring for people with carotid artery rupture. *British Journal of Nursing*, 15(2), 100–103.

Freifeld, A.G., Bow, E.J., Sepkowitz, K.A., et al. (2011) Clinical practice guideline for the use of antimicrobial agents in neutropenic patients with cancer: 2010 update by the Infectious Disease Society of America. *Clinical Infectious Diseases*, 52(4), e56–e93.

Fuccio, L., Guido, A & Andreyev, H.J.N. (2012) Management of intestinal complications in patients with pelvic radiation disease. *Clinics in Gastroenterology and Hepatology*, 10(12), 1326–1334.e4.

Fulop, T. (2016) Hypomagnesemia. Available at: http://emedicine.medscape.com/article/2038394-overview#a4 (Accessed: 6/4/2018)

Furlan, J.C., Robinson, L.R. & Murry, B.J. (2016) Clinical reasoning: stepwise paralysis in patient with adenocarcinoma of lung. *Neurology*, 86(12), e122–e127.

Gagnon, B., Mancini, I., Pereira, J. & Bruera, E. (1998) Palliative management of bleeding events in advanced cancer patients. *Journal of Palliative Care*, 14(4), 50–54.

Gibson, R.J. & Stringer, A.M. (2009) Chemotherapy-induced diarrhoea. *Current Opinions in Supportive Palliative Care*, 3, 31–35.

Gibson, R., Keefe, D., Lalla, R., et al. (2013) Systematic review of agents for the management of gastrointestinal mucositis in cancer patients, *Supportive Care in Cancer*, 21(1), 313–326.

Glare, P., Miller, J., Nikolova, T. & Tickoo, R. (2011) Treating nausea and vomiting in palliative care: a review. *Clinical Interventions in Aging*, 6, 243–259.

Gorski, L., Perucca, R. & Hunter, M. (2010) Central venous access devices: care, maintenance, and potential problems. In: Alexander, M., Corrigan, A., Gorski, L., Hankins, J. & Perucca, R. (eds) *Infusion Nursing: An Evidence-Based Approach*, 3rd edn. St Louis, MO: Saunders Elsevier, pp. 495–515.

Grahn, E., Bogan, A., Cullen, L. & Schardien, K. (2008) Development of a comprehensive evidence based management and professional education strategy for oncology patients at risk for carotid artery rupture. *Oncology Nursing Forum*, 35(3), 518.

Grandjean, C. & McMullen, P. (2010) Hypercalcemia: what constitutes reasonable follow-up? *The Journal for Nurse Practitioners*, 6(9), 691–693.

Green, A.T. (2016) Hypercalcemia in emergency medicine. Medscape. Available at: http://emedicine.medscape.com/article/766373 (Accessed: 6/4/2018)

Grenon, N. & Chan, J. (2009) Managing toxicities associated with colorectal cancer chemotherapy and targeted therapy: a guide for nurses. *Clinical Journal of Oncology Nursing*, 13(3), 285–296.

Guerrera, M.P., Volpe, S.L. & Mao, J.J. (2009) Therapeutic uses of magnesium. *American Family Physician*, 15(80(2)), 157–162.

Guilfoyle, M.R., Weerakkody, R.A., Oswal, A., et al. (2011) Implementation of neuro-oncology service reconfiguration in accordance with NICE guidance provides enhanced clinical care for patients with glioblastoma multiforme. *British Journal of Cancer*, 104(12), 1810–1815.

Gupta, H., Araki, Y., Davidoff, A.M., et al. (2007) Evaluation of paediatric oncology patients with previous multiple central catheters for vascular access: is Doppler ultrasound needed? *Paediatric Blood Cancer*, 48, 527–531.

Hacker, R.I., De Marco Garcia, L., Chawla, A. & Panetta, T. (2012) Fibrin sheath angioplasty: a technique to prevent superior vena cava stenosis secondary to dialysis catheters. *International Journal of Angiology*, 21(3), 129–134.

Harris, D.G. (2010) Nausea and vomiting in advanced cancer. *British Medical Bulletin*, 96(1), 175–185.

Harris, D.G. & Noble, S.I.R. (2009) Management of terminal haemorrhage in patients with advanced cancer: a systematic literature review. *Journal of Pain and Symptom Management*, 38(6), 913–927.

Harrison, P. (2000) *Managing Spinal Injury: Critical Care. The Initial Management of People with Actual or Suspected Spinal Cord Injury in High Dependency and Intensive Care*. Milton Keynes: Spinal Injury Association.

Heskeeth, P.J. (2008) Chemotherapy-induced nausea and vomiting. *New England Journal of Medicine*, 388(23), 2482–2492.

Hickey, J.V. (2002) Intracranial hypertension: theory and management of increased intracranial pressure. In: Hickey, J.V. (ed.) *The Clinical Practice of Neurological and Neurosurgical Nursing*, 5th edn. Philadelphia, PA: Lippincott Williams & Wilkins, pp. 285–318.

Higdon, M. & Higdon, J. (2006) Treatment of oncologic emergencies. *American Family Physician*, 74(11), 1873–1880.

Hjermstad, M.J., Kolflaath, J., Lokken, A.O., Hanssen, S.B., Norman, A.P. & Aass, N. (2016) Are emergency admissions in palliative cancer care always necessary? Results from a descriptive study. *British Medical Journal*, 3, 1–8.

Hodi, F.S., O'Day, S.J., McDermott, D.F., et al. (2010) Improved survival with ipilimumab in patients with metastatic melanoma. *New England Journal of Medicine*, 363, 711–723.

Hoit, B.D. (2011) Pericardial disease. In: Fuster, V., Walsh, R.A., Harrington, R.A. (eds) *Hurst's The Heart*, 13th edn. New York: McGraw-Hill Professional.

Hosttetter, R., Marincola, F. & Schwartzentruber, D. (2005) Malignant ascites. In: Devita, V., Hellman, S. & Rosenberg, S. (eds) *Cancer Prin-*

ciples and Practice of Oncology, 7th edn. Philadelphia: Lippincott Williams & Williams, pp. 2392–2398.

Hou, W. & Sanyal, A.J. (2009) Ascites: diagnosis and management. Medical Clinics of North America, 93(4), 801-817.

HSE (1992) Manual Handling Operations Regulations 1992. London: HMSO.

Hughes, W.T., Armstrong, D., Bodey, G.P., et al. (2002) 2002 guidelines for the use of antimicrobial agents in neutropenic patients with cancer. Clinical Infectious Diseases, 34(6), 730–751.

Imazio, M. & Adler, Y. (2013) Management of pericardial effusion. European Heart Journal, 34, 1186–1197.

Itzkovich, M., Gelernter, I., Biering-Sorensen, F., et al. (2007) The Spinal Cord Independence Measure (SCIM) version III: reliability and validity in a multi-center international study. Disability and Rehabilitation, 29(24), 1926–1933.

Jakobsson, S., Ahlberg, K., Taft, C. & Ekman, T. (2010) Exploring a link between fatigue and intestinal injury during pelvic radiotherapy. Oncologist, 15, 1009–1015

Janelsins, M.C., Tejani, M., Kamen, C., Peoples, A., Mustian, K.M. & Morrow, G.R. (2013) Current pharmacotherapy for chemotherapy-induced nausea and vomiting in cancer patients. Expert Opinion in Pharmacotherapy, 14(6), 757–766.

Johantgen, M.A. (1998) Carotid artery rupture. In: Advanced and Critical Oncology Nursing. Managing primary complications. Pennsylvania, PA: W.B. Saunders.

Johnston, R.L., Lutzky, J., Chodhry, A. & Barkin, J.S. (2009) Cytotoxic T-lymphocyte-associated antigen 4 antibody induced colitis and its management with infliximab. Digestive Disease Science, 54, 2538–2540.

Joint Formulary Committee (2018) British National Formulary. London: BMJ Group, Pharmaceutical Press and RCPCH Publications. Available at: http://www.medicinescomplete.com (Accessed: 19/4/2018)

Joshi, D., Centre, J.R. & Eisman, J.A. (2009) Investigation of incidental hypercalcaemia. British Medical Journal, 339, 4613.

Kane, K.K. (1983) Carotid artery rupture in advanced head and neck cancer patients. Oncology Nursing Forum, 10(1), 14–18.

Kaplow, R. & Iyere, K. (2016) Understanding spinal cord compression. Nursing, 46(9), 44–51.

Karam, N., Patel, P. & deFilippi, C. (2001) Diagnosis and management of chronic pericardial effusions. American Journal of Medical Science, 322(2), 79–87.

Kayley, J. (2008) Intravenous therapy in the community. In: Dougherty, L. & Lamb, J. (eds) Intravenous Therapy in Nursing Practice, 2nd edn. Oxford: Blackwell Publishing, pp. 352–374.

Kearon, C., Kahn, S., Agnelli, G., et al. (2008) Antithrombotic therapy for venous thromboembolic disease: American College of Chest Physicians evidence-based clinical practice guidelines (8th edition). Chest, 133, 454–545.

Keefe, D.M. (2007) Intestinal mucositis: mechanisms and management. Current Opinion in Oncology, 19, 323–327.

Keefe, D. & Anthony, L. (2008) Tyrosine kinase inhibitors and gut toxicity: a new era in supportive care. Current Opinion in Supportive and Palliative Care, 2(1), 19–21.

Keefe, D.M., Brealey, J., Goland, G.J. & Cummins, A.G. (2000) Chemotherapy for cancer causes apoptosis that precedes hypoplasia in crypts of the small intestine in humans. Gut, 47, 632–637.

Keen, A., Fitzgerald, D., Bryant, A. & Dickinson, H.O. (2010) Management of drainage for malignant ascites in gynaecological cancer. Cochrane Database of Systematic Reviews. Available at: http://onlinelibrary.wiley.com/doi/10.1002/14651858.CD007794.pub2/full (Accessed: 6/4/2018)

Kim, S-H., Hyang, M.H., Sohee, P., et al. (2010) Clinical characteristics of malignant pericardial effusion associated with recurrence and survival. Cancer Research and Treatment: official journal of Korean Cancer Association, 42(4), 210–216.

Koch, W.M. (2009) Complications of surgery to the neck. In: Eisele, D. & Smith, R.V. (eds) Complications in Head and Neck Surgery, 2nd edn. St Louis: Mosby, pp. 439–465.

Kornblau, S., Benson, A.B., Catalano, R., et al. (2000) Management of cancer treatment-related diarrhea. Issues and therapeutic strategies. Journal of Pain and Symptom Management, 19(2),118–129.

Krassioukov, A., Eng, J.J., Warburton, D.E., et al. (2009) A systematic review of the management of orthostatic hypotension after spinal cord injury. Archives of Physical Medicine and Rehabilitation, 90(5), 876–885.

L'Esperance, A., Vincent, F., Gaudreault, M., et al. and the Comité de l'évolution des pratiques en oncologie (2012) Treatment of metastatic spinal cord compression: CEPO review and clinical recommendations. Current Oncology, 19(6), e478–e490.

Lee, A. & Grap, M.J. (2008) Care and management of the patient with ascites. Medsurg Nursing, 17(6), 376–381.

Lee, A., Lau, T.N. & Yeong, K.Y. (2000) Indwelling catheters for the management of malignant ascites. Supportive Care in Cancer, 8(6), 493–499.

Lefebvre, C.W. (2016) Tumours of the central nervous system. In: Aghababian, R.V. (ed.) Essentials in Emergency Medicine, 2nd edn. Sudbury, MA: Jones Bartlett Learning.

Legrand, S.B. (2011) Modern management of malignant hypercalcaemia. American Journal of Hospital Palliative Care, 28(7), 5151–5517.

Lesage, C. (1986) Carotid artery rupture. Prediction, prevention and preparation. Cancer Nursing, 9(1), 1–7.

Lestuzzi, C. (2010) Neoplastic pericardial disease: old and current strategies for diagnosis and management. World Journal of Cardiology, 2(9), 270–279.

Levack, P., Graham, J. & Collie, D. (2002) Don't wait for a sensory level – listen to the symptoms: a prospective audit of the delays in diagnosis of malignant cord compression. Clinical Oncology, 14, 472–480.

Lewington, A. & Kanagasundaram, S. (2011) Renal Association clinical practice guidelines on acute kidney injury. Nephron Clinical Practice, 118(suppl 1), c349–c390. Available at:https://www.karger.com/Article/Pdf/328075 (Accessed: 27/4/2018)

Libshitz, H.I. (1993) Radiation changes in the lung. Seminars in Roentgenology, 28, 303–320.

Limper, A.H. (2004) Chemotherapy-induced lung disease. Clinics in Chest Medicine, 25(1), 53–64.

Little, W.C. & Freeman, G.L. (2006) Pericardial disease. Circulation, 113, 1622–1632.

Lobo, B.L., Vaidean, G., Broyles, J., Reaves, A.B. & Shorr, R.I. (2009) Risk of venous thromboembolism in hospitalised patients with peripherally inserted central catheters. Journal of Hospital Medicine, 4(7), 417–422.

Loblaw, D.A., Laperriere, N.J. & Mackillop, W.J. (2003) A population-based study of malignant spinal cord compression in Ontario. Clinical Oncology, 15(4), 211–217.

London Cancer Alliance (2015) LCA Acute Oncology Guidelines September 2013 (updated March 2016). Available at: http://www.london-canceralliance.nhs.uk/media/124008/lca-revised-acute-oncology-clinical-guidelines-september-2013-updated-march-2016-.pdf (Accessed: 27/4/2018)

Longmore, M., Wilkinson, I.B., Baldwin, A. & Wallin, E. (2014) Oxford Handbook of Clinical Medicine, 9th edn. Oxford: Oxford University Press.

Loveday, H.P., Wilson, J.A., Pratt, R.J., et al. (2014) epic3: National evidence-based guidelines for preventing healthcare-associated infections in NHS hospitals in England. Journal of Hospital Infection, 86(S1), S1–S70.

Lovel, T. (2000) Palliative care and head and neck cancer. Editorial. British Journal of Oral and Maxillofacial Surgery, 38, 253–254.

Lundy-Ekman, L. (2007) Motor neurons. In: Neuroscience: Fundamentals for Rehabilitation, 3rd edn. St Louis, MO: Saunders Elsevier, pp. 188–242.

Luo, C.B., Chang, F.C., Mu-Huo Teng, M., Chi-Chang Chen, C.M., Feng Lirng, J. & Cheng, Y. (2003) Endovascular treatment of the carotid artery rupture with massive haemorrhage. Journal of Chinese Medical Association, 66, 140–147.

Macmillan, K. & Struthers, C. (1987) Algorithm for the emergency nursing management of spontaneous carotid artery rupture. Canadian Critical Care Nursing Journal, 4(1), 20–21.

Magan, C.M. (1992) Malignant pericardial effusions: pathology and clinical corrolates. Oncology Nursing Forum, (19(8), 1215–1221.

Malet-Martino, M. & Martino, R. (2002) Clinical studies of three oral prodrugs of 5-fluorouracil (capecitabine, UFT, S-1): a review. Oncologist, 7, 288–323.

Mallik, S., Mallik, G., Macabuloa, S.T. & Dorigo, A. (2016) Malignancy associated hypercalcaemia-responsiveness to IV bisphosphonates and prognosis in a palliative population. *Supportive Care in Cancer*, 24(4), 1771–1777.

Mamada, Y., Yoshida, H., Tania, N., et al. (2007) Peritoneovenous shunts for palliation of malignant ascites. *Journal of Nippon Medical School*, 74(5), 355–358.

Mannix, K.A. (2002) Palliation of nausea and vomiting. *CME Cancer Medicine*, 1, 18–22.

Manzi, N.M., Pires, N.N., Vasques, C.L., Custodio, C.S., Simino, G.P.R. & Reis, P.E.D. (2012) Nursing interventions related to the treatment of syndromic oncological emergencies. *Journal of Nursing UFPE on line*, 6(9), 2307–2311.

Marincola, F.M. & Schwartzentruber, D.J. (2001) *Cancer: Principles and Practice of Oncology*, 6th edn. Philadelphia: Williams & Wilkins, pp. 2745–2752.

Marrs, J.A. (2006) Care of patients with neutropenia. *Oncology Nursing*, 10(2), 164–166.

Martin, K.J., Gonzalez, G.A. & Slatopolsky, E. (2009) Clinical consequences of management of hypomagnesemia. *Journal of the American Society of Nephrology*, 20(11), 2291–2295.

Masi, G., Falcone, A., Di Paolo, A., et al. (2004) A phase I and pharmacokinetic study of irinotecan given as a 7-day continuous infusion in metastatic colorectal cancer patients pretreated with 5-fluorouracil or raltitrexed. *Clinical Cancer Research*, 10, 1657–1663.

Mason, T.M., Ferral, S.M., Boyington, A.R. & Reich, R.R. (2014) Central venous access devices: an investigation of oncology nurses' troubleshooting techniques. *Clinical Journal of Oncology Nursing*, 18(14), 421–425.

Matsuno, O. (2012) Drug-induced interstitial lung disease: mechanisms and best diagnostic approaches. *Respiratory Research*, 13, 39. Available at: https://respiratory-research.biomedcentral.com/articles/10.1186/1465-9921-13-39 (Accessed: 6/4/2018)

Mattison, G., Bilney, M., Haji-Michael, P. & Cooksley, T. (2016) A nurse-led protocol improves the time to first dose intravenous antibiotics in septic patients post chemotherapy. *Supportive Care in Cancer*, 24(12), 5001–5005.

Mayo, D.J. (2000) Catheter-related thrombosis. *Journal of Intravenous Nursing*, 5(2), 10–20.

McCollum, A.D., Catalano, P.J., Haller, D.G., et al. (2002) Outcomes and toxicity in African-American and Caucasian patients in a randomized adjuvant chemotherapy trial for colon cancer. *Journal of the National Cancer Institute*, 94, 1160–1167.

McCurdy, M.T. & Shanholtz, C.B. (2012) Oncologic emergencies. *Critical Care Medicine*, 40(7), 2212–2222.

McDonald, S., Rubin, P., Phillips, T.L. & Marks, L.B. (1995) Injury to the lung from cancer therapy: clinical syndromes, measurable endpoints, and potential scoring systems. *International Journal of Radiation Oncology, Biology and Physics*, 31(5), 1187–1203.

McGibbon, A., Chen, G.I., Peltekian, K.M. & van Zanten, S.V. (2007) An evidence-based manual for abdominal paracentesis. *Digestive Diseases and Sciences*, 52(12), 3307–3315.

McGrath, A. (2005) Anatomy and physiology of the bowel and urinary systems. In: Porett, T. & McGrath, A. (eds) *Stoma Care*. Oxford: Blackwell Publishing, pp. 1–16.

McVay, P.A. & Toy, P.T. (1991) Lack of evidence of increased bleeding after paracentesis and thoracentesis in patients with mild coagulation abnormalities. *Transfusion*, 31(2), 164.

Mercandante, S., Intravaia, G., Ferrera, P., Villari, P. & David, F. (2008) Peritoneal catheter for continuous drainage of ascites in advanced cancer patients. *Supportive Cancer Care*, 16(8), 975–978.

Mestecky, A.M. (2007) Management of severe traumatic brain injury: the need for the knowledgeable nurse. *British Journal of Neuroscience Nursing*, 3(1), 7–13.

Meyerhardt, J.A., Tepper, J.E., Niedzwiecki, D., et al. (2004) Impact of body mass index on outcomes and treatment-related toxicity in patients with stage II and III rectal cancer: findings from Intergroup Trial 0114. *Journal of Clinical Oncology*, 22, 648–657.

Miller, J. & Cooper, J. (2010) The contribution of occupational therapy to palliative medicine. In: Doyle, D., Cherny, N.I., Christakis, N.A., Fallon, M., Kasasa, S. & Portenoy, R.K. (eds) *Oxford Textbook of Palliative Medicine*, 4th edn. Oxford: Oxford University Press, pp. 206–213.

Milligan, J., Lee, J., McMillan, C. & Klassen, H. (2012) Autonomic dysreflexia. *Canadian Family Physician*, 58(8), 831–835.

Minisola, S., Pepe, J., Piemonte, S. & Cipriani, C. (2015) The diagnosis and management of hypercalcaemia. *British Medical Journal*, 350, h2723.

Misra, V. (2016) Use of complementary therapies in the care of patients with spinal cord compression. The Christie NHS Foundation Trust. Available at: www.christie.nhs.uk/MSCC (Accessed: 6/4/2018)

Molassiotis, A. & Borjeson, S. (2006) Nausea and vomiting. In: Kearney, N. & Richardson, A. (eds) *Nursing Patients with Cancer: Principles and Practice*. Edinburgh: Elsevier, Churchill Livingstone, Chapter 20, pp. 415–437.

Monagle, P., Chan, A., Goldenberg, N.A., et al. (2012) Antithrombotic therapy in neonates and children: American College of Chest Physicians evidence-based clinical practice guidelines (9th edition) *Chest*, 141(2 Suppl): e737s–e801s.

Moore, K. & Aithal, G. (2006) Guidelines in the management of ascites in cirrhosis. *Gut*, 55(1), 12.

Morrissey, D.D., Andersen, P.E., Nesbit, G.M., Barnwell, S.L., Events, E.C. & Cohen, J.I. (1997) Endovascular management of haemorrhage in patients with head and neck cancer. *Archives of Otolaryngology, Head and Neck Surgery*, 123, 15–19.

Mort, D., Lansdown, M., Smith, N., Protopapa, K. & Mason, M. (2008) *For Better, For Worse*? London: NCEPOD.

Moyses-Neto, N., Guimaraes, F.M., Ayaub, F.H., Vieria-Neto, O.M., Costa, J.A. & Dantas, (2006) Acute renal failure and hypercalcaemia. *Renal Failure*, 28(2), 153–159.

Muehlbauer, P.M., Thorpe, D., Davis, A., Drabot, R., Rawlings, B.L., & Kiker, E. (2009). Putting evidence into practice: evidence-based interventions to prevent, manage, and treat chemotherapy- and radiotherapy-induced diarrhea. *Clinical Journal of Oncology Nursing*, 13, 336–340.

Nasir, S.S. & Schwartzberg, L.S. (2016) Recent advances in preventing chemotherapy-induced nausea and vomiting. *Oncology Journal*, 30, 750–762.

National Audit Office (2010) Department of Health – Delivering the Cancer Reform Strategy. Available at: www.nao.org.uk/wp-content/uploads/2010/11/1011568.pdf (Accessed: 6/4/2018)

National Cancer Institute (2016) Pneumonitis. Available at: https://www.cancer.gov/publications/dictionaries/cancer-terms/def/pneumonitis (Accessed: 27/4/2018)

National Cancer Intelligence Network (2010) Routes to diagnosis – NCIN data briefing. Available at: http://www.ncin.org.uk/publications/data_briefings/routes_to_diagnosis (Accessed: 26/4/2018)

National Chemotherapy Advisory Group (2009) *Chemotherapy Services in England: Ensuring Quality and Safety*. London: Department of Health.

National Comprehensive Cancer Network (2016) Clinical practice guidelines in oncology: antiemesis. Version 2. Available at: http://www.nccn.org/professionals/physician_gls/pdf/antiemesis.pdf

NCAT (2011) Manual for Cancer Services: acute oncology – including metastatic spinal cord compression measures. Available at: https://www.gov.uk/government/publications/manual-for-cancer-services-acute-oncology-including-metatastic-spinal-cord-compression-measures (Accessed: 6/4/2018)

Newton, H.B. (1999) Neurologic complications of systemic cancer. *American Family Physician*, 15(59), 878–886.

NHS Employers (2011) Needlestick injury. Available at: http://www.saferneedles.org.uk/news/pdf_articles/Needlestick_2011.pdf (Accessed: 6/4/2018)

NHS England (2013) *Sepsis management as an NHS clinical priority*. NHS England. Available at: https://www.england.nhs.uk/wp-content/uploads/2015/08/Sepsis-Action-Plan-23.12.15-v1.pdf (Accessed: 27/4/2018)

NICE (2007a) *Head injury: triage, assessment, investigation and early management of head injury in infants, children and adults*. Clinical guideline 56. London: NICE. Available at: https://www.nice.org.uk/guidance/cg56 (Accessed: 6/4/2018)

NICE (2007b) *Acutely ill adults in hospital: recognising and responding to deterioration*. Clinical guideline 50. London: NICE. Available at: www.nice.org.uk/guidance/cg50 (Accessed: 6/4/2018)

NICE (2008) *Metastatic spinal cord compression in adults: risk assessment, diagnosis and management.* Clinical guideline 75. London: NICE. Available at: www.nice.org.uk/guidance/cg75 (Accessed: 6/4/2018)

NICE (2012a) *Epilepsies: diagnosis and management.* Clinical guideline 137. London: NICE. Available at: www.nice.org.uk/guidance/cg137 (Accessed: 6/4/2018)

NICE (2012b) *Neutropenic sepsis: prevention and management in people with cancer.* Clinical guideline 151. London: NICE. Available at: https://www.nice.org.uk/guidance/cg151 (Accessed: 6/4/2018)

NICE (2013) *Acute kidney injury: prevention, definition and management.* Clinical guideline 169. London: NICE. Available at: www.nice.org.uk/guidance/cg169 (Accessed: 6/4/2018)

NICE (2014) *NICE Support for commissioning metastatic spinal cord compression.* Available at: https://www.nice.org.uk/guidance/qs56/resources/support-for-commissioning-metastatic-spinal-cord-compression-pdf-253725661 (Accessed: 27/4/2018)

NICE (2016) *Sepsis: recognition, diagnosis and early management.* NICE guideline 51. London: NICE. Available at: https://www.nice.org.uk/guidance/ng51 (Accessed: 6/4/2018)

NICE (2018) *PleurX peritoneal catheter drainage system for vacuum-assisted drainage of treatment-resistant, recurrent malignant ascites.* Medical technologies guidance [MTG9] Published date: March 2012 Last updated: February 2018. London: NICE.

Nieto, C.S., Solano, J.M.E., Martinez, C.B., Martin, E.F., Colunga, J.C.M. & Garcia, A.A. (1980) The carotid artery in head and neck oncology. *Clinical Otolaryngology*, 5, 403–417.

Nightingale, J.M. (2015) Applied anatomy and physiology of the gastrointestinal tract. Available at: http://clinicalgate.com/applied-anatomy-and-physiology-of-the-gastrointestinal-tract-git/ (Accessed: 6/4/2018)

Nightingale, J.M., Lennard-Jones, J.E. & Walker, E.R. (1992) A patient with jejunostomy liberated from home intravenous therapy after 14 years; contribution of balance studies. *Clinical Nutrition*, 11, 101–105.

NMC (2015) *The Code.* London: Nursing & Midwifery Council. Available at: https://www.nmc.org.uk/globalassets/sitedocuments/nmc-publications/nmc-code.pdf (Accessed: 27/4/2018)

Notter, R.H., Finkelstein, J.N. & Holm, B.A. (2005) *Lung Injury: Mechanisms, Pathophysiology, and Therapy.* New York: Taylor & Francis.

Novartis (2012) *Certican.* Malaysia: Zuellig Pharma.

O'Brien, C. (2008) Nausea and vomiting. *Canadian Family Physician*, 54(6), 861–863.

Odor, P. & Bailey, A. (2013) Cardiac Tamponade. World Federation of Societies of Anaesthesiologists. Available at: http://www.frca.co.uk/Documents/283%20Cardiac%20Tamponade%20.pdf (Accessed: 6/4/2018)

Oie, Y., Saito, Y., Kato, M., et al. (2013) Relationship between radiation pneumonitis and organizing pneumonia after radiotherapy for breast cancer. *Radiation Oncology*, 38, 56–61.

Okamura H., Kamiyama, R. & Takiguchi, Y. (2002) Histopathological examination of ruptured carotid artery after irradiation. *ORL: journal for oto-rhino-laryngology and its related specialties*, 64, 226–228.

Ozkan, O., Akinci, D., Gocman, R., et al. (2007) Percutaneous placement of peritoneal port-catheters in patients with malignant ascites. *Cardiovascular and Interventional Radiology*, 30(2), 232–236.

Pagès, C., Gornet, J.M., Monsel, G., et al. (2013) Ipilimumab-induced acute severe colitis treated by infliximab. *Melanoma Research*, 23(3), 227–230.

Pan, X.C., Morrison, R.S., Ness, J., Fugh-Berman, A. & Leipzig, R.M. (2000) Complementary and alternative medicine in the management of pain, dyspnea, and nausea and vomiting near the end of life: a systematic review. *Journal of Pain and Symptom Management*, 20, 374–387.

Peebles, C.R., Shambrook, J.S. & Harden, S.P. (2011) Pericardial disease – anatomy and function. *British Journal of Radiology*, 84(spec iss 3), s324–s337.

Peguero, J., Khanfar, A., Mannem, S., Willis, M. & Markowitz, A. (2015) Impending carotid blowout syndrome. *Journal of Clinical Oncology*, 33(23), e97–e98.

Pemberton, L. & Waterhouse, C. (2006) The unconscious patient. In: Alexander, M.F., Fawcett, J.N. & Runciman, P.J. (eds) *Nursing Practice: Hospital and Home*, 3rd edn. Edinburgh: Churchill Livingstone, pp. 965–988.

Pericleous, M., Sarnowski, A., Moore, A., Ijten, R. & Zamon, M. (2016) The clinical management of abdominal ascites, spontaneous bacterial peritonitis and hepatorenal syndrome: a review of current guidelines and recommendations. *European Journal of Gastroenterology and Hepatology*, 28(3), e10–e18.

Peterson, M.E. (2013) Management of adverse events with hormone receptor-positive breast cancer treated with everolimus: observations from a phase 3 trial. *Supportive Cancer Care*, 21(8), 2341–2349.

Petrofsky, M. (2014) Management of malignant pericardial effusion. *Journal of the Advanced Practitioner in Oncology*, 5(4), 218–289.

Pettifer, A. & Grant, S. (2013) The management of hypercalcaemia in advanced cancer. *International Journal of Palliative Nursing*, 19(7), 327–331.

Pfennig, C.L. & Slovis, C.M. (2014) Electrolyte disorders. In: Marx, J.A., Hockberger, R.S., Walls, R.M., et al. (eds) *Rosen's Emergency Medicine: Concepts and Clinical Practice*, 8th edn. Philadelphia, PA: Elsevier Mosby, Chapter 125.

Pittiruti, M. (2015) What the world needs now is an insertion bundle to prevent catheter related thrombosis. Presentation at 29th Annual Association of Vascular Access conference, Dallas, USA, September 26–29.

Pleuvry, B.J. (2012) Physiology and pharmacology of nausea and vomiting. *Anaesthesia and Intensive Care Medicine*, 13(12), 598–602.

Pockros, P.J., Esrason, K.T., Nguyen, C., Duque, J. & Woods, S. (1992) Mobilization of malignant ascites with diuretics is dependent on ascitic fluid characteristics. *Gastroenterology*, 103, 1302–1306.

Porta, C., Osanto, S., Ravaud, A., et al. (2011) Management of adverse events associated with the use of everolimus in patients with advanced renal cell carcinoma. *European Journal of Cancer*, 4(9), 1287–1298.

Prowle, J.R., Echeverri, J.E., Ligabo, V., Ronco, C. & Bellomo, R. (2011) Fluid balance and acute kidney injury: the rationale for fluid therapy. Available at: http://www.medscape.org/viewarticle/715130_2 (Accessed: 6/4/2018)

Putt, L. & Jones, P. (2014) The role of the specialist acute oncology nurse in the new acute oncology services. *Clinical Oncology*, 26(3), 125–127.

Qinming, Z. (2012) Thrombosis. In: Di Carlo, I. & Biffi, R. (eds) *Totally Implantable Venous Access Devices*. Milan: Springer, pp. 173–182.

Quint, D.J. (2000) Indications for emergent MRI of the central nervous system. *Journal of American Medical Association*, 283, 853–860.

Rades, D., Huttenlocher, S., Dunst, J. et al. (2010) Matched pair analysis comparing surgery followed by radiotherapy and radiotherapy alone for metastatic spinal cord compression. *Journal of Clinical Oncology*, 28, 3597–3604.

Rahman, M., Shad, F. & Smith, C.S. (2012) Acute kidney injury: a guide to diagnosis and management. *American Family Physician*, 86(7), 631–639.

Ralston, S.H., Gallacher, S.J., Patel, U., Campbell, J. & Boyle, I.T. (1990) Cancer-associated hypercalcemia: morbidity and mortality. Clinical experience in 126 treated patients. *Annals of Internal Medicine*, 112,499–504,

Rangel-Castillo, L., Gopinath, S. & Robertson, C.S. (2008) Management of intracranial hypertension. *Neurological Clinics*, 26(2), 521–541.

Raslan, A. & Bhardwaj, A. (2007) Medical management of cerebral oedema. *Neurosurgery Focus*, 22, 1–12.

RCN (2016) *Standards for Infusion Therapy*, 4th edn. London: Royal College of Nursing. Available at: https://www.rcn.org.uk/professional-development/publications/pub-005704 (Accessed: 6/4/2018)

Reilly, J.P., Anderson, B.J., Hudock, K.M., et al. (2016) Neutropenic sepsis is associated with distinct clinical and biological characteristics: a cohort study of severe sepsis. *Critical Care*, 20, 222–231.

Remington, M., Fleming, C.R. & Malagelada, J.R. (1982) Inhibition of postprandial pancreatic and biliary secretion by loperamide in patients with short bowel syndrome. *Gut*, 23, 98–101.

Rhodes, V. & Manzullo, E. (1997) Oncologic emergencies. In: Pazdur, R. (ed.) *Medical Oncology: A Comprehensive Review*, 2nd edn. Huntington, NY: PRR.

Richardson, G., & Dobish, R. (2007). Chemotherapy induced diarrhoea. *Journal of Oncology Pharmacy Practice*, 13(4), 181–198.

Ripamonti, C., Twycross, R., Baines, M., et al. for Working Group of the European Association for Palliative Care (2001) Clinical-practice recommendations for management of bowel obstruction in patients with end-stage cancer. *Supportive Care in Cancer*, 9(4), 223–233.

Ripamonti, C., Easson, A.M. & Gerdes, H. (2008) Management of malignant bowel obstruction. *European Journal of Cancer*, 44(8),1105–1115.

308

Rivers, E., Nguyen, B., Havstad, S., et al. and the Early Goal Directed Therapy Collaborative Group. (2001) Early goal-directed therapy in the treatment of severe sepsis and septic shock. *New England Journal of Medicine*, 345,1368–1377.

Rodriguez, F., Carmeci, C., Dalman, R.L. & Lee, A. (2001) Spontaneous late carotid-cutaneous fistula following radical neck dissection: a case report. *Vascular Surgery*, 35(5), 409–413.

Roila, F., Molassiotis, A., Herrstedt, J., et al. on behalf of the participants of the MASCC/ESMO Consensus Conference Copenhagen 2015 (2016) 2016 MASCC and ESMO guideline update for the prevention of chemotherapy- and radiotherapy-induced nausea and vomiting and of nausea and vomiting in advanced cancer patients. *Annals of Oncology*, 27(suppl 5), v119–v133.

Roodenburg, J. & Davies, A. (2005) Head and neck cancer. In: Davies, A. & Finley, I. (eds) *Oral Care in Advanced Disease.* Oxford: Oxford University Press.

Royal College of Obstetricians and Gynaecologists (2014) Management of Ascites in Ovarian Cancer Patients. Scientific Impact Paper No. 45. Available at: https://www.rcog.org.uk/globalassets/documents/guidelines/scientific-impact-papers/sip45ascites.pdf (Accessed: 6/4/2018)

Rull, G. (2013) Ascites Tapping. Available at: https://patient.info/doctor/ascites-tapping (Accessed: 27/4/2018)

Runyon, B.A. (1986) Paracentesis of ascetic fluid. A safe procedure. *Archives of Internal Medicine*, 146(11), 2259.

Runyon, B.A. (2015) Diagnostic and therapeutic abdominal paracentesis. Available at: http://www.uptodate.com/contents/diagnostic-and-therapeutic-abdominal-paracentesis (Accessed: 6/4/2018)

Runyon, B.A., Hoefs, J.C. & Morgan, T.R. (1988) Ascitic fluid analysis in malignancy-related ascites. *Hepatology*, 8, 1104–1109.

Sajid, M.S., Ahmed, N., Desai, M., Baker, D. & Hamilton, G. (2007) Upper limb deep vein thrombosis: a literature review to streamline the protocol for management. *Acta Haematologica*, 118, 10–18.

Sangisetty, S.L. & Miner, T.J. (2012) Malignant ascites: a review of prognostic factors, pathophysiology and therapeutic measures. *World Journal of Gastrointestinal Surgery*, 4(4), 87–95.

Sargent, J.T.S. & Smith, O.P. (2010) Haematological emergencies managing hypercalcaemia in adults and children with haematological disorders. *British Journal of Haematology*, 149, 465 477.

Sargent, S. (2006) Management of patients with advanced liver cirrhosis. *Nursing Standard*, 21(11), 48–56.

Schafer, S. (1997). Oncologic complications. In: Otto, S. (ed.) *Oncology Nursing*, 3rd edn. St. Louis: Mosby, pp. 406–476.

Schiech, L. (2000) Carotid artery rupture. *Clinical Journal of Oncology Nursing*, 4, 93–94.

Seccareccia, D. (2010) Cancer-related hypercalcaemia. *Canadian Family Physician*, 56, 244–246.

Seike, M., Maetani, I. & Sakai, Y. (2007) Treatment of malignant ascites in patients with advanced cancer: peritoneovenous shunt versus paracentesis. *Journal of Gastroenterology and Hepatology*, 22(12), 2161–2166.

Shariat-Madar, B., Jayakrishnan, T.T., Gamblin, T.C. & Turaga, K.K. (2014) Surgical management of bowel obstruction in patients with peritoneal carcinomatosis. *Journal of Surgical Oncology*, 110(6), 666–669.

Shedd, D.P. & Shedd, C. (1980) Problems of terminal head and neck cancer patients. *Head and Neck Surgery*, 2, 476–482.

Shumrick, D.A. (1983) Carotid artery rupture. *Laryngoscope*, 83(7), 1051–1061.

Sippell, R. (2011) EMS Recap: Intracranial Pressure and the Cushing Reflex. *EMSWorld. Available at*: https://www.emsworld.com/article/10453662/ems-recap-intracranial-pressure-and-cushing-reflex (Accessed: 27/4/2018)

Slusser, K. (2014) Malignant ascites. In: Yarbro, C., Wucjik, D. & Gobel, B.H. (eds) *Cancer Symptom Management*, 3rd edn. Sudbury, MA: Jones and Bartlet Publishers, pp. 241–262.

Smith, J., National Back Exchange & BackCare (2011) *The Guide to the Handling of People: A Systems Approach*, 6th edn. Teddington, Middlesex: BackCare.

Spinal Injuries Association (SIA) (2000) *Managing Spinal Injury: Critical Care.* www.spinal.co.uk/

Stein, A., Voigt, W. & Jordan, K. (2010) Chemotherapy-induced diarrhoea: pathophysiology, frequency and guideline-based management. *Therapeutic Advances in Medical Oncology*, 2, 51–63.

Stephenson, J. & Gilbert, J. (2002) The development of clinical guidelines on paracentesis for ascites related to malignancy. *Palliative Medicine*, 16, 213–218.

Strimel, W.J. (2016) Pericardial Effusion Workup. Available at: http://emedicine.medscape.com/article/157325-workup (Accessed: 6/4/2018)

Surviving Sepsis (2015) Sepsis Bundles. Available at: http://www.survivingsepsis.org/bundles/Pages/default.aspx (Accessed: 6/4/2018)

Svoboda, M. (2010) Malignant pericardial effusion and cardiac tamponade (cardiac and pericardial symptoms). In: Olver I.N. (ed.) *The MASCC Textbook of Cancer Supportive Care and Survivorship.* New York: Springer, pp. 83–91.

Thibodeau, G. & Patton, K. (2010) Anatomy of the digestive system. In: Thibodeau, G. & Patton, K. (eds) *Anatomy and Physiology*, 7th edn. St Louis, MO: Mosby, pp. 837–876.

Timp, J.F., Braekkan, S.K., Versteeg, H.H. & Cannegieter, S.C. (2013) Epidemiology of cancer-associated venous thrombosis. *Blood*, 122(10), 1712–1723.

Tiplady, B., Jackson, S.H., Maskrey, V.M., et al. (1998) Validity and sensitivity of visual analogue scales in young and older healthy subjects. *Age and Ageing*, 27(1), 63–66.

Tong, H., Isenring, E. & Yates, P. (2009) The prevalence of nutrition impact symptoms and their relationship to quality of life and clinical outcome in medical oncology patients. *Supportive Care in Cancer*, 17(1), 83–90.

Tortora, G.J. & Derrickson, B.H. (2014) *Principles of Anatomy and Physiology*, 14th edn. Hoboken: John Wiley & Sons.

Tradounsky, G. (2012) Palliation of gastrointestinal obstruction. *Canadian Family Physician*, 58(6), 648–652.

Troughton, R.W., Asher, C.R. & Klein, A.L. (2010) Pericarditis. *Lancet*, 363(9410), 717–727.

Tuca, A., Guell, E., Martinez-Lasada, E. & Codornui, N. (2012) Malignant bowel obstruction in advanced cancer patients: epidemiology, management and factors influencing spontaneous resolution. *Cancer Management and Research*, 4, 159–169.

Tveit, K.M., Guren, T., Glimelius B., et al. (2012) Phase III trial of cetuximab with continuous or intermittent fluorouracil, leucovorin, and oxaliplatin (Nordic FLOX) versus FLOX alone in first-line treatment of metastatic colorectal cancer: the NORDIC VII study. *Journal of Clinical Oncology*, 30, 1755–1762.

Twycross, R. & Black, I. (1998) Nausea and vomiting in advanced cancer. *European Journal of Palliative Care*, 5, 39–45.

Twycross, R., Wilcock, A., & Howard, P. (2014) *Palliative Care Formulary*, 5th edn. Abingdon: Radcliffe Medical Press.

Twycross, R.G., Wilcock, A. & Toller (2009) *Symptom Management in Advanced Cancer*, 4th edn. Palliativedrugs.com.

UK Oncology Nursing Society (UKONS) (2016) Oncology/Haematology 24 hour triage rapid assessment and access tool kit. Available at: http://www.ukons.org/ (Accessed: 27/4/2018)

UK Oncology Nursing Society (UKONS) (2018) The Acute Oncology Initial Management Guidelines. V.2.0. Marlow, Bucks: UKONS. Available at: https://az659834.vo.msecnd.net/eventsairwesteuprod/production-succinct-public/a4b550031a3c45d28b69cb7eea55c24f (Accessed: 26/4/2018)

Upile, T., Triaridia, S., Kirkland, P., et al. (2005) The management of carotid artery rupture. *European Archives of Otorhinolaryngology*, 262, 555–560.

US Department of Health and Human Services (2010) Common terminology criteria for adverse events (CTCAE) version 4.0. Available at: https://www.eortc.be/services/doc/ctc/CTCAE_4.03_2010-06-14_QuickReference_5x7.pdf (Accessed: 27/4/2018)

Vander, E., Nichols, J. & Stover, D.E. (2004) Chemotherapy-induced lung disease. *Clinical Pulmonary Medicine*, 11(2), 84–91.

Vaughan, J. (2013) Developing a nurse-led paracentesis service in an ambulatory care unit. *Nursing Standard*, 28(4), 44–50.

Viele, C.S. (2003). Overview of chemotherapy-induced diarrhoea. *Seminars in Oncology Nursing*, 19(4 Suppl 3), 2–5.

Viscoli, C. (1998) The evolution of the empirical management of fever and neutropenia in cancer patients. *Journal of Antimicrobial Chemotherapy*, 41(suppl D), S65–S80.

309

Walji, N., Chan, A.K. & Peake, D.R. (2008) Common acute oncological emergencies: diagnosis, investigation and management. *Postgraduate Medical Journal*, 84(994), 418–427.

Walker, J. (2015) Diagnosis and management of patients with hypercalcaemia. *Nursing Older People*, 27(4), 22–26.

Warr, D.G. (2008) Chemotherapy- and cancer-related nausea and vomiting. *Current Oncology*, 15(suppl 1), S4–S9.

Watson, M., Barrett, A., Spence, R. & Twelves, C. (2006) *Oncology*, 2nd edn. Oxford: Oxford University Press.

Whiteman, K. & McCormick, C. (2005) When your patient is in liver failure. *Nursing*, 35, 58–63.

Wilkes, G.M. (2011) Chemotherapy: principles of administration. In: Yarbro, C.H., Wujcik, D. & Gobel, B.H. (eds) *Cancer Nursing: Principles and Practice*, 7th edn. Sudbury, MA: Jones & Bartlett, pp. 390–457.

Williams, J.P., Johnston, C.J. & Finkelstein, J.N. (2010) Treatment for radiation-induced pulmonary late effects: spoiled for choice or looking in the wrong direction? *Current Drug Targets*, 11(11), 1386–1394.

Wilson, L.D., Detterbeck, F.C. & Yahalom, J. (2007) Superior vena cava syndrome with malignant causes. *New England Journal of Medicine*, 356, 1862–1869.

Witte, M.H. & Witte, C.L. (1983) Ascites in hepatic cirrhosis: a view from lymphology. In: Foldi, M. & Casley-Smith, J.R. (eds) *Lymphangiology*. Stuttgart: Schattauer Verlag, p. 629–644.

Woodrow, P. (2006) *Intensive Care Nursing: A Framework for Practice*, 2nd edn. Abingdon: Routledge.

World Health Organization (WHO) (2013) Diarrhoeal disease. Available at: http://www.who.int/mediacentre/factsheets/fs330/en/ (Accessed: 6/4/2018)

Yang, J.C., Hirsh, V., Schuler, M., et al. (2013) Symptom control and quality of life in LUX-Lung 3: a phase III study of afatinib or cisplatin/pemetrexed in patients with advanced lung adenocarcinoma with EGFR mutations. *Journal of Clinical Oncology*, 31, 3342–3350.

Young, A., Begum, G., Billingham, L., et al. (2005) WARP-A multicentre prospective randomised controlled trial (RCT) of thrombosis prophylaxis with warfarin in cancer patients with central venous catheters (CVCs). *Journal of Clinical Oncology*, 23(16 suppl), LBA8004.

Zhang, X., Roan, Y.G. & Wang, K.J. (2016) Risk of mTOR inhibitors induced severe pneumonitis in cancer patients: a meta-analysis of randomised controlled trials. *Future Oncology*, 12(12), 1529–1539.

Chapter 8

Living with and beyond cancer

Procedure guidelines

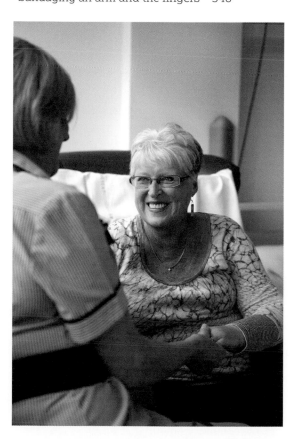

The Royal Marsden Manual of Cancer Nursing Procedures. Edited by Sara Lister and Lisa Dougherty, with Assistant Editor Louise McNamara.
© 2019 The Royal Marsden NHS Foundation Trust. Published 2019 by John Wiley & Sons, Ltd.

Overview

This chapter focuses on the support that may be needed by those living with and beyond cancer. This reflects the understanding that the consequences of treatment can be multidimensional and varied in intensity and individual impact. These effects commonly embrace a wide range of physical consequences interlinked to significant psychological and social consequences (Brem & Kumar 2011). In acknowledging this multidimensional experience, the chapter focuses on the practical processes and procedures related to such problems, including communication for those with laryngectomies and issues associated with day-to-day living including welfare advice. It also includes procedures that address physical issues so nutritional support, living with lymphoedema, managing breathlessness, coping with physical activity and fatigue are addressed. It also includes procedures related to emotional problems including assessment of sexual and body image concerns and nipple tattooing.

SECTION 8.1 INTRODUCTION

This opening section focuses on the needs and care of those living with and beyond a cancer diagnosis. It introduces the recovery package, outlining its structure, content and value. This is followed by a consideration of holistic needs assessment (HNA) and how it can establish the concerns of those affected by cancer.

The experience of living with or beyond cancer

A diagnosis of cancer and the experience of active treatment can give rise to a range of issues and challenges that can affect every aspect of people's lives (Corner and Wagland 2012). This includes continuing physical, emotional, psychological and spiritual distress which, in turn, negatively impacts on quality of life (Grunfeld et al. 2011). Cancer can also disrupt relationships and family life, working and financial stability (Arora et al. 2007, Kim and Given 2008, Kim et al. 2006, Macmillan Cancer Support 2013a, Pitcealthy and Maguire, 2003). For many people, the consequences of the disease and its treatment may be permanent (Macmillan Cancer Support 2013a).

Whilst many people are *surviving* following treatment for cancer, this is quite distinct from the experience of *survivorship* or living with and beyond cancer. For many, this is a life-changing experience that begins on diagnosis but evolves over time. Survivorship will have both positive and negative aspects, simultaneously being unique to each individual but with universal characteristics. Most significantly, though, it will involve constant uncertainty, particularly after the completion of hospital-based treatment (Doyle 2008).

In the UK there are about two million people living with or beyond a cancer diagnosis, including 1.8 million people currently living with cancer and at least one other long-term condition such as heart disease or chronic kidney disease (Macmillan Cancer Support 2016). This number is expected to increase by approximately one million per decade until 2040 (Maddams et al. 2012). It has been established that people who are living with and beyond cancer, cancer survivors, have significant unmet needs and often experience worse health than those who have never had the disease (Armes et al. 2009, Elliot et al. 2011).

The National Cancer Survivorship Initiative

In order to help and support the increasing number of people living with and beyond cancer and to offer them better care, the National Cancer Survivorship Initiative (NCSI) was set up in 2007 and has been complemented and updated by the recommendations of the Independent Cancer Taskforce (2015). The original NCSI report aimed to develop an understanding of the services required and to identify best practice (DH 2007). Its vision placed the focus on recovery, health and well-being; the provision of individual and personalised holistic assessment; care based on a model of self-management; follow-up and support tailored to

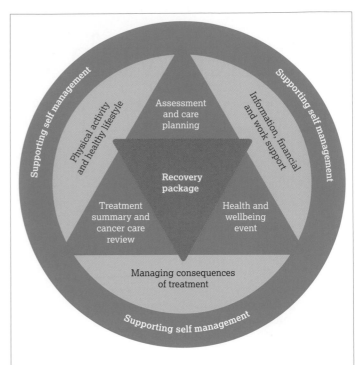

Figure 8.1 The recovery package. *Source:* Macmillan Cancer Support (2013b). © Macmillan Cancer Support 2013.

individual need; and patient-reported outcome measures (DH 2010). This vision of a fundamental shift in care and support for those living with and beyond cancer resulted in the development of the recovery package (NCSI 2013).

The recovery package

The recovery package is designed to address the needs of people living with and beyond cancer at the right time and place and with the support of the right person and incorporates four distinct components (Figure 8.1):

1 holistic needs assessment and care planning
2 treatment summary
3 health and well-being event
4 cancer care review.

These components form the basis of a personalized plan of care for each individual affected by cancer and are designed to encourage the adoption of healthier lifestyles whilst facilitating supported self-management. The recovery package should be a result of the effective partnership of the clinical team and the person living with cancer, having jointly decided on the most appropriate form of stratified care for the individual.

Stratified follow-up and supported self-management

Stratified care means that the clinical team and the person affected by cancer jointly decide on the most effective form of aftercare (see Figure 8.2). The three forms of aftercare are:

1 Supported self-management: this involves the provision of information on self-management support programmes, signs and symptoms to look out for, details of scheduled tests and who to contact if help, information or advice is needed.
2 Shared care: the person affected by cancer continues to have regular contact with healthcare professionals. This may be face to face or by telephone or email.
3 Complex care management: intensive support is given to the person with cancer in order that they might manage their cancer and other conditions.

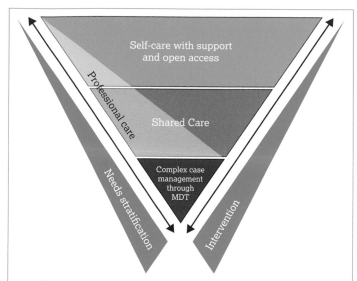

1. Affording people dignity, respect and compassion
2. Offering coordinated care, support or treatment
3. Offering personalized care, support or treatment
4. Being enabling

Figure 8.2 Stratified pathways of care. MDT, multidisciplinary team. *Source:* NHS Improvement (2011). © NHS Improvement 2011. This information is licensed under the Open Government Licence v3.0. To view this licence, visit http://www.nationalarchives.gov.uk/doc/open-government-licence/

Person-centred care

The success of initiatives such as the recovery package ultimately depends upon the adoption of person-centred practices. This means that the needs and goals of people with cancer become central to the process of care with an emphasis being placed on what matters to them rather than what is the matter with them (Health Foundation 2014). This requires healthcare professionals to work with each person's definition of their situation and acknowledge that the practice of person-centred care is predicated on supporting people to participate in decision-making and to self-manage their condition wherever possible. This requires that the person with cancer should be regarded as a partner rather than a passive recipient of care. In addition, healthcare professionals need to comprehend the psychosocial challenges faced by people living with and beyond cancer and what motivates them. The complexity of this is captured by Collins (2014) when he stresses the importance of an interplay of philosophy, principles and activities. He lists the principles of person-centred care as (Collins 2014):

1 affording people dignity, respect and compassion
2 offering co-ordinated care, support or treatment
3 offering personalized care, support or treatment
4 being enabling.

The needs of those affected by cancer

Armes et al. (2009) noted that people can have five or more moderate or severe unmet needs following treatment for cancer and that these needs can remain unchanged for 6 months. It is known that those with unmet needs are 20% more likely to visit their GP and can be expected to attend A&E departments twice as often as their healthy counterparts.

The evidence suggests that healthcare professionals frequently fail to appreciate the extent of the impact and effects of cancer and its treatment (Brennan et al. 2012, Fallowfield et al. 2001, Sanson-Fisher et al. 2000, Soellner et al. 2001, Werner et al. 2012). Consequently, concerns are often unrecognized

or inadequately addressed with the result that people living with and beyond cancer may fail to get the support that they need from the multiprofessional team. This ultimately results in poorer overall health and dissatisfaction with care (Demark-Wahnefried et al. 2005, McDowell et al. 2010).

The needs of those living with and beyond cancer are everybody's business (Brennan 2012) and in this spirit the NCSI (2013) recommends that effective cancer care should commence at the point of diagnosis and should focus on:

- information and support from diagnosis
- promoting recovery
- sustaining recovery
- managing consequences
- supporting people with active and advanced disease.

This theme has been included in *Achieving World-Class Cancer Outcomes: A Strategy for England 2015–2020* in which the Independent Cancer Taskforce (2015) recommends that the recovery package and stratified follow-up pathways should be rolled out expediently.

Holistic needs assessment and care planning

Holistic needs assessment (HNA) is an integral part of the recovery package. It can be defined as 'a process of gathering information from the patient and/or carer in order to inform discussion and develop a deeper understanding of what the person understands and needs' (National Cancer Action Team [NCAT] 2007). It incorporates the physical, psychosocial, spiritual and emotional well-being of the person affected by cancer into the assessment process.

The HNA has been shown to be effective in identifying a person's individual concerns (Doyle and Henry 2014). Its value is that it:

- identifies people who need help
- provides opportunities for people to think through their needs
- helps people self-manage
- helps teams to target support.

When to undertake a holistic needs assessment?

There are a number of key points when a holistic assessment of needs should be conducted. These coincide with significant milestones in the pathway where the person's needs might reasonably be expected to change:

- around the time of diagnosis
- at commencement of treatment
- on completion of the primary treatment plan
- at the point of recognition of incurability
- at the beginning of the end of life
- at the point at which dying is diagnosed
- at any other time that the patient may request
- at any other time that a professional carer may judge necessary
- at each new episode of disease recurrence.

Because it might be difficult to establish a categorical link between high levels of distress and specific phases of the patient experience, assessments should also be undertaken at the request of the patient (NCAT 2007). Biddle et al. (2016) suggest that the appropriate frequency of administration of HNA is the key to its success and this should be determined by the dynamic nature of distress and the context of care delivery. However, it should be noted that it may not be appropriate to conduct a HNA when the individual:

- has severe mental illness
- lacks capacity
- elects not to participate.

Legal and professional considerations

The three primary considerations for healthcare professionals undertaking HNA are:

- Ensuring autonomy: this refers to respecting the person's right to make decisions about their own lives without interference from the healthcare professional.
- Ensuring confidentiality: this assumes that health information is given with the expectation that it will not be divulged except in ways that have been previously agreed upon.
- Recognizing a duty of care: this refers to the legal obligation to take reasonable care to avoid causing harm.

Procedural considerations

The HNA can take the form of a face-to-face meeting or a telephone conversation. It should be conducted in a quiet, private area in which disturbance or interruption can be avoided and confidentiality can be achieved. It should be noted that the benefits of HNA can only be fully realized by allocating adequate time to the process (Biddle et al. 2016). The healthcare professional should open the session by introducing him/herself to the person living with and beyond cancer and ascertain how they would like to be addressed. The healthcare professional should outline the purpose of the HNA and gain verbal consent to proceed.

The HNA and care plans are commonly recorded on proformas which are supplied in the clinical setting. However, there is increasing interest in the use of electronic devices (e.g. tablets) for conducting these assessments. The advantage is that the eHNA allows the individual affected by cancer to complete the HNA questionnaire on a touch screen tablet. This information can then be sent to the healthcare professional through a secure website to facilitate the process of care and support planning. The London HNA tool is available in print and electronic formats. The tool can be accessed at http://www.londoncanceralliance.nhs.uk/news,-events-publications/news/2013/11/london-wide-hna-now-available/

Conducting a holistic needs assessment

Skilled practitioners should undertake HNA. They ought to have a good understanding of biological, psychological and emotional development and have an appreciation of how cancer can impinge on the needs of the population whilst possessing an intimate knowledge of the practice of caring and working with individuals.

The HNA can take many forms and the London Cancer Alliance (LCA) has developed a version in collaboration with London Cancer. The pan-London tool includes a concerns checklist, a distress thermometer and a care plan. The concerns checklist allows the individual to specify which issues are of most concern to them.

In order to facilitate this process, the LCA has also developed a series of prompt tools (LCA 2016) for use during the HNA. These address a wide range of issues including fatigue, breathlessness, constipation, memory, worry and sexual consequences of treatment.

The top ten issues people with cancer of all types are concerned about (Macmillan Cancer Support 2015) are:

1. worry, fear or anxiety
2. tiredness/exhaustion or fatigue
3. sleep problems/nightmares
4. pain
5. eating or appetite
6. anger or frustration
7. getting around (walking)
8. memory or concentration
9. hot flushes/sweating
10. sore or dry mouth.

Some issues can be resolved following discussion and/or sharing of information. Simply allowing the person the opportunity and space to talk may, in itself, be sufficient to ameliorate any concerns. However, other issues may involve prompting or encouraging the individual to take a specific action themselves to address their concern or lead to intervention by a healthcare professional. Finally, there are issues for which the appropriate response must always be to make onward referral to specialist services. Following the discussion, a care plan is agreed that documents the agreed actions and provides a record of the discussion (Doyle and Henry 2014).

It should be noted that there may be occasions when the specialist services that are deemed appropriate are not available. This should be acknowledged and support offered because discussing the issue can, in itself, be helpful.

Members of the Consequences of Cancer and its Treatment collaborative group (CCaT) have developed a series of tips encapsulating concise, pragmatic advice for people who have had cancer treatment (Macmillan Cancer Support 2012). The ten top tips are:

1. Discuss your needs with a healthcare professional at the end of treatment.
2. See a copy of your assessment and care plan.
3. Find out who is your ongoing 'key contact'.
4. Be aware of any post-treatment symptoms.
5. Get support with day-to-day concerns.
6. Talk about how you feel.
7. Take steps towards healthier living.
8. Find out more about what to look for if you are worried about treatment side-effects or the cancer coming back.
9. Monitor your own health and keep up to date with ongoing check-ups.
10. Make suggestions based on your experiences of treatment and care.

Making an assessment is an opportunity to establish a connection with the person and their family and to start to develop ideas around collaboration and engaging motivation to self-care. This requires the healthcare professional to shift slightly away from their traditional role of caring and treatment to one of nurturing and empowerment. This means involving and ideally enabling the patient to lead the conversation about their needs and the best solutions. A well-executed HNA assessment should stimulate

---

Procedure guideline 8.1 Conducting a holistic needs assessment (HNA)

Action	Rationale
1 Identify a quiet, private area in which to conduct the assessment.	To ensure that the environment is conducive to confidential and private discussion (Doyle and Henry 2014, **C**).
2 Introduce self to the individual living with and beyond cancer.	To establish professional and clinical rapport (Doyle and Henry 2014, **E**).
3 Outline the purpose of holistic needs assessment and gain consent to proceed.	To gain the consent and cooperation of the individual affected by cancer (Hughes et al. 2014, **C**).
4 Explain the holistic needs assessment screening tool, e.g. distress thermometer.	To ensure that the individual has an in-depth understanding of the processes being followed (Brennan et al. 2012, **E**).

5	Encourage the individual to indicate their level of distress using the distress thermometer.	To ascertain the degree of distress being experienced by the individual (Brennan et al. 2012, **E**).
6	Encourage the individual to indicate those factors which are causing/contributing to his/her experience of distress using the concerns checklist.	To ascertain the sources of distress being experienced by the individual (Brennan et al. 2012, **E**).
7	Explore highlighted issues if this is deemed appropriate.	To clarify the extent of distress being experienced by the individual (Doyle and Henry 2014, **E**).
8	Develop a care plan in collaboration.	To facilitate the development of an appropriate response in partnership to the extent and sources of distress (Doyle and Henry 2014, **E**).

Procedure guideline 8.1a Developing and actioning a care plan

Action	Rationale
1 Explain the rationale for a personalized care plan (this should include the importance of the individual's perspective).	To gain the consent, cooperation and feeling of ownership of the individual affected by cancer (Hughes et al. 2014, **E**).
2 Resolve issues that lend themselves to discussion and/or sharing of information (simply allowing the person the opportunity and space to talk may, in itself, be sufficient to ameliorate any concerns).	To empower the individual by helping him/her resolve issues unaided (Doyle and Henry 2014, **E**).
3 For specific issues, prompt or encourage the individual to take a specific action him/herself to address his/her concern or lead to intervention by a healthcare professional.	To empower the individual by guiding and supporting him/her to resolve issues by utilizing the resources that are available to him/her (supported self-management) (Doyle and Henry 2014, **E**).
4 For complex or specialist issues, make a referral to other members of the multiprofessional team.	To enable a specialist assessment of need (Hughes et al. 2014, **C**). To ensure the provision of specialist support and care (Hughes et al. 2014, **C**).
5 Record all discussions and agreed action points.	To ensure an accurate record of all discussion/decisions/actions. To clarify and confirm agreed actions (Doyle and Henry 2014, **C**).
6 Provide the individual with a copy of their action plan.	To empower the individual and encourage ownership of the care plan (Hughes et al. 2014, **C**).
7 Share the action plan with other healthcare professionals as appropriate.	To ensure continuity in provision of effective multidisciplinary support and care (Hughes et al. 2014, **C**).

Procedure guideline 8.1b Closure and follow-up

Action	Rationale
1 Meet the individual to review before discharging them.	To demonstrate progress to the individual (Doyle and Henry 2014, **C**). To provide ownership to the individual affected by cancer (Doyle and Henry 2014, **C**).
2 Review the individual's perception of the process.	To provide outcome measures for clinical practice and feedback to the individual on his/her progress (Doyle and Henry 2014, **C**).
3 Review of actions agreed.	To demonstrate progress to the individual and ensure onward referrals for further support are completed (Doyle and Henry 2014, **C**).

the patient to take action to help themselves with the support of healthcare professional and allied services.

SECTION 8.2 WELFARE ADVICE

Overview

Cancer not only affects patients physically, emotionally, socially and psychologically, but also makes a significant impact on their financial circumstances. When someone is initially diagnosed with cancer, their finances might not be at the forefront of their mind, however 70% of cancer patients suffer loss of income and/or increased expenses as a direct consequence of their cancer diagnosis (Macmillan Cancer Support 2012).

Someone with cancer makes on average 53 trips to the hospital, which alone costs around £325 during their treatment (Macmillan Cancer Support 2012). There is also considerable under-claiming of financial benefits by people who are eligible for them. People with cancer may experience barriers to obtaining welfare benefits at three levels (Macmillan Cancer Support 2012):

1 they may not be aware that they could be entitled
2 they may not know how to obtain benefits information and guidance
3 they might not understand how to apply.

Definitions

Benefit – a payment made by the state or an insurance scheme to someone who is entitled to receive it.

This section aims to define the different types of benefits, but is not exhaustive. There are three distinct groups of benefits:

1 contribution benefits
2 means tested benefits
3 non-means tested benefits.

Contribution benefits

Contribution benefits are available to workers who have paid enough National Insurance contributions. These include (Cancer Research UK 2016):

- *Employment and Support Allowance (ESA)* – for people who are ill or disabled, to give them financial support if they cannot work or help to work if they are able to.
- *Pension Credit (PC)* – income support for people over pension age.
- *Bereavement Benefits* – people may be able to get some financial help if someone close to them dies. To collect most of these bereavement benefits, they must either be married or a (same sex) civil partner of the person who has died. The benefits available are a one-off bereavement payment, a bereavement allowance paid for 52 weeks to a surviving spouse (or civil partner) aged between 45 and pension age, and a widowed parent allowance if the claimant is under pension age and gets child benefit for dependent children. Claimants may also get help with funeral costs if a partner, close relative, close friend or child dies. They have to be on a low income and get certain benefits or tax credits.
- *Statutory Sick Pay (SSP)* – a payment for employed people who become sick and who are unable to work. It is not means tested. To qualify, people must be employed and earn enough to pay National Insurance contributions. If people are still ill after 28 weeks, they could be eligible to claim Employment Support Allowance.

Means tested benefits

Means tested benefits are for a claimant who has no income and no or few savings to support themselves and requires the state to help them. These include (Cancer Research UK 2016):

- *Income Support (IS)* – people aged between 16 and pension age can claim IS if they are on a low income, working less than 16 hours a week and not signed on as unemployed. If they have a partner, the partner must work less than 24 hours a week.
- *Housing Benefit (HB)* – for people whose income is low, either because they are on other benefits or they do not earn very much.
- *Council Tax Reduction (CTR)* – replaced Council Tax Benefit from April 2013. People can claim if they are on a low income or on benefits.
- *Universal Credit (UC)* – was introduced in 2013 and is paid to people who are employed on a low income, as well as to those who are out of work. UC is intended to adapt to people's changing circumstances: those on low incomes should get ongoing support as they move in and out of work, rather than benefits stopping and starting and new claims having to be made. UC replaces the following: income-based Job Seeker's Allowance; income-related Employment and Support Allowance; Income Support; Child Tax Credits; Working Tax Credits and Housing Benefit.

Non-means tested benefits

Non-means tested benefits do not take into account the claimant's income and savings in the same way as means tested benefits do, but they do have their own rules which must be met. These include:

- *Disability Living Allowance (DLA)* – a benefit for children under 16 who have difficulties in walking or need more help than a child of a similar age because of a disability or health condition. There are two parts to this benefit: care and mobility. Individuals can claim either or both. The care component consists of lower, middle and higher rate and the mobility component has a higher and lower rate.
- *Personal Independence Payment (PIP)* – benefits for people aged 16–64 that help with some of the extra costs caused by long-term ill-health or a disability. Some of these needs can include personal care or help with getting around. PIP replaced DLA in 2013 for people aged 16–64. Since then, new claims are for PIP, not DLA. There are two parts to these benefits, *the daily living component* and *the mobility component*. Individuals can claim for either or both. If they qualify for the middle or higher rate, they may be entitled to a higher rate of Income Support, Employment Support Allowance, Housing Benefit, Tax Credits, Job Seeker's Allowance or Universal Credit because of their needs.
- *Attendance Allowance (AA)* – for people aged 65 or over who need help with personal care because of illness or disability. There is no mobility addition for this benefit. They must have needed help for at least 6 months unless they are terminally ill, in which case they can claim the higher rate of AA straight away.
- *Carer's Allowance (CA)* – a benefit for carers aged 16 and over who look after a relative or friend for at least 35 hours a week. To get CA, the claimant must be caring for someone who claims either PIP, DLA or AA.

Terminally ill patients, defined in benefit terms as 'patients with a progressive disease and as a result of that disease will have less than 6 months to live', can be awarded the highest rate of benefit for the care component of DLA, enhanced payment of the daily living component for PIP and the highest award of AA. The mobility element will still need to be assessed.

Doctors or specialist nurses will need to complete form DS1500 to accompany the benefit application; this will ensure that these benefit claims are fast tracked and are paid at the higher rate.

The types of benefits available may change dependent on government policy review. Further detailed information can be found at https://www.gov.uk/browse/benefits

Related theory

Government welfare policy

The degree of change arising from the government's welfare reform programme is likely to have an impact on people living with cancer in the UK (Macmillan Cancer Support 2012). The welfare system can be confusing and nurses should keep abreast of any changes to help patients navigate the system.

Immigration control. Some patients who are treated for cancer within the UK may not qualify for benefits as they are not considered to be UK nationals. This may be because they:

- may need permission to enter or remain in the UK but do not yet have it (e.g. they are an asylum seeker waiting for a decision on their application)
- may have permission to enter or remain in the UK on the condition that they do not have 'recourse to public funds' (e.g. foreign workers, students and family members of UK nationals).

This will usually be written in their passports and it means they are unable to claim certain benefits such as PIP (see Figure 8.3).

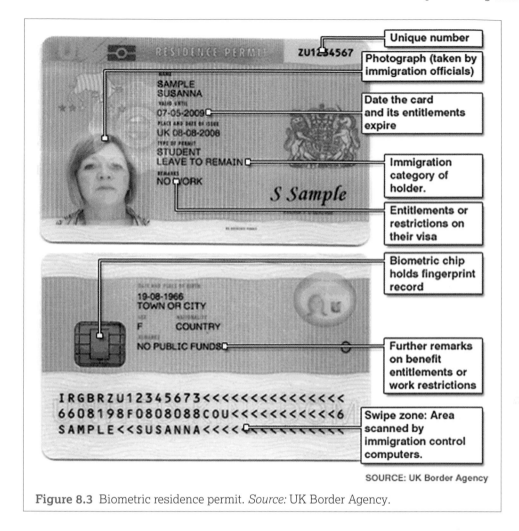

Figure 8.3 Biometric residence permit. *Source:* UK Border Agency.

Evidence-based approaches

Rationale

More than four in ten people who are working when diagnosed with cancer must make changes to their working lives, with almost half changing jobs or leaving work altogether. However, patients do not seem to be getting enough information and advice from healthcare professionals on working during, or returning to work after, cancer treatment (Macmillan Cancer Support 2012).

There are many benefits that could help patients after they have been given a cancer diagnosis, but the system can be confusing. The benefits patients may be entitled to depend on factors such as age, income and where they live (Macmillan Cancer Support 2018a). Research shows that the amount that patients with cancer in the UK are not claiming amounts to around £90 million per year (see Table 8.1).

It is important for cancer nurses to know what benefits are available so they can highlight this to their patients. If patients are unsure of what they are entitled to, nurses should refer them to a benefits adviser.

Although treatment on the NHS is free at the point of delivery, there may still be some costs (e.g. a patient's journey to hospital). However, much of the cost can be reclaimed, which should ease some of the burden (NHS Choices 2016). There are many benefits, grants and help with health costs to which patients with cancer may be entitled. Some of these are outlined in Box 8.1 (Macmillan Cancer Support 2018b). Free prescriptions, wigs and fabric supports are discussed in further detail later in this section.

Free prescriptions

Prescription charges for cancer patients were abolished on April 1 2009 (NHS Choices 2016). Exemption certificates are now issued to those patients who, in their doctor's judgement, are receiving treatment for:

- cancer
- the effects of cancer
- the effects of current or previous cancer treatment.

Table 8.1 Percentage of patients dying from cancer not claiming Disability Living Allowance or Attendance Allowance in the UK and what this means in monetary amounts

Country	Percentage	Amount not claimed by patients
England	39%	Worth ±£81 million
Scotland	32%	Worth ±£8 million
Wales	9%	Worth ±£1.2 million
Northern Ireland	7%	Worth ±£450,000

Box 8.1 Financial support and other benefits

1 Help with children's costs
- Financial assistance is available to help with the care and education of children and young people

2 Help with bills and housing costs
- Council tax reduction schemes are available to help people who are struggling to pay their council tax
- Help to pay mortgage interest payments may be available
- Patients on a low income or already on benefits may be able to get help to pay for their accommodation
- There is help for patients with cancer who are struggling with their energy costs

3 Help with health costs
- Patients may be eligible for free prescriptions if they have cancer. There are also other ways to help with the cost of medications
- Some patients may be able to get free eye tests if they meet certain criteria
- Patients may be able to get free wigs and fabric supports
- The Low-Income Scheme may help patients who still have to pay healthcare costs but may be on a low income
- Patients may qualify for free dental treatment

4 Help with transport and parking
- Patients may be able to get financial help for mobility equipment or nursing home charges
- Patients may be able to get help with their travel costs to and from hospital for treatment
- Patients may qualify for schemes that help them to buy or rent a car, scooter or powered wheelchair
- Patients may be eligible for special travel rates or community transport services in their area
- Older people and people with disabilities can often get free or discounted travel fares
- The Blue Badge Scheme can help with parking costs if patients have severe mobility problems

5 Financial information for people whose cancer cannot be cured
- There may be benefits that the patient can claim towards the end of life
- Some charities and organizations offer grants to people with cancer to help with financial problems
- Patient can get help to sort out their bank accounts and pensions towards the end of life

Source: This information is based on content originally produced by Macmillan Cancer Support and is adapted with its permission. Details are correct at the time of publication.

To apply for a medical exemption certificate (MedEx), patients must ask their doctor for an FP92A form. Their GP, hospital or doctor will sign the form to confirm that the information provided is correct.

- The certificate is valid from 1 month before the date that the NHS Business Authority receives the application form.
- The MedEx lasts for 5 years and then needs to be renewed, which is the patient's responsibility.
- Further information about the application process and refunds can be found on the NHS Business Authority's website (www.nhsbsa.nhs.uk/).

Wigs and fabric supports

Wigs and fabric supports are free of charge on the NHS (Cancer Research UK 2014) if patients:

- are treated as an inpatient
- are under 16 years old, or between 16 and 19 years old and in full-time education
- have a partner who is getting Universal Credit, Income Support, income-based Jobseeker's Allowance or the guarantee credit of Pension Credit
- have an NHS tax credit exemption certificate
- are named on a valid 'help with health costs' (HC2) certificate.

There are no nationally set limits on the number of wigs a patient can have from the NHS. However, there is nothing preventing local NHS organizations from setting their own limit (NHS Choices 2016).

If patients are on a low income but do not qualify for a free wig, they may still be able to get some assistance. This is explained in the Department of Health leaflet called 'Help with health

costs' (HC11; https://www.nhsbsa.nhs.uk/sites/default/files/2017-12/HC11%20%28V7%29%20online%2011.2017.pdf). The leaflet is available from the hospital or at post offices. If the patient is entitled to help, they will receive either a full help certificate (certificate HC2 means they do not need to pay for their wig) or a limited help certificate (certificate HC3 means they may get some help with the cost).

If the patient is being treated as an outpatient and does not otherwise qualify for a free wig, they must pay for one (NHS Choices 2016).

If the patient decides to buy a wig privately, it is worth noting that they do not have to pay Value Added Tax (VAT) on a wig that is bought for hair loss caused by cancer treatment. However, they must fill in a VAT form at the time they buy their wig. The supplier should provide this form because they cannot claim the VAT back later (Cancer Research UK 2014).

In addition to wigs, cancer patients are also entitled to VAT-free products and services if they are designed and/or adapted for a disability. These include certain types of adjustable beds, alarms, wheelchairs and stair lifts. An exhaustive list can be found on the gov.uk website (https://www.gov.uk/financial-help-disabled/vat-relief).

Scope

It is not within the scope of this chapter to explore all benefits available within the welfare system. The following focuses on the benefits that are most relevant to patients with cancer:

1 Personal Independence Payment
2 Attendance Allowance
3 Carer's Allowance
4 Employment and Support Allowance
5 Universal Credit.

Eligibility/non-eligibility

Most patients with cancer will need help and support from people who know about the different benefits. They may need to fill in several forms and make phone calls. It can be time consuming and very stressful at what is already a difficult time (Cancer Research UK 2016). Cancer nurses should explore with patients what their social and occupational needs are as part of the holistic needs assessment (National Cancer Action Team 2007) and from this they will get an indication of what support is needed. See Section 8.1 for more information about the HNA for patients with cancer.

Table 8.2 sets out what the eligibility criteria are for Personal Independence Payment, Attendance Allowance, Carer's Allowance and Employment and Support Allowance (Department for Work and Pensions [DWP] 2018).

Table 8.2 Eligibility/non-eligibility for Personal Independence Payment (PIP), Attendance Allowance (AA), Carer's Allowance (CA), Employment and Support Allowance (DWP 2018a, b, c, d, e)

Benefit	Eligible	Not eligible
Personal Independence Payment (PIP)	• Aged 16–64 (DLA remains for children up to age 16 and DLA recipients aged 65 or over on 8 April 2013 [the day that PIP was introduced]) • Have a long-term health condition or disability and difficulties with 'daily living' or getting around (see Table 8.4) • Be in Great Britain when making a claim. There are some exceptions, for example members and family members of the Armed Forces • Have been in Great Britain for at least 2 of the last 3 years • Be habitually resident in the UK, Ireland, Isle of Man or the Channel Islands	• Those subject to immigration control (unless a sponsored immigrant) • Those who do not satisfy the residence conditions
Attendance Allowance (AA)	• Aged 65 or over • Have a physical disability • The disability is severe enough for the claimant to need help caring for themselves or someone is needed to supervise them, for their own or someone else's safety • Be in Great Britain when making a claim. There are some exceptions, e.g. members and family members of the Armed Forces • Have been in Great Britain for at least 2 of the last 3 years • Be habitually resident in the UK, Ireland, Isle of Man or the Channel Islands • There are some exceptions to these conditions if the patient is living in another European Economic Area (EEA) country or Switzerland	• Those subject to immigration control • Those who do not satisfy the residence conditions • Those in hospital/residential care
Carer's Allowance (CA)	**The person cared for** must already get one of these benefits: • Personal Independence Payment – daily living component • Disability Living Allowance – the middle or highest care rate • Attendance Allowance • Constant Attendance Allowance at or above the normal maximum rate with an Industrial Injuries Disablement Benefit • Constant Attendance Allowance at the basic (full day) rate with a War Disablement Pension • Armed Forces Independence Payment **The claimant** might be able to get CA if all the following apply: • Aged 16 or over • Spend at least 35 hours a week caring for someone • Have been in England, Scotland or Wales for at least 2 of the last 3 years • Normally live in England, Scotland or Wales, or live abroad as a member of the Armed Forces • Not in full-time education • Not studying for 21 hours a week or more • Earn no more than £116 a week (after taxes, care costs while claimant is work and 50% of what claimant pays into pension) – pension is not counted as income • Might still be eligible if moving to or already living in another EEA country	• Those over pensionable age • Those subject to immigration control • Those who do not satisfy the residence conditions

Employment and Support Allowance (ESA)	• Be under State Pension age
	• Not getting Statutory Sick Pay or Statutory Maternity Pay and have not gone back to work
	• Not getting Jobseeker's Allowance
	• Claimant may apply if employed, self-employed, unemployed or a student on Disability Living Allowance or Personal Independence Payment
	• Claimant may get ESA if they have lived or worked abroad and paid enough UK National Insurance (or the equivalent in an EEA or other country with which the UK has an agreement)
		• Those found capable of doing some work after their 'Work Capability Assessment'. The main exceptions are:
		  – where their current condition has become a lot worse
		  – where they are claiming for a new condition
		  – those receiving Universal Credit

(continued)

Table 8.2 Eligibility/non-eligibility for Personal Independence Payment (PIP), Attendance Allowance (AA), Carer's Allowance (CA), Employment and Support Allowance (DWP 2018a, b, c, d, e) *(continued)*

Benefit	Eligible	Not eligible

Universal Credit	• Can currently claim Universal Credit if either:
	  – a single person anywhere in England, Wales and Scotland
	  – a couple or family living in certain areas
	• To get Universal Credit, claimant must:
	  – be 18 or over
	  – be under State Pension age
	  – not be in full-time education or training
	  – not have savings over £16,000
	• Less Universal Credit if claimant has savings over £6000 or earns enough money to cover basic living costs. If living with partner will need to make a joint claim as a couple. Partner's income and savings will be taken into account, even if they are not eligible for Universal Credit
	• If claimant wants to claim a benefit without their savings, partner's savings or their income being taken into account, can apply for either:
	  – 'new style' Jobseeker's Allowance (JSA)
	  – 'new style' Employment and Support Allowance (ESA)
	• Claimant can apply for these if entitled to apply for Universal Credit
	• If claimant has children he/she can make a new Universal Credit claim either:
	  – if claimant has two children or fewer and lives in a Universal Credit area
	  – received Universal Credit in the previous 6 months and payments have stopped
	    – it does not matter how many children there are.
	  – If claimant has three or more children and has not claimed Universal Credit before, he/she can apply for Child Tax Credit
	  – If claimant has a disability or illness that affects his/her work
	  – Claimant may need to have a work capability assessment to see how disability or health condition affects his/her ability to work. If an assessment is needed, claimant will get a letter telling them where to go and what to do
	  – Depending on the outcome of assessment, claimant could be eligible for an extra payment on top of standard allowance
		• Unable to claim Universal Credit if in receipt of the following benefits:
		  – Income Support
		  – income-based Jobseeker's Allowance
		  – income-related Employment and Support Allowance
		  – income-related Incapacity Benefit
		Subject to immigration control

DLA, Disability Living Allowance.

Principles of care

Cancer nurses should ensure that they (Macmillan Cancer Support 2012):

- Refer patients to wider information about work and financial support.
- Encourage patients to share their domestic, social, work and financial situation as part of a needs assessment and in drawing up their written care plan. This needs regular review, particularly at key points in the pathway. This enables clinicians to talk to patients about work and refer them to further support whether they are employed, unemployed or self-employed.
- Refer patients to hospital benefits services as well as benefits services offered by cancer charities. Some reasons for referring patients for additional support include:
  - the patient needs financial support
  - housing/homeless issues
  - advice about appealing a DWP decision
  - the patient needs advice about applying for higher rate benefits
  - the patient's benefit has been stopped
  - reassessment from DLA benefit to PIP
  - applications to charities.

Method of claiming and receiving benefits

It is important the claimant visits the DWP website to access up-to-date information about how to submit claims as these do differ depending on the benefit:

- Personal Independence Payment – the preferred method is by telephone.
- Attendance Allowance – the preferred method is by post.
- Carer's Allowance – can be made through an online application.
- Employment and Support Allowance – the quickest method is by telephone.
- Universal Credit – can be made through an online application.

How payment is made

Benefits are usually paid straight into the patient's bank, building society or credit union account (DWP 2018a, b, c, d, e). See Table 8.3 for how often they are usually paid.

Patients who qualify for Attendance Allowance, Disability Living Allowance and Personal Independence Payment under the special rules (terminally ill) are usually paid weekly.

Anticipated patient outcomes

Patients with cancer will be fully aware of what benefits they and, where applicable, their carers may qualify for. Appropriate

Table 8.3 How often benefits are paid (DWP 2018 a, b, c, d, e)

Benefit	How often it is paid
Personal Independence Payment	Usually every 4 weeks
Attendance Allowance	Usually every 4 weeks
Carer's Allowance	Weekly in advance, or every 4 or 13 weeks
Employment and Support Allowance	Usually every 2 weeks
Universal Credit	Usually every month

referrals will be made to welfare support officers when patients require additional help in navigating the system and making claims. Patients will claim for the benefits they qualify for.

Legal and professional issues

Equality Act 2010
People with cancer are included in the remit for the Equality Act (2010) (Government Equalities Office 2015) and have legal protection from the point of first diagnosis of their cancer. The Equality Act defines a 'disabled person' as an individual with a 'physical (including sensory) impairment or mental impairment which has a substantial and long-term adverse effect on his/her ability to carry out normal day-to-day activities'. 'Long-term' means that the effect of the impairment has lasted or is likely to last for at least 12 months, and cancer is covered from the point of diagnosis (NHS Scotland 2015).

Flexible working
Depending on circumstances, sometimes an employee will need to take care of a family member who becomes ill. Under the Work and Families Act (The National Archives 2006), carers now have the right to request flexible working.

Pre-procedural considerations

Assessment and recording tools

Benefit calculators
Benefit calculators have replaced DWP Benefits Advisers. They are free to use, anonymous and help claimants find out what benefits they could get, how to claim and how their benefits will be affected if they start work. Different calculators are available dependent on what benefit is being considered and can be accessed through the DWP website. The website also sets out what information the claimant needs to have to hand before utilizing them and who should not use them, including those under 18 years of age or living abroad. The benefit calculators are described in Boxes 8.2 and 8.3.

Personal Independence Payment assessment criteria tool
There are ten daily living activities and two mobility activities. Each activity has descriptors that represent varying levels of ability needed to carry it out. For a descriptor to apply, the claimant must be able to carry out the activity safely, to an acceptable

Box 8.2 Use *entitledto* (https://www.entitledto.co.uk/) for information on:

- Income-related benefits
- Tax credits
- Contribution-based benefits
- Council Tax reduction
- Carer's Allowance
- Universal Credit
- How your benefits will be affected if you start work

Box 8.3 Use *turn2us* (https://www.turn2us.org.uk/) for information on:

- Income-related benefits
- Tax credits
- Council tax reduction
- Carer's Allowance
- Universal Credit
- How your benefits will be affected if you start work or change your working hours

Table 8.4 Personal Independence Payment assessment criteria tool

Activity	Possible points
Daily living component (activities 1–10)	
Standard rate=8 points Enhanced rate=12 points	
1 Preparing food	0–8
2 Taking nutrition	0–10
3 Managing therapy or monitoring a health condition	0–8
4 Washing and bathing	0–8
5 Managing toilet needs or incontinence	0–8
6 Dressing and undressing	0–8
7 Communicating verbally	0–12
8 Reading and understanding signs symbols and words	0–8
9 Engaging with other people face-to-face	0–8
10 Making budgeting decisions	0–6
Mobility component (activities 11–12)	
Standard rate=8 points Enhanced rate=12 points	
11 Planning and following journeys	0–12
12 Moving around	0–12

standard, repeatedly and in a reasonable time period. The ability to carry out an activity will be considered over a period of time to take account of the effects of a fluctuating health condition or disability. The assessment takes into account where claimants need the support of another person or persons to carry out an activity and where individuals need aids to complete activities. Individuals will receive a point score for each activity which determines whether a component is payable and at what rate. For each component, individuals will get the standard rate if they score a total of 8–11 points, or the enhanced rate if their scores add up to 12 points or more (DWP 2018d).

Table 8.4 shows the PIP assessment criteria tool.

Specific patient preparation
It is important that patients have their relevant personal information to hand before contacting the DWP to ensure the submission of claims is not delayed. Information required may vary dependent on the respective benefit; however, examples include the following:

- contact details and date of birth
- National Insurance number
- bank or building society details
- doctor's or health worker's name
- details of any time spent abroad, or in a care home or hospital.

There is additional support available to patients who may need it.

- Patients who have a hearing difficulty can access the British Sign Language (BSL) Video Relay Service trial.
- The PIP claims number can be called to ask the DWP to use an alternative format when they contact the claimant, such as braille, large print or audio CD.

- The telephone call can be made by someone supporting the claimant.
- Patients who do not speak English as their first language can access provision made for this.

- It is possible to request a paper claim form for someone who is unable to deal with DWP by telephone and has no one to support them with the claim.

Procedure guideline 8.2 How a patient should make a claim for Personal Independence Payment (DWP 2018d)

Essential equipment and information
- A computer with internet access
- A telephone
- Personal information such as contact details, date of birth, National Insurance number, bank or building society details, doctor's or health worker's name, details of any time spent abroad, or in a care home or hospital

Pre-procedure

Action	Rationale
1 Visit gov.uk/pip	For more information about how to claim. **E**
2 Determine if it is necessary to use the British Sign Language (BSL) Video Relay Service trial. To use this service, the claimant must: (a) first check they can use the service (b) go to the Video Relay Service.	To assist claimants with hearing difficulties. **C**
3 Gather the required information to hand as set out at gov.uk/pip before telephoning DWP.	To ensure the claim is submitted efficiently and there are no unnecessary delays in receiving the benefit. **E**
4 Decide if it is necessary for the telephone call to be made by someone supporting the claimant. Note: the claimant must be present.	To ensure patients who require additional support are not disadvantaged. **E**
5 Decide if it is necessary to access the provisions for people who do not speak English as their first language.	To ensure patients who require additional support are not disadvantaged. **E**
6 Decide if it is necessary to request a paper claim form. This can be requested for someone who is unable to deal with DWP by telephone and has no one to help them make the telephone call.	To ensure patients who require additional support are not disadvantaged. **E**

Procedure

Action	Rationale
7 The claimant **telephones** DWP on 0800 917 2222 or textphone 0800 917 7777.	To start a claim for PIP. **C**
8 *Go directly to number 20 if making a claim under the special rules for terminal illness.*	There are special rules that allow people who are terminally ill to get help quickly when they claim PIP. **C**
9 The date of claim is the date of the telephone call once the claimant has agreed a declaration which will be read out to them by the agent.	To ensure the date benefits are paid from is correct. **C**
10 The **claimant will be sent a form** for them to explain how their condition affects their daily life.	To assess whether PIP is payable and at what rate. **C**
11 The form will be personalized to the claimant and can only be used for them.	To ensure benefits are paid to the correct claimant. **C**
12 The form includes questions about the claimant's ability to carry out key everyday activities.	To assess the claimant's ability to carry out daily living and mobility activities. **C**
13 Claimants should read the information booklet that comes with the form before they start to fill the form in.	To ensure they complete the form accurately and are correctly assessed. **E**
14 The claimant should return the completed form within one calendar month.	To allow for a timely decision on the claim that accurately reflects the claimant's current needs. **C**
15 Claimants can send copies of supporting information with the completed form.	To avoid unnecessary delays and make the process as swift as possible. **E**
16 The claimant will be asked to **attend a PIP assessment** which is delivered by healthcare professional assessment providers working in partnership with DWP.	DWP has outsourced this function to appropriately trained providers. **C**

17	Sometimes a decision is made by using just the written information a claimant sends but some people may be asked to go to a 'face-to-face consultation' with a healthcare professional.	If it is not possible to decide based on the written information, additional assessment may be needed. **C**
18	The healthcare professional will complete the assessment and will send a report back to DWP.	DWP processes the claims and makes the final decision based on the information provided. **C**
19	A DWP decision-maker will then use all this information to **decide entitlement to PIP**.	To ensure benefits are paid correctly per DWP policy. **C**
20	*To claim under the special rules for terminal illness, telephone 0800 917 2222 – callers should select option 1 for a new claim and then option 3.*	Claims made under the special rules for terminal illness criteria follow a different process than standard PIP claims. **C**
21	A dedicated special rules team will take the call and complete the claim.	To ensure the claim is processed swiftly and the claimant receives support in a timely manner. **C**
22	If the claim is being made under these rules, the call can be made by someone supporting the claimant (such as a support organization or family member) without the claimant needing to be present.	It is recognized that the claimant's poor health may not allow them to be present during the telephone call. **C**
23	It is important that the claimant or the person making the phone call has the required information ready before calling DWP.	To avoid any delay in progress of the claim. **E**
24	The claimant will not be sent the form 'How your disability affects you' if they meet the criteria for an award under the special rules.	Claims made under the special rules for terminal illness criteria follow a different process than standard PIP claims. **C**
25	Claimants who meet the criteria for claiming under the special rules will not need a face-to-face consultation.	Claims made under the special rules for terminal illness criteria follow a different process than standard PIP claims. **C**
26	Claimants are encouraged to get a DS1500 medical report from their healthcare professional to support the claim.	To support their application and avoid any delay in progress of the claim. **C**
27	DWP cannot treat a DS1500 as a claim to PIP. It is important that a claim to PIP is made in addition to providing the DS1500.	The DS1500 is a supporting document and the claimant's ability to carry out mobility activities must still be assessed. **C**
28	During the telephone call, if the telephony agent identifies that the claimant needs additional support with completing the claim, they can arrange for a DWP visiting officer to assist the claimant.	To ensure patients who require additional support are not disadvantaged. **C**

Post-procedure

29	The actual length of time to get a decision on a claim depends on individual circumstances, however it is usually 3 weeks.	Some claims may be more complex than others and need additional time to assess. **E**
30	Any delays experienced by the claimant will not affect the date their benefit is paid from.	To ensure patients who qualify for benefits receive these fairly. **C**
31	Claimants will receive a letter giving the decision on the PIP claim and a clear explanation of how that decision has been reached. The decision letter will include the point score for each descriptor and it will show how the evidence has informed the decision that has been made.	To ensure transparency and clear communication. **C**
32	The decision letter will advise the claimant that they can contact the DWP if they wish to discuss the decision further.	To ensure that claimants have an opportunity to seek clarity on any matter. **C**
33	Payment will usually be made every 4 weeks in arrears. Payment will be made weekly in advance for awards made under the special rules for terminal illness.	To ensure patients who qualify for benefits receive these fairly in a manner that best meets their needs. **C**

Procedure guideline 8.3   How a patient should make a claim for Attendance Allowance (DWP 2018a)

Essential equipment and information

- A computer with internet access
- Attendance Allowance application form (Form AA1)
- Personal information such as contact details, date of birth, National Insurance number, bank or building society details, doctor's or health worker's name, details of any time spent abroad, or in a care home or hospital

(continued)

Procedure guideline 8.3 How a patient should make a claim for Attendance Allowance (DWP 2018a) *(continued)*

Pre-procedure

Action	Rationale
1 Visit gov.uk/attendance-allowance	For more information about how to claim. **E**

Procedure

Action	Rationale
2 Download form AA1. The form comes with notes telling the claimant how to fill it in and where to send it. It is also possible to get a copy of the form from the AA helpline.	To apply for AA by post. **C**
3 Telephone: 0345 605 6055 Textphone: 0345 604 5312 Monday to Friday, 8am to 6pm	
4 Determine if it is necessary to use the British Sign Language (BSL) Video Relay Service trial. To use this service, the claimant must: (a) first check they can use the service (b) go to the Video Relay Service.	To assist claimants with hearing difficulties. **E**
5 Call the Attendance Allowance helpline to ask for alternative formats, such as braille, large print, or audio CD.	To assist claimants with sight difficulties. **C**
6 There are 'special rules' to get AA more quickly if the claimant is not expected to live more than 6 months. They must: (a) complete an AA1 form (b) include a DS1500 medical condition report or send it soon after – these are free and can only be obtained from a doctor, specialist nurse or consultant.	To ensure the claim is submitted efficiently and there are no unnecessary delays in receiving the benefit. **C**
7 It is possible for someone to submit the claim under 'special rules' on behalf of someone else without their permission. The letter about the money awarded will not mention 'special rules'.	In recognition that the patient may require the additional support, but not be in a position, for whatever reason, to do request this personally. **C**

Procedure guideline 8.4 How a patient should make a claim for Carer's Allowance (DWP 2018b)

Essential equipment and information

- A computer with internet access
- Personal information such as the claimant's National Insurance number, the date of birth and address of the person being cared for, claimant's bank or building society details
- Information about course details if the claimant is studying, and any employment details including dates and how much they were paid

Pre-procedure

Action	Rationale
1 Visit gov.uk/carers-allowance	For more information about how to claim and to submit the claim form online. **E**

Procedure

Action	Rationale
2 Complete the online application and submit electronically.	To ensure the claim is submitted efficiently and there are no unnecessary delays in receiving the benefit. **C**
3 Claims can be backdated by up to 3 months.	To ensure claimants are awarded benefits fairly. **C**
4 If the claimant cannot apply online, they can apply by post. The address to send the application to is at the end of the online form.	To assist claimants who are not able to access the online application. **C**

Procedure guideline 8.5   How a patient should make a claim for Employment and Support Allowance (DWP 2018c)

Essential equipment and information

- A telephone
- A computer with internet access
- Personal information such as the claimant's National Insurance number, medical certificate, GP's address and phone number, home and mobile telephone numbers, mortgage or landlord details, council tax bill, employer's address and telephone number and dates of employment or last day worked, bank account details, details of any other money they are getting, e.g. benefits or sick pay
- Information about course details if the claimant is studying, and any employment details including dates and how much they were paid

Pre-procedure

Action	Rationale
1 Visit gov.uk/employment-support-allowance	For more information about how to claim and to submit the claim form online. **E**

Procedure

Action	Rationale

2 The quickest way to apply for ESA is by phone. Claimants should contact DWP as follows:
(a) **Contact centre numbers**
    Telephone: 0800 055 6688
    Textphone: 0800 023 4888
    Welsh language telephone: 0800 012 1888
    Monday to Friday, 8am to 6pm
	To ensure the claim is submitted efficiently and there are no unnecessary delays in receiving the benefit. **C**

3 Claimants can also fill in and print out the ESA1 form and send or take it to their local Jobcentre Plus office.	To assist claimants who are unable/prefer not to use the telephone to submit their claim. **C**
4 If the claimant cannot apply online, they can apply by post. The address to send the application to is at the end of the online form.	To assist claimants who are not able to access the online application. **C**

Problem-solving table 8.1 Prevention and resolution (Procedure guidelines 8.2, 8.3, 8.4 and 8.5)

Problem	Cause	Prevention	Action
A claimant disagrees with a decision made by DWP.	• A claimant does not believe DWP have fairly assessed their claim. • A claimant has submitted documentation that has not been interpreted in the same way by DWP.	• Ensure all information submitted is accurate. • Ensure copies are kept of all documents submitted. • Visit the DWP website to read the instructions for making a claim before proceeding.	• Discuss the decision with DWP. • Make a formal request to have the decision looked at again (known as 'mandatory reconsideration') if the claimant is still unhappy. • An appeal can be made to the Social Security and Child Support Tribunal.
A claimant is unhappy with the service they have received from DWP.	• A claimant believes that DWP have not followed their procedures and guidelines. • A claimant believes they have not been fairly assessed or treated. • A claimant believes they have not been treated with respect or courtesy. • There is a misunderstanding or communication breakdown between DWP and the claimant.	• Ensure all information submitted is accurate. • Ensure copies are kept of all documents submitted. • Visit the DWP website to read the instructions for making a claim before proceeding. • Education and training of DWP staff.	• A complaint can be submitted to DWP through the complaints process.

Post-procedural considerations

Ongoing care
Claimants should let DWP know of any change in their needs as soon as possible because the change may affect their entitlement (DWP 2018a, b, c, d, e).

Documentation
It is advisable for patients and claimants to keep copies of all the documentation that they have submitted as well as any reference numbers. They may need this to follow up their claim.

Education of patient and relevant others
Patients and their relevant others may need assistance in completing the application process for benefits and it is important that the nurse or benefits adviser explains clearly what steps have been taken, what the documentation means and answers any questions they may have.

Websites

www.ageuk.org.uk
www.gov.uk
www.macmillan.org.uk
www.cancerresearchuk.org

Useful addresses

Age UK helpline
Age UK was formed from the merger of Age Concern and Help the Aged.
Phone: 0800 169 6565

Attendance Allowance
Warbreck House
Warbreck Hill Road
Blackpool
FY2 0YE
Phone: 0345 605 6055 Monday to Friday, 8.00am to 6.00pm
Textphone: 0345 604 5312

Disability Living Allowance (over 16 years)
Warbreck House
Warbreck Hill Road
Blackpool
FY2 0YE
Phone: 0345 712 3456 Monday to Friday, 8.00am to 6.00pm
Textphone: 0345 722 4433

Disability Living Allowance (child under 16 years)
Disability Benefit Centre
4 Post Handling
Site B
Wolverhampton
WV99 1BY

Personal Independence Payment helpline
Phone: 0345 850 3322
Textphone: 0345 601 6677

DWP Carer's Allowance enquiry service
Disability Carers Service
Palatine House
Lancaster Road
Preston
PR1 1HB
Phone: 0845 608 4321
Textphone: 0845 604 5312
Website: www.gov.uk/carers-allowance

Citizen's Advice Bureau
There is no longer a single national number. You can search for your local office at www.citizensadvice.org.uk

DWP medical examinations complaints
Customer relations
ATOS healthcare
4th floor SE Quarry House
Quarry Hill
Leeds
LS2 7UA
Now known as Independent Assessment Services, www.mypipassessment.co.uk
If the claimant is unhappy with the outcome of the claim, phone the Department of Work and Pensions, 0345 850 3322

Job Centre Plus
Phone: 0800 0556688 (please note, this is free from BT landlines. If using a mobile or other service, the claimant may have to pay).

Macmillan Cancer Support
Provides information about claiming benefits for people with cancer and gives one-off grants to people with low income and savings.
Information line: 0808 808 00 00 (Monday to Friday, 9am to 8pm) – information is available in other languages.
Website: www.macmillan.org.uk

National Insurance enquiries
HM Revenue and Customs
Benton Park View
Newcastle upon Tyne
NE98 1ZZ
Phone: 0300 200 3500
Textphone: 0300 200 3519

Pensions enquiries
For UK residents aged 60 and over:
Phone: 0800 731 7898
Textphone: 0800 731 7339
For pension and benefit enquiries if the claimant lives overseas:
The Pension Service 11
Mail Handling Site A
Wolverhampton
WV98 1LW
Phone: 0191 218 7777
Textphone: 0191 218 7280

Pension Credit enquiries claim line
Phone: 0800 99 1234 Monday to Friday, 8.00am to 6.00pm (except public holidays)
Textphone: 0800 169 0133

SECTION 8.3 SUPPORTING INDIVIDUALS WITH SEXUAL CONCERNS AS A CONSEQUENCE OF CANCER

This section begins with a consideration of sexual concerns in general and how to assess needs. It then continues with a focus on females' concerns followed by males. Each section will consider the effects of specific cancers and their treatment on sexual health and then continue to provide an overview of interventions.

Sexual consequences related to cancer treatment are common (Kennedy and Leiserowitz 2015). These consequences may be physical, psychological, social and spiritual or a combination of these. The manifestation of these concerns and subsequent optimal management will depend on the type of cancer, cancer treatment, patient's age and relational status.

Sexual consequences are caused by a variety of physical and psychological factors. Sexual inactivity may not indicate a sexual problem, however reduced sexual satisfaction, distress or intimacy/sexual avoidance may indicate sexual health concerns. Sexual difficulties may include loss of sexual interest/desire, arousal and sexual pain difficulties, orgasmic difficulties and reduced sexual satisfaction/confidence. These consequences may develop during or soon after treatment, or in some cases many years later. An understanding of oncological sexual consequences, assessment and early and multifaceted interventions can support individuals living with sexual consequences from cancer diagnosis and treatment (LCA 2016).

Definition

The World Health Organization (2006) defines sexual health as:

a state of physical, emotional, mental and social wellbeing in relation to sexuality; it is not merely the absence of disease, dysfunction or infirmity. Sexual health requires a positive and respectful approach to sexuality and sexual relationships as well as the possibility of having pleasurable and safe sexual experiences, free of coercion, discrimination, and violence. For sexual health to be attained and maintained, the sexual rights of all persons must be respected, protected and fulfilled.

Related theory

Sexuality is one of the four primary domains of quality of life (mental, physical, social, sexual) in which sexual quality of life generally refers to body image, sexual desire and sexual functioning (Buchholz et al. 2015). Traditional models define sexual functioning mechanistically in terms of the human sexual response cycle: arousal, plateau, climax (orgasm), and resolution (Masters and Johnson 1966). Newer sexual functioning models incorporate psychological parameters defining sexual dysfunction as an interference in the ability to engage in sexual activity or disruption of the full sexual response cycle (Boquiren et al. 2015).

The interactive biopsychosocial model (IBM) (Lindau et al. 2015) is a theoretical framework of sexuality in the context of ageing and illness (Figure 8.4). The three main characteristics of an individual's sexual expression within the framework include sexual opportunity (defined as the social possibility for partnership), sexual capacity (including the type and frequency of physical behaviours both partnered and unpartnered) and sexual function (relating to the human sexual response cycle encompassing desire, arousal and orgasm) (Masters and Johnson 1966).

The bi-directional relationship between health and sexuality in this framework is theorized across the life span.

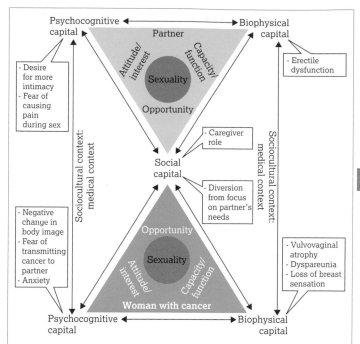

Figure 8.4 Interactive biopsychosocial model of sexuality in the context of cancer, with examples in each domain that influence sexuality. *Source:* Lindau et al. (2015). Reproduced with permission of Johns Hopkins University Press and Elsevier.

Bober and Varela's integrative biopsychosocial model for intervention proposes that sexuality is composed of psychological, relational, biological and cultural factors and therefore an understanding and consideration of all these elements is required when appraising a cancer survivor's experience. Planned interventions must reach beyond the traditional mechanistic approach of sexuality to also consider available resources that can assist mental health, relationship and cultural concerns (Varela et al. 2013).

Evidence-based approaches

Holistic Needs Assessment can enable effective identification of patients' concerns and when partnered with accurate care planning can facilitate early interventions, diagnosis of consequences of treatment, improved communication and better equity of care (Macmillan Cancer Support 2012). It can be helpful to explore with the patient their sexual health before treatment or surgery to obtain a baseline. This is particularly important if it is known that the planned treatment will have significant consequences for sexual health.

Procedure guideline 8.6 Assessing a patient's sexual health concerns

Action	Rationale
1 Invite the patient to a confidential place and ensure they have time to engage with the assessment and conversation.	Respect, confidentiality and dignity; create an environment where the patient feels they can talk about a subject that may be sensitive or embarrassing (Oguchi et al. 2011, **C**).
2 (a) Use the Holistic Needs Assessment (see Section 8.1) or one of the tools described in this section to guide a conversation with the patient about their sexual health.	To obtain baseline assessment to set expectations regarding the likelihood of sexual consequences arising from cancer treatments.
If this is done to establish a baseline it is important to explain this to the patient.	Using a recognized assessment tool can help structure and guide sensitive conversations (LCA 2016). **E, C**

(continued)

Procedure guideline 8.6 Assessing a patient's sexual health concerns *(continued)*

Action	Rationale
(b) Reassess using the same assessment tool post cancer treatment to initiate a focused conversation around any changed sexual health needs.	Early treatment for sexual health concerns can manage expectations, reduce anxiety and improve some functional outcomes. Use of a short survey can initiate a productive exchange including options for improvement (Kennedy and Leiserowitz 2015). **E**
3 If necessary, explore concerns further. Neutral non-judgemental questions may be helpful, taking account of cultural, religious and personal beliefs. It can help to begin with closed easy-to-answer questions: • Is sexual function important to you at the moment?" • Are you able to achieve the same level of sexual function after your surgery/treatment that you had beforehand? • How is this affecting your relationship at the moment?	Begin a conversation to assess the patient's identified needs. Allow them the opportunity to feel at ease and talk. **E** Presenting an opportunity to discuss sexual health concerns is more effective than waiting for the individual to ask for help (Ussher et al. 2012).
4 Communicate to the patient's medical or surgical team the concerns raised and discuss preferred treatments options and referrals to appropriate services.	To ensure the most appropriate individuals are involved in supporting the patient's needs. **E**
5 Refer to specialist services or teams. This could include: • the patient's GP for monitoring and follow-up • local post-treatment effects clinics, including erectile dysfunction/hormone management • a psychosexual counsellor.	To ensure suitable professionals are involved to meet the patient's identified needs. **C, E** Provide the patient with information to enable them to make an informed decision. **P**
6 Document on the holistic needs assessment/care plan or in the patient's hospital notes the concerns raised and the agreed plan of care.	Nurses/healthcare professionals should keep clear and accurate records (NMC 2009, **C**).

Assessment and recording tools

The assessment of sexual problems by nurses is thought to be essential for timely advice and support (Dean 2008). The absence of this discussion or information may potentially lead to the patient misconception that sexual difficulties are unique following cancer and may result in feelings of isolation (Perz and Ussher 2015). Reported barriers to effective communication regarding cancer-related sexual difficulties by healthcare professionals include a lack of time and formal training, and poor grounding to assess sexuality and treat sexual functioning (Zhou et al. 2015). Communication and sexuality discussions can be facilitated with sexuality intervention models (Quinn and Hapell 2012). However, these specialist assessments may be more frequently used in services seeing a large volume of people or where specialist management is undertaken (LCA 2016).

The PLISSIT model

This model provides a framework for healthcare professionals that can allow for engagement of discussion of sexual changes, provide sexual information, and offer support at various levels of increasing concern with corresponding levels of intervention. The intervention levels within the PLISSIT model include: Permission, Limited Information, Specific Suggestions or Intensive Therapy (Perz and Ussher 2015).

The BETTER model

This model is a structured approach that can be useful in supporting nurses in discussions about sexuality. This sexuality intervention model has six individual stages (Quinn and Happell 2012):

B = Bring Up. The nurse simply raises the subject of sexuality, showing that there is a willingness to address this now or in the future.

E = Explain. The nurse normalizes the discussion, explaining that sexuality is an important quality of life issue for many people.

T = Tell. The nurse tells the patient that if there are concerns and they are unable to be immediately addressed a referral for specialist review can be made.

T = Time. The nurse offers the possibility of a future time for further discussion.

E = Educate. The nurse educates regarding the sexual side-effects of treatment.

R = Record. The assessment, treatment and outcome are recorded by the nurse.

Sexual functioning assessment scales

There are multiple validated sexual functioning assessment scales available. These include:

Body Image Scale (BIS)

This scale comprises of 10 items for which a total score is calculated, ranging from 0 to 30; a higher score indicates a higher frequency of body image problem (Bredart et al. 2011).

Sexual Activity Questionnaire (SAQ)

This comprises of questions on sexual status and reasons for a possible absence of sexual activity. It includes an evaluation of sexual pleasure and discomfort during sexual intercourse (e.g. vaginal dryness, pain during sexual intercourse) (Bredart et al. 2011).

Tools specifically for use with women

The Female Sexual Functioning Index (FSFI)

The FSFI organizes sexual function data across six scales: desire, arousal, lubrication, orgasm, satisfaction, and pain (Raggio et al. 2014).

The Female Sexual Distress Scale – Revised

This is a 5-point rating scale (0 = never, 4 = always) with higher scores indicating sexual distress. It evaluates the frequency of negative emotions related to sexual problems over the previous month (Raggio et al. 2014).

Table 8.5 SHIM/IIEF-5 screening tool

Over the past 6 months:	Score				
	1	2	3	4	5
How do you rate your confidence that you could get and keep an erection?	Very low	Low	Moderate	High	Very high
When you had erections with sexual stimulation, how often were your erections hard enough for penetration?	Almost never or never	A few times	Sometimes	Most times	Almost always or always
During sexual intercourse, how often were you able to maintain your erection after you had penetrated (entered) your partner?	Almost never or never	A few times	Sometimes	Most times	Almost always
During sexual intercourse how difficult was it to maintain your erection to the completion of intercourse?	Extremely difficult	Very difficult	Difficult	Slightly difficult	Not difficult
When you attempted sexual intercourse, how often was it satisfactory for you?	Almost never or never	A few times	Sometimes	Most times	Almost always or always
Total score questions 1–5 =					

1–7, severe erectile dysfunction; 8–11, moderate erectile dysfunction; 12–16, mild–moderate erectile dysfunction; 17–21, mild erectile dysfunction; 22–25, no erectile dysfunction.

Source: Adapted from Rosen et al. (1997). Reproduced with permission from Elsevier.

329

Assessment tool for use with men

The International Index of Erectile Function (IIEF)
The IIEF addresses the relevant domains of male sexual function: erectile function, orgasmic function, sexual desire, intercourse satisfaction and overall satisfaction. The abridged Sexual Health Inventory for Men (SHIM) or five-item version of the IIEF (Table 8.5) can be used as a screening tool to identify the presence or absence of erectile dysfunction (Rhoden et al. 2002).

Women's sexual concerns following cancer

Females (in number and proportion) are the largest population group to experience cancers that directly affect the sexual organs. The malignancies that commonly originate in the sexual organs include ovarian, cervical, uterine and breast cancer (see Figure 8.5). The treatment of these malignancies typically involves local or systemic therapies that result in the removal, compromise or destruction of the sexual organs. Additionally, these therapies can cause abrupt or premature menopause, either directly or indirectly by disruption of female sex hormones (Lindau et al. 2015).

Menopause triggered by cancer treatment often results in abrupt, intense and/or prolonged oestrogen depletion with associated symptoms of sexual dysfunction (specifically vaginal dryness, dyspareunia and hot flushes) worse than those typically occurring in natural menopause (Carter et al. 2011). Women with vasomotor menopausal symptoms (hot flushes and night sweats) are twice as likely to experience sexual function problems (Panjari et al. 2011).

Breast cancer
Breast cancer management can involve a variety of treatment modalities including surgery, chemotherapy, radiotherapy and

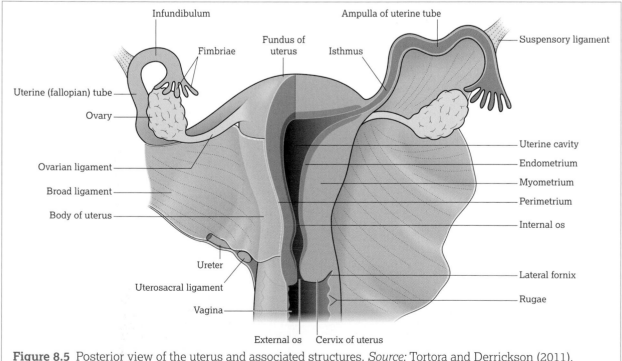

Figure 8.5 Posterior view of the uterus and associated structures. *Source:* Tortora and Derrickson (2011). Reproduced with permission of John Wiley & Sons.

endocrine therapies. Any of these treatments, alone or combined, can impact on sexual function. Sexual difficulties related to breast cancer treatment can include changes in body image, self-esteem, desire, arousal and vaginal function (dryness and atrophic changes), and intimacy and relationship problems (Katz 2011).

The surgical management of breast cancer may consist of breast conservation (lumpectomy, wide local excision) or mastectomy with or without breast reconstruction (autologous tissue reconstruction or implant). All of these procedures cause scars and can result in sensation changes. Sexual function can be negatively affected due to the development of body image concerns and changes to sexual satisfaction related to impaired erogenous zones in the body and pain (Schlenz et al. 2000).

Chemotherapy can cause significant body image changes due to chemotherapy-induced alopecia and weight gain. The impact of cytotoxic drugs on ovarian function or the inclusion of ovarian suppression during chemotherapy can result in changes in desire, arousal, vaginal lubrication, pain, sexual satisfaction and orgasm (Ochsenkuhn et al. 2011).

Radiation treatment can impact on sexual function due to fatigue and pain that can affect desire and arousal. Skin changes and tattoos can lead to body image concerns and lowered self-esteem (Varela et al. 2013).

Endocrine therapy is an important treatment modality in patients with hormone-sensitive breast cancers, working by blocking oestrogen receptors or eliminating oestrogen production. These therapies can result in significant sexual difficulties as a consequence of treatment-related menopausal symptoms including loss of desire, vaginal dryness and atrophy, pain and hot flushes (Derzko and Elliott 2007).

Gynaecological cancers

Sexual dysfunction is common in gynaecological cancers as these cancers directly affect a woman's sexual organs. Treatment for these cancers may vary depending on the specific cancer site (i.e. endometrium, vulva and cervix, ovary).

Surgery may include vulvectomy, radical hysterectomy, bilateral salpingo-oophorectomy and pelvic exenteration. Sexual problems such as body image changes, pain, loss of sensation, vaginal dryness and orgasm difficulties can occur in patients who have undergone vulvectomy and hysterectomy. Following salpingo-oophorectomy the development of sexual difficulties early after treatment may be related to hot flushes, mood changes and sleep disturbance resulting from the abrupt onset of menopause with the later developing symptoms of vaginal dryness, dyspareunia and low libido further resulting in sexual function disturbance (Carter et al. 2013).

The inclusion of chemotherapy or radiotherapy or both increases the risk of severe sexual problems. Radiotherapy can cause damage to the pelvic organs including the vagina, bladder, rectum and uterus (if present), making these women vulnerable to vaginal stenosis and bowel problems (Varela et al. 2013).

Graft-versus-host reaction

Women who undergo haematopoietic transplantation from a donor may develop graft-versus-host reactions (especially when transplant involves stem cells and colony-stimulating factor). This may result in complications including severe vaginal scarring and stenosis (Carter et al. 2011).

Inherited cancers

Women proven to carry gene mutations for inherited cancer syndromes may elect to have risk-reducing surgeries that can cause abrupt premature menopause. Risk-reducing salpingo-oophorectomy is often encouraged in women with the hereditary breast–ovarian cancer syndrome (BRCA1 or BCRA2 gene mutation) at around the age of 40 to reduce the risk of future development of breast or ovarian cancer. For women with hereditary non-polyposis colorectal cancer associated with mutations in the DNA mismatch repair genes, risk-reducing hysterectomy and salpingo-oophorectomy may be recommended (Carter et al. 2011).

The impacts of cancer treatment on sexuality

Contraception

Review of contraception practices with female cancer patients is important at cancer diagnosis, throughout the treatment pathway and into survivorship. The importance of contraceptive measures should be explained and a referral for specialist contraceptive advice may be required (Royal College of Obstetricians and Gynaecologists 2011a). Avoidance of pregnancy may be advised due to the risks of cancer treatments teratogenic to the developing fetus.

The presence of menstrual cycles after treatment with chemotherapy and/or radiation or surgery may be an indicator of fertility potential only. Resumption of cyclic menses is not a reliable indicator of fertility and the need for contraception measures. Following cancer therapy treatment-induced amenorrhoea may be transient or permanent. Some women with regular menstruation are unable to conceive and others without menses may still have oocytes and be able to reproduce (Quinn and Vadaparampil 2012).

Appropriate birth control choices should be discussed because hormonal contraception may be contraindicated with certain tumour types, particularly hormone-responsive tumours. Provision of information regarding non-hormonal contraception such as barrier methods, intra-uterine devices and surgical/radiation sterilization may be advised (Royal College of Obstetricians and Gynaecologists 2018).

Fertility preservation

Various cancer treatment modalities may impact on female fertility. Surgery may result in the removal of reproductive organs or damage to structures needed for reproduction. Radiotherapy can cause gonadal failure and induce tissue fibrosis. Chemotherapy-induced gonadotoxicity can cause permanent amenorrhoea with complete loss of germ cells, transient amenorrhoea, menstrual irregularity and subfertility. The severity of gonadal failure depends on the specific chemotherapy agents used, the cumulative dose administered and the woman's age. The impact of biological therapy on reproduction is largely unknown (Quinn and Vadaparampil 2012).

Following a cancer diagnosis, the subject of fertility-sparing treatment should be raised with all women of reproductive age who want to maintain their ability to conceive. Fertility preservation options will be based on cancer diagnosis, time available between diagnosis and the start of therapy, the treatments that have already taken place, the availability of sperm from a partner or donor and the patient's current fertility status and age (Quinn and Vadaparampil 2012).

Body image concerns

Surgical impact (scars, altered sensation), radiotherapy, alopecia, weight gain and lymphoedema may influence body image, self-esteem and sexual well-being (Varela et al. 2013).

Persistent vasomotor symptoms

Premature or abrupt ovarian failure and menopause onset may result in distressing vasomotor symptoms such as hot flushes and night sweats. These may disrupt sleep, resulting in fatigue and a poorer quality of life, which may impact negatively on sexual interest and sexual functioning (Carter et al. 2011).

Use of systemic hormone replacement therapy (HRT) to manage vasomotor symptoms may be contraindicated in some cancer types. Consideration of referral to a menopause clinic may be necessary (NICE 2015).

Vulvo-vaginal symptoms

Vaginal health management related to cancer or cancer treatment is an important aspect of cancer recovery for many women and may help to reduce or eliminate vaginal discomfort that may cause chronic vulval irritation, reduced sexual pleasure or non-adherence to gynaecological examination as part of cancer surveillance. The primary goals in improving vaginal health subsequent to cancer treatment are the restoration of vaginal lubrication and a natural pH to the vulva and vagina (Carter et al. 2011).

Loss of sexual desire/anorgasmia

Loss of sexual desire is a common sexual problem following cancer treatment in female cancer survivors. Body image concerns related to cancer and cancer treatments may interfere with a cancer survivor's connection with a partner both emotionally and intimately (Boquiren et al. 2015). Any treatment that produces chronic pain, fatigue, nausea or weakness can reduce interest in sex (Schover 1997). Reduced sex hormones related to premature menopause can lower sexual desire. Oestrogen deficiency can disrupt physiological sexual arousal responses, including smooth muscle relaxation, vasocongestion and lubrication (Buchholz et al. 2015). Prescription medications such as narcotics and medications that increase the levels of the neurotransmitter serotonin, in particular selective serotonin reuptake inhibitor (SSRI) antidepressants, can impact negatively on sexual desire and climax (Schover 1997).

Interventions

Pharmacological support

Hormone replacement therapy

HRT is a complex issue in cancer survivors. The NICE guideline *Menopause: Diagnosis and Management* (2015; short version) recommends an individualized approach at all stages of cancer diagnosis, investigation and management of menopause.

Women who are likely to go through menopause because of medical or surgical treatment (including women at high risk because of hormone-sensitive cancer or having gynaecological surgery) should be offered information about menopause and fertility before they commence their treatment.

Referral to a healthcare professional with an expertise in menopause should be considered if the patient has menopausal symptoms and contraindications to HRT or there is uncertainty about the most suitable treatment options for their menopausal symptoms (NICE 2015).

Vaginal oestrogen treatments

Vagifem tablets, Estring (silicon ring) and topical oestrogen creams are the most common vaginal oestrogen treatments. These preparations re-oestrogenize the vaginal epithelium (Goldfarb et al. 2013). Topical local oestrogen preparations are preferred to systemic oestrogen therapy for the symptoms of vulvo-vaginal atrophy as these formulations result in less systemic absorption (Wiggins and Dizon 2008). However, intravaginal oestrogens can cause a transient oestradiol elevation and their use is controversial in women with breast cancer or hormone-sensitive cancers (Goldfarb et al. 2013). Non-hormonal approaches are the first-line choice for the management of urogenital symptoms in women during or after treatment for breast cancer (American and Farrell 2016).

Oncological review and referral to a healthcare professional with menopause expertise should be considered prior to commencement of vaginal oestrogen treatments (NICE 2015).

Pharmacological interventions

Vaginal moisturizers

The fall in oestrogen levels associated with menopause can cause vaginal atrophy and thinning of the vaginal walls and vulval tissues resulting in decreased vaginal lubrication (Edwards and Panay 2016).

The use of vaginal moisturizers is aimed at improving the balance of intracellular fluids in the vaginal epithelium and restoring a premenopausal vaginal pH. Vaginal moisturizers are non-hormonal preparations available in gels, tablets or liquid beads and can be administered in an applicator or as a vaginal suppository. They need to be used several times per week and last 2–3 days before reapplication. Best absorption occurs when used prior to bedtime (Carter et al. 2011).

The two vaginal moisturizer products widely available in the UK are:

* Replens: a polycarbophil-based polymer. It contains purified water, glycerine, mineral water, hydrogenated palm oil and sorbic acid (Wiggins and Dizon 2008).
* Hyaluronic acid (HLA): Hyalofemme. HLA sodium salt is a high molecular weight glycosaminoglycan. It retains high amounts of water, provides an extracellular water film and maintains extracellular swelling, creating a moisturizing effect on the epithelium (Goldfarb et al. 2013).

Vaginal lubricants

Vaginal lubricants provide lubrication to minimize dryness and pain during sexual activity and in gynaecological examinations. They are available over the counter in liquid or gel form and are applied in the vagina and around the genitals prior to sexual activity. There is no evidence that they have any long-term therapeutic benefit (Sunha and Ewies 2013).

Water- and silicon-based lubricants are recommended; water-based lubricants are more easily washed away. Petroleum-based lubricants are more difficult to wash away and can be incompatible with latex condoms. Perfumed or flavoured lubricants may irritate or be atrophic to delicate tissues (Carter et al. 2011).

Non-pharmacological support

See Box 8.4 for practical strategies.

Vaginal dilators

The use of vaginal dilators for the management of sexual dysfunction related to pelvic radiotherapy (cervical, endometrial or rectal cancers) is promoted and evidence based. However, dilator therapy benefits may not be limited to patients undergoing this treatment. This intervention may also be useful in managing vaginal atrophy subsequent to treatment-induced hormonal deprivation, for use in vaginal reconstruction patients, and for women with vaginal graft-versus-host disease (Carter et al. 2011).

Vaginal dilators (Figure 8.6), available in sets of increasing size, provide a gradual vaginal stretching process for managing vaginal pain, stenosis and adhesions (Goldfarb et al. 2013) as well as improving control over pelvic floor muscles (Carter et al. 2013).

Box 8.4 Practical strategies in the management of sexual dysfunction in women following cancer treatment

* Encouragement of regular sexual intercourse (as appropriate) can be beneficial to vaginal health as this is presumed to stimulate increased blood flow and improve vaginal atrophy (Carter et al. 2011). Alternative sexual positions should also be explored if intercourse is uncomfortable due to pressure or functional limitations following surgery (Dean 2008).
* Discourage use of scented soaps, lotions or panty liners which may dry the vulvo-vaginal tissues. Unperfumed emollient products may be advised if dryness and irritation is severe or persistent.
* Exercise has been shown to be beneficial in reducing feelings of fatigue which may contribute to a reduction in sexual functioning.
* Practical advice for management of vasomotor symptoms (hot flushes and night sweats) includes wearing layered and cotton clothing using cotton bedding and regular exercise. Reduction in caffeine, spicy foods, alcohol and smoking may help in reducing the frequency and severity of hot flushes and night sweats (NICE 2015).
* Smoking cessation is an important aspect of vaginal health as smoking is associated with accelerated vaginal atrophy.

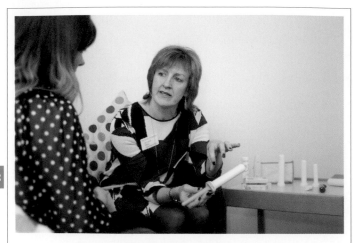

Figure 8.6 Nurse explaining use of vaginal dilator.

Pelvic floor exercises

The pelvic floor muscles provide structural support to the pelvic organs (the vagina, urethra and rectum). Dysfunction of the pelvic floor may result from disruption of the pelvic anatomy and local nerve supply to the pelvic floor muscles caused by cancer or various cancer treatments. This disruption may lead to problems such as urinary incontinence and sexual arousal difficulties (Candy et al. 2016).

Pelvic floor exercises (Box 8.5) can increase pelvic floor strength and draw blood flow to the pelvic floor, improving circulation. Pelvic floor control can aid in maintaining relaxation of pelvic and vaginal muscles, reducing reflexive tightening (and associated pain) during penetration. Pelvic floor exercises may be prescribed to aid incontinence issues by strengthening the pelvic floor muscles (Goldfarb et al. 2013).

Complementary and psychological therapies

Relaxation therapies, acupuncture, cognitive behavioural therapy (CBT) and psychosexual counselling may be considered and may offer improvement for sexual difficulties as a consequence of cancer and cancer treatments (Royal College of Obstetricians and Gynaecologists 2011a). Specifically, the frequency and severity of vasomotor symptoms may be improved with relaxation techniques such as yoga, relaxation massage and mindfulness techniques and evidence-based complementary therapies such as acupuncture (Candy et al. 2016, NICE 2015).

Box 8.5 Pelvic floor exercises

One example of pelvic floor exercises are the Kegel's exercises, named after Arnold Kegel, the gynaecologist who invented them. This exercise involves the voluntary tightening and relaxing of the pubococcygeal muscle close to the vaginal entrance. The muscle surrounds the outer third of the vaginal canal and connects to a sheet of muscle that also fulfils the on/off function for urination and bowel movements. Voluntary control of these muscles can be learned by squeezing to stop urine flow during urination. Once the pubococcygeal muscle has been found, the Kegel's exercise routine of squeezing and relaxing the muscle can be practised daily. A simply routine may involve:

1 squeezing the pubococcygeal muscle while counting to three
2 relaxing the muscle as loosely as possible
3 performing ten Kegels in a row.

It should only take a few minutes to do ten Kegels, and practice will help in sensing the difference between tension and relaxation of the pubococcygeal muscle (Schover 1997).

Men's sexual concerns following cancer

For men living with or beyond cancer, sexual dysfunction is a common consequence of their treatment and can have a negative impact on their quality of life, irrespective of their relationship status or sexual preferences (Dizon and Katz 2015). Treatment-induced male sexual dysfunction includes erectile dysfunction, loss of or reduced sexual interest/desire, anejaculation (also known as dry ejaculation), retrograde ejaculation, climacturia (leakage of urine at climax) (Cunningham et al. 2011), anorgasmia (ejaculation is maintained but orgasmic sensation is lost), and sexual pain, specifically ejaculatory pain after surgery or radiotherapy or because of peripheral neuropathy following chemotherapy. Sexuality, however, encompasses much more than intercourse; it involves body image, masculine identity, attraction and sexual thoughts (Dizon and Katz 2015). These can be affected by changes associated with illness and treatment and may have a negative impact on men's sexual expression following cancer treatment (LCA 2016), particularly if the man also experiences anxiety or depression.

Men experience social, psychological and structural barriers to seeking help, particularly for emotional support (George and Fleming 2004). Men often feel that they need to be given an opportunity and allowed to discuss these concerns through a conversation initiated by someone else; they do not tend to initiate conversations and seek help unless an opportunity is created (LCA 2016).

Anatomy and physiology

The physiology of male sexual function necessitates interactions between vascular, neurological, hormonal and psychological systems. The initial obligatory event required for male sexual activity, the acquisition and maintenance of penile erection, is primarily a vascular phenomenon triggered by neurological signals and facilitated only in the presence of a sufficient hormonal level and psychological mindset (Cunningham et al. 2011). Figure 8.7 shows the anatomical structure of the male sex organs that are affected either by cancer or its treatments. The structure and/or function of the male sexual organs can be affected by the following cancers: bowel, bladder, and other male-specific cancers such as prostate, testicular and, less commonly, penile.

While sexual dysfunction can be directly related to a primary diagnosis of cancer, aspects of male sexuality are often impacted to a greater extent by treatment than by the disease (Dizon and Katz 2015). One-third of men report that they need help with changes in sexual feelings and relationships and their sense of masculinity following treatment (Hyde et al. 2016). Treatment can have wide-ranging effects:

- Systemic treatments such as chemotherapy can temporarily or permanently damage testicular function and this may affect the man's fertility. Although sterility is not associated with many drugs, chemotherapy may reduce the number of sperm or their motility (Royal Marsden 2017). Chemotherapy can also temporarily lower testosterone and have a direct or indirect effect on sexual desire (Cancer Research UK 2015).
- Surgical treatments have differing impacts on sexual function depending on the organs involved. This is not an exhaustive list of surgeries but examples of those that can result in altered sexual function and reduced sexual well-being for men who are treated for cancer.
  - A radical prostatectomy for prostate cancer involves the removal of the whole prostate gland, seminal vesicles and the draining nodes; this is performed through an incision in the lower half of the abdomen (BAUS 2016).
  - Retroperitoneal lymph node dissection for testicular cancer involves a midline incision of the abdomen, pushing the bowels aside so that the lymph nodes located within the retroperitoneum on the side of the testicular cancer that drains the testicle can be removed; the blood supply to the affected testicle and

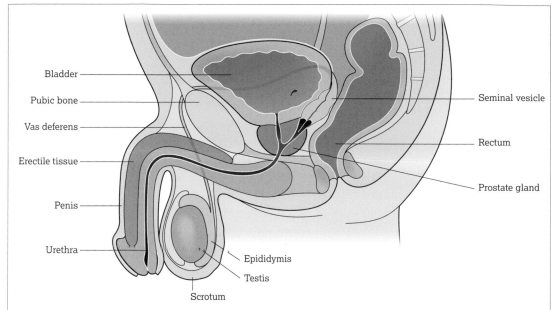

Figure 8.7 Male organs of reproduction and surrounding structures. *Source:* Adapted from Tortora and Derrickson (2011). Reproduced with permission of John Wiley & Sons.

spermatic cord are also removed. This can cause retrograde ejaculation (Testicular Cancer Awareness Foundation 2016).
– Surgical interventions such as cystectomy for muscle-invasive bladder cancer or pelvic exenteration for rectal cancer where the bladder, rectum, anus and prostate gland are all removed also cause altered sexual function as the nerves that supply the penis are either removed or permanently damaged (Macmillan Cancer Support 2016).

It is important when assessing men's sexual health to understand also their pre-existing health conditions, exacerbated by to their cancer treatment.

Sexual inactivity is not in itself problematic as long as the person is not dissatisfied, distressed or avoiding sex because of sexual difficulties. If they are, early identification of problems and simple strategies put in place in partnership with the man and/or couple may be effective (LCA 2016).

Impact of cancer treatment on sexual health

Infertility
Infertility results from reduced (or loss of) sperm production with or without altered ejaculation (retrograde/anejaculation). Prior to treatment/surgery, ensure a discussion has taken place of the potential impact of treatment on fertility. If the man desires, make a referral to onco-fertility/reproductive health or andrology services for sperm cryopreservation.

Body image and threat to masculinity
Changes to physical appearance from chemotherapy (e.g. hair loss or skin and nail changes), surgical scars and altered anatomy (e.g. orchidectomy for testicular cancer, stoma formation in bladder and bowel cancers) can have a profound impact on a man's sense of self which in turn impacts his sexual health. The impact can be reduced by ensuring the man is informed in advance of treatment of the side-effects. A prosthesis can be offered post orchidectomy. If necessary, refer the patient to psychological support or a psychosexual therapist.

Loss of sexual desire (libido)
This can occur as a direct result of cancer treatments such as hormone therapy, chemotherapy and/or surgery, or cranial or pelvic radiotherapy. Information in advance can help men manage their expectations and prepare them to cope with the changes. Referral to psychosexual counselling can help support the man and his partner adjust to the changes.

Ejaculatory changes
These can occur as a result of treatment. Testosterone supplementation may be considered for some men (those with testicular, bowel or bladder cancer) but not for men beginning treatment for prostate cancer. Giving information to men prior to treatment can help manage their expectations and prepare them to cope with the changes. Referral to a psychosexual therapist for support with ejaculatory difficulties should also be considered.

Interventions

Pharmacological treatments
There are different pharmacological interventions that can support men with sexual dysfunction after a full patient assessment has been carried out. For erectile dysfunction, phosphodiesterase type 5 inhibitors such as vardenafil, sildenafil, avanafil and tadalafil can be prescribed. If these medications prove to be ineffective, alprostadil is commonly used and administered either by intracavernosal or intraurethral routes. These medicines work by relaxing the blood vessels in the penis, allowing blood to flow into it, causing an erection (Sexual Advice Association 2016). They need to be prescribed by a trained healthcare professional with experience in men's sexual health who can teach the man to self-administer. The patient will need to be assessed regularly for side-effects and the efficacy of the selected treatment.

Non-pharmacological interventions
Early erectile dysfunction rehabilitation usually involves a combination of treatments used to improve blood flow to the penis and reduce cavernous tissue damage, thereby preventing penile atrophy. This may help improve long-term erectile function and enable an earlier return of assisted or unassisted erections sufficient for intercourse (Macmillan Cancer Support 2016). Vacuum erection devices can achieve this and are often used in combination with pharmacological treatments after radical prostatectomy and other radical pelvic surgeries. Men should be given the opportunity to be assessed by a specialist and be taught how to use these devices safely.

Websites

Cancer.Net
Sexuality and cancer treatment: women.
http://www.cancer.net/navigating-cancer-care/dating-sex-and-reproduction/sexuality-and-cancer-treatment-women

COSRT
The College of Sexual and Relationship Therapists (COSRT), the UK's leading organization for therapists specializing in sexual and relationship issues.
http://www.cosrt.org.uk/

London Cancer Alliance
Sexual Consequences of Cancer Treatment: Management Pathway.
http://www.londoncanceralliance.nhs.uk/media/125886/lca-sexual-consequences-of-cancer-treatment-management-pathway-march-2016-v2-final.pdf

HNA Prompt Sheet: Sexual Consequences for Women
http://www.londoncanceralliance.nhs.uk/media/118602/lca-hna-sex-consequences-women-prompt-sheet-march-2016.pdf

Menopause Matters UK
https://menopausematters.co.uk

NICE
NICE guideline 23: Menopause: diagnosis and management
https://www.nice.org.uk/guidance/NG23

Relate
Offers a range of services for couple and family relationships
https://www.relate.org.uk

The Royal College of Obstetricians and Gynaecologists UK
https://www.rcog.org.uk

The Sexual Advice Association
A charitable organization that aims to help improve the sexual health and well-being of men and women and raise awareness of the extent to which sexual problems affect the general population.
https://sexualadviceassociation.co.uk/

Product websites

https://www.astroglide.co.uk
https://www.durex.co.uk
https://www.pjurmed.com
http://www.hyalofemme.co.uk/
https://www.replens.co.uk/professionals

Patient resources

Macmillan Cancer Support
Side effects and symptoms:
http://www.macmillan.org.uk/information-and-support/coping/side-effects-and-symptoms/fertility-in-women
Macmillan Learn Zone: Sexual relationships and cancer:
http://learnzone.org.uk/courses/course.php?id=68
Relationships and sex:
http://www.macmillan.org.uk/information-and-support/coping/relationships/your-sex-life-and-sexuality
Fertility in women:
http://www.macmillan.org.uk/information-and-support/coping/side-effects-and-symptoms/fertility-in-women

Breast Cancer Care
Your body, intimacy and sex:
https://www.breastcancercare.org.uk/information-support/publication/your-body-intimacy-sex-bcc110
Fertility and breast cancer treatment:
https://www.breastcancercare.org.uk/information-support/publication/fertility-breast-cancer-treatment-bcc28

SECTION 8.4 NUTRITIONAL STATUS

Definition
The term 'nutritional status' refers to the condition and function of the human body with respect to body composition and the balance of minerals, vitamins and trace elements. It is influenced by nutritional intake, absorption of nutrients from food, physical activity, disease states and cancer treatment (Arends et al. 2017).

Related theory
Good nutrition, the supply of optimal nutrients and fluid to meet requirements, is an essential component of health, with poor nutrition contributing to ill health and prolonged recovery from illness or disease. It is therefore crucial that the nutritional status of all patients is assessed and considered during the whole of the person's care. Treatment for cancer can contribute to long-term consequences which may ultimately impact on nutritional status. Examples of this include dysphagia, reduced appetite, early satiety or altered bowel function leading to poor digestion and absorption of nutrients. As a result, people may experience weight loss and deficiencies of specific nutrients such as iron and vitamins D and B_{12}. The risk of these nutritional inadequacies can be predicted in some people, for example those who have undergone surgery to the gastrointestinal tract or who have received pelvic radiotherapy. However, in others they may be less predictable and arise due to late effects of cancer treatment or other co-morbid conditions.

Gastrointestinal symptoms can arise because of cancer treatment. These can be both upper and lower gastrointestinal symptoms and may arise because of surgery to the gastrointestinal tract, chemotherapy or, more commonly, radiotherapy, particularly when given to the head, neck or pelvis. Persistent symptoms are likely to impact on quality of life with those affected potentially having problems swallowing or altered bowel habits. The latter can result in them being less confident to leave the house, travel or return to work. Symptoms may also impact on nutritional status as people make dietary changes in an attempt to control symptoms or experience malabsorption of macro- or micronutrients (Abayomi et al. 2009a, b).

Treatment of hormone-dependent cancers such as breast and prostate cancer can result in changes in body composition with weight gain, additional fat deposition and a decrease in bone density. These changes arise due to a combination of treatment (hormonal) and nutritional factors and can influence body image, ability to exercise, morbidity and mortality outcomes with respect to both cancer and other diseases.

There is now also strong emerging evidence that patients with head and neck cancer treated by radical or adjuvant (chemo-) radiation may present with late dysphagia (Hutcheson et al. 2012, Szczesniak et al. 2014). These patients are disease free and can present up to 9 years post treatment. The most common presenting symptoms include dysarthria, dysphonia, cranial nerve neuropathy (especially X and XII), trismus and mandibular osteoradionecrosis.

The following signs may help identify those at risk of dysphagia and necessitate a referral to the speech and language therapist.

Please note that these are red flags for recurrence and patients should be referred to their oncologist/surgeon.

- Reports of swallowing problems (including gradual deterioration in swallowing function).
- Coughing during or after eating.
- Voice changes, especially a wet/hoarse voice quality.
- Recurrent chest infections.
- Taking longer to eat meals.
- Avoiding certain foods and altering diet.

Presenting at such a late stage may mean that therapy exercises will not be of benefit (Hutcheson et al. 2012, Langmore et al. 2015) but the speech and language therapist can advise regarding postures and techniques to make the swallow safer. All head and neck cancer patients are given prophylactic swallowing exercises prior to commencing their chemo/radiotherapy and are advised to continue these forever.

While the focus of survivorship is often on patients, the impact on carers of supporting an individual with oropharyngeal dysphagia cannot be underestimated (Nund et al. 2014, Patterson et al. 2012).

It is essential that issues with eating, drinking and ultimately nutritional status are identified both during and after cancer treatment. This enables people to be signposted to appropriate advice, support services or specialist services as appropriate.

Evidence-based approaches

Screening of nutritional status is a method for identifying those at nutritional risk. It is generally aimed at identifying those who are at risk of under-nutrition. It is a requirement for all patients on admission to hospital and at their first outpatient appointment (NICE 2012). Information obtained from nutritional screening then allows a suitable nutritional assessment to be undertaken on those who are at medium or high risk with the aim of providing the appropriate advice and support to improve or maintain nutritional status. Nutritional assessment is usually undertaken by a healthcare professional who has the relevant expertise, such as a registered dietitian or nutrition nurse.

Nutrition screening usually involves the use of a nutrition screening tool, which focuses on aspects such as weight loss and comparison with normal body weight, for example the Malnutrition Universal Screening Tool (MUST) (British Association of Parenteral and Enteral Nutrition [BAPEN] 2003). Some screening tools are cancer specific such as the Royal Marsden Nutrition Screening Tool (Shaw et al. 2015) and these may include questions on symptoms that affect dietary intake. Screening for over-nutrition can be undertaken using calculation of body mass index (BMI) from measurements of height and weight and the measurement of waist circumference (NHS Choices 2016). Waist circumference can indicate central (abdominal) adiposity, a risk factor for metabolic syndrome and associated conditions including type 2 diabetes.

Indications

Use of the holistic needs assessment gives people an opportunity to identify if they have any particular needs with respect to eating or drinking. If specific questions or issues are raised with respect to eating and drinking it may be appropriate to address these without the need for nutrition screening. For example, the person may have specific questions about foods or the optimal balance of their diet. However, if it is uncertain what support is required then screening tools can be used to identify risk of under- or over-nutrition. In addition, it may be helpful to screen for bowel symptoms arising as a consequence of cancer treatment.

Pre-procedural considerations

Methods for measuring height and weight of an adult patient

Taking an accurate height and weight of a patient is an essential part of nutrition screening. In addition, for those who are

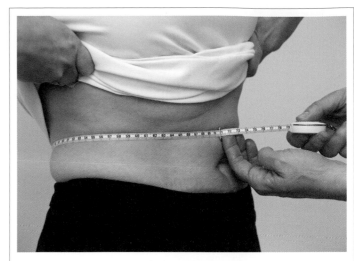

Figure 8.8 Measurement of waist circumference.

overweight it is helpful to have an accurate measurement of waist circumference (Figure 8.8).

Check that the patient can stand or sit on the appropriate scales. The patient should remove outdoor clothing and shoes before being weighed and having height measured. When obtaining a height measurement and waist circumference, check that the patient can stand upright while the measurement is taken. For patients who are unable to stand, height may be determined by measuring ulna length and using conversion tables. If neither height nor weight can be measured or obtained, BMI can be estimated using the mid upper arm circumference (MUAC) (BAPEN 2003). It may not be possible to weigh patients who cannot be moved or are unable to sit or stand. Alternative methods to obtain weight should be explored, for example bed scales that can be placed under the wheels of the bed, scales as an integral part of a bed, or a patient hoist with weighing facility.

Equipment

Scales

Scales (either sitting or standing) must be calibrated and positioned on a level surface. If electronic or battery scales are used, then they must be connected to the mains or have appropriate working batteries prior to the patient getting on the scales.

Stadiometer

This is a device for measuring height. It may be mounted on weighing scales or wall mounted.

Tape measure

A tape measure is required if estimating height from ulna length or MUAC and for measurement of waist circumference. The tape measure should measure in centimetres and either be disposable or made of plastic that can be cleaned with a detergent wipe between patient uses.

Assessment tools

Identification of patients who are malnourished or at risk of malnutrition is an important step in nutritional care. There are a number of screening tools available that consider different aspects of nutritional status. National screening initiatives demonstrated that 28% of patients admitted to hospital were found to be at risk of malnutrition – high risk (22%) and medium risk (6%) (BAPEN 2009). Particular diagnoses, such as cancer, increase the risk of malnutrition (Shaw et al. 2015).

Procedure guideline 8.7 Measuring the weight, height and waist circumference of the patient

Essential equipment
- Scales
- Stadiometer (preferably fixed to the wall)

Optional equipment
- Tape measure

Pre-procedure

Action	Rationale
1 Position the scales for easy access and apply the brakes (if appropriate).	To ensure that the patient can get on and off the scales easily and to avoid accidents should the scales move. **E**
2 Ask the patient to remove shoes and outdoor garments. The patient should be wearing light indoor clothes only (see Figure 8.9).	Outdoor clothes and shoes will add additional weight and make it difficult to obtain an accurate bodyweight. **E**

Procedure

Action	Rationale
3 **Weight:** Ensure that the scales record zero then ask the patient to stand on the scales (or sit if using sitting scales). Ask the patient to remain still and check that the patient is not supporting any weight on any object, for example leaning on the wall, or having stick or feet resting on the floor.	To record an accurate weight (NMC 2009).
4 Note the reading on the scale and record immediately, taking care that it is legible. Check with the patient that the weight reflects their expected weight and that the weight is similar to previous weights recorded. This may require conversion of weight from kg to stones and pounds or vice versa.	To check that the weight is correct. If the weight is not as expected, then the patient should be re-weighed. **E**
5 **Height:** Ensure that the patient has removed their shoes and then ask them to stand straight with heels together. If the stadiometer is wall mounted, the heels should touch the heel plate or the wall. With a freestanding device, the person's back should be toward the measuring rod.	Shoes will provide additional height and make the measurement inaccurate. Standing with feet apart will make the measurement inaccurate. **E** To ensure that the patient is standing upright. If the person does not have their back against the measuring rod, then the measuring arm may not reach the head. **E**
6 The patient should look straight ahead, arms by their side and with the bottom of the nose and the bottom of the ear in a parallel plane. The patient should be asked to stretch upwards to reach maximal height.	To ensure an accurate height is measured. **E**
7 Record height to the nearest millimetre.	To record an accurate measurement of the patient's height (NMC 2009). **C**
8 To estimate the height of a patient from ulna length, ask the patient to remove any long-sleeved jacket, shirt or top.	To be able to access their left arm for measurement purposes. **E**
9 Measure between the point of the elbow (olecranon process) and the midpoint of the prominent bone of the wrist (styloid process) on the left side if possible (Figure 8.10).	To obtain measurement of the length of the ulna. **E**
10 Estimate the patient's height to the nearest centimetre, using a conversion table.	To estimate the patient's height (BAPEN 2003). **C**
11 **Body mass index:** Estimate the patient's BMI using a conversion table or online BMI calculator	To estimate the patient's BMI (BAPEN 2003). **C**
12 **Waist circumference:** To measure waist circumference, ensure that a tape of adequate length is available. The correct position for measuring waist circumference is midway between the uppermost border of the iliac crest and the lower border of the costal margin (rib cage). The tape should be placed around the abdomen at the level of this midway point and a reading taken when the tape is snug but does not compress the skin (see Figure 8.8).	To obtain accurate measurement of waist circumference (National Obesity Forum 2016). **C**
13 Document the measurement.	To record an accurate measurement of waist circumference. **C**

Post-procedure

Action	Rationale
14 Document height, weight and waist circumference in the patient's notes.	To record the accurate measurement of patient's height and weight (NMC 2009). **C**

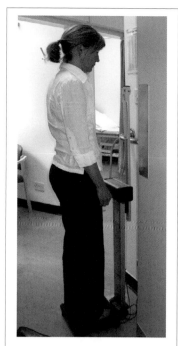

Figure 8.9 Weighing a patient. *Source:* Dougherty and Lister (2015).

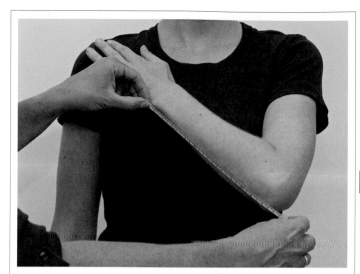

Figure 8.10 Measure between the point of the elbow (olecranon process) and the midpoint of the prominent bone of the wrist (styloid process). *Source:* Dougherty and Lister (2015).

Problem-solving table 8.2 Prevention and resolution (Procedure guideline 8.7)

Problem	Cause	Prevention	Action
Patient unable to stand on scales.	Poorly positioned scales. Patient balance not sufficient.	Check with patient prior to asking them to stand on scales if they are able to do so. Offer sitting scales if necessary.	Ensure both sitting and standing scales are available in the hospital.
Weight obtained appears too low.	Patient may have put pressure on scales prior to them reaching zero.	Ensure zero is visible before patient touches scales.	Check weight with patient once obtained. Re-weigh patient to check correct weight.
Weight obtained appears too high.	a. Patient may be wearing outdoor clothes, shoes or be carrying a bag, have a full drainage bag or other medical fluid collecting device. b. Patient may have fluid retention, for example oedema or ascites.	Ensure that the patient is wearing light indoor clothes before standing on the scales. Ask patient to empty any drainage bags. Check whether patient has fluid retention.	Check weight with patient once obtained. Re-weigh patient to check correct weight.
Patient is unable to stand.	Patient is unwell or has physical disability.	Discuss the procedure with patient before undertaking height measurement.	Consider estimating height from ulna measurement.
Difficulty measuring waist circumference in obese patients.	Tape measure may not be long enough. Difficulty identifying the correct position to measure waist circumference.	Calculate BMI and if it exceeds 35 kg/m^2 then do not measure waist circumference.	Use BMI alone.

Post-procedural considerations

After taking a measurement of height it is useful to check with the patient that the figure obtained is approximately the height that is expected. However, it is important to consider that patients may report a loss in height with increasing years. Cumulative height loss from age 30 to 70 years may be about 3 cm for men and 5 cm for women; by age 80 years it increases to 5 cm for men and 8 cm for women (Sorkin et al. 1999).

Consideration must be given to the patient's weight and whether this reflects a change in their clinical condition. The weight may be being used as part of a nutritional screening or assessment of BMI.

After taking a measurement of weight it is useful to check with the patient that the figure obtained is what they would expect or whether there have been significant changes over time.

A person identified at risk of malnutrition should be referred to a registered dietitian and undergo a full nutritional assessment. Subjective global assessment (SGA) and patient generated subjective global assessment (PG-SGA) are comprehensive assessment tools that need more time and expertise to carry out than most screening tests. The most important feature of using any screening tool is that patients identified as requiring nutritional assessment or intervention have a nutritional care plan initiated. People can be signposted to reliable, evidence-based published and online resources to support them in making dietary changes to improve their nutritional intake (Shaw 2015).

If the person is assessed as being overweight or obese then this can be discussed with the patient with respect to appropriate lifestyle changes. Advice and ongoing support may be needed for the patient to successfully lose weight and increase physical activity. Ideally body weight should be in the optimal range. This range varies depending on age and ethnicity so individuals may need specific advice regarding their own target (NHS Choices 2016).

Assessment and recording tools

Nutrition screening

The Royal Marsden Nutrition Screening Tool (RMNST) (Table 8.6).

Calculation of body mass index

Body mass index (BMI) or comparison of a patient's weight with a chart of ideal bodyweight gives a measure of whether the patient has a normal weight, is overweight or underweight, and may be calculated from weight and height using the following equation:

$$BMI = \frac{Weight\ (kg)}{Height\ (m)^2}$$

Tables and online programs are available to allow the rapid and easy calculation of BMI (NHS Choices 2016). Calculation of BMI allows comparison with desirable ranges of BMI, indicating whether people are under- or overweight. These comparisons, however, are not a good indicator of whether the patient is at risk nutritionally, as an apparently normal weight can mask severe muscle wasting, for example in sarcopenia and cachexia. Changes in food intake and disease state also influence nutritional risk.

Measurement of waist circumference

The waist circumference measurement for men and women at which there is an increased relative risk for heart disease, type 2 diabetes and cancer is defined in Table 8.7.

In some populations (e.g. in persons of Asian descent), waist circumference may be a better indicator of risk than BMI. In very obese patients (those with a BMI > 35 kg/m²), waist circumference has added little to the predictive power of disease risk (National Obesity Forum 2016).

Table 8.6 The Royal Marsden Nutrition Screening Tool (RMNST)

Question	If the answer to the question is yes then score
1 Has the patient experienced unintentional weight loss in the last 3 months?	
(>7 kg in men or >5.5 kg in women)	10
If not, unintentional weight loss less than the above	5
2 Does the patient look underweight?	5
3 Has the patient had a reduced food intake (less than 50% of meals) in the last 5 days (this may be due to mucositis, dysphagia, nausea, bowel obstruction, vomiting)?	5
4 Is the patient experiencing symptoms that are affecting food intake, e.g. mucositis, nausea, vomiting, diarrhoea, constipation?	3
Total score	Maximum 23

Score	Action
0–4	Low risk of malnutrition. Reassure.
5–9	Moderate risk of malnutrition. Explore difficulties and provide appropriate support and resources.
Over 10	High risk of malnutrition. Refer to a registered dietitian for full assessment and care plan.

© The Royal Marsden NHS Hospital Foundation Trust

Assessment of bowel habits following treatment for cancer

Some key questions about bowel function can be used to assess whether a person requires a referral to a gastroenterologist for further investigation and management. The questions in Box 8.6 have been devised to identify people with persistent gastrointestinal symptoms following pelvic radiotherapy who would benefit from specialist assessment and advice from a gastroenterologist (Pelvic Radiation Disease Association 2016).

Table 8.7 Waist circumference measurement for men and women at which there is an increased relative risk for heart disease, type 2 diabetes and cancer

	Increased risk	Substantially increased risk
Men	≥94 cm	≥102 cm
Women	≥80 cm	≥88 cm

Box 8.6 Questions to identify people with persistent gastrointestinal symptoms following pelvic radiotherapy

Following pelvic radiotherapy does your patient:
- need to open their bowels at night
- need to rush to the loo, or not make it in time
- have bleeding, or
- other gastrointestinal symptoms that interfere with an active full life?

If the answer to any of these questions is YES then a referral to a gastroenterologist is essential.

Source: Pelvic Radiation Disease Association (2016).

Websites

Undernutrition/weight loss

Macmillan Cancer Support: The building-up diet
Practical advice on increasing dietary intake to address weight loss.
http://www.macmillan.org.uk/information-and-support/coping/maintaining-a-healthy-lifestyle/preventing-weight-loss/the-building-up-diet.html

A Practical Guide for Lung Cancer Nutritional Care
Aimed at healthcare professionals with a focus on nutritional management of people with lung cancer.
http://lungcancernutrition.com/A%20Practical%20Guide%20to%20Lung%20Cancer%20Nutritional%20Care.pdf

Overnutrition/weight gain

World Cancer Research Fund UK
Evidence-based dietary guidelines and useful tips and recipes
http://www.wcrf-uk.org/

NHS choices: Obesity
Includes a BMI calculator, diagnosis and management of obesity.
http://www.nhs.uk/Conditions/Obesity/Pages/Introduction.aspx

Macmillan Cancer Support: Maintaining a healthy lifestyle
Aimed at patients and includes information on healthy eating and tips for losing weight.
http://www.macmillan.org.uk/information-and-support/coping/maintaining-a-healthy-lifestyle/managing-weight-gain

Symptoms

Macmillan Cancer Support
What to do after cancer treatment ends: 10 top tips
http://www.macmillan.org.uk/Documents/Cancerinfo/Living-withandaftercancer/Whattodoaftertreatment.pdf

Macmillan guidance on long term consequences of treatment for gynaecological cancer: Part 1: pelvic radiotherapy
Aimed at healthcare professionals.
http://www.macmillan.org.uk/Documents/AboutUs/Health_professionals/MAC14942_GYNAE_GUIDE.pdf

Pelvic Radiation Disease Association
Information and support for those who have late effects of pelvic radiotherapy.
http://www.prda.org.uk/

SECTION 8.5 COMPRESSION THERAPY IN THE MANAGEMENT OF LYMPHOEDEMA

Overview

This section describes the management of lymphoedema using compression therapy. Lymphoedema can develop because of treatment for cancer when lymph nodes have been surgically removed or irradiated. It can also occur when cancer obstructs lymph drainage routes. Lymphoedema is a chronic, life-long condition, therefore early identification and treatment is crucial. After initial patient education and the development of an agreed treatment plan to reduce and control the swelling, patients are encouraged to self-manage their condition with support when required.

Lymphoedema

Definition

Lymphoedema is a form of chronic oedema caused either by damage to the lymphatic system (termed 'secondary lymphoedema') or congenital defects in the lymphatic system (termed 'primary lymphoedema') (Todd 2013). This section will focus only on cancer-related lymphoedema.

Anatomy and physiology

The lymphatic system works closely with the cardiovascular system to maintain fluid balance within the body. The cardiovascular system transports nutrients and oxygen to the body's cells via blood vessels. As the blood flows through the vessels, nutrients and water pass into the spaces between the cells, known as the interstitial spaces, to form interstitial fluid (Partsch and Moffatt 2012).

The lymphatic system moves this interstitial fluid, now known as 'lymph', via a network of superficial and deep lymphatic vessels forming a one-way drainage system towards the two main ducts, the thoracic duct and the right lymphatic duct, which empty lymph back into the venous system.

Lymph drainage commences with the superficial vessels, called initial lymphatics, which are found in the connective tissue spaces. Movement of lymph in the initial lymphatics is dependent upon muscle activity and changes in tissue pressure (Partsch and Moffatt 2012). The larger, deeper lymph vessels act as collecting vessels and contain smooth muscle and valves enabling them to contract and propel lymph in a unidirectional flow. Lymph nodes are situated in groups within the larger lymph vessels and act as filters to collect and destroy bacteria and viruses (Drake et al. 2015). See Figure 8.11 for a simplified diagram of the lymphatic system.

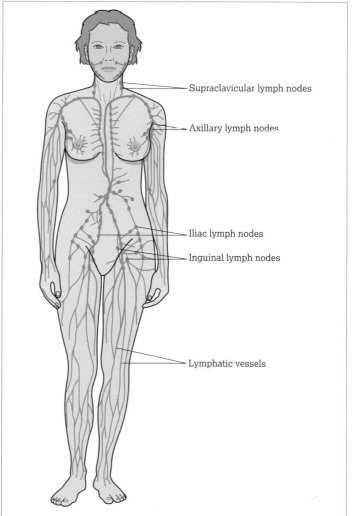

Figure 8.11 Simplified diagram of the lymphatic system.

339

The balance between tissue fluid formation and reabsorption is dependent upon pressures across the capillary wall, known as Starling's forces. Any change can affect fluid levels in the tissues and result in the appearance of oedema (Partsch and Moffatt 2012).

A reduction in the drainage routes of the lymphatic system can occur following cancer-related treatment in lymph node areas, and oedema can appear in the adjacent limb or truncal quadrant of the body.

In summary, the lymphatic system has the following main functions:

- to regulate homeostasis by returning large molecules to the circulation and draining excess fluid from the interstitium
- to dispose of unwanted cellular by-products
- to defend the body from infection by absorbing micro-organisms and generating an autoimmune response when necessary.

Related theory

Oedema and lymphoedema may be caused by a wide range of conditions, both cancer and non-cancer related (Williams 2012a). When the lymphatic system fails due to damage, obstruction or congenital abnormality, fluid cannot be drained and builds up in the interstitial spaces causing lymphoedema (Nazarko 2015, Partsch and Moffatt 2012). Other causes of peripheral oedema include venous, renal or hepatic disease, obesity, lipo-oedema and some medications (Bianchi et al. 2012). In these cases, the lymphatic system has not failed and treatment may differ (Nazarko 2015). Dependency or gravitational oedema may develop in the immobile patient when failure to activate the muscle pump causes an increase in capillary filtration and reduced lymph drainage in the dependent limb (Milne 2015).

As described previously, there are two types of lymphoedema, primary or secondary, depending on aetiology. Primary lymphoedema occurs when there is an abnormality in the lymphatic system and may be present from birth (Nazarko 2015). Secondary lymphoedema arises from external factors affecting the function of the lymphatic system. This includes treatment for cancer involving the removal or irradiation of lymph node areas and other causes which include infection, venous disease, inflammation and trauma to the lymphatic channels or vessels (International Society of Lymphology 2013).

Lymphoedema is most commonly seen in patients with cancer because of damage to lymph nodes following surgery and/or radiotherapy, but it can also occur as a result of local tumour obstruction in lymph node areas. The reported incidence of lymphoedema following cancer treatment varies widely between studies. However, in breast cancer patients, the prevalence of chronic arm oedema is reported as being between 14.9% and 29.8%, average 20% or one in five patients (DiSipio et al. 2013), and in patients treated for gynaecological cancers it is between 28% and 47% (Lymphoedema Framework 2006). Lymphoedema can also develop after treatment for other malignancies: melanoma, sarcoma, genitourinary and head and neck cancers (Fu et al. 2014). Cancer-related lymphoedema often develops within 5 years of treatment, however lymphoedema can develop at any time after treatment and patients face a lifetime risk of developing it (Fu et al. 2014).

Lymphoedema can affect any part of the body, including the face and head, but it most commonly affects a limb. The swelling can have physical, psychological and psychosocial implications for the patient and is associated with a number of complications arising from its development (Cooper 2014). Limb heaviness may lead to impaired function, reduced mobility and musculoskeletal problems (Woods 2010). Skin and tissue changes develop with increased lymph stasis in the oedematous limb and give rise to the characteristic deepened skin folds and skin thickening. Over time, complex skin conditions can occur (Todd 2013). There is an increased risk of local and systemic infection because of poor lymph drainage, and recurrent episodes of cellulitis are common (Cooper 2014).

Evidence-based approaches

Rationale

Compression therapy in the management of lymphoedema involves the use of compression garments, low-stretch bandages (Fu et al. 2014), and more recently the use of adjustable wrap compression systems (Damstra and Partsch 2013). Compression therapy initiates physiological effects within the arterial, venous, lymphatic and microcirculation (Partsch and Moffatt 2012).

Compression reduces oedema by (Partsch 2012, Partsch and Moffatt 2012):

- increasing lymphatic drainage from oedematous tissues to non-oedematous tissues
- reducing the formation of excess tissue fluid by reducing capillary filtration and decreasing lymphatic load
- containing the tissues of the swollen limb and promoting the maintenance of a normal shape to the limb
- increasing blood flow in the microcirculation, initiating a softening of fibrotic tissue and maintaining skin integrity
- maximizing the effect of the muscle pump.

Compression therapy influences the principles of Starling's hypothesis by increasing local tissue pressure, counteracting capillary fluid filtration and enhancing lymph reabsorption (Partsch and Moffatt 2012).

The type of material from which the bandages or garments are made can determine the degree of pressure exerted on the tissues below (Partsch 2012), although the level of pressure achieved is also dependent upon a complex combination of other factors including the size and shape of the limb and the activity of the wearer (Partsch and Mortimer 2015).

The characteristics of compression garments, bandages and adjustable wrap compression systems have been summarized by the acronym PLaCE (Partsch and Moffatt 2012, Partsch and Mortimer 2015) (see Box 8.7).

Box 8.7 PLaCE: characteristics of compression garments, bandages and adjustable wrap compression systems

- *Pressure.* This is mainly determined by the manual force with which the bandage is applied, and is not determined by the bandage itself.
- *Layers.* Bandages are applied with some overlap, therefore even one bandage will be multilayer. A single compression arm sleeve will be single layer.
- *Components.* A bandaging application will be comprised of different components (e.g. liner and padding as well as the textile components of the bandage itself).
- *Elastic property/stiffness.* Compression bandages and garments are categorized according to their elastic property, traditionally as elastic (long stretch) and inelastic (short stretch/low stretch). Elastic compression garments (also called round knit) are seam free, made from finer fabric and suitable for managing mild, uncomplicated swelling, where skin is intact and there is no limb distortion (Todd 2015). Inelastic bandages, garments or adjustable wrap systems produce a more ridged structure around the limb which does not yield. This produces high pressure peaks when muscles are contracted, but tolerable lower resting pressure. These are referred to as compression systems with a high static stiffness index (SSI). Compression with high SSI will not yield during exercise leading to a massaging effect and oedema reduction (Elwell 2015, Partsch and Moffatt 2012, Partsch and Mortimer 2015).

Indications and contraindications

Indications for the most suitable type of compression therapy will depend on the patient and the extent of their swelling and will be made after full assessment, see text on bandaging and compression garments.

Principles of care

Compression therapy in the management of lymphoedema can be approached in two phases: the intensive phase and the maintenance phase (Tidhar et al. 2014).

The intensive phase

The intensive phase of treatment is a short period of therapist-led treatment, usually planned over a 2- to 3-week period, in which specific aims are identified, discussed and agreed between the patient and the therapist. Depending upon the oedema present, however, the treatment may be planned over a longer or shorter period. During the intensive or reduction phase of treatment, short-stretch, inelastic bandages are applied to the swollen limb each day and left in place for a period of 23 hours as part of a multilayer system to provide a semi-rigid encasement to the limb (Muldoon 2010). Alternatively, other bandaging systems (generally comprising two layers – a foam layer and an adhesive top layer) are applied twice weekly (Moffatt et al. 2012). This aspect of treatment is combined with other elements of treatment including (International Lymphoedema Framework 2012, Tidhar et al. 2014):

- a skincare regimen to minimize the risks of infection and optimize skin condition
- specific exercises to promote lymph drainage and maintain joint mobility
- information, support and advice on self-management
- manual lymphatic drainage (MLD) administered by a specially trained therapist to stimulate lymph drainage by moving fluid to an area with functioning lymphatics.

The maintenance phase

During the maintenance phase, the concept of self-care is promoted to encourage the patient to become independent in the long-term management and control of their swelling. Compression garments suitable for the nature and extent of swelling are selected and there is now a wide range of styles depending on the individual needs and preferences of patients. Co-morbidities, mobility and dexterity limitations will also have to be considered in garment selection (Elwell 2016). Compression garments are worn for a period each day and the therapist evaluates progress at regular intervals initially to ensure that the garments remain appropriate and that any problems can be identified at an early stage (Linnitt 2011). Once the swelling is stable and maximum reduction has been achieved, the patient is encouraged to commence long-term control through self-supported management. This aspect of treatment is also combined with other elements including:

- a skincare regimen to minimize the risks of infection and optimize skin condition
- specific exercises to promote lymph drainage and maintain joint mobility
- simple lymphatic drainage (SLD), a simplified version of MLD taught to the patient by a therapist to stimulate normal draining lymphatics (Todd 2013).

Not all patients will follow both phases of treatment, and many may only need to follow the maintenance phase. The decision concerning the most appropriate phase of treatment for the patient should be made by a skilled therapist taking the patient's wishes into consideration.

Assessment of the patient with lymphoedema and calculation of limb volume

Evidence-based approaches

Rationale

When the use of compression therapy is being considered, a full and careful assessment will highlight the patient's main problems and any co-existing complications. This information is then used to set realistic treatment goals and to determine the most suitable approach to compression therapy treatment. Clinical and physical indications determined during a full assessment of the patient will facilitate the most appropriate choice of compression therapy for the individual patient. Several treatments are used in combination during the management of lymphoedema; their choice and usefulness can be determined by the therapist and patient at the time of assessment. The experience of living with lymphoedema as a long-term chronic condition is unique for each patient and can have an impact on many areas of the individual's life (Ridner et al. 2012). The physical and psychological effects are not short-lived, and enormous motivation and perseverance coupled with adaptation are demanded to achieve control or reduction of the swelling (Nazarko 2014, Woods 2010).

Clarifying the influence of the lymphoedema on the patient's lifestyle, occupation and chosen social activities will help to identify patient-focused problem areas that may require adjustment. By gaining an understanding of the impact that the swelling may be having upon personal feelings and emotions, relevant supportive strategies can be identified (Woods 2010).

Principles of care

Assessment should encompass a person-centred framework (McCormack and McCance 2010) and include the following elements:

- *Details of the patient's medical history*: to determine the cause of swelling and whether compression therapy can be used safely. Arterial insufficiency of the lower limb must always be excluded prior to the use of compression therapy. Palpation of the pedal pulses alone is an unreliable predictor of adequate arterial supply. The measurement of the ankle to brachial pressure index (ABPI) is recommended if there is any doubt about the patient's peripheral arterial status (International Society of Lymphology 2013). If the patient has a history of diabetes or cardiac failure, a medical assessment should also be completed prior to the commencement of treatment and there should be close supervision during its progress to prevent complications caused by fluid shift exacerbating cardiac failure or risk of damage to the skin in a diabetic patient (International Society of Lymphology 2013).
- *Physical assessment*: to determine the extent of the oedema and palpation of oedema to identify if it is pitting, non-pitting or fibrosed and to assess the skin condition and limb shape, the patient's disease status and the presence of any pain or altered sensations within the limb (Bianchi et al. 2012, Quéré and Sneddon 2012). The patient's ability to follow a treatment plan, including compression therapy, should also be assessed. The patient should be observed putting on and removing their garment to ensure they can safely do so; consider appliance aids if necessary (see Table 8.8). Weight should be recorded and monitored as obesity increases the risk of developing lymphoedema (Milne 2015). Figure 8.12a is an example of mild, uncomplicated lymphoedema of the arm and Figure 8.12b is an example of severe, uncomplicated lymphoedema of the arm. Figure 8.13 is an example of moderate uncomplicated lymphoedema of the leg.
- *Psychosocial assessment*: to determine the influence of the swelling upon the patient's life. This includes the influence upon limb function and mobility, employment, hobbies, activities and personal roles, and also includes the patient's thoughts on wearing compression garments (Cooper 2014, Woods 2010).

Table 8.8 Examples of application aids

Aid	Description	Supplier
Acti glide	An application to allow open or closed toe compression stockings to glide onto leg	L&R: www.activahealthcare.co.uk

Aid	Description	Supplier
Easy pad	A rectangular piece of non-slip foam to assist with the application of compression garments	Juzo: www.juzo.com
Easy-slide	A limb-shaped slide sheet designed to ensure easy application of the garment with the right amount of pressure	Credenhill: www.credenhill.co.uk

Aid	Description	Supplier
Easy-slide Magnide	A limb-shaped slide sheet with magnets to ease application for closed toe garments	Credenhill: www.credenhill.co.uk

Aid	Description	Supplier
Ezy-As	A rigid 'C' shaped plastic structure designed to assist with fitting of compression garments	Ezy-as: www.ezyasabc.com

Aid	Description	Supplier
Foot slide	A shaped piece of silky material to assist with the application of open toe compression garments over the foot	Supplied with most compression stockings
Medi Butler	A specially designed metal frame that holds the garment in place so that the foot or hand can slide into it. The frame has handles that are used to pull the garment up the limb 	medi: www.mediuk.co.uk
Mediven 2 in 1	A limb-shaped slide sheet that assists with the putting on and taking off of garments 	medi: www.mediuk.co.uk
Rubber gloves	Cotton-lined rubber gloves to provide a better grip on garments to assist in donning and doffing	Widely available in retail shops and also through Haddenham Healthcare: www.hadhealth.com
Sleeve on	A metal applicator with a suction pad to secure the applicator to a firm surface during the application and removal of garments	Haddenham Healthcare: www.hadhealth.com
Slide On Stocking (SOS)	Metal frame designed to hold the garment in place so that the foot can slide into it	Sigvaris: www.sigvaris.com/global/en
Rolly	A flexible plastic band that rolls compression garments on to the limb 	Sigvaris www.sigvaris.com/global/en

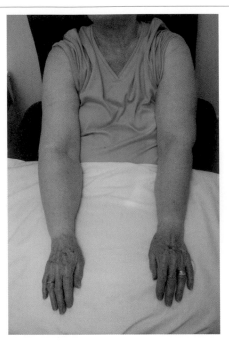

Figure 8.12a Mild uncomplicated arm lymphoedema.

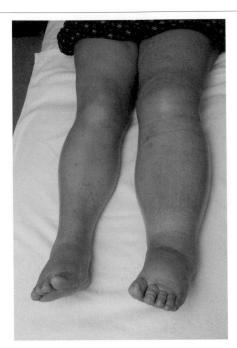

Figure 8.13 Moderate uncomplicated lymphoedema of the leg.

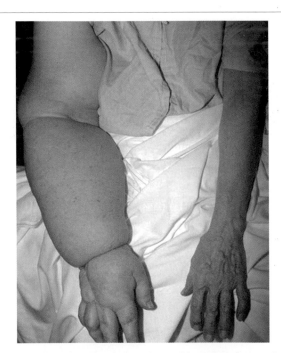

Figure 8.12b Severe uncomplicated lymphoedema of the arm. *Source:* Dougherty and Lister (2011).

- *Implementation*: to determine the appropriateness of interventions and modify them where required. An individualized, holistic approach will incorporate education and support, particularly if personal changes are required to minimize the risk of complications developing. Success will be achieved when the patient possesses positive motivational factors and is an active participant in the management of their lymphoedema (Cooper 2014).
- *Evaluation*: to assess progress, modify and stop the intervention if necessary. To evaluate the outcome of a plan of treatment, suitable outcome indicators are required (Frisby 2010). No standardized method of evaluating the outcome of a plan of treatment has been determined but the measurement of limb volume using surface measurement is the most frequently used means of assessing response to treatment in lymphoedema management (Williams and Whitaker 2015). The effect of treatment on the patient's psychological and psychosocial well-being should, however, also be monitored, and this is frequently achieved in a more subjective manner where the patient's views are sought (Keeley et al. 2010).

Methods of measuring limb size, shape and volume

The measurement of both limbs assists in determining the presence of early lymphoedema in a limb. When swelling is present, limb measurements can objectively identify the degree of swelling to assist in making decisions concerning appropriate treatment. Repeated limb measurements over time can evaluate response to treatment and facilitate motivation with self-management (Williams and Whitaker 2015). Simple measurements of a limb assist in the choice of the correct size of compression garment.

Simple surface measurements of a limb

A frequently used method of establishing alterations in limb size and shape is the circumferential measurement of limb size (Williams and Whitaker 2015). This can be established by recording and comparing measurements taken of both limbs with a tape measure positioned at fixed points on a limb, usually the wrist and 10 cm above and below the point of the elbow (olecranon process) or 15 cm above and below the superior pole of the patella (Piller 1999). Although this method is easy and quick to complete, its use is primarily to track only broad changes in limb

Assessment should also include the following:

- *Planning*: to improve problems and utilize patient strengths. The healthcare professional should work in partnership with the patient to enable them to take appropriate action to manage their lymphoedema and work towards long-term control. Planning should focus on the patient's objectives so that immediate problems can be addressed. Long- and short-term goals can then be identified and agreed with the patient.

circumference. The method is prone to error if the tape measure is not positioned in the same place on each consecutive occasion.

Limb volume measurements of a limb

A more accurate method of assessing response to treatment is the measurement of limb volume (Figure 8.14). Multiple circumferential measurements of both limbs at 4 cm intervals, applied to the formula for the volume of a cylinder, provide a reliable method of determining the size of the limb and a useful, objective means of determining response to treatment. This is the most widely used method of establishing limb volume (Williams and Whitaker 2015). Reproducibility is accurate if care is taken with the procedure and a standard format for the recording of the measurements is used (Ng and Munnoch 2010).

Pre-procedural considerations

The sequential circumferential measurement of a limb for the calculation of limb volume should not be confused with simple limb measurements used in the choice of compression garment for a patient. These are recorded at set points on the limb and used to guide the therapist in choosing the correct size garment for the patient.

The principles in Table 8.9 and points in Table 8.10 should be considered when using sequential circumferential measurements to calculate limb volume (Williams and Whitaker 2015).

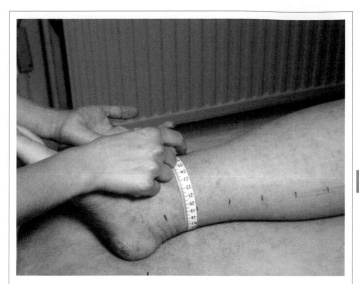

Figure 8.14 Measurement of limb volume. *Source:* Dougherty and Lister (2011).

Table 8.9 Using sequential circumferential measurements to measure limb volume

Indications	Contraindications
To determine the total excess volume of the swollen limb compared with the patient's contralateral normal limb	In palliative care, the tracking of limb volume changes in a limb may not be appropriate and simple circumferential limb measurements can provide an alternative means of assessment
To establish the distribution of the swelling along the limb	In the presence of infection or open wounds
To provide information to assist in the choice of compression therapy	To detect early lymphoedema. Consideration should be given to other symptoms including patterns of transient swelling and any sensation changes (Finlay et al. 2013)
To provide an objective method of determining response to treatment by indicating: • changes in the size and shape of the limb over time • changes in the excess volume • the distribution of any volume loss or gain in the limb (Williams and Whitaker 2015)	

Table 8.10 Points for consideration when recording sequential circumferential measurements to calculate limb volume

Principle	Rationale
Ensure that the same position is used for the same patient each time the limb is measured	The position of the limb will affect the measurements taken because the degree to which muscles are flexed or relaxed will influence the shape and size of the limb
The limb should be marked afresh on each measuring occasion with a washable ink, even when measuring on consecutive days	Any increase or decrease in limb volume will influence the position of the marks on the limb
Tension should not be exerted on the tape measure during measuring	If tension is applied it will vary between measurers and recordings will not be consistent
The tape measure should be positioned so that it is horizontal around the limb, taking care to ensure that it is not pulled tightly	To minimize inaccuracies in measurement
The same number of measurements should be taken on both limbs each time measurements are taken	The normal limb acts as a control in patients with unilateral swelling
The starting point for the taking of measurements should be clearly identified by measuring and clearly recording the distance from the tip of the middle finger to the wrist or base of heel to point above ankle where the tape measure lies flat	This starting point on the wrist/ankle should be used each time
A standard format for the recording of measurements should be adopted	To ensure that key points can be referred to

Procedure guideline 8.8 Compression therapy limb volume calculation: lower limb

Essential equipment
- Ruler, preferably 30 cm or longer
- Tape measure: avoid those made from fabric which tends to stretch and cannot be adequately cleaned; use plastic or disposable paper
- Washable skin marker for marking the limb
- Record chart and pen

Pre-procedure

Action	Rationale
1 Explain and discuss the proposed procedure with the patient.	To ensure that the patient understands the procedure and gives their valid consent (NMC 2015). **C**
2 Place the patient in a sitting position with the legs outstretched horizontally, preferably on a firm couch with adjustable height.	To ensure the lower limbs are relaxed and supported. The adjustable height means that the measurer can work without straining their back. **E**

Procedure

Action	Rationale
3 Standing to the outside of the leg, ask the patient to flex the foot to a right angle. Measure the distance from the base of the heel to the ankle, along the inside of the leg; mark the ankle, allowing at least 2 cm of leg to lie below the mark, and record the distance on the chart.	To establish and clearly record a reproducible fixed starting point for all subsequent measurements (Lymphoedema Framework 2006, **C**). Note: the marks represent a point midway through each cylinder segment, they do not represent the base of the cylinder, therefore at least half the segment (i.e. 2 cm) must lie below the mark.
4 Ask the patient to relax the foot. From the starting point, using a ruler, mark the inside of the leg at 4-cm intervals along the length of the leg up to the groin.	Reducing the limb to 4-cm segments improves the accuracy of measurement since these segments resemble a cylinder more closely than does the whole limb. The formula used here assumes that the measurements are 4 cm apart (Williams and Whitaker 2015, **E**).
5 Place the tape measure around the limb and measure the circumference at each marked point, recording the measurement on the chart. Make sure that the tape lies smoothly around the relaxed limb and that it does not lie at an angle. (Decide at the outset whether the tape is to be placed above, below or on the mark and keep to the same position every time: document position.)	Ensuring that there are no gaps between the limb and the tape and that the procedure is the same each time reduces error (Williams and Whitaker 2015, **E**).
6 Repeat the process on the other leg, whether or not it is swollen.	If only one limb is affected the normal limb acts as the patient's own control (Williams and Whitaker 2015, **E**).
7 If desired, a circumference measurement may be taken of the foot but this is not included in the calculation of volume.	The foot cannot be considered to be a cylinder and it is therefore inappropriate to include it in the calculation of volume.

Post-procedure

Action	Rationale
8 Ensure that the same number of measurements are made and clearly recorded on the record sheet for each leg.	Accurate documentation will ensure accuracy during limb volume calculation for each limb (Williams and Whitaker 2015, **E**).
9 Remove the marks from the patient's skin using warm water and a mild soap preparation.	Removing the marks maintains patient dignity. Mild soap ensures that the skin is not irritated.

Procedure guideline 8.9 Compression therapy limb volume calculation: upper limb

Essential equipment
- Ruler, preferably 30 cm or longer
- Tape measure; avoid those made from fabric which tends to stretch
- Washable skin marker for marking the limb
- Record chart and pen

Pre-procedure

Action	Rationale
1 Explain and discuss the proposed procedure with the patient.	To ensure that the patient understands the procedure and gives their valid consent (NMC 2015, **C**).

2	Sit the patient in a chair with their arms extended in front and resting on the back of a chair. The arms should be as close to an angle of 90° to the body as possible.	To ensure the arms are supported and accessible at a standard height. Changing the angle of the arms to the body will result in changes in the measurements. **E**
3	If only one arm is swollen, start with the unaffected arm.	To establish the normal limb as a control (Williams and Whitaker 2015, **E**).

Procedure

4	Measure the distance from the tip of the middle finger to the wrist. Mark the wrist, allowing at least 2 cm above the ulnar styloid, and note down the distance.	To establish and clearly record a reproducible fixed starting point for all subsequent measurements (Lymphoedema Framework 2006, **E**).
		Note: The marks represent a point midway through each cylinder segment, they do not represent the base of the cylinder, therefore at least half the segment (i.e. 2 cm) must lie below the mark.
5	From the starting point, using a ruler, mark along the ulnar aspect of the arm at 4-cm intervals up to the axilla.	Reducing the limb to 4-cm segments improves the accuracy of measurement since these segments resemble a cylinder more closely than does the whole limb (Williams and Whitaker 2015, **E**).
6	Place the tape measure around the limb and measure the circumference at each marked point, recording each measurement on the chart. Make sure that the tape lies smoothly around the relaxed limb and that it does not lie at an angle. Decide at the outset whether the tape is to be placed above, below or on the mark and keep to the same position every time.	Ensuring that there are no gaps between the limb and the tape and that the procedure is the same each time reduces error (Williams and Whitaker 2015, **E**).
7	Repeat the process on the other arm.	If only one limb is affected, the normal limb acts as the patient's own control (Williams and Whitaker 2015, **E**).
8	If desired, a circumference measurement may be taken of the hand but this is not included in the calculation of volume.	The hand cannot be considered to be a cylinder and it is therefore inappropriate to include it in the calculation. **E**
9	Ensure that the same number of measurements are made and clearly recorded on the record sheet for each arm.	Accurate documentation will ensure accuracy during limb volume calculation for each limb (Williams and Whitaker 2015, **E**).

Post-procedure

10	Remove the marks from the patient's skin using warm water and a mild soap preparation.	Removing the marks maintains patient dignity. Mild soap ensures that the skin is not irritated. **E**

Problem-solving table 8.3 Prevention and resolution (Procedure guidelines 8.8 and 8.9)

Problem	Cause	Prevention	Action
The tape measure will not lie evenly on the surface of the skin because of the shape of the limb and development of deepened skin folds.	The effect of the lymphoedema on the tissues and the distribution of swelling.	The limb shape can be artificially corrected.	Wrap the limb in cling film to create a more cylindrical shape. Mark the cling film and measure at these points.
Loose areas of skin, making it difficult to place the tape measure smoothly around the limb.	Age-related loss of skin turgor or weight loss causing excess skin.	The limb shape can be artificially corrected.	Elevation of the limb distributes the excess skin and a more accurate measurement of the limb can be obtained.
Limited range of movement of upper limb, making limb positioning difficult.	Brachial plexopathy.	Work within the patient's ability.	Position the limb comfortably and seek assistance if necessary to support the limb.
Skin lesions, open wounds, pain or tenderness resulting in the omission of some measuring points and inaccurate calculation of limb volume.	Measurements cannot be taken where there is a breach of skin integrity or pain.	Carefully examine the skin for breaks in skin integrity prior to measuring and check that the patient is comfortable so that action can be taken if necessary.	Cover any open wounds with cling film to ensure measurements can be taken in the required place. Avoid pulling the measuring tape tightly to avoid trauma to the area.

Post-procedural considerations

Once a sequential circumference measurement of both limbs has been recorded, a few formulas may be used to calculate the limb volume of each limb (Williams and Whitaker 2015).

The formula for the volume of a cylinder (Box 8.8) considers the limb as a series of cylinders, each with a height of 4 cm.

To calculate the volume of the limb, each measurement needs to be converted into a volume for that segment of the cylinder and then totalled. This is illustrated in Table 8.11.

The volume difference between the limbs is then usually expressed as a percentage. The calculation for this is shown in Table 8.12.

Compression bandaging

Definition

Short-stretch, inelastic bandages are used during the intensive or reduction phase of treatment for lymphoedema.

Related theory

The bandages used in compression therapy are termed 'short-stretch bandages'. They have a high resistance to stretch. When applied to a limb, they provide it with a firm external encasement. During joint movement and muscular contraction of the limb, pressure against the firm external encasement leads to a temporary increase in pressure within the tissues (working pressure), providing a massaging effect on the lymphatics as well as the

Box 8.8 Procedure for calculating volume from circumferences

> The formula for calculating the volume of a cylinder is $\frac{circumference^2}{\pi}$. The formula must be applied to each circumference measurement ($circ_1$, $circ_2$, ..., $circ_n$) in order to calculate the volume of each segment; the volumes are then totalled to give the total limb volume.
>
> $$So \left(\frac{circ_1 \times circ_1}{3.1415}\right) + \left(\frac{circ_2 \times circ_2}{3.1415}\right) + \left(\frac{circ_3 \times circ_3}{3.1415}\right) + ...etc.$$
>
> Using a programmable calculator to calculate the volume of a cylinder will speed up the process of calculation.

Table 8.11 Example calculation of the total volume of a limb using the formula in Box 8.8

Circumference measurement (cm)	C^2/π (3.14)	Volume of each cylinder (mL)
18.4	=	107.7
19.1	=	116.1
21	=	140.3
23.2	=	171.3
24.9	=	197.3
25.7	=	210.2
26.6	=	225.2
29.6	=	278.8
30.3	=	292.2
31.7	=	319.8
32.7	=	340.3
33.5	=	357.2
Total volume	=	**2757**

Table 8.12 Calculating the volume difference between the limbs as a percentage

Formula for calculation

Divide 100 by unaffected limb volume and multiply by the volume difference between the limbs

Worked example

Swollen limb volume	Unaffected limb volume	Difference between the limbs
2757	Minus 2459	Equals 298
100 divided by 2459 (unaffected limb volume)	Multiplied by 298 (volume difference between the limbs)	Equals 12.11

The swollen limb is 12% bigger than the normal limb

venous system to stimulate lymph drainage (Partsch and Mortimer 2015, Williams 2012b). Conversely, when the muscle is inactive during rest, short-stretch bandages support the tissues and provide a relatively low resting pressure. This ensures that the patient remains comfortable and encourages compliance with the planned course of treatment (Williams 2012b).

Long-stretch bandages with a high degree of elasticity are unsuitable for the management of lymphoedema. These bandages exert a high working and high resting pressure on the tissues of the limb and can be uncomfortable when left in place for long periods of time.

The pressure exerted by the short-stretch bandage on the limb is influenced by a number of factors:

- *The circumference of the limb*: the highest pressure is achieved where the limb is narrowest (Partsch 2012). When a bandage is applied to a limb of normal proportions, therefore, the highest pressure will be achieved at the ankle or wrist, with graduated, reducing pressure along the length of the limb as the circumference increases (Quéré and Sneddon 2012). Limbs that are thin and areas where there are bony prominences will need careful protection to avoid high pressure on these exposed areas which can lead to skin or tissue damage (Linnitt 2011).
- *The number of layers*: every bandage is applied with a degree of overlap. Several layers applied over each other increase the stiffness and pressure applied to the limb (Partsch and Mortimer 2015).
- *The components of the bandage system*: the use of padding and foam beneath the bandages increases the sub-bandage pressure and stiffness of the assembled bandage (Partsch and Mortimer 2015).

Evidence-based approaches

Rationale

Indications
- *Large limbs*. Elastic compression garments used on large swollen limbs may be ineffective due to the difficulties of applying sufficient tension to compress the limb (Linnitt 2011).
- *Mis-shapen limbs*. Elastic compression garments cannot accommodate extreme shape distortion (Linnitt 2011). Elastic compression garments can tourniquet in skin folds if the limb is awkwardly shaped, and can cause discomfort or skin damage (Todd 2013). Foam or soft padding placed under short-stretch bandages will smooth out the folds and restore normal shape to the limb. (See Figures 8.15 and 8.16 for examples of a misshapen limb before and after bandaging.)

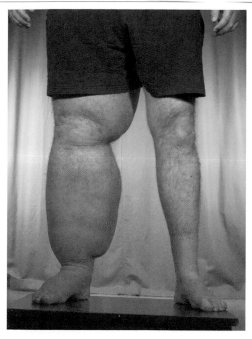

Figure 8.15 Example of a misshapen limb before bandaging. *Source:* Dougherty and Lister (2011).

- *Severe lymphoedema.* Large limbs with long-standing oedema require high pressures to break down tissue fibrosis. Short-stretch bandages provide a low resting and high working pressure which promotes a softening of hardened tissues (Partsch and Moffatt 2012).
- *Lymphorrhoea.* The leakage of lymph fluid from the skin responds readily to external pressure provided by short-stretch bandages (Board and Anderson 2013).
- *Damaged or fragile skin.* Elastic compression garments can cause damage to fragile skin. Short-stretch bandages should be used until the skin condition improves (Linnitt 2011).

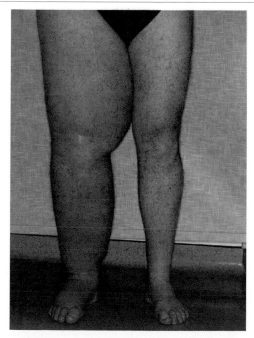

Figure 8.16 Example of a misshapen limb after bandaging. *Source:* Dougherty and Lister (2011).

Contraindications

Short-stretch bandages should not be used if (Todd 2013):

- there is arterial disease; tissue ischaemia can occur
- there is infection in the swollen limb; pain may occur
- there is uncontrolled cardiac failure; fluid overload can occur
- there is deep vein thrombosis; anticoagulation therapy should be commenced prior to the use of bandages
- the patient lacks manual dexterity and would be unable to remove bandages if they became uncomfortable.

Principles to be followed in multilayer bandaging

This discussion of multilayer bandaging will focus on the use of short-stretch, inelastic bandages using a standard approach to application. The application of alternative bandaging systems available (usually comprising two layers: a foam padding layer for comfort and a self-adhesive compression layer) will not be discussed in this section. Short-stretch bandages are available in a range of widths and provide a low resting pressure to the swollen limb when the muscle is inactive and a high working pressure during activity when the muscle is pumping against the resistance created by the bandage (Partsch and Mortimer 2015).

For bandaging to be effective, the following principles must be considered:

- *An even pressure should be provided around the circumference of the limb.* Where the limb shape is irregular or distorted by swelling, an even profile can be achieved with the use of padding or foam to add bulk to an area where shape requires correcting (Schuren 2012).
- *The pressure from the bandages must be graduated along the length of the limb to ensure that the greatest pressure is achieved distally and the least proximally.* Graduated pressure will be achieved naturally in a regularly shaped limb where the circumference of the wrist or ankle is smaller than the circumference of the root of the limb. Graduated pressure can also be achieved by selecting the correct bandage width for the size of the limb and controlling the amount of bandage tension and overlap used (Hegarty-Craver et al. 2014). Moderate tension only should be used and the bandages should never be stretched to their maximum length.
- *The pressure applied to the limb should be adequate to counter the limb circumference.* Greater pressure is required when the circumference of the limb is large. This can be achieved by using more than one layer of bandages and selecting the correct width of bandage for the circumference of the limb (Hegarty-Craver et al. 2014).
- *The bandages should be left in place day and night and removed once every 24 hours.* This enables skin hygiene to be attended to and the condition of the skin to be checked. Reapplication of the bandages then ensures that effective compression is maintained on the changing limb shape (Quéré and Sneddon 2012).
- *The bandages should be comfortable for the patient and removed at any time if they cause any pain, numbness or discoloration (blueness) in the fingers or toes.* This may indicate a variety of causes, including too great a compression on the limb. A satisfactory outcome of treatment should be achieved within 2–3 weeks. More advanced stages of lymphoedema may require up to 4–6 weeks of treatment. The patient may then begin the maintenance phase of treatment in which containment compression garments are fitted.

Palliative care

Compression bandaging can be versatile and extremely useful in the palliative care setting when volume reduction may be unrealistic or not indicated and the emphasis is on optimizing the patient's quality of life.

The burden of treatment should not exceed the benefit to be gained from providing support and comfort to a limb with a low level of pressure using a modified technique of bandaging designed around the patient's needs. The therapist should have expertise to apply the correct degree of pressure to the limb and avoid forcing fluid into adjacent areas (Towers 2012). Many hospices now employ a lymphoedema therapist to support palliative care patients.

Legal and professional issues

Ensure the patient understands the procedure and all it entails and has given consent (NMC 2015). Written information should also be supplied. Compression bandaging should only be carried out by a skilled therapist with the necessary skills and experience to apply bandages to the swollen limb (Quéré and Sneddon 2012), ensuring that pressure is graduated towards the root of the limb and evenly applied. Poor technique can lead to serious consequences with damage to the skin and tissues if the bandages are incorrectly or inappropriately applied (Linnitt 2011). The therapist has a professional responsibility to ensure the safety of the patient and should therefore always ensure that there are no contraindications to the use of low-stretch compression bandages. Therapists also have a duty to maintain the knowledge and skills they need for safe and effective practice (NMC 2015).

Appropriate courses are available for therapists throughout the UK, however there is no one specific body that accredits therapists.

Pre-procedural considerations

Specific patient preparations

Arterial blood flow

If there is any concern regarding the patient's arterial blood flow, an ABPI should be measured using a hand-held Doppler before undertaking any compression therapy. An ABPI reading of 0.8 or below should be referred for medical opinion (Cooper 2015).

Appropriate clothing

The bandaging materials used on a swollen limb can be bulky and patients will therefore require appropriate information and advice concerning suitable loose-fitting, easily applied clothing and, if the leg is being bandaged, appropriate wide-opening footwear that will accommodate the bulk of the bandages during treatment.

Timing of appointments

As the bandages are worn for 23 hours a day, the timing of appointments for the bandages to be replaced will need to consider opportunities to attend to personal hygiene, travel arrangements and family and work commitments. The bandages can be removed at home before the appointment to allow for personal hygiene but it is advisable for the patient to wear a suitable compression garment on the journey to the appointment.

Driving

It is not recommended that patients drive themselves in a car to or from appointments. The bandages will mean that the affected limb will be bulkier than usual, making reaction times slower. Safety can therefore be compromised. If the patient chooses to drive, they must be advised to check with their motor insurance company before doing so.

Activities of daily living

Activities of daily living may have to be adapted because of the bulk of the bandages. The therapist should discuss and outline with the patient an appropriate exercise regimen to be followed during treatment, to ensure that maximum effectiveness is gained from the course of bandaging.

Information

Verbal information given should be supported by written information and include details of what the patient should do if problems develop with the bandages and whom to contact (Fu et al. 2014).

Procedure guideline 8.10   Compression bandaging (multilayer short-stretch): bandaging an arm and the fingers

Essential equipment
- Tubular stockinette: this can be purchased in a long roll and a length cut to suit the limb size. Different widths are available
- Light retention bandages: 6 and 10 cm to bandage digits and to hold foam padding in place
- Synthetic orthopaedic padding rolls: 6 cm, 10 cm to pad and reshape the limb
- Shaped/contoured foam pieces to apply compression to areas of fibrosis
- Pieces of low-density foam cut to shape to pad out uneven areas
- Low-stretch bandages, 6 and 8 cm. A variety of widths is required to suit the shape of the limb
- Tape

Pre-procedure

Action	Rationale
1 Explain and discuss the procedure with the patient.	To ensure that the patient understands the procedure and gives their valid consent (NMC 2015, **C**).
2 If possible, the patient should be seated in a chair with the limb relaxed and supported on the back of a chair or appropriate limb support. The therapist should be positioned in front of the patient.	To ensure the comfort of both the patient and therapist. To ensure that the skin and muscles are positioned correctly to avoid inappropriate areas of pressure. **E**
3 The swollen limb should be clean and well moisturized with a bland emollient (e.g. E45) before being bandaged.	To promote skin hygiene and integrity. **E**

Procedure

4 Cut a length of tubular stockinette long enough to fit the patient's arm. Cut a small hole for the thumb and slip over the patient's arm.	To protect the skin from chafing and from any sensitivity caused by the synthetic materials of the padding and foam (Quéré and Sneddon 2012, **E**).

5 The fingers must be bandaged (**Action figure 5a** and Figure 8.17a). Using a narrow light retention bandage, anchor the bandage loosely at the wrist and bring it across the back of the hand to the thumb. Bandage around the thumb from the tip downwards (start at the level of the nail bed). Do not pull the bandage tight but go gently and firmly. Take the bandage under the wrist and back over the back of the hand to the index finger (**Action figure 5b**). Again, bandage from the nail bed down to the webs of the finger. Repeat the same procedure for all fingers. Finish by tucking in the end of the bandage (**Action figure 5c** and Figure 8.17b).

To reduce or prevent swelling (Quéré and Sneddon 2012, **E**).

6 Check the colour and temperature of the tips of the fingers.

To ensure that the blood supply is not compromised (Quéré and Sneddon 2012, **E**).

7 Check that the patient can move the fingers and make a fist.

To check that the bandage is not too tight (Quéré and Sneddon 2010, **E**).

8 Flat, ridged or contoured foam can be cut to size and used over stockinette in areas of fibrosis or for additional compression (see Figure 8.17c).

To produce a massaging effect over fibrotic tissue to soften tissue (Quéré and Sneddon 2012, **E**).

9 Using the roll of padding, cover the hand in a figure of eight, padding out the palm and back of the hand (**Action figure 9** and Figure 8.17d).

Padding out the hand ensures even pressure distribution and protects the bony areas of the hand (Quéré and Sneddon 2012, **E**).

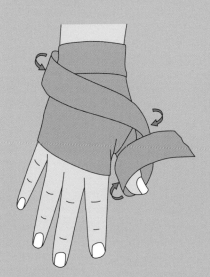

Action Figure 5a Bandaging swollen fingers.

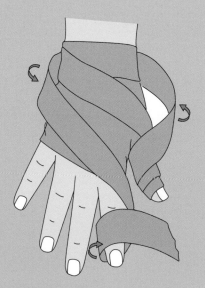

Action Figure 5b Bandage is taken under wrist, back over hand, to index finger.

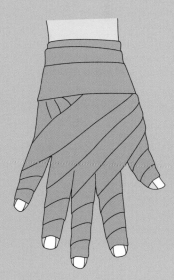

Action Figure 5c Finished bandage.

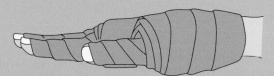

Action Figure 9 Palm and back of hand are padded out.

(continued)

Procedure guideline 8.10 Compression bandaging (multilayer short-stretch): bandaging an arm and the fingers *(continued)*

Action	Rationale
10 Continue the padding up to the axilla, doubling it over at the elbow (**Action figure 10** and Figure 8.17d).	Doubling it over at the elbow crease protects the delicate skin at the elbow. **E**
11 Take a 6-cm compression bandage and start by anchoring it loosely at the wrist. Advise the patient to hold their fingers apart while the hand is bandaged and take the bandage across the dorsum of the hand to wrap it twice around the hand close to the base of the fingers. Continue bandaging the hand firmly in a figure of eight until all the hand is covered (see **Action figure 11**). Continue the rest of the bandage up the forearm in a spiral, covering half of the bandage with each turn. Keep the bandage as smooth as possible (Figures 8.17e and f).	The bandage width must relate to the circumference of the limb with the narrowest bandage used on the smallest circumference (Quéré and Sneddon 2012, **E**).
12 Take an 8- or 10-cm bandage and, starting at the wrist, bandage in a spiral, still covering half of the bandage with each turn, up to the top of the arm (**Action figure 12** and Figure 8.17g).	Two layers are used on the forearm to ensure that pressure is highest distally (Quéré and Sneddon 2012, **E**).
13 A top layer of bandages can be applied in a spiral.	Applying a top layer can even out and maintain optimal pressure. **E**
14 Secure the end of the bandage with tape.	Tape is used instead of fastening clips due to risk of injury. **E**

Post-procedure

15 Once again, check the colour and sensations of the finger tips and check that the patient can move all joints.	To check that the blood flow is not compromised (Quéré and Sneddon 2012, **E**).
16 Remind the patient to use the limb as normally as possible, to exercise as advised and to remove the bandages if any pain, tingling or numbness is experienced.	To ensure good lymph flow and to prevent complications developing. **E**
17 Record the details of the procedure followed in the patient's relevant documentation.	To maintain accurate records and provide a point of reference for subsequent treatment (NMC 2015, **C**).

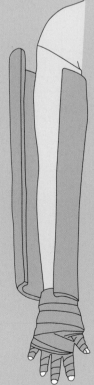

Action Figure 10 Rolls of padding are applied firmly in a spiral up the arm, starting around the hand. Extra padding is applied to the elbow crease.

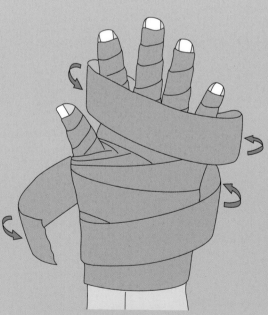

Action Figure 11 Hand is bandaged firmly in a figure of eight using a 6 cm compression bandage.

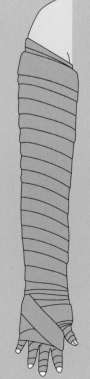

Action Figure 12 Starting at the wrist, an 8 or 10 cm bandage is used to cover to the top of the arm, in a spiral fashion.

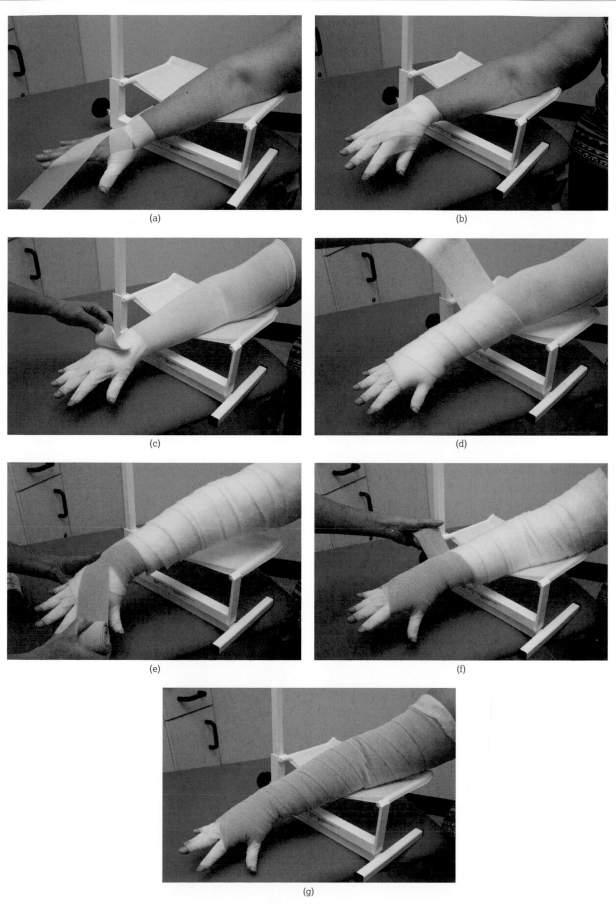

Figure 8.17 a–g Bandaging an arm and the fingers.

Procedure guideline 8.11   Compression bandaging (multilayer short-stretch): bandaging a leg and the toes

Essential equipment

- Tubular stockinette: this can be purchased in a long roll and a length cut to suit the limb size. Different widths are available
- Light retention bandages: 4-cm width to bandage the toes, 6-cm or 10-cm to hold foam in place
- Synthetic orthopaedic padding rolls: 6-cm, 10-cm and 12-cm width rolls to pad and reshape the limb
- Sheet of low-density foam to cut to shape and pad out uneven areas
- Low-stretch compression bandages, 8, 10 and 12 cm. A variety of widths is required to suit the shape of the limb
- Tape scissors

Pre-procedure

Action	Rationale
1 Explain and discuss the procedure with the patient.	To ensure that the patient understands the procedure and gives their valid consent (NMC 2015, **C**).
2 If possible, the patient should be seated upright on a bed or treatment couch. Raise the bed or couch to a comfortable height.	To ensure the comfort of both the patient and nurse. **E**
3 The swollen limb should be clean and well moisturized with a bland emollient (e.g. E45) before being bandaged.	To promote skin hygiene and integrity (Cooper 2012, **E**).

Procedure

Action	Rationale
4 Cut a length of tubular stockinette long enough to fit the patient's leg. Slip over the leg.	To protect the skin from chafing (Quéré and Sneddon 2012, **E**).
5 If the toes are swollen or tend to swell, they must be bandaged. The little toe can be omitted. Using a narrow light retention bandage, anchor the bandage around the foot and bring across the top of the foot to the big toe (**Action figure 5a** and Figure 8.18a). Bandage around the toe from the tip downwards (start at the level of the nail bed). Do not pull the bandage tight, but proceed gently and firmly. Take the bandage under the foot and back over the top of the foot to the next toe (**Action figure 5b**). Repeat the same procedure for each toe that needs to be bandaged. Finish by tucking in the end of the bandage (**Action figure 5c**).	To reduce or prevent swelling (Quéré and Sneddon 2012). To prevent friction to and around the little toe. **E**
6 Foam pads can be cut to size and placed over the dorsum of the foot, around the ankle and behind the knee (**Action figures 6a, 6b**).	To protect bony prominences and joint flexures (Quéré and Sneddon 2012, **E**).
7 Secure the pads firmly in place with light retention bandages.	
8 Using padding, even out any exaggerated contours of the limb. Corrugated or contoured foam can be used over areas of fibrotic tissue.	To create a smooth profile on which to apply the bandages. To apply additional compression or to treat fibrotic areas (Cooper 2012, **E**).

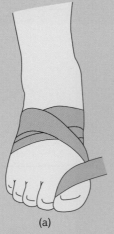
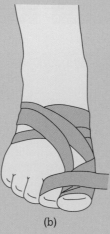
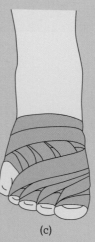

(a)   (b)   (c)

Action Figure 5 (a) A narrow light retention bandage is anchored around the foot and brought across the foot to the big toe. (b) The toes are bandaged in turn from the nail bed along the length of the toe. (c) The bandage is taken under the foot and back over the top of the foot to bandage the next toe.

9 Using a 10-cm roll of padding, apply firmly in a spiral up the leg, starting around the foot. Use the 20-cm padding over the thigh (**Action figure 9** and Figures 8.18b and c).	To protect the skin and create a smooth profile on which to bandage (Quéré and Sneddon 2012).
10 Advise the patient to hold their foot at a 90° angle while it is bandaged. Use 8-cm compression bandage and begin by anchoring it with a double layer wrapped around the foot close to the base of toes (**Action figure 10**, Figures 8.19d and e). Continue bandaging the foot firmly, forming a figure of eight to cover the heel and ankle without leaving any gaps. Any surplus bandage should be taken up the leg in a spiral.	To avoid constriction at the ankle. Fluid will accumulate in any unbandaged areas (Quéré and Sneddon 2012, **E**).
11 Using a 10-cm bandage, continue from where the first bandage finished, using a spiral up the leg and covering half of the bandage with each turn (50% overlap). Remember to bandage firmly. Use the widest bandage over the thigh. Secure the end of the last bandage with tape (Figure 8.19f).	The bandage width must relate to the circumference of the limb with the narrowest bandage used on the smallest circumference (Quéré and Sneddon 2012, **E**).
12 Apply a second layer of bandage, from ankle to thigh, using a spiral or figure of eight. Secure the end with tape (**Action figure 12**, Figures 8.18g and h).	To keep the bandages in place and provide additional pressure along the length of the leg (Quéré and Sneddon 2012, **E**).

Post-procedure

13 Check the colour and temperature of the patient's toes. It may be difficult for the patient to flex the knee at first but this should get easier as the bandages loosen slightly.	To check that the blood flow is not compromised (Quéré and Sneddon 2012, **E**).
14 Remind the patient to use the limb as normally as possible, to exercise as advised and to remove the bandages if any pain, tingling or numbness is experienced.	To ensure good lymph flow and to prevent complications developing (Quéré and Sneddon 2012, **E**).
15 Record the details of the procedure in the relevant patient documentation.	To maintain accurate records and provide a point of reference for subsequent treatment (NMC 2015, **C**).

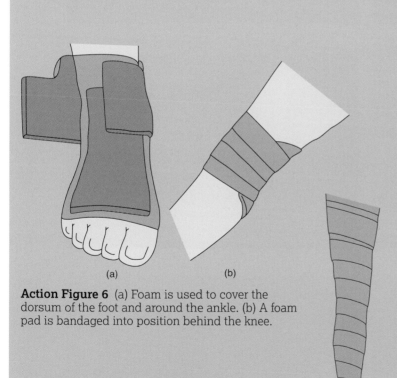

(a)   (b)

Action Figure 6 (a) Foam is used to cover the dorsum of the foot and around the ankle. (b) A foam pad is bandaged into position behind the knee.

Action Figure 9 Rolls of padding are applied firmly in a spiral up the leg, starting around the foot.

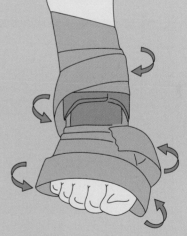

Action Figure 10 Bandaging the foot using an 8-cm compression bandage and starting close to the toes.

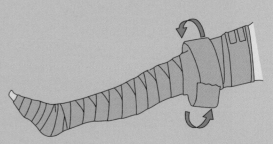

Action Figure 12 Applying a second layer of bandage, from ankle to thigh.

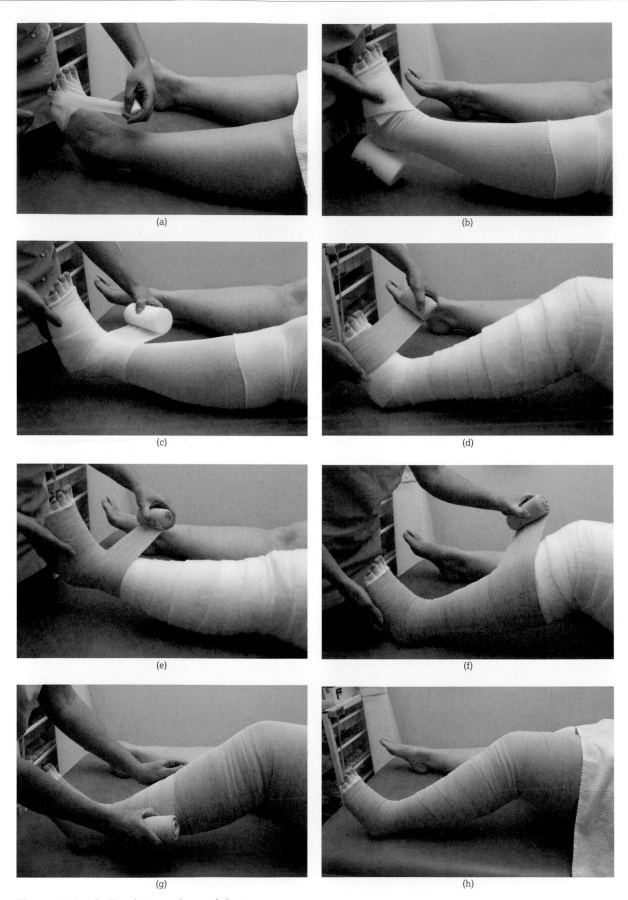

Figure 8.18 a–h Bandaging a leg and the toes.

Problem-solving table 8.4 Prevention and resolution (Procedure guidelines 8.10 and 8.11)

Problem	Cause	Prevention	Action
Patient becomes breathless.	An unknown cardiac pathology may lead to fluid overload as the lymphatic fluid moves from the swollen limb.		Initiate immediate first aid and seek medical attention if the patient becomes breathless during compression bandaging. Compression bandaging should be stopped until the patient's condition is stabilized.
Pain, discomfort, numbness and/or tingling of digits when bandages are in place.	Incorrect pressure gradient.	Ensure patient gives feedback throughout the procedure. Observe the skin each day for signs of inflammation where excess pressure may have been applied.	Check the pressure gradient after each bandage application. Ensure overlap of bandages is even along the length of the limb. Feel the pressure of the bandages regularly to ensure the consistency of the gradient.
Pain and tenderness over bony prominences noted when the bandages are removed, for example wrist and ankle.	Inadequate padding over bony prominences.	Careful assessment of the limb shape prior to application of bandages.	Use foam and padding to protect bony prominences and even out the shape of the limb.
Skin irritation developing in sensitive areas, for example elbow crease and popliteal crease, during the course of bandaging.	Areas of excess movement resulting in friction from the bandages.	Ensure there are no skin allergies to the materials being used.	Use appropriate moisturizer for the patient. Protect the limb with stockinette. Use extra padding in areas of sensitivity.
Poor compliance with bandaging causing premature removal of bandages each day.	Lack of information given to patient. Lifestyle commitments.	Ensure the patient is given appropriate information verbally and in writing prior to commencement of treatment.	Explore the problems the patient is experiencing. Explain the procedure thoroughly and its intended benefits.
Congestion developing at the root of the limb during bandaging.	Too much pressure throughout the limb causing an overload of fluid at the root of the limb.		Reduce the pressure of the bandage throughout the limb. Teach simple lymphatic drainage (SLD). Carry out manual lymphatic drainage (MLD).

357

Post-procedural considerations

Immediate care

Evaluation of each stage of the bandaging procedure is essential to ensure that the bandage and padding have been used appropriately and correctly. This ensures that the best results are being achieved and that resources are being used to the maximum.

The process of evaluation must be thorough and should include the following.

- *Continuous attention to the colour of the digits.* Too much pressure will result in compromised circulation.
- *Continuous attention to the sensations experienced in the bandaged limb.* The bandages should not cause pain, numbness or tingling.
- *The shape of the limb.* A cylindrical contour should be achieved with the use of soft foam and padding.
- *The overlap of the bandages.* This should be even and consistent with no gaps in the bandages.
- *The pressure achieved.* This should feel even to the patient and there should be no creases in the bandages. Layers should be used appropriately (Quéré and Sneddon 2012). The therapist should feel the bandages regularly during the procedure to ensure the consistency of the gradient.

Ongoing care

The patient should feel comfortable and be able to move their limb. Information should be given concerning when and how to remove the bandages if necessary. The patient should be made aware that if the bandages do have to be removed, a compression garment must be worn until their next appointment. It is vital that the patient reports any concerns to the therapist at each visit.

Compression garments

Definition

Elastic compression garments are used in the long-term management of lymphoedema. Patients are required to wear their garments daily, with most patients wearing their garments all day and removing them at night. For some patients, their treatment plan may include the flexibility to wear the garment just for exertive activities or for a few hours each day, depending upon their needs.

Evidence-based approaches

Rationale

Choosing the correct garment for the patient can be a difficult decision and should always follow a detailed assessment of the patient (Todd 2015). It should only be undertaken by a healthcare professional with knowledge and appropriate skills to ensure patient safety.

The size of the required garment can be determined by following the manufacturer's individual size chart and recording three or four circumferential measurements at set points along the length of the limb. It is important to remember that size charts provide a guide only, and the patient's evaluation of the comfort of the fitted garment is essential. An alternative style or a larger or smaller size may be required.

Indications

- Mild, uncomplicated swelling with a normal limb shape (Nazarko 2014).
- The maintenance of limb shape and size following a course of intensive therapy (Quéré and Sneddon 2012).
- To control swelling and provide support in the palliative treatment of oedema (Norton and Towers 2010).

Contraindications

- *Arterial disease.* Blood supply may be further compromised (Elwell 2016).
- *Acute heart failure.* Symptoms may be exacerbated (Elwell 2016).
- *Distortion of limb shape.* The garment will not fit (Todd 2013).
- *Skin folds.* The garment will cause ridges and a tourniquet effect to the limb (Todd 2013).
- *Open wounds.* The garment will become soiled and pose an infection risk.
- *Fragile skin.* Application and removal of the garment may cause further damage to the skin (Todd 2013).
- *Lymphorrhoea.* The garment will become wet and may cause skin excoriation (Todd 2013).
- *An acute infective episode (cellulitis).* Application and removal of the garment may be painful and cause damage to the friable skin (Elwell 2016).
- *Severe peripheral neuropathy.* The patient will not be able to tell if the garment is causing damage to the skin (Elwell 2016).

Legal and professional issues
Ensure the patient understands how to use compression garments and has given consent (NMC 2015).

Pre-procedural considerations
Several factors need to be taken into consideration before deciding to fit a patient with an elastic compression garment. The patient should be motivated and compliant with the use of garments and have the physical skills to apply and remove the garment safely. A full physical assessment of the patient will determine the condition of the skin and tissues and the shape and size of the limb in order to determine the style, size and appropriate compression class of garment suitable for the patient.

Equipment
A wide range of elastic compression garments for the treatment of lymphoedema is now available on the drug tariff, making it easier for patients to establish a long-term supply of their garments.

Elastic compression garments apply an external force to the limb which pulls in to exert pressure on the tissues below (Partsch 2012). The pressure can be sustained over long periods of time during both activity and inactivity of the limb, providing a high working pressure while the muscle is active and a high resting pressure during inactivity of the muscle at rest (Elwell 2015).

It is important to acknowledge that different classifications of compression exist. These are determined by testing methods, yarn specification, compression gradient and garment durability (Elwell 2016). In the UK, elastic compression garments are

Table 8.13 Compression classes and indications for their use

Indications	Suggested compression level
Mild lymphoedema	Class 1
• Excess limb volume <20% • No shape distortion • Maintenance • Palliation	*Low compression* British Standard: 14–21 mmHg French Standard: 10–15 mmHg German Standard: 18–21 mmHg
Moderate lymphoedema	Class 2
• Excess limb volume 20–40% • Mild shape distortion • Maintenance	*Medium compression* British Standard: 18–24 mmHg French Standard: 15–20 mmHg German Standard: 22–32 mmHg
Severe lymphoedema	Class 3
• Excess limb volume >40% • Moderate shape distortion • Fibrosed tissues • Skin changes; hyperkeratosis and papillomatosis	*High compression* British Standard: 25–35 mmHg French Standard: 22–32 mmHg German Standard: 34–46 mmHg

available in the British Standard BS 6612, French Standard ASQUAL and German Standard RAL-GZ 387:2000. Each standard adopts different testing techniques to determine the degree of pressure measured at the ankle when the garment is in place, and the pressure range used to define the compression class of the garment differs between each of these standards (Partsch 2012, Todd 2015). The compression levels used are generally higher than those used to treat venous disease and are classified according to the range of pressure exerted at the ankle by the garment. Table 8.13 outlines the indications for compression garments and the suggested compression classification. Although the differing standards may appear confusing, it is useful to be able to select garments from a range of manufacturers to find the most suitable garment and to allow patients a wider choice.

The use of elastic compression garments (Partsch and Mortimer 2015):

- increases interstitial tissue pressure and reduces production of lymph
- promotes lymph movement along superficial and deep lymphatics
- increases lymph reabsorption
- provides an external counterforce during activity which enhances muscle pump action.

A wide range of garments are available which differ in construction, compression class and style, in addition to size and colour.

- *Construction.* Garments are manufactured as either round-knit or flat-knit. Round-knit garments are produced in one piece from synthetic fibres and are readily available in a variety of sizes 'off the shelf' to accommodate the needs of most patients. Although more cosmetically acceptable to patients, these garments tend to roll or gather in areas along the limb if the limb is mis-shapen (Todd 2013). They are more suitable therefore for patients whose limbs have maintained a regular shape. Some round-knit garments are manufactured with inelastic materials, creating a stiffer garment. The pressure under these garments will be higher while the muscle is active. Flat-knit garments are manufactured from one piece of material sewn together with a seam. The shape can be adjusted during manufacture to suit patients' specific needs and the provision of accurate measurements before manufacture ensures a good fit. Flat-knit garments offer the highest working pressure relative to their resting pressure and are more suitable for patients with moderate to severe lymphoedema (Todd 2015).

- *Compression class*. The degree of pressure exerted by the garment on the surface of the skin it surrounds determines its compression class (Todd 2015). The highest compression provided by a garment when fitted can be found at the wrist or the ankle. The compression is then graduated along the length of the limb to encourage movement of the fluid out of the limb.
- *Style*. All areas affected by swelling must be contained within the compression garment or further swelling will develop. The patient should be instructed concerning the application, removal and care of the garment to ensure that maximum effectiveness is achieved through its use. The patient's physical ability must be taken into account when choosing a garment as a high degree of dexterity and strength may be required during its application and removal and this may be impractical for the patient (Todd 2015).
- *Size*. The correct garment is one that fits well and is comfortable for the patient with no loose pockets of material where swelling can develop and no areas of constriction where a tourniquet effect can occur. The manufacturer's guidance for choosing the correct size is based on simple limb measurements and particular attention should be given to the fit at the ankle or wrist where high levels of compression can occur (Todd 2015).

The application of elastic garments can be greatly eased by the wearing of household rubber gloves during application; gloves facilitate control of the garment and prevent damage to its fabric. Application aids are also available commercially and may assist some patients who experience difficulties (see Table 8.8). Moisturizing cream should be applied at night-time rather than in the morning before putting the garment on. A very fine layer of talcum powder applied to hot sticky skin can ease application. If this is the first time that the patient has worn elastic compression garments, the therapist should explain to the patient that the feeling of pressure may seem strange for the first few hours, but that it should not cause pain in the limb or numbness in the digits or toes.

Procedure guideline 8.12   Elastic compression garments: application to the leg

Essential equipment
- Appropriate application aids if required (see Table 8.8)
- A compression garment that is appropriate for the patient's lymphoedema (see Figure 8.19)

Pre-procedure

Action	Rationale
1 Explain and discuss the procedure with the patient.	To ensure that the patient understands the procedure and gives their valid consent (NMC 2015, **C**).
2 If possible, position the patient seated upright on a bed or couch and raise the height to a comfortable level.	To ensure the comfort of both the patient and nurse. **E**

Procedure

Action	Rationale
3 Turn the stocking inside out to the heel.	This makes it easier to ease the stocking up. **E**
4 Pull the foot of the stocking over the patient's foot.	
5 Turn the rest of the stocking back over the foot and up the leg.	To prevent a tourniquet effect developing at the ankle and to enable the stocking to be eased up the leg. **E**
6 Ask the patient to keep the leg straight and if possible to push against the nurse.	To ensure that a good grip can be gained on the stocking. **E**
7 Starting at the foot, gradually ease the stocking into place over the heel and up the leg a bit at a time, until it is in its final position.	Since it is the material of the stocking that provides the pressure, it must be distributed evenly to ensure an even distribution of pressure. **E**
8 Do not pull from the top.	This will cause the stocking top to become overstretched and will lead to an uneven distribution of the stocking material (manufacturer's instructions, **C**).
9 Once the stocking is in place, check that there are no creases or wrinkles, particularly around the joints.	Wrinkles cause chafing of the skin and constricting bands of pressure. **E**

Post-procedure

Action	Rationale
10 Check that the patient finds the stocking comfortable and ask that any feelings of pain, tingling or numbness be reported. Check the toes for any visible signs of altered circulation.	Pain, tingling or numbness indicates that the stocking has been either inappropriately applied or fitted. **E**
11 To remove the stocking, peel it off the limb from the top downwards. Do not roll it down.	Rolling the stocking can result in tight bands of material forming, which are difficult to move. **E**
12 Document the manufacturer and style and size of garment that the patient has been provided with.	To maintain accurate records (NMC 2015, **C**).

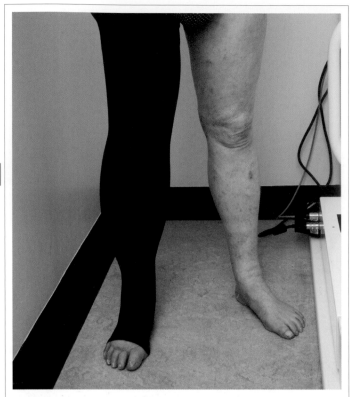

Figure 8.19 Example of elastic compression garment for the leg.

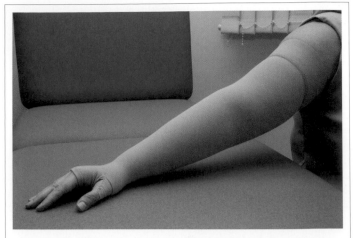

Figure 8.20 Example of elastic compression garment for the arm.

Procedure guideline 8.13 Elastic compression garments: application to the arm

Essential equipment
- Appropriate application aids if required (see Table 8.8)
- A compression garment that is appropriate for the patient's lymphoedema (see Figure 8.20)

Pre-procedure

Action	Rationale
1 Explain and discuss the procedure with the patient.	To ensure that the patient understands the procedure and gives their valid consent (NMC 2015, **C**).
2 The patient may be seated or standing.	

Procedure

Action	Rationale
3 Turn the sleeve inside out to the wrist. Pull over the patient's hand. *Note*: if a glove or separate handpiece is worn, always put the sleeve on *after* the glove or handpiece.	To avoid increasing swelling in the hand. **E**
4 Turn the rest of the sleeve back over the hand and up the arm.	To prevent a tourniquet effect developing at the wrist and to enable the sleeve to be eased up the arm. **E**
5 Ask the patient to grip something stable, such as a towel rail or the back of a chair.	This steadies the arm and gives the patient something to pull against. **E**
6 Working from the hand or wrist, gradually ease the sleeve up the arm.	Since it is the material that provides the pressure, it must be evenly distributed to ensure an even distribution of pressure. **C**
7 Do not pull up from the top.	To prevent the top becoming overstretched which will result in an uneven distribution of pressure. **C**
8 Once the sleeve is in place, check that there are no creases or wrinkles, particularly around the joints.	Wrinkles and creases cause chafing of the skin and constricting bands of pressure. **E**

Post-procedure

Action	Rationale
9 Check that the patient finds the sleeve comfortable and ask that any signs of pain, tingling or numbness be reported. Check the fingers for any visible signs of altered circulation.	Pain, tingling or numbness indicates that the sleeve has been either inappropriately applied or fitted. **E**

10 To remove the sleeve, peel it off the limb from the top. Do not roll it down.	Rolling the sleeve down can lead to tight bands of material forming which are difficult to move. **E**
11 Document the manufacturer and style and size of garment that the patient has been provided with.	To maintain accurate records (NMC 2015).

Problem-solving table 8.5 Prevention and resolution (Procedure guidelines 8.12 and 8.13)

Problem	Cause	Prevention	Action
Wrinkling of the garment along the length of the limb.	Poor application and positioning of the garment.	Supply written instructions with diagrams/pictures concerning the application and removal of the garment.	Demonstrate application and removal of the garment and observe the patient's technique when the garment is provided. The use of donning aids may be required.
Slippage of garment during wear.	Poorly fitting garment.	Ensure the correct measurements are taken to guide the therapist in the selection of the correctly sized garment.	Review size of garment. Consider the use of a grip top or skin glue to minimize slippage at the top of the garment.
Change of sensation in the limb during wear of the garment.	Garment too tight.	Ensure the correct measurements are taken to guide the therapist in the selection of the correctly sized garment.	Assess for other possible reasons for a change in sensation, e.g. musculoskeletal or circulatory impairment. Review the size of garment and consider alternative garments.
Skin sensitivity or reaction when wearing compression garment.	Possible allergic reaction to the material of the garment.	Check the patient's allergy status prior to fitting a garment.	Treat any allergy appropriately. Remove the garment until skin reaction clears. A cotton stockinette lining can be worn underneath the garment to protect the skin. An alternative garment may be required.
Poor compliance with use of the garment.	Limited information given to patient with regard to the importance of wearing the garment. Lifestyle commitments.	Ensure the patient is given sufficient information to become compliant with treatment.	Explore the problems the patient is experiencing. Explain the purpose of the garments thoroughly and the intended benefits.
Swelling extending beyond the edge of the garment: fingers or toes, upper thigh or upper arm.	Inappropriate style of garment for the patient's needs.	Thorough assessment to establish the history and extent of swelling.	If fingers or toes are swollen, use a compression glove or toe caps. If upper thigh or upper arm is swollen, the garment must extend into the adjacent truncal quadrant.

Post-procedural considerations

Immediate care
Evaluate the overall fit of the garment. There should be an even pressure throughout the garment, with no areas of loose-fitting material. The garment should be comfortable so that the patient can use their limb without restriction.

Ongoing care
The shape and size of the limb may change due to an increase in swelling. This can cause the garment to become ill fitting and cause trauma or damage to the skin. Compression garments should be checked regularly to ensure they remain appropriate in size, style and fit.

Education of patient and relevant others
- Ensure the patient knows for how long the garment needs to be worn each day. As each patient is different, the therapist should advise appropriately. Ideally garments should be worn during waking hours and removed at night (Todd 2015).
- Advise the patient on the care of the garment. The garment should be washed after every wear at 40°C. Hand washing is also acceptable. A biological detergent can be used but fabric softener should be avoided. The garment should be air dried and not tumble dried.
- Advise the patient about how to acquire replacement or additional garments. Many garments are available on drug tariff from the patient's doctor. It is advisable to replace the garments every 6 months.

Adjustable wrap compression systems

Definition
Adjustable wrap compression systems (also referred to as Velcro wraps) are generally made from short-stretch or inelastic, flexible

362

felt-like fabric which wraps around the limb and is secured with multiple overlapping Velcro straps (Noble-Jones 2016). Adjustable wrap compression systems are designed to be easier to apply than standard compression bandages and to be adjustable by a clinician, patient or carer.

Evidence-based approaches

Rationale

Adjustable wrap compression systems are used as an alternative to compression bandaging to reduce swelling during the initial treatment phase or worn daily for long-term management (Noble-Jones 2016). Adjustable wrap compression systems can be used on their own or in addition to compression garments where swelling is not being adequately managed with compression garments alone (Mullings 2012, Noble-Jones 2016). A range of garments is available on drug tariff including hand wraps, arm wraps, ankle–foot wraps, and lower leg, knee and thigh pieces (see Figures 8.21 and 8.22). The adjustable wrap compression systems are reusable and should be replaced after 6 months of daily wear. They are supplied with a liner to be worn under the wrap system. Choice of the most suitable adjustable wrap compression system should be decided after a detailed assessment of the patient (Linnitt 2011).

Adjustable wrap compression systems are useful for patients who are unable to apply and remove a compression garment due to limited dexterity and mobility. They are also useful for patients in the palliative stages of disease or those who have fragile skin that may be damaged during the application and removal of a compression garment (Wigg 2012). The patient or carer can adjust these systems without removing the device in response to changing swelling and to ensure sustained compression (Linitt 2015, Mullings 2012).

Indications

- Reduction in swelling in intensive phase of treatment (Damstra and Partsch 2013).
- Maintenance of limb shape and size in patients unable to apply and remove compression garments (Partsch and Mortimer 2015).
- To control swelling and provide support to patients with fragile skin who would not tolerate the application of a compression garment (Partsch and Mortimer 2015).
- Useful in distorted limbs as the wrap system can be wrapped and readjusted to the limb shape. Made to measure wraps are also available (Linitt 2015, Mullings 2012).

- Useful in patients unable to travel to the clinic daily for multi-layer bandaging.
- Useful for patients with reduced mobility as the adjustable wrap system is lightweight and less bulky than multilayer bandages (Linnitt 2011, Mullings 2012).

Contraindications (similar to multilayer short-stretch bandaging)

- *Acute cellulitis.* The skin may be too tender to tolerate compression.
- *Severe peripheral neuropathy.* The patient will not be able to feel if the wrap system is causing damage to the skin.
- Allergy to compression materials.
- *Arterial disease.* Tissue ischaemia can occur.
- *Infection in the swollen limb.* Pain may occur.
- *Uncontrolled cardiac failure.* Fluid overload can occur.
- *Deep vein thrombosis.* Anticoagulation therapy should be commenced prior to the use of any compression.
- *Physical or psychological limitations of the patient to comply safely with treatment.* For example, lack of manual dexterity or cognitive impairment (Todd 2013).

Legal and professional issues

Ensure the patient understands the use of the adjustable wrap compression system and has given consent (NMC 2015). Healthcare professionals must work within their scope of practice (NMC 2015).

Pre-procedural considerations

Several factors need to be taken into consideration before deciding to fit a patient with an adjustable wrap compression system. The patient should be motivated and compliant with the use of garments and have the physical skills to apply and remove the garment safely. A full physical assessment of the patient will determine the condition of the skin and tissues and the shape and size of the limb so that a style and size of garment suitable for the patient can be selected. Patients should be involved where possible in the choice of adjustable wrap compression system. Some have a choice of colour and fabric which will assist with acceptability to the patient and aid concordance (Gray 2013).

Figure 8.21 Adjustable wrap compression system for the lower leg.

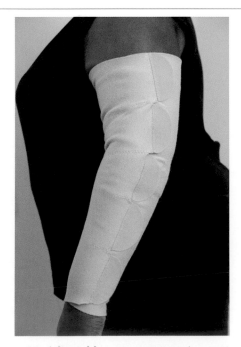

Figure 8.22 Adjustable wrap compression system for the arm.

Equipment

The aim of an adjustable compression wrap system is to achieve a tolerable resting pressure and a pressure sufficient to counteract gravity when standing (Partsch and Mortimer 2015). This is best achieved by using stiff compression products which result in high pressure when needed in the upright position. The pressure can be sustained over long periods of time during both activity and inactivity of the limb, providing a high working pressure while the muscle is active and a high resting pressure during inactivity of the muscle at rest (Todd 2011). Adjustable wrap compression systems are designed to be easy to use and apply (Wigg 2012). All of them come with the manufacturer's instructions, often with on-line support and training. These adjustable wrap compression systems support patient self-management in controlling lymphoedema (Noble-Jones 2016).

The use of adjustable compression wrap systems (Todd 2011):

- increases interstitial tissue pressure and reduces production of lymph
- promotes lymph movement along superficial and deep lymphatics
- increases lymph reabsorption
- provides an external counterforce during activity which enhances muscle pump action.

Construction

Garments are manufactured from synthetic fibres and are readily available in a variety of sizes and lengths 'off the shelf' to accommodate the needs of most patients. Some manufacturers offer a range of inelastic materials, from softer 'lite' wrap systems to firmer, stiffer compression wrap systems. The pressure under these adjustable wrap compression systems will be higher while the muscle is active. Made to measure adjustable wrap compression systems are also available. These can be adjusted during manufacture to suit patients' specific needs, and the provision of accurate measurements before manufacture ensures a good fit. Some adjustable wrap compression systems can also be trimmed for optimal fit.

Compression class

It is important to follow the manufacturer's instructions for using the adjustable wrap compression system to achieve correct compression over the correct circumference of the limb (Wigg 2012). Laplace's law dictates that the highest compression provided by a garment when fitted can be found at the wrist or the ankle. The compression is then graduated along the length of the limb to encourage movement of the fluid out of the limb (Wigg 2012).

Style

All areas influenced by swelling must be contained within the adjustable compression wrap system or further swelling will develop. The patient should be instructed concerning the application, removal and care of the adjustable wrap compression system to ensure that maximum effectiveness is achieved through its use. The patient's physical ability must be considered when choosing an adjustable wrap compression system as some degree of dexterity will be required during its application and removal (Wigg 2012).

Size

The manufacturer's guidance for choosing the correct size is based on simple limb measurements.

363

Procedure guideline 8.14   Adjustable wrap compression system: application to the lower leg

Essential equipment

- An adjustable wrap compression system that is appropriate for the patient's lymphoedema

Pre-procedure

Action	Rationale
1 Explain and discuss the procedure with the patient.	To ensure that the patient understands the procedure and gives their valid consent (NMC 2015, **C**).
2 If possible, position the patient seated upright on a bed or couch and raise the height to a comfortable level.	To ensure the comfort of both the patient and nurse. **E**

Procedure

Action	Rationale
3 Apply a liner to the leg, or apply the patient's compression garment if the adjustable wrap compression system is being used as adjunct to a compression garment.	To protect the skin. **E**
4 Unfasten all of the straps of the adjustable wrap compression system and fold back each strap securing the Velcro pads.	To ensure the wrap is open and flat and to ensure Velcro pads do not stick and tangle, making application difficult. **E**
5 Position the adjustable wrap compression system under the lower leg with the position of the top of the wrap below the knee crease and base of the wrap above the ankle.	To ensure correct fitting and that the wrap is not rubbing behind the knee or at the ankle. **E**
6 Follow the manufacturer's instructions for securing the Velcro straps until all of the straps are securely fastened.	To ensure that the wrap is applied securely and that straps overlock without gaps. To ensure the correct compression is applied and is even (Wigg 2012, **E**).
7 Check compression as per manufacturer's instructions; some recommend inserting your index, middle and ring fingers between the straps. If fingers do not fit comfortably the wrap may be too tight.	To check correct compression is being applied and to reduce the risk of applying too much compression. **E**
8 Once the adjustable wrap compression system is in place, check that there are no creases or wrinkles, particularly around the joints.	Wrinkles cause chafing of the skin and constricting bands of pressure. **E**

(continued)

Procedure guideline 8.14 Adjustable wrap compression system: application to the lower leg *(continued)*

Post-procedure

Action	Rationale
9 Check that the patient finds the adjustable wrap compression system comfortable and that they are not experiencing any feelings of pain, tingling or numbness. Check the toes for any visible signs of altered circulation.	Pain, tingling or numbness indicates that the adjustable wrap compression system has been inappropriately applied or fitted. **E**
10 To remove the adjustable wrap compression system, unfasten each Velcro strap, folding back and fastening it on itself.	To prevent the wrap sticking to itself or becoming tangled, so that the wrap is ready for future application. **E**
11 Inspect the skin; a mild indent where the straps have been is normal.	To ensure skin is not reddened and ensure compression is not too tight; the patient may need a thicker liner if their skin is fragile. **E**
12 Document the manufacturer and style and size of the adjustable wrap compression system that the patient has been provided with.	To maintain accurate records (NMC 2015, **C**). To ensure continuity of care when subsequent garments are required. **E**

Procedure guideline 8.15 Adjustable wrap compression system: application to the arm

Essential equipment
- An adjustable wrap compression system that is appropriate for the patient's lymphoedema

Pre-procedure

Action	Rationale
1 Explain and discuss the procedure with the patient.	To ensure that the patient understands the procedure and gives their valid consent (NMC 2015, **C**).
2 The patient should be seated. Extend their arm out; rest on a flat surface if required.	To support the arm. **E**

Procedure

Action	Rationale
3 Apply a liner or apply the patient's compression garment if the adjustable wrap compression system is being used as adjunct to a compression garment.	To protect the skin. **E**
4 Unfasten all the straps of the adjustable wrap compression system and fold back each strap securing the Velcro pads.	To ensure the wrap is open and flat and to ensure Velcro pads do not stick and tangle, making application difficult. **E**
5 Position the arm wrap on the arm with the base of the wrap above the wrist and the top below the axilla.	To prevent rubbing at the axilla. **E**
6 Secure the top strap near the axilla.	To hold the arm wrap in the correct position. **E**
7 Beginning at the wrist, secure the straps, following the manufacturer's instructions. Straps are usually pulled at 75% stretch (not full stretch on arm).	To ensure equal consistent compression is applied. **E**
8 Apply elbow straps before surrounding straps.	To ensure wrinkle-free application and allow movement of the elbow joint. **E**
9 Continue to the axilla then undo the original strap and secure again.	To ensure consistent application of compression. **E**
10 Visually inspect the arm wrap.	To ensure all straps are secure. **E**

Post-procedure

Action	Rationale
11 Check that the patient finds the adjustable wrap compression system comfortable and that they are not experiencing any feelings of pain, tingling or numbness.	Pain, tingling or numbness indicates that the sleeve has been inappropriately applied or fitted. **E**
12 To remove the adjustable wrap compression system, unfasten each Velcro strap, folding it back and fastening it on itself.	To prevent Velcro sticking to itself and make reapplication easier. **E**
13 Inspect the skin. A mild indent where the straps have been is normal.	To check for areas of redness and ensure straps have not been applied with too much stretch. **E**
14 Document the manufacturer and style and size of the arm wrap that the patient has been provided with.	To maintain accurate records (NMC 2015, **C**).

Problem-solving table 8.6 Prevention and resolution (Procedure guidelines 8.14 and 8.15)

Problem	Cause	Prevention	Action
Wrinkling of the adjustable compression wrap along the length of the limb.	Poor application and positioning of the garment.	Supply written instructions with diagrams/pictures showing the application and removal of the garment.	Demonstrate application and removal of the compression wrap and observe the patient's technique; the patient may need assistance from a carer, especially for an arm wrap.
Change of sensation in the limb during wear of the compression wrap.	Compression wrap straps applied too tight/incorrect size.	Ensure the correct measurements are taken to guide the therapist in the selection of the correctly sized wrap.	Assess for other possible reasons for a change in sensation, e.g. musculoskeletal or circulatory impairment. Reduce stretch of straps during application to reduce compression. Review the size of the wrap and consider alternative garments.
Poor compliance with the use of the compression wrap.	Limited information given to patient about the importance of wearing the compression wrap. Lifestyle commitments.	Ensure the patient is given sufficient information to become compliant with treatment.	Explore the problems the patient is experiencing. Explain the purpose of the compression wrap thoroughly and the intended benefits.
Swelling extending beyond the edge of the compression wrap: fingers or toes, upper thigh or upper arm.	Inappropriate style of garment for the patient's needs.	Thorough assessment to establish the history and extent of swelling.	If fingers or toes are swollen, use a compression garment. If the upper thigh or upper arm is swollen, the garment must extend into the adjacent truncal quadrant.

365

Post-procedural considerations
Immediate care
Evaluate the overall fit of the compression wrap system. There should be an even pressure throughout the compression wrap, with no areas of loose-fitting material. The compression wrap should be comfortable so that the patient can use their limb.

Ongoing care
The shape and size of the limb may change due to an increase or decrease in swelling. Compression wrap systems should be checked regularly to ensure they remain appropriate in size, style and fit.

Education of patient and relevant others
- Ensure the patient knows for how long the adjustable wrap compression system should be worn each day. As each patient is different, the therapist should advise appropriately. Adjustable wrap compression systems used to maintain swelling reduction are generally worn during waking hours and removed at night. If the adjustable wrap compression system is being used as an alternative to multilayer bandaging, it should remain in place day and night (Wigg 2012).
- Advise the patient on the care of the garment. Instructions vary so care instructions should be followed. The adjustable wrap compression system should be worn over a liner or compression garment and should not need daily washing. Most adjustable wrap compression systems can be machine washed, but some thicker, stiffer wraps need to be hand washed; all should be air dried flat.
- Advise the patient about how to acquire replacement or additional garments. Many garments are available on drug tariff from the patient's doctor. It is advisable to replace adjustable wrap compression systems after 6 months of daily wear.

Websites

British Lymphology Society: www.thebls.com
Lymphoedema Support Network: www.lymphoedema.org/lsn
International Lymphoedema Framework: www.lympho.org
Australasian Lymphology Association: www.lymphoedema .org.au
Lymphedema People: www.lymphedemapeople.com
National Lymphedema Network: www.lymphnet.org
Free online product information and training can be sourced from individual companies:
www.bsnmedical.co.uk/education.html
www.mediuk.co.uk/service/support-vascular/
www.hadhealth.com
http://lohmann-rauscher.co.uk/educationwww.altimed.co.uk/ help/theory-of-compression/
www.sigvaris.com/uk/en-uk/

SECTION 8.6 NON-PHARMACOLOGICAL MANAGEMENT OF BREATHLESSNESS

This section will discuss the symptom of breathlessness in people with cancer and will outline some evidence-based non-pharmacological approaches that may help in the management of this symptom. It is often a difficult symptom to manage effectively and management should be modified frequently in response to changes in the person and their progress. The aims of management are to reduce the distress of breathlessness and support people to feel more in control of their breathing so they can be as independent and active as possible.

This section will not outline the pathophysiology of the causes of breathlessness or the pharmacological management of breathlessness.

Definition

Breathlessness is a term used to describe a subjective experience of breathing discomfort that consists of qualitatively distinct sensations that vary in intensity. It is a common, often debilitating symptom that is distressing for both the person and their carers (Parshall et al. 2012). It is a problem where there is a complex interplay between physical, psychological, emotional and functional factors because the impairment of breathing has life-threatening connotations. Because of this interplay the underlying pathology may not correlate with the patient's perception of their symptoms (Jolley and Moxham 2016). Box 8.9 lists some of the impacts that may be expressed by people who experience breathlessness.

Anatomy and physiology

A good working knowledge of normal human anatomy and physiology influencing breathing mechanics is required (Pryor and Prasad 2008). The sensation of breathlessness results from the multiple sensory inputs from chemical, mechanical and neural receptors that are interpreted in the central nervous system. This is a complex, multifaceted process. It may be influenced by, and impact on, bodily functions, activities and participation and environmental factors such as social support and financial resources. The physiological changes occurring as a result of deconditioning and inactivity are described in Section 8.7, Physical activity for people with cancer.

Presenting symptoms

Many people with cancer experience breathlessness. The prevalence and severity often increase as their disease progresses and

Box 8.9 Some of the impacts that may be experienced by people with breathlessness

Fear of suffocation and death
Panic
Distress
Anxiety
Debilitation and restricted mobility
Inability to care for self
Restricted social functioning
Loss of role (work, family)
Reduced self-esteem
Sleep disturbance including fear of falling asleep
Fatigue from the effort of breathing
Fatigue from the emotional impacts of breathlessness
Disruptions to relationships and sexual functioning
Unique experience specific to the individual (hard for others to understand and seemingly disproportionate to the presenting pathophysiology)

towards the end of life. People's experience of breathlessness is unique to them; they often report it as a distressing symptom and it frequently occurs in a symptom cluster together with fatigue and pain (Thomas et al. 2011).

Related theory (causative or influencing factors)

Breathlessness may be caused by a wide range of clinical conditions affecting the stimulus to breathe (neural respiratory drive) or altering the mechanics of breathing. As can be seen in Figure 8.23, effective management is dependent on a multisystems assessment and detailed analysis of the potential causative factors before a good management plan can be developed with the patients and carers. Best practice consists of both non-pharmacological and pharmacological interventions (Chin and Booth 2016).

Breathing

At rest, breathing in (inspiration) is an active process in which the diaphragm muscle contracts, increasing the volume of the thoracic cavity and drawing air in. Breathing out (expiration) is passive in normal resting conditions; on exertion, the internal intercostal muscles and abdominal wall muscles are used to push the diaphragm upwards, reducing the volume of the thoracic cavity and pushing air out. If the chest wall mechanics are altered

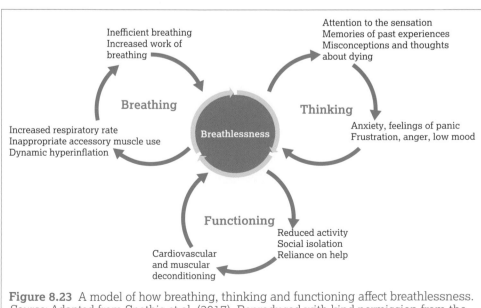

Figure 8.23 A model of how breathing, thinking and functioning affect breathlessness. *Source:* Adapted from Spathis et al. (2017). Reproduced with kind permission from the Cambridge Breathlessness Intervention Service.

due to the effects of cancer or other co-morbidities the threshold for breathlessness will be lower. This is further explained in *The Royal Marsden Manual of Clinical Nursing Procedures, Ninth Edition*: Chapter 6 Moving and positioning.

Thinking

Difficulty breathing may cause strong emotional responses, releasing hormones that stimulate the neural respiratory drive centrally. Panic, anxiety, gloomy thoughts and worry may increase overall muscular tension, which reduces the efficiency of breathing and increases the metabolic rate and energy requirements. The worry and anxiety of carers may contribute to this and inadvertently add to the drive to breathe (Bausewein et al. 2010).

Functioning

Breathlessness may also be a result of poor cardiovascular fitness that may develop as people become less active following a cancer diagnosis and treatment (Parshall et al. 2012). This deconditioning may cause a reduced ability to participate in previously undertaken activities. (Deconditioning is addressed in Section 8.7, Physical activity for people with cancer.) Poor nutritional status may contribute to reduced muscle strength and output (Section 8.4, Nutritional status). Poor sleep and fatigue may also contribute to breathlessness. Poor pacing or rushing activity may also contribute to reduced functioning (Section 8.8, Cancer-related fatigue and sleep). The loss of functioning experienced by those with breathlessness contributes to the 'thinking' aspects and can compound breathlessness.

Evidence-based approaches

There is a robust evidence base for the beneficial effect and cost-effectiveness of a multidisciplinary approach to the management of this complex symptom (Booth et al. 2011b, Higginson et al. 2014). Non-pharmacological approaches may form a higher proportion of this management earlier in the disease trajectory, with pharmacological interventions playing an increasing role as the symptom advances (Higginson et al. 2014).

Rationale

Optimal management of breathlessness combines a sensory–nociceptive model (focusing on the causes due to the neural pathways and mechanisms that can be relieved by pharmacological interventions) and the biopsychosocial model (focusing on physical and behavioural modification and psychological intervention) to achieve an integrated approach where the individual's emotional experience of breathlessness is considered inseparable from its physical symptoms (Corner et al. 1996).

Diagnosis and treatment of underlying causes is the first approach to managing this symptom; however, despite optimal treatment, breathlessness persists in many patients and the use of non-pharmacological approaches and a multidisciplinary approach is required (Booth et al. 2011a). Optimal breathlessness management for each person may be achieved by a detailed assessment and a thorough understanding of the triggers of the episodes of breathlessness; a problem-solving approach to managing the causative factors or triggers; and the management of the remaining symptoms with non-pharmacological and pharmacological treatment.

Any possible solutions or treatments will be discussed and tested with the person and their carers for best effect, so that the person is able to manage the symptoms by themselves. Involvement of carers is important to empower both the person and their carer with techniques that may be effective. This will reduce anxiety for both parties as it will also improve the use of techniques in the situations triggering breathlessness and improve the ability to cope at home. This also gives the opportunity for both parties to discuss their own needs in managing this frightening symptom.

Indications

- When the assessment has demonstrated the causes and triggers that limit participation or activity for the patient and/or their carers.
- Where the assessment has indicated a lack of understanding, education or coping strategies to manage the symptom.
- Where the patient has indicated a willingness to try the procedures.

Contraindications

- Where there is no indication for the procedure.
- Where the person and family experience no benefit from the procedures.
- Where the person and family perceive it as burdensome.

Principles of care

The principles of non-pharmacological management address any underlying causes of breathlessness, identifying the breathing, thinking and functioning components. It is important that all reversible causes for breathlessness have been ruled out or treated appropriately before trialling these procedures. Carer training and support is integral to the success of these procedures and consideration should be given as to how this may be best achieved before starting.

Legal and professional issues

Practitioners should be trained and confident in using these procedures as this will reassure the patient. This requires a good knowledge of the practice of caring and working with individuals and their carers. The intervening professional must have undergone relevant competency training in the area to cover their practice. Clear and accurate records relevant to the clinician's practice must be kept at all times (NMC 2015).

Assessment and recording tools

A dual approach to measurement of the effect of the intervention and recording should be taken to capture the magnitude and impact of the sensation of breathlessness for the individual. An objective measure of how the breathlessness felt to the patient before and after the intervention in response to a simple question 'How does it make you feel when you are breathless?' should be used. The sensation of breathlessness can be quantified using a measurement scale, for example a visual analogue scale (Adams et al. 1985), the modified Borg (1970) scale (see Section 8.7, Physical activity for people with cancer) or a numerical rating scale as shown in Figure 8.24 (Gift and Narsavage 1998, Guyatt et al. 1987).

Non-pharmacological support

Functioning

Refer to a physiotherapist for consideration of a course of pulmonary rehabilitation to educate and to manage breathlessness caused by deconditioning. These courses often include strategies that promote functioning. These strategies should all be considered even if a course is not accessible.

The strategies include:

- Testing any benefit from appropriate walking aids to increase the patient's base of support. Offer a resting place during the activity (e.g. wheeled walker or a gutter rollator) (Booth et al. 2011a, Pryor and Prasad 2008).
- Assessing the influence of environmental factors (e.g. set-up of home situation, poor sleep hygiene or poor pacing of activities; see Sections 8.7, Physical activity for people with cancer and 8.8, Cancer-related fatigue and sleep).
- Assessing nutritional status and energy requirements. Nutritional supplements should be provided if needed (see Section 8.4, Nutritional status).
- Teaching resting positions that improve the mechanics of breathing and lower the required energy expenditure (Figure 8.25).

Please indicate what level you feel your breathlessness is now, at rest, today, by placing a pen mark on the line below.

0 ———————————————————————————————— 10

no problems with breathlessness   worst breathlessness ever

Figure 8.24 Numerical rating scale.

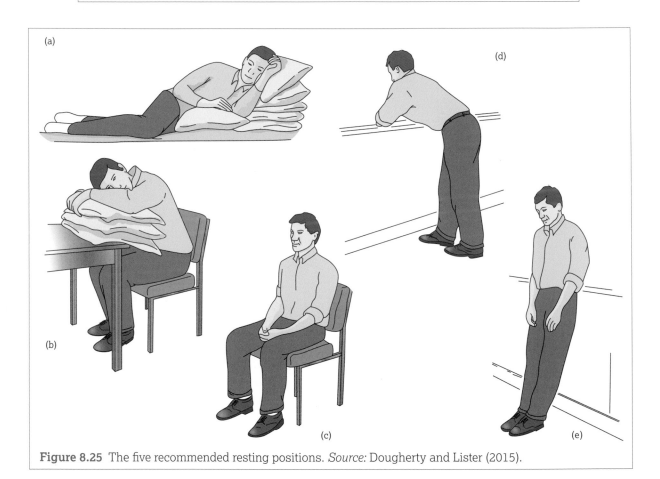

Figure 8.25 The five recommended resting positions. *Source:* Dougherty and Lister (2015).

Breathing

Refer to a physiotherapist or a trained respiratory nurse for education about the causes of breathlessness, breathing control, breathlessness management and advice for optimal positioning at rest and during activity. Physiotherapists may also give advice on airway clearance and cough techniques as well as specific inspiratory muscle training (Booth et al. 2011a, Pryor and Prasad 2008).

A handheld fan (Figure 8.26) with the draft directed to the face reduces the sense of breathlessness. It can be introduced to the patient and tested for effect as set out in Procedure guideline 8.16 (Galbraith et al. 2010).

Procedure guideline 8.16   Breathlessness management: using a handheld fan

Essential equipment
- A light, battery-driven handheld fan
- A valid outcome measure for breathlessness

Pre-procedure

Action	Rationale
1 Introduce self to patient and carers.	To establish professional and clinical rapport and comply with professional codes of conduct (NMC 2015, **C**).

2 Gain consent from the patient to assess their medical and psychosocial history.	To understand the background for the presentation and any treatments undergone to treat the reversible causes of breathlessness. **E**
3 Carry out an assessment of breathlessness including taking a measure of breathlessness at baseline (e.g. visual analogue scale, VAS, or numerical rating scale, NRS [Figure 8.24]) and a subjective descriptor from the patient if indicated.	To obtain a baseline objective and subjective assessment of breathlessness to measure change against (Booth et al. 2011a, **R**).
4 Discuss the use of the handheld fan. Explain and discuss the procedure with the patient.	To ensure that a trial of the intervention is acceptable and could be effective for the patient and that they understand the procedure and give their valid written consent (NMC 2013, **C**).
5 Gain agreement to discontinue the intervention if it is not found to be clinically effective on that day.	To ensure that the patient is not left with equipment of no benefit. **E**
6 Introduce the basic principles of resting positions as shown in Figure 8.25.	To promote an energy-efficient position for the duration of the intervention (Galbraith et al. 2010, **R**).

Procedure

7 Introduce the handheld device and regulate the speed and direction so that a flow is directed against the patient's face at the level of the cheek.	To stimulate the area innervated by the second and third branches of the trigeminal nerve (Galbraith et al. 2010, **R**).
8 Ask the patient what they felt the effect of the intervention was and record the measure of breathlessness again (e.g. VAS or NRS).	To establish any clinical effect due to the intervention (Galbraith et al. 2010, **R**).
9 If the fan was thought to be effective by the patient subjectively or objectively and they want to continue to use the intervention, teach them how to place the fan for best effect.	To enable the patient to continue the intervention as a tool to self-manage their breathlessness as they require on exercise or at rest (Booth et al. 2011a, **R**; Galbraith et al. 2010, **R**).
10 Leave written instructions and teach any family or carers to use the device.	To provide ownership of the sessions to patients and their carers and enable ongoing practice (Schneiders et al. 1998, **C**).
11 If the intervention was not subjectively or objectively effective for the patient, discuss this with the patient and gain agreement to discontinue the intervention.	In order not to increase any treatment burden for the patient or their carers. **E**

Post-procedure

12 Document the intervention and its effect in the patient record.	Legal requirement of professional body and employing institution (NMC 2015, **E**).
13 Review of the session as per procedure after an agreed interval to modify or discontinue the intervention as required.	To enable informed expert review and modification of the intervention as required. **E**

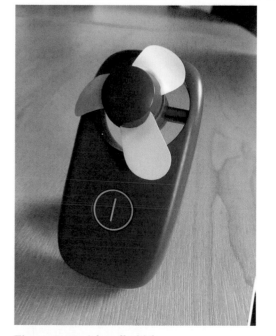

Figure 8.26 A handheld fan.

Thinking

To moderate the effect of thinking or emotion on the neural respiratory drive, it is important to identify any related triggers and educate about breathlessness triggered by anxiety. Management of these psychological triggers may be supported by referral to other therapies to develop and use coping strategies. These strategies may include education about the relationship between emotions and breathlessness; cognitive behavioural therapy; mindfulness; self-hypnosis; visual aids; acupuncture or acupressure; aromatherapy massage; or referral to learn relaxation (see Procedure guideline 8.17) (Booth et al. 2011a, Dyer et al. 2008, Powell 2009, Thomas et al. 2011).

Rationale

To reduce the effect of the symptoms of breathlessness, patients may be offered individually chosen aroma stick inhalers as part of the care offered by complementary therapists.

Indications

When a patient has reported that their breathlessness has been eased during the aromatherapy massage sessions.

Equipment

It is an individual plastic inhaler device. The inner wick is blank/unscented, permitting the addition of essential oils (Dyer et al. 2008). The wick absorbs the essential oils (up to 20 drops are applied); the device is then sealed and can be used until there is no longer a smell (Figure 8.27).

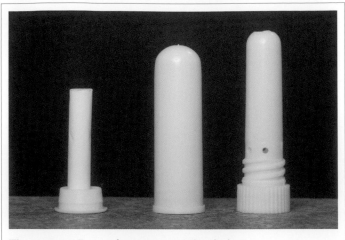

Figure 8.27 Parts of an aroma stick inhaler.

Procedure guideline 8.17 Breathlessness management: essential oil administration via an aroma stick inhaler

Essential equipment
- High-grade essential oils to include: menthol, eucalyptus and peppermint
- A 10-point VAS breathlessness scale

Pre-procedure

Action	Rationale
1 Introduce self to patient and carers.	To establish professional and clinical rapport and comply with professional codes of conduct (CSP 2011, **C**).
2 Gain consent from the patient to assess their medical and psychosocial history.	To understand the background for the presentation and any treatments undergone to treat the reversible causes of breathlessness. **E**
3 Carry out an assessment of breathlessness including taking a measure of breathlessness at baseline using a 10-point visual analogue scale and a subjective descriptor from the patient if indicated.	To obtain a baseline objective and subjective assessment of breathlessness so change can be measured (Booth et al. 2011a, **R**).
4 Discuss the use of aroma stick inhalers in the cancer setting. Explain and discuss the procedure with the patient.	To ensure that a trial of the intervention is acceptable and could be effective for the patient. That they understand the procedure and give their valid written consent (NMC 2013, **C**).
5 Gain agreement to discontinue the intervention if it is not found to be clinically effective on that day.	To ensure that the patient is not left with equipment of no benefit. **E**
6 Introduce the basic principles of resting positions as shown in Figure 8.26.	To promote an energy-efficient position for the duration of the intervention (Galbraith et al. 2010, **R**).

Procedure

Action	Rationale
7 Introduce the aroma stick inhaler pre-loaded with the essential oil mixture and demonstrate its use by removing the outer casing, holding the stick beneath the nose and inhaling. Replace the casing after use.	To give a cooling sensation and stimulate the area innervated by the second branch of the trigeminal nerve (Booth et al. 2011a, **R**).
8 Ask the patient what they felt the effect of the intervention was and record the measure of breathlessness again (e.g. VAS).	To establish any clinical effect due to the intervention (Dyer et al. 2008, **R**).
9 If the essential oils delivered by the aroma stick inhaler were thought to be effective by the patient subjectively or objectively and they want to continue to use the intervention, teach them to use the device for the best clinical effect.	To enable the patient to continue the intervention as a tool to self-manage their breathlessness (Dyer et al. 2008, **R**).
10 Teach the patient, family or carers to use and clean the device. Provide written instructions.	To provide ownership of the intervention to patients and their carers and enable ongoing practice (Schneiders et al. 1998, **C**). To ensure that the patient can continue to use the device safely.

11 If the intervention was not subjectively or objectively effective for the patient, discuss this with the patient. If appropriate, suggest the intervention is discontinued.	In order not to increase any treatment burden for the patient or their carers. **E**

Post-procedure

12 Document the intervention and its effect in the patient's record.	Legal requirement of professional body and employing institution (NMC 2015, **C**).
13 Review the session as per procedure after an agreed interval to modify or discontinue the intervention as required.	To enable informed expert review and modification of the intervention as required. **E**

Websites

www.cuh.nhs.uk/breathlessness-intervention-service-bis/resources

www.cancerresearchuk.org/about-cancer/coping/physically/breathing-problems/shortness-of-breath

www.macmillan.org.uk/information-and-support/coping/side-effects-and-symptoms/breathlessness

SECTION 8.7 PHYSICAL ACTIVITY FOR PEOPLE WITH CANCER

This section will discuss physical activity and how to help support people with cancer to be physically active both during and after treatment. Physical activity is beneficial to everyone including people who have had a cancer diagnosis. Achieving 150 minutes a week of moderate intensity activity can help prevent or manage more than 20 chronic conditions including coronary heart disease, stroke, type 2 diabetes, cancer, obesity, mental health problems and musculo-skeletal conditions (Department of Health 2012). Cancer diagnosis and treatment has an impact on the body leading to many changes, both physical and psychological. Physical activity is known to decrease as a direct result of cancer diagnosis and treatments (Irwin et al. 2003). As a result of treatment, people frequently become de-conditioned and lose cardiovascular fitness which can lead to other consequences including fatigue and reduced physical function. Cancer treatment can also have a negative effect on muscle mass and joint mobility which can also affect functional ability and ultimately quality of life. Figure 8.28 illustrates the components of health-related fitness (Saxton and Daley 2010).

In recent years there has been an increasing amount of research demonstrating the benefits of physical activity and exercise for people with cancer, such that it is now becoming practice to incorporate it into standard models of care as Figure 8.29 shows (DH 2011). Physical activity also has the advantage that it gives people

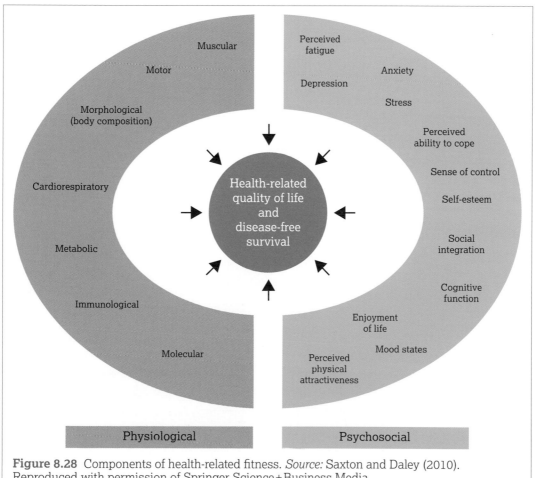

Figure 8.28 Components of health-related fitness. *Source:* Saxton and Daley (2010). Reproduced with permission of Springer Science+Business Media

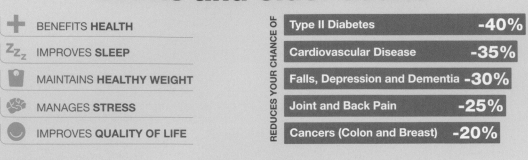

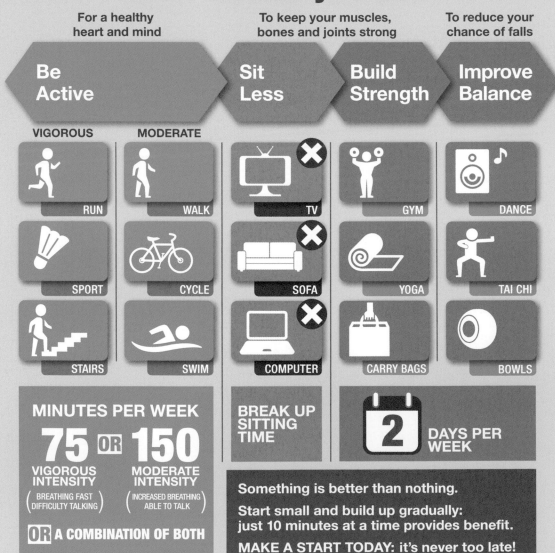

Figure 8.29 A model of the benefits of physical activity. *Source:* DH (2011). © Crown copyright. Reproduced under the Open Government Licence v3.0, https://www.nationalarchives.gov.uk/doc/open-government-licence/version/3/

the opportunity to empower themselves by regaining fitness and consequently improve their quality of life at a time when there is often a feeling of loss of control. However, although the message is that physical activity is an important adjunct to treatment, there are still challenges regarding how to integrate this into practices of care (Davies et al. 2011). One way to assist self-management is to tailor it to the individual and this can often lead to liaising with and onward referral to specialists in exercise provision.

Definition

Physical activity is defined as any bodily movement produced by the skeletal muscles that results in a substantial increase in energy expenditure (Bouchard et al. 1994). It is important to recognize that all activities involving movement during our daily life such as housework or walking to work are forms of physical activity.

In contrast, exercise is a specific form of physical activity where the goal is to achieve some increase in fitness. It is usually carried out in a more purposeful fashion and at a more intense level and over an extended period of time (Courneya and Friedenreich 2010). The terms physical activity and exercise are often used interchangeably but, whichever term is used, the intensity of the activity is important when considering the extent of physiological changes.

Definition of exercise levels

There are many tools to help gauge the intensity of exercise and physical activity, but one that is commonly used for people with cancer is the Borg scale, which rates the perceived level of breathlessness on exertion (Borg 1998). A modified Borg scale (Figure 8.30) uses numbers 0 to 10, with 10 being maximal exertion.

Moderate intensity aerobic exercise (5–6 on the modified Borg scale) is at an intensity that raises the heart rate but it is possible to still talk.

Vigorous intensity aerobic exercise (about 9 on the modified Borg scale) is at a level where the heart rate is significantly increased, which makes it difficult to speak more than a few words without pausing for breath.

Anatomy and physiology

In order to assist with regards to physical activity, it is important to have some knowledge of the physiological changes as a result of activity. Prolonged periods of rest will cause the body to become deconditioned, resulting in a decrease in maximum oxygen consumption, cardiac output and muscle mass. All of this compromises fitness and exercise tolerance, which can result in a negative impact on function.

0	
1	Very weak
2	Weak (light)
3	Moderate
4	Somewhat strong
5	Strong (heavy)
6	Strong
7	Very Strong
8	Very Strong
9	Very, very strong
10	Maximal

Figure 8.30 Modified Borg scale of perceived exertion. Source: https://www.cdc.gov/physicalactivity/basics/measuring/exertion.htm.

Increasing the levels of physical activity or doing exercise training can lead to positive physiological changes in both the cardiovascular system and the body musculature over time (changes can be measured within 10–12 weeks).

Physiological changes of exercise

Aerobic exercise will lead to increased efficiency of the:

- cardiovascular system
- respiratory system
- metabolic rate
- lymphatic system.

Weight-bearing exercise will also increase bone density (Winters-Stone et al. 2010). Patients who are risk of metastatic bone disease should still be encouraged to be physically active. However new onset bone pain or pain that has changed in nature or intensity should always be investigated for fracture risk (Macmillan 2018).

Muscle-strengthening exercise will lead to an improvement in the muscles' ability to use energy due to:

- increased levels of oxidative enzymes in the muscles
- increased mitochondrial density and size
- increase in number of capillary vessels within the mucsles allowing them to work more efficiently.

Endurance

This term relates to the ability of the body to carry out an exercise over time, whether it is a specific muscle contraction or cardiovascular endurance. Regular physical activity can also assist in building up endurance.

Measuring fitness

Exercise can be measured by looking at three main components: the frequency, intensity and duration of carrying out physical activity (Saxton and Daley 2010). Measuring these three components will help to determine the activity level of the individual. More specific measurements can be taken to look at specific cardiovascular fitness indicators such as VO_2 max. The most accurate way of measuring VO_2 max is by using a treadmill or a specially designed calibrated cycle. This is known as cardiopulmonary exercise testing or CPET.

VO_2 max (maximum oxygen consumption during exercise)

Fitness levels are often described on the basis of energy expenditure used during activity. VO_2 max is a common method of assessing the level of energy used and measuring fitness. VO_2 max is the measurement of the maximum amount of oxygen that an individual can utilize during intense, or maximal exercise. It is measured as millilitres of oxygen used in one minute per kilogram of body weight (mL/kg/min) (Quinn 2018)

Related theory

Although there is uncertainty regarding the type and quantity of exercise, evidence supports that exercise can be beneficial in improving quality of life after cancer treatment (Mishra et al. 2012). The advantages of physical activity in the short term have also been shown to have enduring long-term effects after treatment (Mutrie et al. 2012). A review of the evidence to support the role of physical activity at all stages of the cancer care pathway was completed by Macmillan Cancer Support (2017). The summary of the evidence showed that physical activity can be beneficial in:

1 *Improving or preventing the decline of physical function without increasing fatigue.* Because the majority of cancer therapies have a range of unwanted side-effects including pain and peripheral neuropathy, cancer patients typically lose cardiovascular fitness, experience fatigue and have a reduced sense of well-being over the course of their treatment. There has

traditionally been an emphasis on the importance of rest and conserving energy which can contribute to a gradual deterioration in function long after treatment has finished. There is good evidence to support the benefit of exercise for cancer fatigue (Cramp and Byron-Daniel 2012). Although adequate rest is very important during treatment, people should be encouraged to minimize the time that they are inactive and to aim to return to normal activity levels as soon as possible (Chartered Society of Physiotherapy 2014, Saxton and Daley 2010).

2 *Recovering physical function after debilitating treatment.* A systematic review of the evidence demonstrates that appropriate levels of exercise during treatment can help to minimize side-effects and limit functional decline as well as improve psychological well-being (Macmillan Cancer Support 2012). The evidence also supports the role of exercise after treatment as an effective way to recover physical and mental health (Macmillan Cancer Support 2012). Both anxiety and depression have been shown to be improved by carrying out physical activity.

Emerging evidence supports the role that exercise may play in positively influencing the risk of recurrence for certain cancers (Fong et al. 2012, Saxton and Daley 2010). There is also some evidence that it assists in reducing mortality for some cancers as well as reducing the risk of developing other long-term conditions. The majority of the research regarding the risk of recurrence and mortality is focused on breast cancer and colon cancer. Exercise has also been found to help decrease the rate of cancer progression for men with prostate cancer (Macmillan Cancer Support 2017).

Evidence-based approaches

- The Department of Health (DH) has set guidelines of 30 minutes of moderate physical activity five times a week for adults aged 19–64 as well as specific strengthening exercises twice a week. The total of 150 minutes of exercise in a week can also be broken down into 10-minute episodes of exercise (DH 2011). Although this is not cancer specific, it is what people should be working towards following their primary cancer treatment (Campbell et al. 2011).
- The American College of Sports Medicine (Schmitz et al. 2010) also looked at the evidence regarding physical activity for people with cancer and concluded that overall the benefits to quality of life outweighed any potential disadvantages. After taking into consideration any precautions regarding exercise, they recommended following the Guidelines on Physical Activity for Americans (U.S. Department of Health and Human Services 2008) which are consistent with the recommendations given by the Department of Health.
- The World Health Organization (WHO 2010) *Global Recommendations on Physical Activity for Health* also set out guidance in line with the Department of Health advice. Again this is not cancer specific.

Rationale

Physical activity can assist physiological changes by increasing muscle bulk and strength and also increasing joint mobility through stretches. It is also important to increase cardiovascular fitness at all stages to help overcome some of the related side-effects such as cancer fatigue. Physical activity has been proven to help with these physiological changes and also to improve mood. Research has highlighted numerous positive effects for the inclusion of physical activity interventions following any cancer diagnosis including minimizing biological processes associated with tumour growth (Betof et al. 2015). It also helps to improve psychosocial factors during and after cancer.

Indications

Physical activity is relevant to all people with cancer at any stage of their disease or treatment. Tailoring physical activity advice and intervention to the individual ensures that it is meaningful to them (Bourke et al. 2013). There is also evidence to support that making a healthy lifestyle change is often triggered at the time of cancer diagnosis (Saxton and Daley 2010). This is referred to as the teachable moment and relates to the time when people with cancer are more receptive to making beneficial lifestyle changes (Demark-Wahnefried et al. 2005). Nurses are in an ideal position to help support and advise people with cancer to be more active both during and after treatment (Hall-Alston 2015). People at risk of osteoporosis due to cancer treatment may benefit from moderate intensity aerobic exercises, including some weight-bearing exercises, to assist bone health (Winters-Stone et al. 2010).

Contraindications

At any stage:

- if the person feels unwell with, for example, dizziness/breathlessness
- red flags – unexplained weight loss or pain, night pain, constant pain, suspected metastatic spinal cord compression (MSCC; see Chapter 7), new unexplained symptoms and signs of cauda equina syndrome (a neurological condition in which there is damage to the cauda equina).

Pre-treatment:

- any co-morbidity, such as arthritis, that may restrict patients from participating in all types of exercise.

During treatment:

- on the day of chemotherapy
- excessive diarrhoea or vomiting
- haematology – check with the medical team
- low white blood cell count
- low haemoglobin – if the patient is anaemic
- insufficient nutritional intake.

After treatment:

- If the patient has osteoporosis or bone metastases they need to avoid exercises such as heavy weights that will put excessive stress on the bones.

People with cancer should check with their medical team before commencing any new physical activity or exercise initiatives.

Principles of care

Encourage people with cancer to keep physically active both during and after treatment (Campbell et al. 2011, Hall-Alston 2015, Schmitz et al. 2010). A growing body of evidence indicates that physical activity has potential value at all stages of the cancer pathway. Physical activity during treatment will optimize cardiopulmonary fitness and can reduce symptom burden including cancer-related fatigue. Physical activity post treatment can also improve health and wellbeing and in palliative patients, quality of life. There is also evidence to show that patients who are physically active after a cancer diagnosis enjoy a longer survival and lower risk of recurrence and disease progression (Macmillan Cancer Support 2017).

Legal and professional issues

It is recommended that any professional giving specific exercise advice or running group exercise sessions should ensure competency through additional training.

Pre-procedural considerations

Equipment

Ensure people are aware that they will need to be suitably dressed in loose comfortable clothes, such as jogging pants, and good

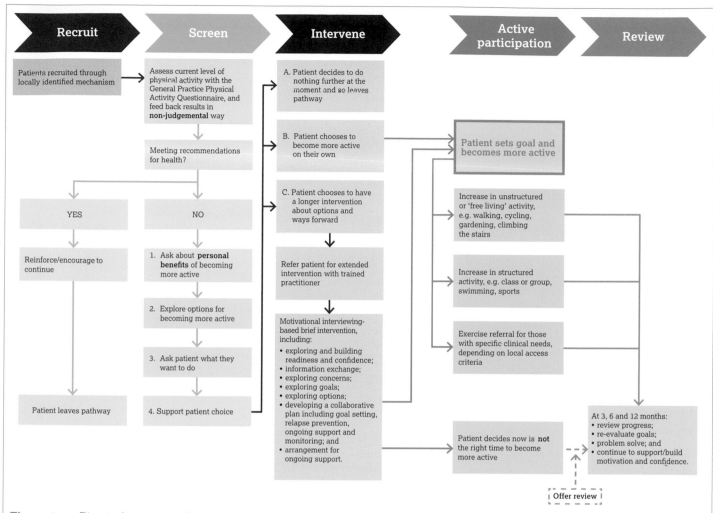

Figure 8.31 Physical activity pathway. *Source:* Department of Health (2012). © Crown copyright 2012. Reproduced under the Open Government Licence v3.0, https://www.nationalarchives.gov.uk/doc/open-government-licence/version/3/

375

supportive footwear, particularly lace-up shoes, when carrying out physical activity.

Assessment and recording tools
There are a variety of ways to provide a baseline assessment of physical activity levels including exercise diaries such as that provided by Macmillan Cancer Support (2016a), self-report or a more validated tool such as the Godin-Shephard Leisure-Time Physical Activity Questionnaire (Godin 2011). The decision on what assessment tool to use will depend on the individual patient's situation.

Pharmacological support
Be aware if patient is on any medication that may restrict or preclude exercise.

Procedure guideline 8.18   Supporting physical activity

Essential equipment
- Suitable footwear and clothing
- Safe environment

Pre-procedure

Action	Rationale
1 Introduce self to patient, in either inpatient or outpatient setting.	To establish professional and clinical rapport. **E**
2 Gain consent from the patient for the intervention.	To ensure the patient understands the procedure and provides verbal consent (NMC 2015).
3 Ensure a safe environment.	To decrease the risk of falls. **E**

Procedure

4 Carry out a holistic needs assessment.	To provide a baseline of the patient's concerns. **E**

Procedure guideline 8.18 Supporting physical activity *(continued)*

Action	Rationale
5 Ensure that the patient does not have additional complex health issues or contraindications (Campbell et al. 2011) prior to supporting and advising on physical activity.	To ensure health and safety. **E**
6 If additional complex health issues or contraindications are identified, ensure medical review prior to proceeding with the consultation.	To ensure health and safety. **E**
7 If appropriate, carry out a valid screening tool such as the Godin-Shephard Leisure-Time Physical Activity Questionnaire (Godin 2011) to evaluate level of physical activity.	To ascertain baseline assessment of physical activity levels. **E**
8 Identify from information gained as to whether the patient is experiencing difficulty in being physically active at the recommended levels.	To identify a patient who requires further information or support in order to improve physical activity levels.
9 Give verbal and written advice (such as the Macmillan booklet on physical activity, 2016) on both the benefits of physical activity and also how to start increasing physical activity levels.	To provide best evidence-based practice (Hall-Allston 2015). **E**
10 Consider recommending use of other resources to support physical activity such as pedometers, apps, fitness bands.	To assist in self-management (Bourke et al. 2013). **E**
11 Consider onward referral for supervised exercise sessions depending on local provision.	To help support patient with achieving increasing physical activity (Bourke et al. 2013). **E**
12 Document the action taken.	To provide best evidence-based practice. **E**

Problem-solving table 8.7 Prevention and resolution (Procedure guideline 8.18)

Problem	Cause	Prevention	Action
Lack of motivation.	During treatment: • side-effects of treatment • low mood • uncertainty about how to be physically active. Long-term consequences of treatment: • long-term side-effects • low mood • unsure about how to be physically active.	Ensure timing of giving information – where possible link to teachable moment.	Consider attending behavioural change training such as motivational interviewing.
Lymphoedema or at risk of lymphoedema.	Removal of lymph nodes leads to risk of lymphoedema.	Inform regarding the benefits of exercise to assist the lymphatic system.	Give advice on slow progression of exercises. Advise to avoid repetitive or sustained exercises.
Bone metastases.	Patient at increased risk of fracture.	Advise to avoid heavy impact exercises.	Refer to specialist services such as physiotherapy.
Concurrent or pre-existing co-morbidities, e.g. heart disease.	Precaution/contraindications to exercise		Liaise/refer to relevant medical team.
Identification of new symptoms, e.g. dizziness or red flags.	Physiological changes as a result of increased energy expenditure.	Screen for any physiological changes or red flags through questioning.	Refer for urgent medical review.
Exacerbation of existing symptoms such as pain or fatigue.	• Exercising at too intensive a level. • Incorrect form of exercise.	Reduce level of intensity. Modify exercise type.	If an ongoing problem, contact medical team for review.

Problem	Cause	Prevention	Action
Risk of falls.	Poor balance, exercise too difficult.	Screen for balance problems through questioning. Encourage supportive footwear. Consider advice to be given on types of exercises.	Request medical review. Consider referral to local community falls team.
Lack of resources for onward referral.	No national standard care of exercise provision/resources.		Online resources such as Macmillan Cancer Support or specific cancer charities, e.g. PCUK/Breast Cancer Care.

377

Post-procedural considerations

Give the patient sufficient time to ask questions to ensure they understand the benefits to being physically active. Discuss an onward plan and follow up if appropriate to assess self-management.

Complications

These may include non-compliance with lifestyle changes at review. Look to identify barriers to exercise and manage them. Consider low mood and refer for psychological support if appropriate.

Websites

Walking for health: www.walkingforhealth.org.uk/
Macmillan Cancer Support: Maintaining a healthy lifestyle: www.macmillan.org.uk/information-and-support/coping/maintaining-a-healthy-lifestyle/keeping-active
Macmillan 2016 Move More: https://be.macmillan.org.uk/be/s-840-move-more.aspx
Rambling groups: www.ramblers.org.uk/go-walking/group-finder.aspx
UK government guidelines on exercise: www.gov.uk/government/publications/uk-physical-activity guidelines

SECTION 8.8 CANCER-RELATED FATIGUE AND SLEEP

This section discusses and describes the cancer-related fatigue (CRF) and sleep disturbances that patients often experience because of their treatment. It recommends approaches and techniques that may help in the management of these symptoms. The key focus is management because there is no one set solution or quick-fix, one-size, fits-all answer. The management of these symptoms requires an approach that assesses, reviews and monitors the individual patient's progress.

This section will discuss first CRF and then sleep.

Cancer-related fatigue

Definitions

CRF is a distressing, persistent, subjective sense of physical, emotional and/or cognitive tiredness or exhaustion related to cancer or cancer treatment that is not proportionate to recent activity and interferes with usual functioning (NCCN 2016). This differs from excessive tiredness which is a common complaint of today's society, some level being found in almost all of the population (Ogilvy et al. 2008).

CRF is a complicated multidimensional symptom and its causes vary (Ritterband et al. 2012). It is one of the most frequent and disturbing complaints in over 75% of both acute and palliative cancer patients (de Raaf et al. 2012).

Presenting symptoms

CRF impacts on a person's ability to function and is not completely improved with rest or sleep (NCCN 2016). It may present as significant fatigue, depressed mood and reduced quality of life (Barsevick et al. 2010, Bjorneklett et al. 2012, Courtier et al. 2013).

CRF is a relentless exhaustion and lack of energy that prevents patients from taking part in everyday activities that they previously managed independently (Chan et al. 2011). CRF may also result in insomnia or disturbed sleep patterns, cognitive deficits, memory difficulties, reduced attention and concentration.

Related theory

Although patients report that CRF is not relieved by sleep, sleep is important to patients' quality of life and their tolerance to treatment (Ancoli-Israel et al. 2001). Psychological well-being may also be affected with impatience and mood swings (Cooper and Kite 2015). CRF can develop into a chronic condition, persisting for months to years after cancer treatment has finished. Various factors can affect sleep such as the biochemical changes associated with the process of neoplastic growth and anticancer treatments (Roscoe et al. 2007).

CRF is multifactorial. It can be caused by cancer treatment such as chemotherapy, radiotherapy, biological therapy and surgery. Side-effects such as poor nutrition, low mood, anxiety, memory difficulties, poor sleep and the medication patients need to take all contribute to CRF. Comprehensive assessment of people experiencing CRF should be completed to identify and treat reversible causes and offer person-centred care. The complex web of possible causes of CRF means that effective treatment is a challenge for cancer care providers (NCI 2015).

Evidence-based approaches

Rationale

The Survivorship movement states that cancer patients are living life beyond cancer, and palliative patients require support in living active meaningful lives with as much urgency as all other cancer survivors (Hwang et al. 2015, NCSI 2013). Assessment and provision of individually tailored exercise and physical activity programmes are recommended for CRF (Cancer Research UK 2017, LCA 2016, NCCN 2016, NCSI 2013).

In combination with physical activity, the individual patient's CRF requires assessment for management of energy conservation (Cooper and Kite 2015, LCA 2016). Simple techniques such as those outlined in Procedure guideline 8.19 may be indicated.

Indications

Aerobic exercise can make a statistically significant improvement in CRF for patients who are undergoing or have completed treatment for cancerous solid tumours (Cramp and Byron-Daniel 2012). Physical activity is recommended for patients with prostate, breast and colon cancer and those having treatment with radiotherapy, chemotherapy and stem cell transplant (Mitchell et al. 2014).

Contraindications

Research has been unable to identify any pattern of physical activity modalities, frequency or intensity of exercise or the best time in the patient's treatment pathway to introduce exercise and physical activity for CRF (Mitchell et al. 2014). No clear theme has emerged regarding specific activities that are beneficial to patients and the longitudinal benefits of exercise for patients with CRF (Cramp and Byron-Daniel 2012). This reinforces the necessity for individual assessment, monitoring and review (Cooper and Kite 2015).

Principles of care

Although there is no uniform solution to this complex problem, fatigue management requires an approach which involves thorough assessment to establish the causes, whether any prescribed medication can help or is, indeed, contributing to the fatigue (LCA 2016), and to establish the optimum programme to support the patient with regular reviews (Lowrie 2006). Education and counselling are required to ensure patient engagement and involvement in the management of CRF (NCCN 2016).

With prolonged insomnia, a skilled practitioner in CRF needs to carry out a programme of fatigue management and may use an outcome measure such as Functional Assessment of Chronic Illness Therapy– Fatigue (FACIT-F) (Gascon et al. 2013). There is a good correlation between the FACIT fatigue and Fatigue Severity Scale (FSS) scores (Cella et al. 2011). FACIT-F consists of five experience and eight impact questions. Practically speaking, this implies that fatigue as an outcome can be expressed as a single number, and the experience of the symptom is more likely to be endorsed at mild levels of fatigue, presumably before the symptom exerts an adverse impact upon function (Cella et al. 2011).

The principles of CRF management include advising the patient to take gentle but regular exercise to increase the heart rate but not cause even worse fatigue. The person must establish their own exercise tolerance and routine as individuals will differ. Similarly, the individual needs to establish their own dietary boundaries, including whether a hot milky drink at bedtime helps with sleep.

Legal and professional issues

- Clear and accurate records relevant to the clinician's practice must always be kept, without falsification. Immediate and appropriate action must be taken if this is not carried out.
- Any risks or problems must be identified as they arise and the steps taken to deal with them recorded.
- Any record must be clearly dated, timed and attributable to the person making the entry.
- Any legal requirements must be met regarding appropriate data sharing and data confidentiality in record keeping (NMC 2015).

Pre-procedural considerations

Assessment tools

An assessment tool such as the FSS (Figure 8.32) may be used to identify key areas of daily life on which the fatigue is having an impact. This concise scale can be filled in again by the patient later to compare how they are coping. It has a reliability which falls within acceptable ranges, its precision and clinically important change estimates provide guidelines for interpreting change in scores from these outcomes in clinical research of intervention and rehabilitation approaches for managing fatigue. The analysis of construct validity further established the meaningful interpretation of the FSS, the scale is simple, economical and efficient at capturing the severity and impact of fatigue in, primarily the physical nature of fatigue (Learmouth et al. 2013).

Procedure guideline 8.19   Fatigue management

Pre-procedure

Action	Rationale
1 Introduce self to patient, either in the inpatient or outpatient setting.	To establish professional and clinical rapport. **E**
2 Gain consent from the patient for the intervention.	To ensure the patient understands the procedure and provides verbal consent (NMC 2015, **E**).

Procedure

Action	Rationale
3 Assess the impact of fatigue on the patient using a tool, e.g. the Fatigue Severity Scale (Figure 8.32).	To obtain a baseline assessment of fatigue and sleep disturbance (Gascon et al. 2013, Minton and Stone 2009; **E**). To enable expert assessment and a relevant treatment programme. **E**
4 Identify what effects the fatigue is having on the individual's ability to carry out daily activities by discussing this with the patient, identifying their daily activity pattern.	To obtain a baseline assessment of fatigue and sleep disturbance (Gascon et al. 2013, Minton and Stone 2009; **E**).
5 Advise on using the 5 Ps for **fatigue management** (Box 8.10).	To introduce basic principles of energy conservation (Ewer-Smith 2006; **C**).

Post-procedure

Action	Rationale
6 Document assessment.	Legal requirement of professional body and employing institution.
7 Make a follow-up appointment.	To ensure engagement in the programme. **C** To review and monitor progress. **C**
8 Review the programme.	To establish how the patient is coping. **C**

FATIGUE SEVERITY SCALE (FSS)

Date _____   Name _____

Please circle the number between 1 and 7 which you feel best fits the following statements. This refers to your usual way of life within the last week. 1 indicates "strongly disagree" and 7 indicates "strongly agree."

Read and circle a number.	Strongly Disagree → Strongly Agree						
1. My motivation is lower when I am fatigued.	1	2	3	4	5	6	7
2. Exercise brings on my fatigue.	1	2	3	4	5	6	7
3. I am easily fatigued.	1	2	3	4	5	6	7
4. Fatigue interferes with my physical functioning.	1	2	3	4	5	6	7
5. Fatigue causes frequent problems for me.	1	2	3	4	5	6	7
6. My fatigue prevents sustained physical functioning.	1	2	3	4	5	6	7
7. Fatigue interferes with carrying out certain duties and responsibilities.	1	2	3	4	5	6	7
8. Fatigue is among my most disabling symptoms.	1	2	3	4	5	6	7
9. Fatigue interferes with my work, family, or social life.	1	2	3	4	5	6	7

VISUAL ANALOGUE FATIGUE SCALE (VAFS)

Please mark an "X" on the number line which describes your global fatigue with 0 being worst and 10 being normal.

0	1	2	3	4	5	6	7	8	9	10

Figure 8.32 The Fatigue Severity Scale (FSS) and Visual Analogue Fatigue Scale (VAFS). *Source:* Learmouth et al. 2013. Reproduced with permission of Elsevier.

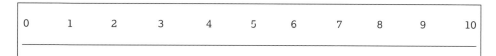

Problem-solving table 8.8 Prevention and resolution (Procedure guideline 8.19)

Problem	Cause	Prevention	Action
Lack of motivation.	During treatment: • side-effects and long-term consequences of treatment • low mood • uncertainty about how much activity to undertake and balance activity and rest.	Ensure timing of giving information. Relate advice on activity to practical tasks so that the patient can learn the advice and use it in a practical way.	Consider attending behavioural change training such as cognitive behavioural training and motivational interviewing.
Concurrent or pre-existing co-morbidities, e.g. heart disease.	Precaution/contraindications to exercise.	Ensure the patient is aware of their own limitations and restrictions.	Liaise/refer to relevant medical team.
Identification of new symptoms, e.g. dizziness or red flags.	Physiological changes as a result of increased energy expenditure.	Screen for any physiological changes or red flags through questioning.	Refer to urgent medical review.
Exacerbation of existing symptoms such as fatigue or anxiety.	Exercising at too intensive a level. Incorrect form of exercise.	Reduce level of intensiveness. Modify exercise type.	If ongoing problem, contact medical team for review.

(continued)

Problem-solving table 8.8 Prevention and resolution (Procedure guideline 8.19 *[continued]*)

Problem	Cause	Prevention	Action
Risk of falls.	Poor balance, exercise too difficult. Too fatigued to tolerate exercise.	Screen for balance problems through questioning and observation. Encourage supportive footwear. Consider advice to be given on types of exercises.	Request medical review. Consider referral to local community falls team.
Lack of resources for onward referral.	No national standard care of exercise provision/resources.		Online resources such as Macmillan Cancer Support or specific cancer charities, e.g. PCUK/Breast.

Post-procedural considerations

Immediate care
Psychological issues may occur affecting quality of life due to ongoing fatigue. These should be addressed by acknowledging this symptom and encouraging the use of fatigue management and energy conservation techniques as described in Box 8.10 (i.e. prioritizing, planning, pacing, posture and permission).

Ongoing care
Ongoing issues relating to fatigue require review of the techniques as described above.

Documentation
Any written advice should be documented in the individual's medical notes.

Education of patient and relevant others
The advice given in Procedure guideline 8.19 can be provided to the patient and their relevant others.

Complications
No complications would be anticipated.

Box 8.10 The five Ps

- **Prioritize:** Consider which activities are important to you each day, and prioritize which activities you would like to conserve your energy for. Try to cut out unnecessary tasks to conserve your energy.
- **Plan:** Organize your activities as effectively as possible to conserve as much energy as you can. Consider which times of the day are best for you to be active or at rest. Try not to do too much in any one day, and plan your activities for the week ahead as much as possible.
- **Pace:** It is important to balance periods of activity with periods of rest. You may need to rest during an activity and allow yourself a little extra time to get things done.
- **Position:** Work out a position that is comfortable for you when you feel breathless and practise this so that you can help yourself. Think about your posture and try to maintain this so that you avoid becoming uncomfortable and conserve your energy.
- **Permission:** Give yourself permission *not* to do activities that result in you becoming breathless and tired. Instead of thinking along the lines of 'I must', 'I ought', try and change the way you think about things and say to yourself 'I choose to do ....' 'I wish to do ....' instead.

Sleep

Definition
Sleep disorders have been recognized for centuries as a frequent complication of medical illness. Human sleep is a complex and dynamic physiological function. It is an active condition affected by waking physiological and psychological states which, in turn, has significant effects on those waking conditions.

Presenting symptoms
Recognized symptoms of sleep disturbance include (Roscoe et al. 2007):

- insomnia, a subjective complaint by the patient of poor sleep, insufficient sleep, difficulty initiating or maintaining sleep, interrupted sleep, poor quality or non-restorative sleep, or sleep that occurs at the wrong time of the day-night cycle
- sleep deprivation resulting in a broad spectrum of physiological and psychological changes, including progressive fatigue, sleepiness, poor concentration, depression and irritability
- excessive daytime sleepiness
- disorders of the sleep-wake schedule, having lengthy daytime naps, difficulty falling asleep.

Related theory
As relaxation focuses on enabling the patient to relax, it improves their quality of life, reduces stress and anxiety, and thus improves mood. Relaxation also aims to reduce the impact of fatigue and improve sleep and the global quality of life and physical functioning (Charalambous et al. 2016, Greenlee et al. 2014).

Daytime fatigue and sleepiness may occur because of tumour effects (e.g. cytokines), chemotherapy, radiotherapy or surgery (Ancoli-Israel et al. 2001). Cytokines are non-antibody polypeptides secreted by inflammatory leukocytes and can be induced by cancer cells. They may play a role in the sleep disturbances of cancer patients due to cytokine-based neuroimmunological mechanisms (Fiorentino and Ancoli-Israel 2007).

There are strong correlations between fatigue and emotional distress (NCCN 2016), sleep disorder being amongst the causes. Sleep disturbances affect between 30 and 75% of newly diagnosed or recently treated cancer patients (Fiorentino and Ancoli-Israel 2007). These vary from difficulties falling asleep to difficulty staying asleep with frequent awakenings. Anxiety over disease recurrence, persisting sleep disturbance and physical deconditioning after a prolonged illness have also been considered important in predicting fatigue (Courtier et al. 2013).

Box 8.11 Breathing technique to assist in relaxation

Instructions:
1 Loosen any tight clothing. Position yourself comfortably, either lying or sitting, but ensuring that your back is supported.
2 Close your eyes if you wish.
3 Keep your shoulders and upper chest relaxed.
4 Place your hand flat on your stomach.
5 Inhale slowly (through your nose if possible).
6 As you breathe in, your stomach should gently swell underneath your hand (this should not be a forced movement using your abdominal muscles).
7 Remember to keep your shoulders and upper chest relaxed.
8 Exhale slowly through your mouth (your stomach will gently flatten beneath your hand).
9 Pause, then repeat steps 2–9.
10 During the exercise, think of a positive word or phrase such as 'I am relaxed' or 'calm'.

Stress management techniques and relaxation exercises (Box 8.11) may help the sleep pattern (Varvogli and Darviri 2011). Cognitive behavioural therapy has been shown to be an effective treatment with this patient population (Ritterband et al. 2012). CBT is a way of changing unhelpful ways of thinking that can result in anxiety and disturb the sleep pattern (The Royal College of Psychiatrists 2012).

Evidence-based stress management techniques including progressive muscular relaxation, autogenic training, biofeedback, guided imagery, mindfulness and CBT may reduce sleep disturbance and daytime related fatigue (Vargas et al. 2014). These techniques need to be carried out by advanced expert clinicians. CBT, for example, is a treatment approach that encompasses assessment strategies, cognitive and behavioural treatment techniques. The clinician and patient work together to set goals and homework. By changing thought patterns, cognitive and behavioural changes can take place to enable the individual to

substitute life-enhancing thoughts and beliefs (Varvogli and Darviri, 2011).

Evidence-based approaches

Rationale

Studies show that relaxation and guided imagery demonstrate a statistically significant reduction in anxiety (Leon-Pizarro et al. 2007) and how instruction in progressive muscular relaxation may help in maintaining activities (Christman and Cain 2004). Patients also feel able to take control of their lives, setting goals and priorities by managing their anxiety levels (Cooper 2014).

As with fatigue management, the management of disturbed sleep requires a multiprofessional approach, including medical, nursing and allied healthcare professionals (e.g. occupational therapy and physiotherapy) to carry out holistic and accurate assessment and screening.

More complex coping strategies need to be tailored to the individual's needs so that they can develop a toolkit that can be used in their daily routine to manage this symptom. These needs can only be established following specific assessment and treatment programmes by skilled and experienced clinicians such as medical and nursing, occupational therapy and physiotherapy specialists in sleep management.

Multidimensional assessment should ideally include a clinical evaluation together with self-report questionnaires and daily sleep diaries (Morin et al. 2011). One example of a sleep diary is shown in Figure 8.33 (National Sleep Foundation 2016).

This information will enable the clinician to analyse the patient's behavioural patterns and establish an appropriate treatment programme. The treatment programme should be reviewed with an outcome measure to enable the patient to gauge their progress (Barsevick et al. 2010).

Indications

Interventions and advice to help individuals with poor sleep are principally needed when sleep-wake disturbances are a persistent problem linked to poor quality of life. Knowledge of the prevalence, severity and correlates of these disturbances provides

381

Day and date	Day 1	Day 2	Day 3	Day 4	Day 5	Day 6	Day 7
I went to bed last night at:							
I got up this morning at:							
Last night, I fell asleep: – Easily – After some time – With difficulty – Not at all							
I woke up during the night: – No. of times – For how long							
Last night I slept for how many hours							
Sleep was disturbed by (name causes)							
When I woke up, I felt: – Refreshed – Slightly refreshed – Fatigued							
Any other causes for poor sleep							

Figure 8.33 Sleep diary. *Source:* National Sleep Foundation (2016). Reproduced with permission of the National Sleep Foundation.

useful information to healthcare providers during clinical evaluations for treatment of these disturbances in cancer survivors (Otte et al. 2010).

Contraindications

Although most people are aware of the common-sense approach to sleep hygiene as shown in Procedure guideline 8.20, failure to adhere to these guidelines is extremely widespread. Engagement and compliance with this advice is a challenge with many sleep disorders.

The individual symptoms of, for example, insomnia are not a diagnosis in themselves. Single and multi-symptom measurements in themselves are of limited usefulness in distinguishing fatigue, depression and insomnia (Donovan and Jacobsen 2007).

Relaxation and guided imagery techniques should not be used with patients known to have psychotic episodes as these techniques promote channelled thoughts and there is a risk of the patient experiencing hallucinations.

Principles of care

When addressing patients' difficulties in sleeping, the following points should be considered (LCA 2016):

- assessing for and treating physical symptoms (e.g. pain)
- checking medication that affects sleep (e.g. steroids, chemotherapies, anticonvulsants and antihypertensives)
- introducing principles of relaxation and anxiety management techniques
- sleep hygiene including:
  - limiting stimulants, caffeine or alcohol, removing the TV from the bedroom to avoid stimulation of flashing images and lights
  - regulating room and body temperature
  - a standard routine of sleep and rest
  - regulating nutrition to avoid hunger or overeating before bedtime
- the role of exercise.

Procedure guideline 8.20   Relaxation and anxiety management

Pre-procedure

Action	Rationale
1 Introduce self to patient, either in the inpatient or outpatient setting.	To establish professional and clinical rapport. **E**
2 Gain consent from the patient for the intervention.	To ensure the patient understands the procedure and provides verbal consent (NMC 2015; **E**).

Procedure

Action	Rationale
3 Assess baseline of the patient's anxiety and sleep pattern using visual analogue scale Insomnia Severity Index Sleep Assessment (Morin et al. 2011): Sleep problem — 5 being most difficult Difficulty falling asleep — 0–5 Difficulty staying asleep — 0–5 Problem waking up early — 0–5	To establish the patient's perception of their anxiety level. **C**
4 Establish triggers for anxiety.	To identify causes for anxiety. **C**
5 Discuss how to use relaxation techniques in daily routine and how to apply them in practice.	To enable the patient to use relaxation techniques as part of a toolkit of skills to cope with fatigue and anxiety. **C**
6 Provide simple advice on managing poor sleep in the form of a written leaflet, in conjunction with a session at which the information is discussed and explained thoroughly (see information in Figure 8.34).	To enable the patient to use the advice at home (RCP 2012).
7 Provide a recording of each session for the patient to continue practising (e.g. on their smart phone, MP3 download or compact disc of the session).	To provide ownership of sessions to patient and enable ongoing practice. **C**
8 Encourage use of a sleep diary (Figure 8.33).	To enable the patient to measure the success of sleep strategies. **C**

Post-procedure

Action	Rationale
9 Document the consultation.	Legal requirement of professional body and employing institution (NMC 2015, **E**).
10 Have one final therapy session to ensure the patient understands all instructions and the healthcare professional can answer any remaining questions before discharging the patient.	To demonstrate progress to the patient and refer on to further support if required. **C**

This fact sheet is to help you to remember what you discussed with the occupational therapist.

Difficulty with sleeping is a common effect of cancer and its treatments. It is often due to a multitude of factors, including physical, emotional and psychological aspects. Lack of or decreased quality of sleep can impact your mood, memory, and ability to learn. It can also decrease your immune system, and does not allow your body and body systems to have necessary rest. This may in turn affect quality of life.

It is important that you discuss this with your medical team, so that it can be addressed in the multidisciplinary team.

For good sleep hygiene, the following strategies may be useful:

* Set a standard rising time routine (e.g. 10pm – 6am – get up regardless if you had poor sleep during the night).
* Avoid excessive time in bed as it may hamper your ability to have a good amount of rest at night.
* Try not to watch television/read/eat in bed – associate bedtime with sleep.
* Try to engage in calming activities for 60 minutes before going to bed – listening to music, relaxation CD or meditation session. Avoid watching TV or other activities with bright lights or sudden noises as these things are stimulating to the brain.
* Limit/avoid daytime napping and don't nap close to bedtime.
* Get out of bed when you cannot sleep – some people find doing mundane tasks, like doing the dishes, helps trigger the need to sleep.
* Exercise regularly.
* Limit caffeine and alcohol in the evening.
* Try a light snack before bed – try not to go to bed hungry as this may keep you up. Similarly, try not to have a heavy meal.
* Use lavender on pillow – known for its sleep-inducing properties. Do check if you have any allergies, or any medical reason not to use this.
* Milky drink before bed.
* Relaxation techniques/music – use the relaxation CD 30 minutes prior to going to bed. You can see your occupational therapists for relaxation therapy sessions to help you with the techniques.
* Ear plugs and eye masks – help create a more peaceful environment.
* A dark room with blackout curtains may help.
* Use white noise if this helps you to relax and can block out noises that frustrate and alert you.

Tips for family and friends

Additional tips specifically for you:

Figure 8.34 Occupational therapy program – tips and strategies for improving sleep. *Source:* The Royal Marsden Hospital NHS Foundation Trust (2015).

SECTION 8.9 COMMUNICATION FOR A PATIENT WITH A LARYNGECTOMY

This section details the procedures associated with supporting a patient who communicates with the assistance of a surgical voice prosthesis following a laryngectomy.

Definitions
* *Laryngectomy*: removal of the larynx and surrounding structures.
* *Stoma*: a hole in the neck through which the laryngectomy patient breathes.
* *Surgical voice restoration (SVR)*: a means to restore communication using a silicone voice prosthesis.
* *Tracheoesophageal puncture (TEP)*: a hole created between trachea and oesophagus to allow voice prosthesis placement.

Anatomy and physiology
Laryngeal carcinoma is the primary reason for total laryngectomy, removal of the larynx. In 2011, 2360 people were diagnosed with laryngeal carcinoma in the UK (Jones et al. 2016). Organ preservation is the first line of treatment using concurrent chemoradiation but if this fails a total laryngectomy may be required. Large hypopharyngeal tumours involving the pyriform sinus, posterior pharyngeal wall and post-cricoid regions may also warrant a laryngectomy if chemoradiation is unsuccessful.

In a small number of non-cancer cases, patients may undergo a laryngectomy if they have severe dysphagia resulting in significant aspiration and multiple chest infections.

The larynx is found in the neck at the level of the third and sixth cervical vertebrae. It lies anterior to the oesophagus, situated at the top of the trachea (Mathieson 2001). It is made of bone and cartilage held together by muscles and membranes. As the upper airway is shared with the food passage, the main function of the larynx is to protect the airway from saliva and food and drink from entering the trachea and lungs. The larynx allows production of a cough to clear unwanted materials from the airway (Corbridge 1998) and is used for voicing. Within the larynx, held between the thyroid cartilage and the arytenoids, lie the vocal folds; as air from the trachea passes up towards the vocal folds, they vibrate to make sound. This is then directed up towards the resonating cavities, pharynx and nasal cavities to the mouth where the lips and tongue articulate to produce voice.

Related theory
Once the vocal cords have been removed, another vibrating source needs to be created. There are a variety of communication options post laryngectomy, including oesophageal speech, artificial larynx and surgical voice restoration.

Box 8.12 lists the variety of ways in which communication is restored post laryngectomy.

SVR has become the most popular form of restoring communication, with success rates of up to 90% reported (Op de Coul et al. 2000). SVR entails creating a fistula between the posterior wall of the trachea and the anterior wall of the oesophagus, into which a one-way voice prosthesis is placed. By closing off the tracheostoma, pulmonary air is diverted through the prosthesis into the oesophagus where the walls vibrate to make sound (van As-Brooks and Fuller 2007).

Box 8.12 Ways in which communication is restored after laryngectomy

- *Oesophageal voice* involves moving air into the oesophagus (Searl and Reeves 2007) either by inhaling or injecting air into the back of the mouth. Instead of the vocal cords vibrating, the walls of the pharynx vibrate. Sound then moves into the mouth where recognizable speech is produced by the articulators, tongue, lips and palate. Patients are asked to imagine gulping air into their mouths, begin to swallow but return it to their mouth in a controlled manner. It has previously been described as 'burped speech' and usually the patient can achieve a small number of words on one breath.
- An *artificial larynx* involves using a battery-powered device that is placed against the neck or cheek or intraorally (Searl and Reeves 2007). When the button is pushed, a vibration occurs in the head of the device and it is this vibration through the tissues that creates sound as the patient mouthes the words.
- *Surgical voice restoration (SVR)* allows communication to be restored by use of a voice prosthesis which may also be referred to as a valve. See Figure 8.35 for the operative site for surgical voice restoration.

The prosthesis is a silicone device that fits into the TEP and acts as a one-way valve, preventing food and drink from entering the trachea from the oesophagus (Figure 8.36). Patients can have the puncture created during their laryngectomy operation, which is called a *primary puncture*. Post-operatively, patients with a primary puncture are fed via a stoma gastric tube, which enables the puncture to remain patent, avoids food contamination around the healing pharynx and decreases the risk of fistula formation (Karlen and Maisel 2001, Rhys-Evans et al. 2003). Once healing has occurred, the stoma gastric tube is removed and the prosthesis can be placed into the TEP.

If patients are required to wait for their puncture following the laryngectomy surgery, for example due to an extended laryngectomy, they are likely to have a *secondary puncture*. Another option involves patients having their voice prosthesis placed into the TEP during the laryngectomy surgery; this is known as *primary placement*.

Voice prostheses

Voice prostheses have been available in Britain for over 25 years (Singer 2004) and there are several devices on the market, mainly Blom-Singer (InHealth Technologies, Carpinteria, California, USA) and Provox (Atos Medical, Malmo, Sweden) products. All work according to the same principle with a one-way valve, two flanges (one anterior and one posterior) to secure the prosthesis *in situ* in the TEP, and a strap to attach to the neck (Figure 8.37). The prostheses come in a variety of diameters and lengths and it is the role of the specialist speech and language therapist to choose the most appropriate model for the patient, taking into account the patient's requirements. Prostheses can be either exdwelling, meaning the patient can be taught to self-change, or indwelling, requiring the input of a specialist clinician, including a specialist speech and language therapist, Ear, Nose and Throat (ENT) doctor or a nurse experienced in fitting and managing voice prostheses.

Voice prostheses are usually kept in Speech and Language Therapy or Ear, Nose and Throat Departments. Patients are provided with all the items that are needed for cleaning their voice prosthesis (see Procedure guideline 8.20), usually by the speech and language therapist or an appropriately trained specialist nurse. Patients need to store the items securely but they do not need to be kept in a sterile environment. Frequently patients receive a sealable bag to store their equipment.

Humidification

All laryngectomy patients need to wear a heat–moisture exchange system (HME) for humidification. As the patient no longer breathes through the nose there is a reduction in filtration, humidification, heat exchange and resistance. Studies have shown that people with laryngectomies have increased mucus production,

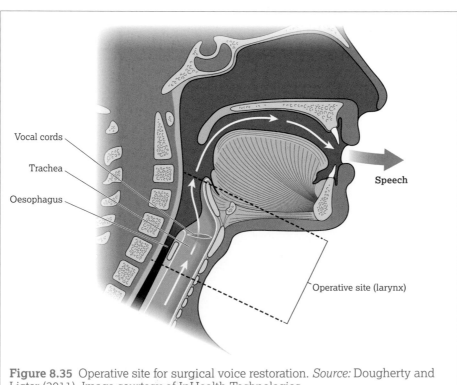

Figure 8.35 Operative site for surgical voice restoration. *Source:* Dougherty and Lister (2011). Image courtesy of InHealth Technologies.

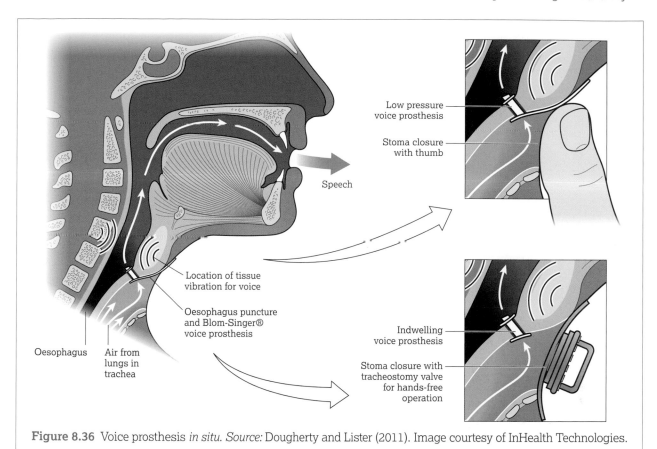

Figure 8.36 Voice prosthesis *in situ. Source:* Dougherty and Lister (2011). Image courtesy of InHealth Technologies.

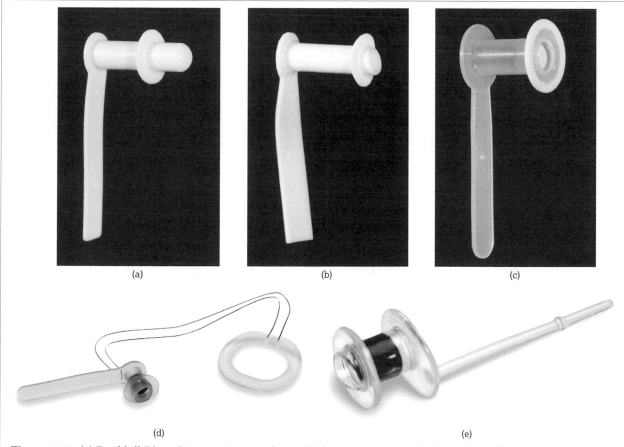

Figure 8.37 (a) Duckbill Blom-Singer voice prosthesis. (b) Low-pressure ex dwelling Blom-Singer voice prosthesis. (c) Indwelling Blom-Singer voice prosthesis. (d) Non-indwelling (NID) voice prosthesis. Photo courtesy of Atos Medical, www.atosmedical.com. (e) Vega voice prosthesis, indwelling. Photo courtesy of Atos Medical, www.atosmedical.com.

386

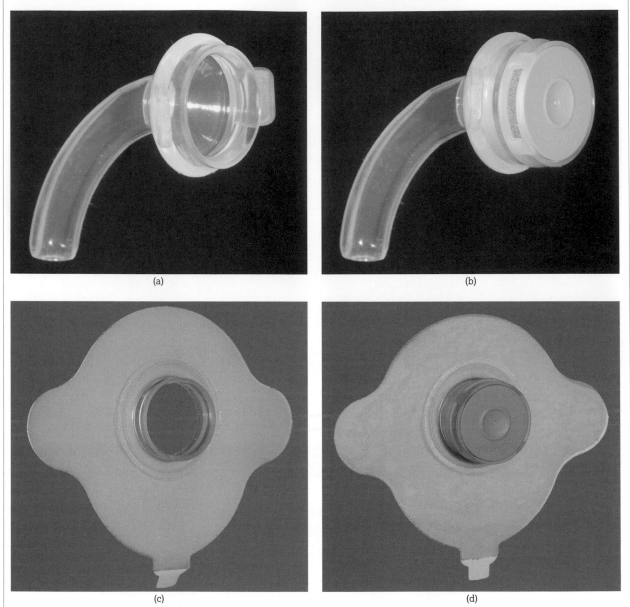

Figure 8.38 (a) Provox laryngectomy tube, (b) Provox laryngectomy tube with HME filter, (c) Provox HME baseplate, (d) Provox HME baseplate with filter *in situ*.

dryness, crusting, coughing, shortness of breath and increased risk of chest infections (Jones et al, 2003, Zurr et al. 2006) Use of an HME will:

- trap moisture on expiration to warm air on inspiration
- filter inhaled air
- provide air stream resistance to encourage lung expansion.

Post-operatively, patients may wear a hypoallergenic baseplate, and a filter cassette will fit into this device (Figure 8.38).

Legal and professional issues
One of the care requirements is placing an HME device. This is an advanced practice role of a specialist nurse who has met the required competencies (see Table 8.14).

Table 8.14 Competencies for use of an HME device in a laryngectomy patient

Knowledge and understanding	Skills
Altered anatomy following a laryngectomy	An ability to recognize a laryngectomy versus a tracheostomy
The function of the HME	Ability to recognize an HME
The importance of placing an HME on a patient	An ability to provide the patient/carer with the relevant physical preparation for attaching the HME
Principles of HME selection	An ability to match the correct HME type to the patient
Complications that may arise post HME placement such as skin reaction, stomal discomfort	An ability to evaluate the HME and recognize patient discomfort

Procedure guideline 8.21   HME placement

Essential equipment
- Skin preparation wipes
- Skin barrier wipes
- Gauze pads
- Light source
- Saline nebulizer
- Sterile water
- Clinically clean tray
- HME baseplate or laryngeal tube
- HME filter
- Single-use disposable tweezers

Pre-procedure

Action	Rationale
1 Explain and discuss the procedure with the patient.	To ensure the patient understands the procedure and gives their valid consent (NMC 2015, **C**).
2 Settle the patient in a chair or upright in bed and arrange lighting to illuminate the stoma.	To ensure the patient is comfortable and well supported. **E**

Procedure

Action	Rationale
3 Ask the patient to use the nebulizer.	To loosen secretions in the trachea (Everitt 2016, **E**).
4 Wet the gauze and wipe around the stoma, wiping away from the stoma.	To ensure the stomal area is clean and prevent water entering the trachea. **E**
5 Using tweezers, carefully remove any dry crusts in the trachea.	To ensure breathing is not impeded. **E**
6 Using the skin preparation barrier, carefully wipe around the stomal area.	To protect stomal skin (Brewster 2004, **E**).
7 *Either* place the correct size of laryngeal tube into the airway.	To provide a holder for the HME filter (Ackerstaff et al. 1995, **R5**).
8 *Or* place the HME baseplate onto stomal skin, ensuring the skin is stretched to allow a firm seal.	To provide a holder for the HME filter (Ackerstaff et al. 1995, **R5**).
9 Place the HME filter into either the laryngeal tube or baseplate, ensuring it is clicked into place.	To ensure the HME is fitted fully into the holder (Ackerstaff et al. 1995, **R5**).
10 Replace the filter throughout the day as it becomes fouled with mucus.	To ensure breathing is not impeded (Ackerstaff et al. 1995, **R5**).
11 Remove and clean the laryngeal tube at least twice a day.	To ensure mucus is removed from the tube and breathing is not impeded (Ackerstaff et al. 1995, **R5**).
12 The HME baseplate can remain in place for 72 hours but daily removal and cleaning is recommended.	Removal allows inspection of the stomal area to ensure skin has not reacted (Ackerstaff et al. 1995, **R5**).
13 Removal of the baseplate requires dampening of the HME baseplate and gentle use of skin removal product, easing the baseplate away from the skin.	Gentle removal ensures skin is not traumatized (Brewster 2004, **E**).

Post-procedure

Action	Rationale
14 Record the procedure including shape and type of HME baseplate and filter type.	To maintain accurate records (NMC 2009, **C**).

Problem-solving table 8.9 Prevention and resolution (Procedure guideline 8.21)

Problem	Cause	Prevention	Action
Skin reaction.	HME baseplate causing skin to react.	Regular use of barrier skin preparation.	Remove baseplate and allow skin to recover.
Ongoing skin reaction.	HME baseplate causing skin to react.	Trial of different baseplates.	Remove baseplate, allow skin to recover and trial a different baseplate.
Stomal shrinkage.	Post-operative complication.	Daily measuring of stoma size.	Consider insertion of a laryngeal tube.

Post-procedural considerations

Ensure the patient is comfortable wearing the baseplate/laryngeal tube and that they can remove and replace the HME filter. Choice of HME in the acute post-operative situation will usually be with a hypoallergenic baseplate. Use of a laryngeal tube as an option is usually recommended by the surgical team.

Immediate care

Once the HME is in place the patient is not required to do anything. If there is a voice prosthesis *in situ* the patient is shown how to occlude the filter to achieve voice.

Ongoing care

Speech and language therapists and nurses are responsible for teaching the patient how to remove and replace the HME device and monitor stoma size.

Cleaning

The voice prosthesis needs to be cleaned at least twice a day, more frequently when it is first inserted. It is also essential to clean it if the prosthesis leaks or if there is no voice (Procedure guideline 8.22).

The cleaning of a voice prosthesis is an advanced practice role of a specialist nurse who has met the required competencies (see Table 8.15).

Table 8.15 Competencies for cleaning a voice prosthesis in a laryngectomy patient

Knowledge and understanding	Skills
Altered anatomy following a laryngectomy	An ability to recognize a laryngectomy versus a tracheostomy
The function of a voice prosthesis	An ability to recognize a voice prosthesis *in situ*
The importance of keeping the prosthesis clean	An ability to provide the patient/carer with relevant physical preparation for cleaning the prosthesis
Principles of brush selection	An ability to perform a safe cleaning technique with the appropriate equipment
Complications that may arise during or after cleaning, their cause and preventive measures	An ability to evaluate cleaning technique with regard to demonstrating knowledge and recognizing difficulties, their cause and future preventive measures

---

Procedure guideline 8.22 Voice prosthesis: cleaning *in situ*

Essential equipment
- Non-sterile gloves and eye protection
- Light source
- Saline nebulizer
- Gauze pads
- Sterile water
- Micropore tape
- Prosthesis brush: non-sterile, reusable single patient use (Figure 8.39)
- Single-use disposable tweezers
- Long cotton buds
- Clinically clean tray

Pre-procedure

Action	Rationale
1 Explain and discuss the procedure with the patient.	To ensure that the patient understands the procedure and gives their valid consent (NMC 2015, **C**).

Procedure

Action	Rationale
2 Settle the patient in a chair or upright in bed and arrange lighting to illuminate the stoma.	To ensure the patient is comfortable and well supported. **E**
3 Ask the patient to use the nebulizer.	To loosen secretions in trachea (Everitt 2016, **E**).
4 Wet the gauze and wipe around the stoma, wiping away from the stoma.	To ensure the stomal area is clean and prevent water entering the trachea. **E**
5 Remove the tape and clean behind the strap; replace with new tape.	To ensure the stomal area is fully cleaned and the prosthesis is secured. **E**
6 Using tweezers, carefully remove any dry crusts from around the prosthesis and trachea.	To ensure breathing is not impeded. **E**
7 Wet the cotton buds and carefully clean the outside of the prosthesis.	To ensure air can enter the prosthesis. **E**
8 Wet the prosthesis brush and carefully insert into the barrel of the prosthesis, turning one way only, and remove. Hold the strap of prosthesis during the procedure. The patient does not need to do anything at this point.	To ensure the barrel of the prosthesis is clean to allow air flow. To ensure the prosthesis does not become dislodged. **E**

Post-procedure

Action	Rationale
9 Record the procedure.	To maintain accurate records (NMC 2015, **C**).

Problem-solving table 8.10 Prevention and resolution (Procedure guideline 8.22)

Problem	Cause	Prevention	Action
Loss of the prosthesis or stoma gastric catheter.	Accidental dislodgement or excessive coughing.	Teach patients how to insert the stent or catheter while on the ward.	Immediately insert either stent or catheter (Fr14 or smaller as needed) and secure with tape. Check that the patient has not inhaled the prosthesis; if they have, call for urgent ENT (Figure 8.41).
Peripheral leak.	Voice prosthesis too long. Enlarged TEP.		Specialist Speech and Language Therapist (SLT) or another trained clinician to downsize as appropriate. Specialist SLT and ENT to manage (Figure 8.41).
Central leakage.	Food debris preventing closure of prosthesis.	Thickener added to all drinks.	Clean with a brush. Specialist SLT or another trained clinician (specialist nurse/ENT doctor) to change.
Loss of voice.	Debris blocking barrel of prosthesis.		Clean with a brush.
	Due to incorrectly sized prosthesis.		Specialist SLT or another trained clinician to change device.
	Due to oedema in the TEP or voicing technique.		Specialized SLT to advise.

389

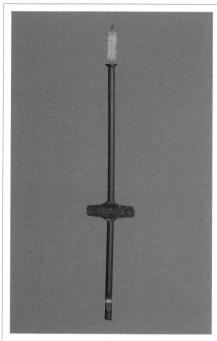

Figure 8.39 Prosthesis brush.

Post-procedural considerations

Immediate care
Once the voice prosthesis has been cleaned the patient should be able to voice and swallow with no difficulty.

Patients are taught, along with their carers, how to independently clean the prosthesis. This is done at least twice daily and if there are concerns about leakage from the prosthesis or voice changes (Figure 8.40).

Education of patient and relevant others
There are a variety of voice prostheses and it is essential that these are only changed by a specialist speech and language therapist or another trained professional. Patients are often able and encouraged to self-change an exdwelling voice prostheses following extensive training and completion of a competency programme.

Websites and useful addresses

National Association of Laryngectomy Clubs
Telephone: 0207 7308585
Website: www.laryngectomy.org.uk

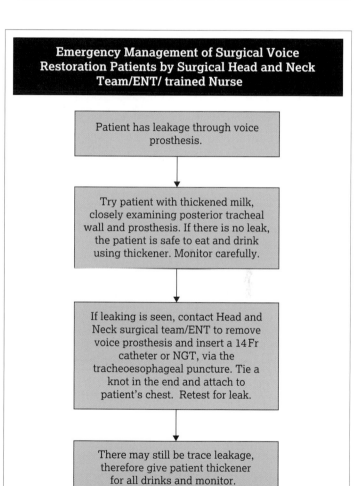

Figure 8.40 Emergency management of a dislodged voice prosthesis. *Source:* Speech and Language Therapy Department, Royal Marsden Hospital NHS Foundation Trust. NG, nasogastric; NGT, nasogastric tube; SLT, Speech and Language Therapy.

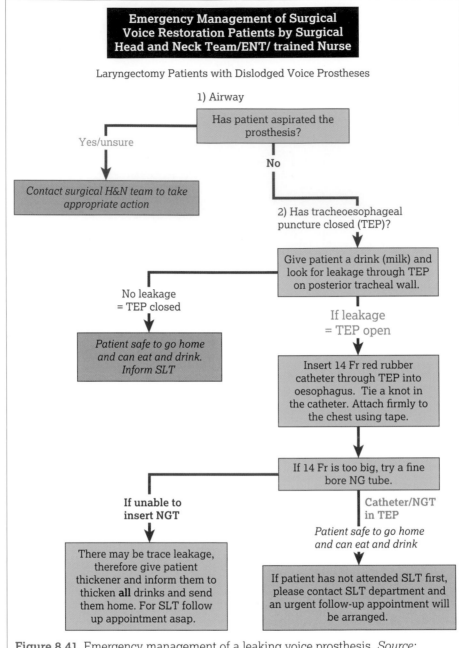

Figure 8.41 Emergency management of a leaking voice prosthesis. *Source:* Speech and Language Therapy Department, Royal Marsden Hospital NHS Foundation Trust. ENT, Ear, Nose and Throat; H&N, head and neck; NBM, nil by mouth; NGT, nasogastric tube.

SECTION 8.10 NIPPLE TATTOOING

This section focuses on the nurse-led procedure of nipple tattooing for women who have had major breast surgery because of cancer.

Breast cancer surgery constitutes a complex treatment pathway for patients and may be combined with adjuvant therapies such as chemotherapy and radiotherapy. Areola tattooing occurs at the end of this surgical journey and improves body image (Goh et al. 2011). This in turn provides a psychological boost to a patient's confidence and can help reduce some of the sexual relationship problems that breast cancer patients face (Piot-Ziegler et al. 2010). Reports suggest that levels of patient satisfaction are high and patients would recommend this procedure to others (Spear and Arias 1995).

Areolar tattooing can create an optical effect that greatly enhances the appearance of a reconstructed nipple–areola complex (NAC) and can help achieve a natural-looking appearance. Fading can occur after a variable time period, particularly if the person has previously had radiotherapy, so the procedure may have to be repeated (Aslam et al. 2015). The procedure of nipple tattooing and areolar reconstitution can be successfully undertaken by clinical nurse specialists and appropriate follow-up carried out in nurse-led clinics (Clarkson et al. 2006, Potter et al. 2007).

Definition

Tattoo

Tattooing is the introduction, by punctures, of permanent colours into the skin. It is more specifically 'the process of implantation of exogenous colour fast pigments into the skin or mucous membranes leading to a discoloration known as a tattoo' (Vassileva and Hristakieva 2007). Tattoos are now widely promoted for many indications including breast reconstruction to provide an areola and/or nipple for the reconstructed breast (Vassileva and Hristakieva 2007).

Tattoo is a composite word derived from the Polynesian word 'ta' (meaning to strike something) and the Tahitian word 'tatau' (meaning to mark something) (Potter et al. 2007). The history of tattooing dates back to more than 5000 years ago, and nipple tattooing represents a modern application of an ancient custom.

Related theory

The reconstruction process

Areolar tattooing is the final part of a long process facing a woman after breast cancer diagnosis and treatment. If immediate reconstruction with expanders is chosen, patients undergo weekly saline injections until the desired overfill amount is achieved. Then they wait approximately 2 months for the skin to stretch adequately to ensure there is enough to cover an implant (Rolph et al. 2016).

The patient then goes back to the operating theatre for implant placement and waits 6 weeks to have nipple flap reconstruction. The nipple flap is not done at the time of implant placement because the patient is placed in a compression bra post surgery to prevent seroma formation. The compression on the nipple flap could compromise the blood flow to the flap, which might diminish its viability.

If patients choose immediate or delayed flap reconstruction, they must wait 6 weeks to 2 months post surgery to be taken back to the operating theatre for revision of the flap and nipple flap reconstruction.

In either scenario, the patient must then wait from 6 weeks to 3 months, based on her surgeon's preference, to have the areolar tattoo done. These time periods are dependent on whether the patient requires adjuvant therapy for her cancer (Sisti et al. 2016).

Evidence-based approaches

Indications

Not all patients wish to have a surgically constructed nipple; some may opt for a prosthetic nipple that is made of silicone and can be moulded from the contralateral nipple. These false nipples are secured with a special adhesive material that can sometimes be difficult to obtain. Moreover, they tend to come off when immersed in water (e.g. when swimming). Nipples that are created from the patients' own tissues rely on a combination of local flaps (e.g. skate flap) or skin grafts from other parts of the body (e.g. inner thigh region). Despite a realistic contour, these surgically formed nipples are often pale in colour relative to a normal NAC. The overall appearance of a surgical nipple can be greatly enhanced using tattooing techniques, which are simple and safe procedures in the final stages of breast reconstruction. The following groups of patients are potential candidates who may benefit from methods of tattooing:

- patients who have had breast reconstructive surgery
- patients who decline formal nipple reconstruction.

Tattooing of the areola in breast reconstruction patients will help promote a realistic outcome in aesthetic terms and a range of skin colour pigments is available.

Contraindications

There are several conditions that are either absolute or relative contraindications to areolar tattooing:

- history of allergy (particularly to adhesive dressings or topical creams)
- cardiac disease (patients with previous rheumatic fever may need antibiotic cover)

- diabetes mellitus (there is a greater risk of rejection of the pigment)
- keloid scars (more difficult to penetrate with needles)
- pregnancy (defer until after the baby is born)
- emotionally unstable patients
- needle phobia (patients may require extra psychological support)
- hepatitis C
- positive HIV status
- methicillin-resistant *Staphylococcus aureus* (MRSA) carriage.

Principles of care

Asepsis

The procedure should be performed in an aseptic manner with meticulous hand washing to reduce any risk of infection. Any equipment that may cause a needlestick injury must be safely disposed of. Local anaesthetic procedure policies should be followed.

Techniques for implantation of pigment

The pointillist technique is a method for application of a series of dots of colour but can produce an unnatural effect. Circular movements around the nipple projection are the most effective, but backward and forward strokes can be employed. Feathering around the edge of the areola gives a natural finish.

Factors determining pigment acceptance

Several factors influence how well the skin accepts pigmentation:

- One of the most important factors is the speed of the technician – the faster and more direct the pigment implantation, the better is the acceptance. With increasing experience, the right touch is developed.
- Another factor determining pigment acceptance is the innate condition of the skin. Oily skin is associated with a thicker dermis, which results in pigment penetrating deeper than for a person with a relatively thin dermis. The dermis becomes thinner with increasing age, which allows the pigment to penetrate more readily.
- Darker pigment colours take more rapidly and persist for longer periods than lighter colours; the former have a higher iron oxide content, which increases the density of the pigment.
- Diabetes and certain other medical conditions can increase the chance of pigment rejection.
- Impaired acceptance of the pigment may be observed in patients who have received radiotherapy to the breast (Aslam et al. 2015).
- When performing the tattooing process, the technician should work with the pen positioned at an angle of 45% to minimize pigment migration.

Anticipated patient outcomes

Patients want to know what the tattooed nipple will look like and it is important that they have realistic expectations. A further area of concern is whether the procedure is painful; patients should be reassured that most reconstructed breasts are insensate. Another key question that is asked by many patients is 'What will my partner think?'. Most women, post mastectomy, do not undress in front of their partner but may feel that nipple reconstruction and tattooing provides the opportunity to show their 'new body' to their partner. Some women will no longer have any form of sexual relationship with their partner and the simple procedure of tattooing can evoke profound emotional feelings (Allen 2017). The nurse-led tattooing service can therefore be very special for these women.

Legal and professional issues

Competencies

All practitioners should be assessed by a competent practice facilitator prior to performing procedures on their own. Nurses must always operate within their scope of practice as set out by their profession (NMC 2015). Learning tools may include competency-based workbooks.

Consent

Those patients who are suitable for areolar tattooing must be consented by an appropriately trained member of the surgical team. Written information is supplied to the patient and they must have the opportunity to read and understand this before signing a standard consent form. Written consent is often undertaken several days in advance of the planned procedure and therefore secondary verbal consent should be obtained immediately prior to carrying out the procedure.

Education

The patient's co-operation is essential to ensure the procedure is undertaken safely. All patients should be given access to information and support in a manner that they understand (DH 2005a, NMC 2013). Written information should be available and patients often access information via the internet at sites such as www.macmillan.org.uk. Consideration must be given to those patients with learning disabilities, language barriers or sensory deficit (DH 2009).

Pre-procedural considerations

Timing

The surgeon has a direct role to play in advising on the timing of any NAC tattooing; usually the optimal time is 6–8 weeks after NAC reconstruction. It is essential that the newly formed NAC is fully healed before any attempt is made at tattooing it.

All non-dissolvable skin sutures should have been removed at this stage. If any sutures remain they should be removed and tattooing rescheduled for one week's time. Caution should be exercised in those patients who are unhappy with the results of surgical nipple reconstruction, or indeed the breast reconstruction in general. These women should be referred back to the surgeon for further consultation. For younger patients with more advanced cancer, areolar tattooing can significantly enhance overall health-related quality of life and help minimize sexual morbidity (Burke et al. 2016).

Photographs

Photographic documentation is very important for the patient's records; all breast reconstruction patients will have signed consent for photography before surgery is undertaken (this is usually an integral section of the standard consent form). These photographic records will assist in choosing an appropriate colour of pigment for tattooing when patients have undergone bilateral mastectomy. Some patients benefit from seeing 'before' and 'after' photographs and this can be an essential component of patient education and information giving (Figures 8.42 and 8.43). Nonetheless, it should always be remembered that patients are individuals and each tattooed NAC is different.

Matching the other nipple

Some have suggested that the manoeuvre of closing one eye and then judging the position of the nipples is useful for assessing balance. Matching the reconstructed NAC to the contralateral side can be challenging; the areola does not always have a completely circular outline and several adjustments may be necessary to achieve symmetry (Figure 8.44). Formal measurements are not always helpful when one breast is slightly higher or of smaller size than the other and indeed can be deceptive when there is any kind of 'optical illusion'. Ultimately, the patient herself must be the final judge of the position, outline, contour and colour of the reconstructed nipple. The practitioner can advise patients, but they are accountable and more extreme requests should be dealt with by suitable compromise and always carefully documented. Tattooing will help to disguise surgical scars and detract the eye

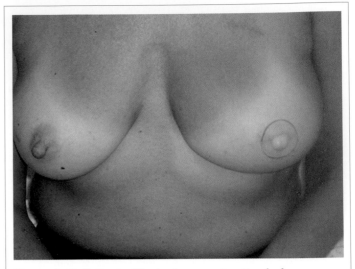

Figure 8.42 Patient with nipple reconstruction before tattooing the NAC.

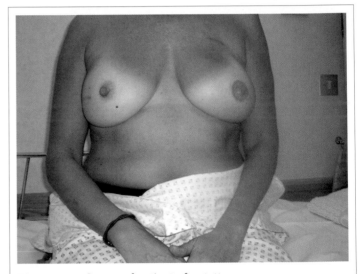

Figure 8.43 Image of patient after tattoo.

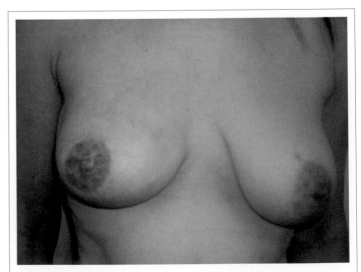

Figure 8.44 Matching the reconstructed NAC to the contralateral side.

from focussing on these. The areola should never be coloured too dark or created too large as a reduction in circumference and tattoo lightening are both very difficult to achieve.

Allergic reactions

Patch testing is performed routinely in all patients with a history of allergy to ensure they will not have an allergic reaction to the pigment. This test should be carried out 3–4 weeks prior to the procedure and can conveniently be performed by a needle scratch to a mutually acceptable area (e.g. behind the ear). This area should be examined after a period of 24 hours.

Choice of colour

A range of pigments are available from several companies. There are two basic colours (light and dark) and it is best to keep things simple and not use too many different colours (Figure 8.45). Universal laws of colour state that blue is the darkest and the only 'cool' primary colour, red is medium and considered to be a 'warm' primary colour, and yellow is the lightest and represents a warm primary colour.

It is important to appreciate that black pigment can migrate or potentially turn blue; this can be avoided by mixing orange pigment with the black. Pigment colours generally change once they are implanted into the skin. Significant changes in shade can occur throughout the month-long healing process.

The colour should be matched in a slightly lighter shade after discussion with the patient. It should be remembered that if a darker colour is selected, then subsequent lightening can be problematic and patients should be warned of this. Mixing flesh-coloured pigments is difficult and can only be learnt through practice and experience. Often the colour of the areola is an excessively vivid shade of flesh and this should be avoided.

Equipment

Needles

The needles employed for tattooing are made of nickel and manufactured in disposable cartridges, which are available in a range of sizes (Figure 8.46). The type of needle used is very much a matter of personal preference. The manner in which needles are grouped or soldered together determines the configuration, which in turn affects the needles' implantation pattern. Typical configurations are round, flat and magnum. Two types of needle are commonly used:

- Round needles: these have a rounded end corresponding to the site of soldering.
- Flat needles: these are flat with either a five- or seven-prong cluster, which permits effective penetration of the dermis and deposits the pigment within the skin yielding the best end-results.

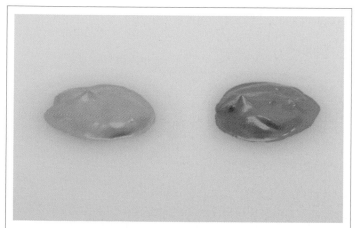

Figure 8.45 Choice of pigment colours.

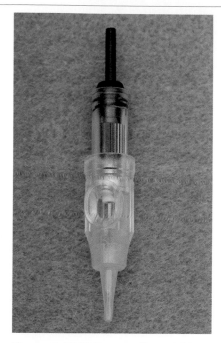

Figure 8.46 Tattoo needle cartridge.

For experienced technicians who wish to work with both speed and accuracy, nine intertwined flat needles can be used for shading and filling in large areas of skin.

The most common configurations of needles used in areolar tattooing are called round magnums. The needle tips are arranged in a fan shape or arch at the points. In use, the round magnums conform better to the deflecting skin so as to give better, more consistent implantation of ink/pigment across the width, and in turn do less damage to the skin. It is recommended that these needles are used for no more than 45 minutes of tattoo time as they can lead to marked pain and discomfort.

Pigment

Pigments are made up of iron oxide, glycerol, distilled water and alcohol. Pigment acceptance is achieved by depositing coloured pigment through the four layers of the epidermis into the first layer of the dermis. The initial inflammatory response due to the penetration of the needles and insertion of the iron oxide pigment causes a migration of macrophages to the area. The macrophages engulf the pigment granules and draw them downward into the second, deeper layer of the dermis. This process takes 1–2 weeks. Pigment granules must be over 6 µm so that macrophages cannot transfer the pigment beyond the second layer of the dermis; these pigment granules are too large to penetrate blood vessels and therefore have minimal tendency to spread or migrate beyond the site of injection. The choice of pigment colours is dependent on individual taste and natural skin colour.

Pharmacological support

EMLA cream can be applied before tattooing to partially numb the skin, but topical cream should not be used when there is any history of lidocaine allergy.

Non-pharmacological support

Special consideration may be needed for those who are extremely anxious. Measures include ensuring that the patient has a family member or friend present and complementary therapies such as relaxation, massage and music.

Procedure guideline 8.23 Nipple tattooing

Essential equipment

- Antiseptic skin cleaning agent (Sterets Tisept Sachets) 0.015% and 0.15% w/v cutaneous solution chlorhexidine gluconate cetrimide
- Sterile dressing pack
- Sterile gloves
- Plastic apron
- Sterile scissors
- Surgical marking pen
- Areolar stencil

- Pigments
- Needle cartridge for tattooing
- Hand piece for holding tattoo needle
- Medical tattoo machine (Figure 8.47)
- Cotton bud
- Mepilex Border Sterile dressing 7×7.5 cm

Medicinal products

- EMLA cream

Pre-procedure

Action	Rationale
1 Explain and provide written information about the nipple tattoo procedure.	To ensure the patient is properly informed about the procedure (DH 2005a, **C**; NMC 2015, **C**).
2 Obtain written informed consent.	To enable patients to actively participate in and comply with their treatment (NMC 2015, **C**).
3 Match colour a slightly lighter shade after discussion with the patient. Mix pigment colour.	To ensure a close match to existing breast. **E**
4 Apply EMLA cream for 40 minutes to tattoo site.	To minimize pain during the areolar tattooing procedure. **E**
5 Prepare the procedure trolley and ensure that all the necessary equipment is readily available (Figure 8.48).	To ensure the procedure is performed efficiently and correctly. **E**
6 Ensure patient privacy by drawing the curtains and making use of a sheet or blanket.	An environment that facilitates the patient's need for privacy and dignity is essential for areolar tattooing (NMC 2015, **C**).
7 Assist the patient into the correct position.	

Procedure

Action	Rationale
8 Open the pack and then open all the equipment onto the sterile field.	To maintain asepsis throughout the procedure to minimize the risk of infection (Fraise and Bradley 2009, **E**).
9 Wash hands and apply sterile gloves.	To maintain asepsis throughout the procedure to minimize the risk of infection (Fraise and Bradley 2009, **E**).
10 Reassure and observe the patient throughout the procedure.	To allay anxiety and facilitate the patient's maximum co-operation. **P**
11 Clean the skin thoroughly at the tattoo site with an antiseptic solution, for example chlorhexidine 0.5% and alcohol solution and allow to dry.	To maintain asepsis throughout the procedure to minimize the risk of infection (Fraise and Bradley 2009, **E**).
12 Commence the procedure with gentle circular movements, stretching the skin with the other hand. Lightly feather around the areolar edge to give a natural finish.	To achieve a natural result. **P**
13 Cover the areola in pigment at least three times.	To give best results. **P**
14 Check the pigment uptake by removing the excess pigment with clean gauze. Repeat as necessary to check area of uptake.	To achieve a consistent result. **P**
15 Apply yellow soft paraffin to areola.	To prevent pigment drying. **E**
16 Apply a sterile dressing.	To achieve haemostasis and decrease the risk of infection at the tattoo site. **E**

Post-procedure

Action	Rationale
17 Dispose of sharps as per local policy.	To ensure the safe handling and disposal of needles and other sharp instruments and to protect staff, patients and visitors from exposure to bloodborne pathogens (DH 2005b, **C**; Loveday et al. 2016, **C**)
18 Record the necessary information in the appropriate documents as per local policy.	To maintain accurate records (NMC 2015, **C**).
19 Ensure the patient has returned to pre-procedure functional status before discharge.	To ensure the safe management and recovery of patients receiving sedation. **E**
20 Give the patient appropriate aftercare instructions (see Education).	To ensure the safe management of patients and to enable them to actively participate in and comply with their treatment (NMC 2013, **C**).

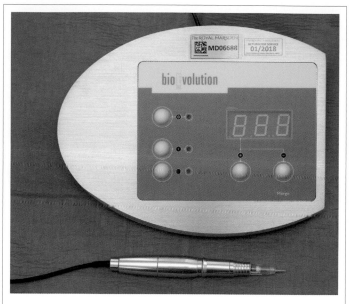

Figure 8.47 Medical tattoo machine.

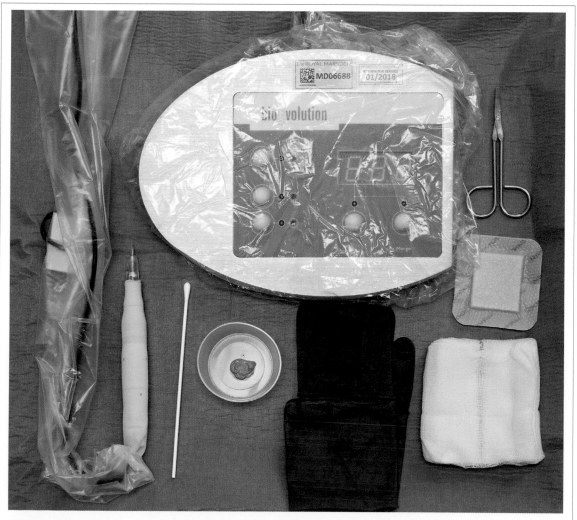

Figure 8.48 Procedure trolley with equipment including: hand piece for holding tattoo needle, needle cartridge for tattooing, cotton bud, sterile gloves, pigment, medical tattoo machine, sterile gauze, sterile dressing.

Problem-solving table 8.11 Prevention and resolution (Procedure guideline 8.23)

Problem	Cause	Prevention	Action
Damage and possible rupture of underlying breast prosthesis.	a. The prosthesis is superficial (that is near the skin surface) the needles may pierce it when applying the pigment b. The practitioner applies too much pressure and goes too deep.	The practitioner must assess the breast in advance and note how close the prosthesis is to the skin surface. If it is close to the surface it maybe indicated by wrinkly skin.	If a rupture occurs the doctor must be called immediately and the prosthesis removed. An incident form should also be completed.
Bleeding secondary to the tattoo needle rupturing small subareolar blood vessels.	Tattooing involves a distinct hovering action, which is very different to the incision of tissues with a scalpel blade.	Avoid visible blood vessels as far as possible, however this problem is very rare.	Apply pressure until the bleeding stops.

References

Section 8.1: Introduction

Armes, J., Crowe, M., Colbourne, L. et al (2009) Patients' supportive care needs beyond the end of cancer treatment: a prospective, longitudinal survey. *Journal of Clinical Oncology*, 27(36), 6172–6179.

Arora, N., Finney Rutten, L., Gustafson, D., Moser, R. & Hawkins, R. (2007) Perceived helpfulness and impact of social support provided by family, friends, and health care providers to women newly diagnosed with breast cancer. *Psycho-Oncology*, 16(5), 474–486.

Biddle, L., Paramasivan, S., Harris, S., Campbell, R., Brennan, J. & Hollingworth, W. (2016) Patients' and clinicians' experiences of holistic needs assessment using a cancer distress thermometer and problem list: a qualitative study. *European Journal of Oncology Nursing*, 23, 59–65.

Brem, S. & Kumar, N. (2011) Management of treatment related symptoms in patients with breast cancer. *Clinical Journal of Oncology Nursing*, 15(1), 63–71.

Brennan, J., Gingell, P., Brant, H. & Hollingworth, W. (2012) Refinement of the distress management problem list as the basis for a holistic therapeutic conversation among UK patients with cancer. *Psycho-oncology*, 21(12), 1346–1356.

Collins, A. (2014) *Measuring what really matters*. The Health Foundation. Available at: http://www.health.org.uk/sites/health/files/MeasuringWhatReallyMatters.pdf (Accessed: 15/3/2018)

Corner, J. & Wagland, R. (2013) *National Cancer Survivorship Initiative: Text analysis of patients' free text comments: Final report*. Southampton: University of Southampton.

Demark-Wahnefried, W., Aziz, N., Rowland, J. & Pinto, B. (2005). Riding the crest of the teachable moment: Promoting long-term health after the diagnosis of cancer. *Journal of Clinical Oncology*, 23(24), 5814–5830.

Department of Health (DH) (2007) *Cancer Reform Strategy*. London: Department of Health.

Department of Health (DH) (2010) *National Cancer Survivorship Initiative Vision*. London: Department of Health

Dougherty, L. & Lister, S. (eds) (2011) *The Royal Marsden Hospital Manual of Clinical Nursing Procedures*, 8th edn. Oxford: Wiley-Blackwell.

Dougherty, L. & Lister, S. (eds) (2015) *The Royal Marsden Hospital Manual of Clinical Nursing Procedures*, 9th edn. Oxford: Wiley-Blackwell.

Doyle, N. (2008) Cancer survivorship: evolutionary concept analysis, *Journal of Advanced Nursing*, 63(4), 499–509.

Doyle, N. & Henry, R. (2014) Holistic needs assessment: rationale and practical implementation. *Cancer Nursing Practice*, 13(5), 15–21.

Elliott, J., Fallows, A., Staetsky, L., et al. (2011) The health and well-being of cancer survivors in the UK: findings from a population-based survey. *British Journal of Cancer*, 105(Suppl 1), S11–S20.

Fallowfield, L., Ratcliffe, D., Jenkins, V. & Saul, J. (2001) Psychiatric morbidity and its recognition by doctors in patients with cancer. *British Journal of Cancer*, 84, 1011–1015.

Grunfeld, E., Julian, J., Pond, G., et al. (2011) Evaluating survivorship care plans: results of a randomized, clinical trial of patients with breast cancer. *Journal of Clinical Oncology*, 29(36), 4755–4762.

Health Foundation (2014) Person-centred care made simple. Available at: http://www.health.org.uk/sites/health/files/PersonCentredCareMadeSimple.pdf (Accessed: 15/3/2018)

Hughes C., Henry, R., Richards, S. & Doyle, N. (2014) Supporting delivery of the recovery package for people living with and beyond cancer. *Cancer Nursing Practice*, 13(10), 30–35.

Independent Cancer Taskforce (2015) *Achieving world-class cancer outcomes: a strategy for England 2015-2020*. Available at: http://www.cancerresearchuk.org/sites/default/files/achieving_world-class_cancer_outcomes_-_a_strategy_for_england_2015-2020.pdf (Accessed: 15/3/2018)

Kim, Y. & Given, B. (2008) Quality of life of family caregivers of cancer survivors. *Cancer*, 112(Suppl 11), 2556–2568.

Kim, Y., Baker, F., Spillers, R. & Wellisch, D. (2006) Psychological adjustment of cancer caregivers with multiple roles. *Psycho-Oncology*, 15(9), 795–804.

London Cancer Alliance (LCA) (2016) Holistic Needs Assessment Prompt Tools. Available at: http://www.londoncanceralliance.nhs.uk/information-for-healthcare-professionals/forms-and-guidelines/lca-patient-experience-programme/holistic-needs-assessment-prompt-tools/ (Accessed: 15/3/2018)

Macmillan Cancer Support (2012) *Improving cancer patient experience: a top tips guide*. Available at: http://www.macmillan.org.uk/documents/aboutus/commissioners/patientexperiencesurvey_toptipsguide.pdf (Accessed: 15/3/2018)

Macmillan Cancer Support (2013a) *Cancer's hidden price tag: revealing the costs behind the illness*. MAC14167. London: Macmillan Cancer Support.

Macmillan Cancer Support (2013b) *The recovery package*. Available at: http://www.macmillan.org.uk/Aboutus/Healthandsocialcareprofessionals/Macmillansprogrammesandservices/RecoveryPackage/RecoveryPackage.aspx (Accessed: 15/3/2018)

Macmillan Cancer Support (2015) *Revealed: the top ten concerns burdening people with cancer*. Available at: http://www.macmillan.org.uk/aboutus/news/latest_news/revealedthetoptenconcernsburdeningpeoplewithcancer.aspx (Accessed: 15/3/2018)

Macmillan Cancer Support (2016) *Cancer then and now*. Available at: http://www.macmillan.org.uk/documents/campaigns/cancer-then-now-report-final-online.pdf (Accessed: 15/3/2018)

Maddams, J., Utley, M. & Møller, H. (2012) Projections of cancer prevalence in the United Kingdom, 2010-2040. *British Journal of Cancer*, 107(7), 1095–1202.

McDowell, M., Occhipinti, S., Ferguson, M., et al. (2010) Predictors of change in unmet supportive care needs in cancer. *Psycho-Oncology*, 19(5), 508–516.

National Cancer Action Team (NCAT) (2007) *Holistic needs assessment for people with cancer*. London: NHS.

National Cancer Survivorship Initiative (NCSI) (2013) *Living with and beyond cancer: taking action to improve outcomes*. London: Department of Health.

Pitcealthy, C. & Maguire, P. (2003) The psychological impact of cancer on patients' partners and other key relatives: a review. *European Journal of Cancer*, 39(11), 1517–1524.

Sanson-Fisher, R., Girgis, A., Boyes, A., Bonevski, B., Burton, L. & Cook, P. (2000) The unmet supportive care needs of patients with cancer. *Cancer*, 88(1), 226–237.

Soellner, W., De Vries, A., Steixner, E., et al. (2001) How successful are oncologists at identifying patient distress, perceived social support, and need for psychosocial counselling? *British Journal of Cancer*, 84, 179–185.

Werner, A., Stenner, C. & Schuz, J. (2012) Patient versus clinician symptom reporting: how accurate is the detection of distress in the oncologic after-care? *Psycho-Oncology*, 21, 818–826.

Section 8.2: Welfare advice

Cancer Research UK (2014) Coping with hair loss. Available at: http://www.cancerresearchuk.org/about-cancer/coping-with-cancer/coping-physically/changes-to-your-appearance-due-to-cancer/hair-loss/coping-with-hair-loss (Accessed: 15/3/2018)

Cancer Research UK (2016) Government benefits. Available at: http://www.cancerresearchuk.org/about-cancer/coping-with-cancer/coping-practically/financial-support/government-benefits#2TcyCpDGEy8x90VB.99 (Accessed: 15/3/2018)

Department for Work and Pensions (DWP) (2018a) Attendance Allowance. Available at: https://www.gov.uk/attendance-allowance (Accessed: 15/3/2018)

Department for Work and Pensions (DWP) (2018b) Carer's Allowance. Available at: https://www.gov.uk/carers-allowance (Accessed: 15/3/2018)

Department for Work and Pensions (DWP) (2018c) Employment and Support Allowance. https://www.gov.uk/employment-support-allowance (Accessed: 15/3/2018)

Department for Work and Pensions (DWP) (2018d) Personal Independence Payment. Available at: https://www.gov.uk/pip (Accessed: 15/3/2018)

Department for Work and Pensions (DWP) (2018e) Personal Independence Payment (PIP) quick guide. Available at: https://www.gov.uk/government/uploads/system/uploads/attachment_data/file/524037/pip-quick-guide.pdf (Accessed: 15/3/2018)

Government Equalities Office (2015) Equality Act 2010. Available at: https://www.gov.uk/guidance/equality-act-2010-guidance (Accessed: 15/3/2018)

Macmillan Cancer Support (2012) Improving cancer patient experience: a top tips guide. Available at: http://www.macmillan.org.uk/documents/aboutus/commissioners/patientexperiencesurvey_toptipsguide.pdf (Accessed: 15/3/2018)

National Cancer Action Team (2007) Holistic needs assessment for people with cancer London, NHS.

NHS Choices (2016) NHS in England – help with health costs. Available at: http://www.nhs.uk/NHSEngland/Healthcosts/Pages/help-with-health-costs.aspx (Accessed: 15/3/2018)

NHS Scotland (2015) Equality and diversity: your legal requirements and reasonable adjustments you can make. Available at: http://www.healthyworkinglives.com/advice/Legislation-and-policy/employee-issues/disability-discrimination-act (Accessed: 15/3/2018)

The National Archives (2006) Work and Families Act 2006. Available at: http://www.legislation.gov.uk/ukpga/2006/18/contents (Accessed: 15/3/2018)

Section 8.3 Supporting individuals with sexual concerns as a consequence of cancer

American, C.P. & Farrell, R. (2016) ACOG Committee Opinion No. 659 Summary: The use of vaginal estrogen in women with a history of estrogen-dependent breast cancer. *Obstetrics and Gynecology*, 127(3), 618–619.

Boquiren, V., Esplen, M., Wong, J., Toner, B., Warner, E. & Malin, N. (2015) Sexual functioning in breast cancer survivors experiencing body image disturbance. *Psycho-Oncology*, 25, 66–76.

Bredart, A., Dolbeault, S., Savignoni, A., et al. (2011) Prevalence and associated factors of sexual problems after early-stage breast cancer treatment: results of a French exploratory survey. *Psycho-Oncology*, 20, 841–850.

British Association of Urological Surgeons (BAUS) (2016) Patients: general information: cancer. Available at: http://www.baus.org.uk/patients/information/cancer.aspx (Accessed: 23/3/2018)

Buchholz, S., Mogele, M., Lintermans, A., et al. (2015) Vaginal-estriol-lactobacilli combination and quality of life in endocrine-treated breast cancer. *Climacteric*, 18, 252–259.

Cancer Research UK (2015) Sex and chemotherapy for men. Available at: http://www.cancerresearchuk.org/about-cancer/cancer-in-general/treatment/chemotherapy/sex/men (Accessed: 23/3/2018)

Candy, B., Jones, L., Vickerstaff, V., Tookman, A. & King, M. (2016) Interventions for sexual dysfunction following treatments for cancer in women (Review). *Cochrane Database of Systematic Reviews*, (2), CD005540.

Carter, J., Goldfrank, D., & Schover, L. (2011) Simple strategies for vaginal health promotion in cancer survivors. *Journal of Sexual Medicine*, 8(2), 549–559.

Carter, J., Stabile, C. & Gunn, A. (2013) The physical consequences of gynaecologic cancer surgery and their impact on sexual, emotional and quality of life issues. *Journal of Sexual Medicine*,10(suppl 1), 21–34.

Cunningham, G.R., Rosen, R.C., Snyder, P.J., O'Leary, M.P. & Martin, K.A. (2011) Overview of male sexual dysfunction. UpToDate. Available at: https://www.uptodate.com/contents/overview-of-male-sexual-dys-function (Accessed: 23/3/2018)

Dean, A. (2008) Supporting women experiencing sexual problems after treatment for breast cancer. *Cancer Nursing Practice*, 7(8), 28–33.

Derzko, C. & Elliott, S. (2007) Management of sexual dysfunction in post-menopausal breast cancer patients taking adjuvant aromatase inhibitor therapy. *Current Oncology*, 14(Suppl 1), S20–S40.

Dizon, D. & Katz, A. (2015) Overview of sexual dysfunction in male cancer survivors, UpToDate. Available at: https://www.uptodate.com/contents/overview-of-sexual-dysfunction-in-male-cancer-survivors (Accessed: 23/3/2018)

Edwards, D. & Panay, N. (2016) Treating vulvovaginal atrophy/genitourinary syndrome of menopause : how important is vaginal lubricant and moisturizer composition? *Climacteric*, 19(2), 151–161.

George, A. & Fleming, P. (2004) Factors affecting men's help-seeking in the early detection of prostate cancer: implications for health promotion. *Journal of Men's Health and Cancer*, 1, 345–352.

Goldfarb, S., Mulhall, J., Nelson, C., Kelvin, J., Dickler, M. & Carter, J. (2013) Sexual and reproductive health in cancer survivors. *Seminars in Oncology*, 40(6), 726–744.

Hyde, M.K., Newton, R.U., Galvao, D.A., et al. (2016) Men's help-seeking in the first year after diagnosis of localised prostate cancer. Available at: https://www.ncbi.nlm.nih.gov/pmc/articles/PMC5347946/ (Accessed 22/6/2018)

Katz, A. (2011) Breast cancer and women's sexuality. *The American Journal of Nursing*, 111(4), 63–67.

Kennedy, V. & Leiserowitz, G. (2015) Preserving sexual function in women and girls with cancer: survivorship is about more than surviving. *American Journal of Obstetrics and Gynecology*, 213(2), 119–120.

Lindau, S., Amramsohn, E. & Matthews, A. (2015) A manifesto on the preservation of sexual function in women and girls with cancer. *American Journal of Obstetrics and Gynecology*, 213(2), 166–174.

London Cancer Alliance (LCA) (2016) Sexual Consequences of Cancer Treatment: Management Pathway. Available at: http://www.londoncanceralliance.nhs.uk/media/125886/lca-sexual-consequences-of-cancer-treatment-management-pathway-march-2016-v2-final.pdf (Accessed: 23/3/2018)

Macmillan Cancer Support (2012) Holistic Needs Assessment and Care Planning – Introduction. Winter 2012. Available at: http://be.macmillan.org.uk/Downloads/CancerInformation/SGPwinter2012hna.pdf (Accessed 18/6/18)

Macmillan Cancer Support (2016) Treating erectile dysfunction after surgery for pelvic cancers. Available at: http://be.macmillan.org.uk/Downloads/ResourcesForHSCPs/InformationResources/MAC15226-2590PostsurgeryEDguideINTERACTIVE.pdf (Accessed: 23/3/2018)

Macmillan Cancer Support (2018a) Financial Support Tool. Available at: https://finance.macmillan.org.uk/benefits/benefits-online (Accessed 3/7/2018)

Macmillan Cancer Support (2018b) Benefits and other financial support. Available at: https://www.macmillan.org.uk/information-and-support/organising/benefits-and-financial-support. (Accessed 3/7/2018)

Masters, W. & Johnson, V. (1966) *Human Sexual Response*. Vol. 1. Boston: Little, Brown & Co.

NICE (2015) *Menopause: diagnosis and management* (NG23). Available at https://www.nice.org.uk/guidance/NG23 (Accessed: 23/3/2018)

NMC (2015) *The Code. Professional standards of practice and behaviour for nurses and midwives*. London: Nursing and Midwifery Council, p.9.

Ochsenkuhn, R., Hermelink, K., Clayton, A., et al. (2011) Menopausal status in breast cancer patients with past chemotherapy determines long-term hypoactive sexual desire disorder. *Journal of Sexual Medicine*, 8, 1486–1494.

Oguchi, M., Jansen, J., Butow, P., et al. (2011) Measuring the impact of nurse cue-response behaviour on cancer patients' emotional cues. *Patient Education Counselling*, 82(2), 163–168.

Panjari, M., Bell, R.J. & Davis, S.R. (2011). Sexual function after breast cancer. *Journal of Sexual Medicine*, 8(1), 294–302.

Perz, J. & Ussher, J. (2015) A randomised trial of a minimal intervention for sexual concerns after cancer: a comparison of self-help and professionally delivered modalities. *BMC Cancer*, 15, 629.

Quinn, C. & Happell, B. (2012) Getting BETTER: Breaking the ice and warming to the inclusion of sexuality in mental health. *International Journal of Mental Health Nursing*, 21, 154–162.

Quinn, G.P. & Vadaparampil, S.T. (2012) Reproductive health and cancer in adolescents and young adults. *Advances in Experimental Medicine and Biology*, 732.

Raggio, G.A., Butryn, M.L., Arigo, D., Mikorski, R. & Palmer, S.C. (2014) Prevalence and correlates of sexual morbidity in long-term breast cancer survivors. *Psychology & Health*, 29(6), 632–650.

Rhoden, E., Teloken, C., Sogari, P. & Vargas Souto, C. (2002) The use of the simplified International Index of Erectile Dysfunction (IIEF-5) as a diagnostic tool to study the prevalence of erectile dysfunction. *International Journal of Impotence Research*, 14(4), 245–250.

Rosen, R.C., Riley, A., Wagner, G., Osterloh, I.H., Kirkpatrick, J. & Mishra, A. (1997) The international index of erectile function (IIEF): a multidimensional scale for assessment of erectile dysfunction. *Urology*, 49(6), 822–830.

Royal College of Obstetricians and Gynaecologists (RCOG) (2011) *Pregnancy and Breast cancer*. Available at: https://www.rcog.org.uk/globalassets/documents/guidelines/gtg_12.pdf (Accessed: 23/3/2018)

Royal College of Obstetricians and Gynaecologists (2018) Treatment for Symptoms of the Menopause. Available at: https://www.rcog.org.uk/globalassets/documents/patients/patient-information-leaflets/gynaecology/pi-treatment-symptoms-menopause.pdf (Accessed: 22/6/2018)

Royal Marsden NHS Foundation Trust (2017) Chemotherapy. Your questions answered. Available at: www.royalmarsden.nhs.uk/patientinformation (Accessed: 29.6.18)

Schlenz, J., Kuzbati, R., Gruber, H. & Holle, J. (2000) The sensitivity of the nipple–areola complex: an anatomic study. *Plastic and Reconstructive Surgery*, 105(3), 905–909.

Schover, L. (1997) *Sexuality and Fertility after Cancer*. Chichester: John Wiley & Sons

Sexual Advice Association (2016) Oral treatment for erectile dysfunction. Available at: http://sexualadviceassociation.co.uk/oral-treatment-erectile-dysfunction/ (Accessed: 23/3/2018)

Sunha, A. & Ewies, A. (2013) Non-hormonal topical treatment of vulvovaginal atrophy: an up-to-date overview. *Climacteric*, 16, 305–312.

Testicular Cancer Awareness Foundation (2016) Retroperitoneal lymph node dissention patient information. Available at: http://www.testicularcancerawarenessfoundation.org/rplnd-surgery (Accessed: 23/32018)

Tortora, G.J. & Derrickson, B.H. (2011) *Principles of Anatomy and Physiology*, 13th edn. Hoboken, NJ: John Wiley & Sons.

Ussher, J., Perez, J. & Gilbert, E. (2012) Information needs associated with changes in sexual well-being after breast cancer. *Journal of Advanced Nursing*, 69(2), 327–337.

Varela, V., Zhou, E. & Bober, S. (2013). Management of sexual problems in patients and survivors. *Current Problems in Cancer*, 37, 319–352.

Wiggins, D. & Dizon, D. (2008) Dyspareunia and vaginal dryness after breast cancer treatment. *Sexuality Reproduction and Menopause*, 6(3), 18–22.

World Health Organization (2002) *Defining sexual health: report of a technical consultation on sexual health*. Available at: http://www.who.int/reproductivehealth/topics/gender_rights/defining_sexual_health.pdf (Accessed: 23/3/2018)

World Health Organization (2006) *Defining sexual health. Report of a technical consultation on sexual health 28–31 January 2002, Geneva.*

Available at: http://www.who.int/reproductivehealth/publications/sexual_health/defining_sexual_health.pdf (Accessed: 3/7/2018)

Zhou, E.S., Falk, S.J. & Bober, S.L. (2015) Managing premature menopause and sexual dysfunction. *Current Opinion in Supportive and Palliative Care*, 9(3), 294–300. (Accessed: 23/3/2018)

Section 8.4 Nutritional status

Abayomi, J.C., Kirwan J. & Hackett A.F. (2009a) Coping mechanisms used by women in an attempt to avoid symptoms of chronic radiation enteritis. *Journal of Human Nutrition and Dietetics*, 22, 310–316.

Abayomi, J.C., Kirwan J. & Hackett A.F. (2009b) The prevalence of chronic radiation enteritis following radiotherapy for cervical or endometrial cancer and its impact on quality of life. *European Journal of Oncology Nursing*, 13, 262–267.

Arends, J., Bachmann, P., Baracos, V. et al. (2017) ESPEN guidelines on nutrition in cancer patients. *Clinical Nutrition*, 36(1), 11–48.

British Association of Parenteral and Enteral Nutrition (BAPEN) (2003) Malnutrition universal screening tool. Available at: http://www.bapen.org.uk/screening-and-must/must/must-toolkit (Accessed: 23/3/2018)

British Association of Parenteral and Enteral Nutrition (BAPEN) (2009). Nutrition screening survey in the UK in 2008. Hospitals, care homes and mental health units. A report by the British Association of Parenteral and Enteral Nutrition. Available at: http://www.bapen.org.uk/pdfs/nsw/nsw_report2008-09.pdf (Accessed: 23/3/2018)

Dougherty, L. & Lister, S. (2015) *The Royal Marsden Manual of Clinical Nursing Procedures*, Professional Edition, 9th. Oxford: John Wiley & Sons.

Hutcheson, K., Lewin, J., Barringer, D. et al. (2012) Late dysphagia after radiotherapy- based treatment for head and neck cancer. *Cancer*, 118(23), 5793–5799.

Langmore, S.E., McCulloch, T.M., Krisciunas, G.P. et al. (2015) Efficacy of electrical stimulation and exercise for dysphagia in patients with head and neck cancer: a randomized clinical trial. *Head & Neck*, 38(S1), E1221–E1231.

National Obesity Forum (2016) Waist circumference. Available at: http://www.nationalobesityforum.org.uk/healthcare-professionals-main-menu-155/assessment-mainmenu-168/171-waist-circumference.html (Accessed: 23/3/2018)

NHS Choices (2016) What's your BMI? Available at: http://www.nhs.uk/Livewell/loseweight/Pages/BodyMassIndex.aspx (Accessed: 23/3/2018)

NICE (2012) Nutrition Support in Adults, Quality statement 1: Screening for the risk of malnutrition. London: NICE.

NMC (2015) *The Code. Professional standards of practice and behaviour for nurses and midwives.* London: Nursing & Midwifery Council, p.9.

Nund, R.L., Ward, E.C., Scarinci, N.A., Cartmill, B., Kuipers, P. & Porceddu S.V. (2014) Survivors' experiences of dysphagia-related services following head and neck cancer: implications for clinical practice. International Journal of Language & Communication Disorders, 49(3), 354–363.

Patterson, J.M., Rapley, T., Carding, P.N., Wilson, J.A. & McColl, E. (2012) Head and neck cancer and dysphagia; caring for carers. *Psycho-Oncology*, 22(8), 1815–1820.

Pelvic Radiation Disease Association (2006). Facts about late effects of pelvic radiotherapy. Available at: http://www.prda.org.uk/wp-content/uploads/2016/09/PRDA-Fact-sheet-download.pdf (Accessed: 27/4/2018)

Shaw, C. (2015) *The Royal Marsden Cancer Cookbook*. London: Kyle Books.

Shaw, C., Fleuret, C., Pickard, J.M., Mohammed, K., Black, G. & Wedlake, L. (2015) Comparison of a novel, simple nutrition screening tool for adult oncology inpatients and the Malnutrition Screening Tool (MST) against the Patient-Generated Subjective Global Assessment (PG-SGA). *Supportive Care in Cancer*, 23(1), 47–54.

Sorkin, J.D., Muller, D.C. & Andres, R. (1999) Longitudinal change in height of men and women: implications for interpretation of the body mass index: the Baltimore longitudinal study of aging. *American Journal of Epidemiology*, 150(9), 969–977.

Szczesniak, M.M., Maclean, J., Zhang, T., Graham, P.H. & Cook, I.J. (2014). Persistent dysphagia after head and neck radiotherapy: a common and under-reported complication with significant effect on non-cancer-related mortality. *Clinical Oncology (Royal College of Radiologists)*, 26(11), 697–703.

Section 8.5 Compression therapy in the management of lymphoedema

Bianchi, J., Vowden, K. & Whitaker, J. (2012) Chronic oedema made easy. *Wounds UK*, 8(2), 1–4.

Board, J. & Anderson, J. (2013) Treatment for lymphorrhoea in limbs and in advanced disease. *British Journal of Community Nursing*, 18(4 Suppl), S20–S25.

Cooper, G. (2012) Lymphoedema treatment in palliative care: a case study. *British Journal of Nursing*, 21(15), 897–903.

Cooper, G. (2014) An overview of lymphoedema for community nurses. *Journal of Community Nursing*, 28(5), 50–59.

Cooper, G. (2015) Compression therapy and the management of lower-limb lymphoedema: the male perspective. *British Journal of Community Nursing*, 20(3), 118–124.

Damstra, R. & Partsch, H. (2013) Prospective, randomised, controlled trial comparing the effectiveness of adjustable compression Velcro wraps versus inelastic multicomponent compression bandages in the initial treatment of leg lymphoedema. *Journal of Vascular Surgery*, 1(1), 13–19.

DiSipio, T., Rye, S., Newman, B. & Hayes, S, (2013) Incidence of unilateral arm lymphoedema after breast cancer: a systematic review and meta-analysis. *Lancet Oncology*, 14(6), 500–515.

Dougherty, L. & Lister, S. (2011) *The Royal Marsden Manual of Clinical Nursing Procedures*, Professional Edition, 8th. Oxford: John Wiley & Sons.

Dougherty, L. & Lister, S. (2015) *The Royal Marsden Manual of Clinical Nursing Procedures*, Professional Edition, 9th. Oxford: John Wiley & Sons.

Drake, R.L., Wayne Vogl, A., Mitchell, A.W.M. (2015) Lymphatic system. In: *Grey's Anatomy for Students*, 3rd edn. Philadelphia: Churchill Livingstone Elsevier; 2015, p.29.

Elwell, R. (2015) Compression bandaging for chronic oedema: applying science to reality. *British Journal of Community Nursing*, 20(5, Suppl), S4–S7.

Elwell, R. (2016) An overview of the use of compression in lower-limb chronic oedema. *British Journal of Community Nursing*, 21(1), 36–42.

Finlay, B., Ullah, S. & Piller, N. (2013) Relationship between pain, tightness, heaviness, perceived limb size, and objective limb size measurements in patients with chronic upper-limb lymphoedema. *Journal of Lymphoedema*, 8(1), 10–16.

Frisby, J. (2010) Assessment; prioritising the goals of palliative care model. In: Glover, D. (ed.) *The Management of Lymphoedema in Advanced Cancer and Oedema at the End of Life*. International Lymphoedema Framework and Canadian Lymphoedema Framework, pp. 8–11. Available at: https://www.lympho.org/wp-content/uploads/2016/03/Palliative-Document.pdf (Accessed: 23/3/2018)

Fu, M., Deng, J. & Armer, J. (2014) Putting evidence into practice: cancer-related lymphoedema. *Clinical Journal of Oncology Nursing, Supplement*, 18(6), 68–79.

Gray, D. (2013) Achieving compression therapy concordance in the new NHS: a challenge for clinicians. *Journal of Community Nursing*, 27(4), 107–110.

Hegarty-Craver, M., Grant, E., Kravitz, S., Reid, L., Kwon, K. and Oxhenham, W. (2014) Research into fabrics used in compression therapy and assessment of their impact on treatment regimens. *Journal of Wound Care*, 23(9, Suppl), S14–S22.

International Lymphoedema Framework (2012) Compression therapy: a position document on compression bandaging. Available at: https://www.lympho.org/portfolio/compression-therapy-a-position-document-on-compression-bandaging/ (Accessed: 27/4/2018)

International Society of Lymphology (2013) The diagnosis and treatment of peripheral lymphedema: 2013 Consensus Document of the International Society of Lymphology. *Lymphology*, 46(1), 1–11.

Keeley, V., Crooks, S., Locke, J., Veigas, D., Riches, K. & Hilliam, R., (2010). A quality of life measure for limb lymphoedema (LYMQOL). *Journal of Lymphoedema*, 5(1), 26–37.

Linnitt, N. (2011) Compression hosiery versus bandaging for chronic oedema. *Nursing and Residential Care*, 13(4), 183–185.

Linnitt, N. (2015) Managing lower limb oedema with compression therapy. *British Journal of Community Nursing*, 20(6), 286–288.

Lymphoedema Framework (2006) Best practice for the management of lymphoedema: International Consensus. London: Medical Education Partnership (MEP).

McCormack, B. & McCance, T. (2010) Person centered processes. In: *Person Centred Nursing: Theory and Practice*. Oxford: Wiley-Blackwell, Chapter 6.

Milne, J. (2015) The causes of oedema and managing any associated complications. *Wound Care Today*, 2(1), 16–25.

Moffatt, C.J., Franks, P.J., Hardy, D., Lewis, M., Parker, V. & Feldman, J.L. (2012) A preliminary randomized controlled study to determine the application frequency of a new lymphoedema bandaging system. *British Journal of Dermatology*, 166(3), 624–632.

Muldoon, J. (2010) Intermittent pressures in compression bandaging for oedema management. *British Journal of Community Nursing*, 15(4, Suppl), S4–S9.

Mullings, J. (2012) Juxta-fit compression garments in lymphoedema management. *British Journal of Community Nursing*, 17(10, Suppl), S32–S37.

NMC (2015) *The Code. Professional standards of practice and behaviour for nurses and midwives*. London: Nursing and Midwifery Council, p.9.

Nazarko, L. (2014) Living with lymphoedema: improving quality of life. *Nursing & Residential Care Journal*, 16(10), 551–557.

Nazarko, L. (2015) Living with lymphoedema: enhancing quality of life. *Nursing & Residential Care Journal*, 17(6), 314–321.

Ng, M. and Munnoch, A. (2010) Clinimetrics of volume measurements in upper limb LE. *Journal of Lymphoedema*, 5(2), 62–67.

Noble-Jones, R. (2016) Compression moves on: advances in care are changing practice. *British Journal of Nursing*, 25(4), 204–206.

Norton, S. & Towers, A. (2010) Adapting CDT for the palliative patient-specifics of management when treating CDT. In: Glover, D. (ed.) *The Management of Lymphoedema in Advanced Cancer and Oedema at the End of Life*. International Lymphoedema Framework and Canadian Lymphoedema Framework, pp.12–19. Available at: https://www.lympho.org/wp-content/uploads/2016/03/Palliative-Document.pdf (Accessed: 23/3/2018)

Partsch, H. (2012) Compression therapy: clinical and experimental evidence. *Annals of Vascular Diseases*, 5(4), 416–423.

Partsch, H. & Moffatt, C. (2012) An overview of the science behind compression bandaging for lymphoedema and chronic oedema (Chapter 2). In: *Compression therapy: a position document on compression bandaging*. International Lymphoedema Framework in Association with World Alliance for Wound and Lymphoedema Care, pp.12–23. Available at: https://www.lympho.org/wp-content/uploads/2016/03/Compression-bandaging-final.pdf (Accessed: 23/3/2018)

Partsch, H. & Mortimer, P. (2015) Compression for leg wounds. *British Journal of Dermatology*, 173, 359–369.

Piller, N. (1999) Gaining an accurate assessment of the stages of lymphoedema subsequent to cancer: the role of objective and subjective information, when to make measurements and their optimal use. *European Journal of Lymphology*, 7(25), 1–9.

Quéré, I. & Sneddon, M. (2012) Adapting compression bandaging for different patient groups (Chapter 4). In: Glover, D. (ed.) *Compression Therapy: A position document on compression bandaging*. International Lymphoedema Framework in Association with World Alliance for Wound and Lymphoedema Care, pp.32–48. Available at: https://www.lympho.org/wp-content/uploads/2016/03/Compression-bandaging-final.pdf (Accessed: 23/3/2018)

Ridner, S.H., Sinclair, V., Deng, J., Bonner, C.M., Kidd, N. & Dietrich, M.S. (2012) Breast cancer survivors with lymphoedema: glimpses of their daily lives. *Clinical Journal of Oncology Nursing*, 16(6), 609–614.

Schuren, J. (2012) Optimising compression bandaging. In: *Compression Therapy: A position document on compression bandaging*. International Lymphoedema Framework in Association with World Alliance for Wound and Lymphoedema Care, pp. 24–31. Available at: https://www.lympho.org/wp-content/uploads/2016/03/Compression-bandaging-final.pdf (Accessed: 23/3/2018)

Tidhar, D., Hodgson, P., Shay, C. & Towers, A. (2014) A lymphedema self-management programme: report on 30 cases. *Physiotherapy Canada*, 66(4), 404–412.

Todd, M. (2011) Use of compression bandaging in managing chronic oedema. *British Journal of Community Nursing*, 16 (10, Suppl), S4–S12.

Todd, M. (2013) Improving oedema management through joined-up working. *Nursing & Residential Care*, 15(10), 650–655.

399

Todd, M. (2015) Selecting compression hosiery. *British Journal of Nursing*, 25(4), 210–212.

Towers, A. (2012) Adapting compression bandaging for the palliative patient. In: Glover, D. (ed.) *Compression Therapy: A position document on compression bandaging*. International Lymphoedema Framework in Association with World Alliance for Wound and Lymphoedema Care, pp. 57–61. Available at: https://www.lympho.org/wp-content/uploads/2016/03/Compression-bandaging-final.pdf (Accessed: 23/3/2018)

Wigg, J. (2012) Supervised self-management of lower limb swelling using FarrowWrap. *British Journal of Community Nursing*, 17(4, Suppl), S22–S29.

Williams, A. (2012a) Surgery for people with lymphoedema. *Journal of Community Nursing*, 26(5), 27–33.

Williams, A. (2012b) Working in partnership with people to promote concordance with compression bandaging. *British Journal of Community Nursing*, 17(10a, Suppl), S1–S16.

Williams, A. & Whitaker, J. (2015) Measuring change in limb volume to evaluate lymphoedema treatment outcome. *EWMA Journal*, 15(1), 27–32.

Woods, M. (2010) Lymphoedema and breast cancer. In: Harmer, V. (ed.) *Breast Cancer Nursing: Care and Management*. Oxford: Wiley-Blackwell, pp.215–231.

Section 8.6 Non-pharmacological management of breathlessness

Adams, L., Chronos, N., Lane, R. & Guz, A. (1985) The measurement of breathlessness induced in normal subjects: validity of two scaling techniques. *Clinical Science*, 69, 7–16.

Bausewein, C., Booth, S., Gysels, M., Kuhnbach, R., Haberland, B. & Higginson, I.J. (2010) Understanding breathlessness: cross-sectional comparison of symptom burden and palliative care needs in chronic obstructive pulmonary disease and cancer. *Journal of Palliative Medicine*, 13(9), 1109–1118.

Booth, S., Moffat, C., Burkin, J., Galbraith, S. & Bausewein, C. (2011a) Nonpharmacological interventions for breathlessness. *Current Opinion in Supportive and Palliative Care* 5(2), 77–86.

Booth, S., Moffat, C., Farquhar, M., Higginson, I.J. & Burkin, J. (2011b) Developing a breathlessness intervention service for patients with palliative and supportive care needs, irrespective of diagnosis. *Journal of Palliative Care*, 27(1), 28–36.

Borg, G. (1970) Perceived exertion as an indicator of somatic stress. *Scandinavian Journal of Rehabilitation Medicine*, 2(2), 92–98.

Chartered Society of Physiotherapy (CSP) (2011) *Code of Members' Professional Values and Behaviour*. London: CSP.

Chin, C. & Booth, S. (2016) Managing breathlessness: a palliative care approach. *Postgraduate Medical Journal*, 92(1089), 393–400.

Corner, J., Plant, H., A'hern, R. & Bailey, C. (1996) Non-pharmacological intervention for breathlessness in lung cancer. *Palliative Medicine*, 10(4), 299–305.

Dougherty, L. & Lister, S. (2015) *The Royal Marsden Manual of Clinical Nursing Procedures*, Professional Edition, 9th. Oxford: John Wiley & Sons.

Dyer, J., McNeil, S., Ragsdale-Lowe, M. & Tratt, L. (2008). A snap-shot of current practice: the use of aromasticks for symptom management. *International Journal of Clinical Aromatherapy*, 5(2), 1–5.

Galbraith, S., Fagan, P., Perkins, P., Lynch, A. & Booth, S. (2010) Does the use of a handheld fan improve chronic dyspnoea? a randomised, controlled, crossover trial. *Journal of Pain and Symptom Management*, 38(5), 831–838.

Gift, A.G. & Narsavage, G. (1998) Validity of the numeric rating scale as a measure of dyspnea. *American Journal of Critical Care*, 7(3), 200–204.

Guyatt, G.H., Berman, L.B., Townsend, M. et al. (1987) A measure of quality of life for clinical trials in chronic lung disease. *Thorax*, 42,773–778.

Higginson, I.J., Bausewein, C., Reilly, C.C., et al. (2014) An integrated palliative and respiratory care service for patients with advanced disease and refractory breathlessness: a randomised controlled trial. *The Lancet. Respiratory Medicine*, 2(12), 979–987.

Jolley, C.J. & Moxham, J. (2016) Dyspnea intensity: a patient-reported measure of respiratory drive and disease severity. *American Journal of Respiratory and Critical Care Medicine*, 193(3), 236–238.

NMC (2013) *Consent*. London: Nursing and Midwifery Council.

NMC (2015) *The Code. Professional standards of practice and behaviour for nurses and midwives*. London: Nursing & Midwifery Council, p.9.

Parshall, M.B., Schwartzstein, R.M., Adams, L., et al.; American Thoracic Society Committee on Dyspnea (2012) An official American Thoracic Society statement: update on the mechanisms, assessment, and management of dyspnea. *American Journal of Respiratory and Critical Care Medicine*, 185(4), 435–452.

Powell, T. (2009) *The Mental Health Handbook: A Cognitive Behavioural Approach*, 3rd edn. Oxford: Speechmark Publications, Routledge, Taylor & Francis Group.

Pryor, J.A. & Prasad, A. (2008) *Physiotherapy for Respiratory and Cardiac Problems*, 4th edn. London: Churchill Livingstone.

Schneiders, A.G., Zusman, M. & Singer, K.P. (1998) Exercise therapy compliance in acute low back pain patients. *Musculoskeletal Science and Practice*, 3(3), 147–152.

Spathis, A., Booth, S., Moffat, C., et al. (2017) The Breathing, Thinking, Functioning clinical model: a proposal to facilitate evidence-based breathlessness management in chronic respiratory disease. *npj Primary Care Respiratory Medicine*, 27(1), 27.

Thomas, S., Bausewein, C., Higginson, I. & Booth, S. (2011) Breathlessness in cancer patients - implications, management and challenges. *European Journal of Oncology Nursing: the official journal of European Oncology Nursing Society*, 15(5), 459–469.

Section 8.7 Physical activity for people with cancer

Betof, A., Lascola, C., Weitzel, D., et al. (2015) Modulation of murine breast tumor vascularity, hypoxia and chemotherapeutic response by exercise. *Journal of the National Cancer Institute*, 107(5).

Borg, G. (1998) *Borg's Perceived Exertion and Pain Scales*. Champaign, IL: Human Kinetics.

Bouchard, C., Shephard, R.J. & Stephens, T. (1994) *Physical Activity, Fitness, and Health: International proceedings and consensus statement*. Champaign, IL: Human Kinetics.

Bourke, L., Homer, K.E., Thaha, M.A., et al. (2013) Interventions for promoting habitual exercise in people living with and beyond cancer. *Cochrane Database of Systematic Reviews*, 9: CD010192.

Campbell, A., Stevinson, C. & Crank, H. (2011) The British Association of Sport and Exercise Sciences Expert statement on exercise and cancer survivorship. *The Sport and Exercise Scientist*, 28,16–17.

Chartered Society of Physiotherapy (2014) So your patient has cancer? A guide to physiotherapists not specializing in cancer. Available at: http://www.csp.org.uk/publications/so-your-patient-has-cancer-guide-physiotherapists-not-specialising-cancer (Accessed: 23/3/2018)

Courneya, K. & Friedenreich, C. (2010) Physical Activity and Cancer. Volume 186 of the series Recent Results in Cancer Research. Springer, pp.1–10.

Cramp, F. & Byron-Daniel, J. (2012) Physical activity for the management of cancer-related fatigue in adults. *Cochrane Database of Systematic Reviews*, 11(131), CD006145.

Davies, N.J., Batehup, L. & Thomas, R. (2011) The role of diet and physical activity in breast, colorectal, and prostate cancer survivorship: a review of the literature. *British Journal of Cancer*, 105, S52–S73.

Demark-Wahnefried, W., Aziz, N.M., Rowland, J.H. & Pinto, B.M. (2005) Riding the crest of the teachable moment: promoting long-term health after the diagnosis of cancer. *Journal of Clinical Oncology: official journal of the American Society of Clinical Oncology*, 23(24), 5814–5830.

Department of Health (DH) (2011) Physical activity guidelines for adults (aged 19-64). Available at: https://www.gov.uk/government/uploads/system/uploads/attachment_data/file/213740/dh_128145.pdf (Accessed: 23/3/2018)

Department of Health (2012) Let's Get Moving. London: Department of Health.

Fong, D., Ho, J.W, Hui, B.H, et al. (2012) Physical activity for cancer survivors: meta-analysis of randomised controlled trials. *British Medical Journal*, 344, e70.

Godin G. (2011) The Godin-Shephard Leisure-Time Physical Activity Questionnaire. *Health and Fitness Journal of Canada*, 4, 18–22.

Hall-Alston J. (2015) Exercise and the breast cancer survivor: the role of the nurse practitioner. *Clinical Journal of Oncology Nursing*, 19(5):E98–E102.

Irwin, M., Crumley, D., McTiernan, A. & Bernstein, L. (2003) Physical activity levels before and after a diagnosis of breast carcinoma. *Cancer*, 97(7), 1746–1757.

Macmillan Cancer Support (2012) Interventions to promote physical activity for people living with and beyond cancer: evidence-based guidance. Available at: https://www.macmillan.org.uk/documents/aboutus/health_professionals/physicalactivityevidencebasedguidance.pdf (Accessed 3/7/2018)

Macmillan Cancer Support (2017) Physical activity and cancer – a concise evidence review. https://www.macmillan.org.uk/_images/the-importance-physical-activity-for-people-living-with-and-beyond-cancer_tcm9-290123.pdf

Macmillan Cancer Support (2018) Physical activity for people with metastatic bone disease. https://www.macmillan.org.uk/_images/physical-activity-for-people-with-metastatic-bone-disease-guidance_tcm9-326004.pdf

Mishra, S.I., Scherer, R.W., Geigle, P.M., et al. (2012) Exercise interventions on health-related quality of life for cancer survivors. *Cochrane Database of Systematic Reviews*, 8: CD007566.

Mutrie, N., Campbell, A., Barry, S., et al. (2012) Five-year follow up of participants in a randomized controlled trial showing benefits from exercise for breast cancer survivors during adjuvant treatment. Are there lasting effects? *Journal of Cancer Survivorship*, 6, 420–430.

NMC (2015) *The Code. Professional standards of practice and behaviour for nurses and midwives.* London: Nursing and Midwifery Council, p.9.

Quinn E (2018) https://www.verywellfit.com/what-is-vo2-max-3120097

Saxton, J. & Daley, A. (eds) (2010) *Exercise and Cancer Survivorship: Impact on Health Outcomes and Quality of Life.* New York: Springer-Verlag.

Schmitz, K., Courneya, K.S., Matthews, C., et al. (2010) American College of Sports Medicine roundtable on exercise guidelines for cancer survivors. *Medicine Science in Sports and Exercise*, 42, 1409–1426.

U.S. Department of Health and Human Services (2008) *2008 Physical Activity Guidelines for Americans.* Washington (DC): U.S. Department of Health and Human Services, ODPHP Publication No. U0036. Available at: http://www.health.gov/paguidelines (Accessed: 23/3/2018)

Winters-Stone, K.M., Schwartz, A. & Nail, L.M. (2010) A review of exercise interventions to improve bone health in adult cancer survivors. *Journal of Cancer Survivorship: research and practice*, 4(3), 187–201.

World Health Organization (2010) *Global Recommendations on Physical Activity for Health.* Geneva: World Health Organization.

Section 8.8 Cancer-related fatigue and sleep

Ancoli-Israel, S., Moore, P.J. & Jones, V. (2001) The relationship between fatigue and sleep in cancer patients: a review. *European Journal of Cancer Care*, 10(4), 245–255.

Barsevick, A., Beck, S.L., Dudley, W.N., et al. (2010) Efficacy of an intervention for fatigue and sleep disturbance during cancer chemotherapy. *Journal of Pain and Symptom Management*, 40(2), 200–216.

Bjorneklett, H.G., Lindemalm, C., Ojutkangas, M.L., et al. (2012) A randomised controlled trial of a support group intervention on the quality of life and fatigue in women after primary treatment for early breast cancer. *Supportive Care in Cancer*, 20(12), 3325–3334.

Cancer Research UK (2017) Tiredness with cancer (Fatigue). Available at: http://www.cancerresearchuk.org/about-cancer/coping/physically/fatigue (Accessed 23/3/2018)

Cella, D., Lai, J.S. & Stone, A. (2011) Self-reported fatigue: one dimension or more? Lessons from the FACIT-F Questionnaire. *Supportive Care in Cancer*, 19(9), 1441–1450.

Chan, C.W., Richardson, A. & Richardson, J. (2011) Managing symptoms in patients with advanced lung cancer during radiotherapy. Results of a psychoeducational randomised controlled trial. *Journal of Pain and Symptom Management*, 41(2), 347–357.

Charalambous, A., Giannakopoulou, M., Bozas, E., Marcou, Y., Kitsios, P. & Paikousis, L. (2016) Guided imagery and progressive muscle relaxation as a cluster of symptoms management intervention in patients receiving chemotherapy: a randomized control trial. *Plos One*, 11(6):c0156911.

Christman, N.J. & Cain, L.B. (2004) The effects of concrete objective information and relaxation on maintaining usual activity during radiation therapy. *Oncology Nursing Forum*, 31(2), E39–45.

Cooper, J. (2014) What is the cancer patient's own experience of participating in an occupational therapy led relaxation programme? *Progress in Palliative Care*, 22(4), 206–211.

Cooper, J. & Kite, N. (2015) Occupational therapy in palliative care. In: Cherny, N., Fallon, M., Kaasa, S., Portenoy, R.K. & Currow D.C. (eds) *The Oxford Textbook of Palliative Medicine*, 5th edn. Oxford: Oxford University Press, pp.177–183.

Courtier, N., Gambling, T., Enright, S., Barrett-Lee, P., Abraham, J. & Mason, M.D. (2013) Psychological and immunological characteristics of fatigue women undergoing radiotherapy for early-stage breast cancer. *Supportive Care in Cancer*, 21(1), 173–181.

Cramp, F. & Byron-Daniel, J. (2012). Exercise for the management of cancer-related fatigue in adults. *Cochrane Database of Systematic Reviews*, 11(131) Available at: http://onlinelibrary.wiley.com/doi/10.1002/14651858.CD006145.pub3/epdf (Accessed: 23/3/2018)

De Raaf, P.J., de Klerk, C., Timman, R., Hinz, A. & van der Rijt, C.C.D. (2012) Differences in fatigue experiences among patients with advanced cancer, cancer survivors and the general population. *Journal of Pain and Symptom Management*, 44(6), 823–830.

Donovan, K.A. & Jacobsen, P.B. (2007) Fatigue, depression and insomnia: evidence for a symptom cluster in cancer. *Seminars in Oncology Nursing*, 23(2), 127–135.

Ewer-Smith C. (2006) Remember the 5 P's. In: Cooper, J. (ed.) *Occupational Therapy in Oncology & Palliative Care*. Chichester: Wiley-Blackwell.

Fiorentino, L. & Ancoli-Israel, S. (2007) Sleep dysfunction in patients with cancer. *Current Treatment Options in Neurology*, 9(5), 337–346.

Gascon, P., Rodriguez, C.A., Valentin, V., et al. (2013) Usefulness of the PERFORM questionnaire to measure fatigue in cancer patients with anaemia: a prospective, observational study. *Supportive Care in Cancer*, 21(11), 3039–3049.

Greenlee, H., Balneaves, L.G., Carlson, L.E., et al. (2014) Clinical practice guidelines on the use of integrative therapies as supportive care in patients treated for breast cancer. *Journal of the National Cancer Institute Monographs*, 50, 346–358.

Hwang, E., Lokietz, N.C., Lozano, R.L. & Parke, M.A. (2015) Functional deficits and quality of life among cancer survivors: implications for occupational therapy in cancer survivorship care. *American Journal of Occupational Therapy*, 69(6), 8–10.

Learmouth, Y., Dlugonski, D., Pilutti, L., Sandroff, B., Klaren, R. & Moti, R. (2013) Psychometric properties of the Fatigue Severity Scale and the Modified Fatigue Impact Scale. *Journal of Neurological Sciences*, 331, 102–107.

Leon-Pizarro, C., Gich, I., Barthe, E., Rovirosa, A., Farrus, B. & Casas, F. (2007) A randomised trial of the effect of training in relaxation and guided imagery techniques in improving psychological and quality-of-life indices for gynaecologic and breast brachytherapy patients. *Psycho-Oncology* 16(11), 971–979.

London Cancer Alliance (LCA) (2016) HNA Prompt Sheet: Fatigue. Available at: http://www.londoncanceralliance.nhs.uk/media/122127/lca-hna-fatigue-prompt-sheet-january-2016.pdf (Accessed: 27/4/2018)

Lowrie, D. (2006) Occupational therapy and cancer related fatigue. In: Cooper, J. (ed.) *Occupational Therapy in Oncology and Palliative Care*, 2nd edn. Chichester: Wiley-Blackwell, pp.61–81.

Minton O. & Stone P. (2009) A systematic review of the scales used for the measurement of cancer-related fatigue (CRF). *Annals of Oncology*, 20(1), 17–25.

Mitchell, S., Hoffman, A.J., Clark, J.C., et al. (2014) Putting evidence into practice: an update of evidence based intervention for cancer-related fatigue during and following treatment. *Clinical Journal of Nursing Oncology*, 18(6), 38–58.

Morin, C.M., Belleville, G., Belanger, L. & Ivers H. (2011) The Insomnia Severity Index: Psychometric indicators to detect insomnia cases and evaluate treatment response. *Sleep*, 34(5), 601–608.

National Cancer Institute (NCI) (2015) Fatigue(PDQ®)-Patient Version: Causes of Fatigue in Cancer patients. Available at: http://www.cancer.gov/about-cancer/treatment/side-effects/fatigue/fatigue-pdq#section/27 (Accessed: 23/3/2018)

National Cancer Survivorship Initiative (NCSI) (2013) *Living With and Beyond Cancer: Taking Action to Improve Outcomes*. London: Department of Health.

National Comprehensive Cancer Network (NCCN) (2016) NCCN Clinical Practice Guidelines in Oncology Version 1.2016: Cancer-Related Fatigue. Available at: https://www.nccn.org/professionals/physician_gls/default.aspx#supportive (Accessed: 23/3/2018)

National Sleep Foundation (2016) Sleep diary. Available at: https://sleep-foundation.org/sleep-diary/SleepDiaryv6.pdf (Accessed: 23/3/2018)

NMC (2015) *The Code. Professional standards of practice and behaviour for nurses and midwives.* London: Nursing & Midwifery Council, p. 9.

Ogilvy, C., Livingstone K. & Prue G (2008) Management of cancer related fatigue. In: Rankin, J., Robb, K., Murtagh, N., Cooper, J. & Lewis, S. (eds) *Rehabilitation in Cancer Care.* Oxford: Wiley-Blackwell, pp. 264–279.

Otte, J.L., Carpenter, J.S., Russell, K.M., Bigatti, S.B. & Champion, V.L. (2010) Prevalence, severity and correlates of sleep-wake disturbances in long-term breast cancer survivors. *Journal of Pain and Symptom Management,* 9(3), 535–547.

Ritterband, L.M., Bailey, E.T., Thorndike, F.P., Lord, H.R., Farrell-Carnahan, L. & Baum, L.D. (2012) Initial evaluation of an internet intervention to improve the sleep of cancer survivors with insomnia. *Psycho-Oncology,* 21(7), 695–705.

Roscoe, J.A., Kaufman, M.E., Matteson-Rusby, S.E., et al. (2007) Cancer-related fatigue and sleep disorders. *The Oncologist,* 12(suppl 1), 35–42.

The Royal College of Psychiatrists (RCP) (2012) *Sleeping Well.* London: The Royal College of Psychiatrists.

The Royal Marsden Hospital (NHS Foundation Trust) (2015) *Occupational Therapy Programme – Tips and Strategies for Improving Sleep.* London: The Royal Marsden (NHS) Foundation Trust.

Vargas, S., Antoni, M.H., Carver, C.S., et al. (2014) Sleep quality and fatigue after a stress management intervention for women with early-stage breast cancer in southern Florida. *International Journal of Behavioural Medicine,* 21(6), 971–981.

Varvogli, L. & Darviri, C. (2011) Stress management techniques: evidence-based procedures that reduce stress and promote health. *Health Science Journal,* 5(2),74–89.

Section 8.9 Communication for a patient with a laryngectomy

Ackerstaff, A.H., Hilgers, F.J., Aaronson, N.K., De Boers, M.F., Meeuwis, C.A. & Balm, A.J. (1995) Heat and moisture exchangers as a treatment option in the post-operative rehabilitation of laryngectomised patients. *Clinical Otolaryngology,* 20, 504–509.

Brewster, L. (2004) Ensuring correct use of skin care products on peristomal skin. *Nursing Times,* 100 (19), 34–35.

Corbridge, R.J. (1998) *Essential ENT Practice.* London: Arnold.

Everitt, E. (2016) Tracheostomy 4: Supporting patients following a laryngectomy. *Nursing Times,* 112: online issue 1, 6–8.

Jones, A.S., Young, P.E., Hanafi, Z.B., Makura, Z.G., Fenton, J.E. & Hughes, J.P. (2003) A study of the effect of resistive heat moisture exchanger (Trachinaze) on pulmonary function and blood gas tensions in patients who have undergone a laryngectomy: a randomised control trial of 50 patients studied over a 6-month period. *Head and Neck,* 25, 361–367.

Jones, T.M., De, M., Foran, B., Harrington, K. & Mortimore, S. (2016) Laryngeal cancer: United Kingdom National Multidisciplinary guidelines. *Journal of Laryngology and Otology,* 130 (Suppl S2), S75–S82.

Karlen, R.G. & Maisel, R.H. (2001) Does primary tracheoesophageal puncture reduce complications after laryngectomy and improve patient communication? *American Journal of Otolaryngology,* 22(5), 324–328.

Mathieson, L. (2001) *The Voice and Its Disorders,* 6th edn. London: Whurr.

NMC (2009) *Record keeping: guidance for nurses and midwives.* London: Nursing and Midwifery Council.

NMC (2015) *The code: Professional standards of practice and behaviour for nurses and midwives.* London: Nursing and Midwifery Council.

Op de Coul, B.M., Hilgers, F.J., Balm, A.J. et al. (2000) A decade of post-laryngectomy vocal rehabilitation in 318 patients: a single Institution's experience with consistent application of provox indwelling voice prostheses. *Archives of Otolaryngology, Head and Neck Surgery,* 126(11), 1320–1328.

Rhys-Evans, P.H., Montgomery, P.Q. & Gullane, P.J. (eds) (2003) *Principles and Practice of Head and Neck Oncology.* London: Taylor and Francis.

Searl, J.P. & Reeves, S. (2007) Nonsurgical voice restoration following total laryngectomy. In: Ward, E.C. & van As-Brooks C.J. (eds) *Head and Neck Cancer – Treatment, Rehabilitation and Outcomes.* San Diego: Plural Publishing.

Singer, M.I. (2004) The development of successful tracheoesophageal voice restoration. *Otolaryngology Clinics of North America,* 37(3), 507–517.

Van As-Brooks, C.J. & Fuller, D.P. (2007) Prosthetic tracheoesophageal voice restoration following total laryngectomy. In: Ward, E.C. & van As-Brooks C.J. (eds) *Head and Neck Cancer – Treatment, Rehabilitation and Outcomes.* San Diego: Plural Publishing.

Zurr, J.K., Muller, S.H., de Jongh, F.H., van Zandwijk, N. & Hilgers, F.J. (2006) The physiological rationale of heat and moisture exchangers in post-laryngectomy pulmonary rehabilitation: a review. *European Archives of Otorhinolaryngology,* 263, 1–8.

Section 8.10 Nipple tattooing

Allen, D. (2017) Moving the needle on recovery from breast cancer: the healing role of postmastectomy tattoos. *JAMA,* 317(7), 672–674.

Aslam, R., Page, F., Francis, H. & Prinsloo, D. (2015) Does radiotherapy affect tattoo fading in breast reconstructive patients? *Journal of Plastic, Reconstructive and Aesthetic Surgery, Open,* 6, 53–55.

Burke, N.J., Orenstein, F., Chaumette, S. & Luce, J. (2016) Assessing the impact of post-surgery areola repigmentation and 3-dimensional nipple tattoo procedures on body image and quality of life among medically underserved breast cancer survivors. *Cancer Research,* 76(4).

Clarkson, J.H., Tracey, A., Eltigani, E., et al (2006) The patient's experience of a nurse-led nipple tattoo service: a successful program in Warwickshire. *Journal of Plastic, Reconstructive and Aesthetic Surgery,* 56, 1058–1062.

DH (2005a) *Creating a Patient-Led NHS – Delivering the NHS Improvement Plan.* London: Department of Health.

DH (2005b) *Hazardous Waste (England) Regulations.* London: Department of Health.

DH (2009) *Reference Guide to Consent for Examination or Treatment,* 2nd edn. London: Department of Health.

Fraise, A.P. & Bradley, T. (eds) (2009) *Ayliffe's Control of Healthcare-associated Infection: A Practical Handbook,* 5th edn. London: Hodder Arnold.

Goh, S.C.J., Martin, N.A., Pandya, A.N. & Cutress, R.I. (2011) Patient satisfaction following nipple-areolar complex reconstruction and tattooing. *Journal of Plastic, Reconstructive and Aesthetic Surgery,* 64(3), 360–363.

Loveday, H.P., Wilson, J.A., Prieto, J. & Wilcox, M.H. (2016) epic3: revised recommendation for intravenous catheter and catheter site care. *Journal of Hospital Infection,* 92(4), 346–348.

NMC (2013) *Consent.* London: Nursing and Midwifery Council.

NMC (2015) *The Code: Professional standards of practice and behaviour for nurses and midwives.* London: Nursing and Midwifery Council.

Piot-Ziegler, C., Sassi, M.L., Raffoul, W. & Delaloye, J.F. (2010) Mastectomy, body deconstruction and impact on identity: a qualitative study. *British Journal of Health Psychology,* 15(Pt 3), 479–510.

Potter, S., Barker, J., Willoughby, L., et al. (2007) Patient satisfaction and time-saving implications of a nurse-led nipple and areola reconstitution service following breast reconstruction. *Breast,* 16(3), 293–296.

Rolph, R., Mehta, S. & Farhadi, J. (2016) Breast reconstruction: options post mastectomy. *British Journal of Hospital Medicine,* 77 (6), 334–342.

Sisti, S., Grimaldi, L., Tassinari, J., et al (2016) Nipple-areolar complex reconstruction techniques: a literature review. *European Journal of Surgical Oncology,* 42(4), 441–465.

Spear, S. & Arias, J. (1995) Long-term experience with nipple-areola tattooing. *Annals of Plastic Surgery,* 35, 232–235.

Vassileva, S. and Hristakieva, E. (2007) Medical applications of tattooing. *Clinics in Dermatology,* 25(4), 367–374.

Chapter 9

End of life care

Procedure guideline

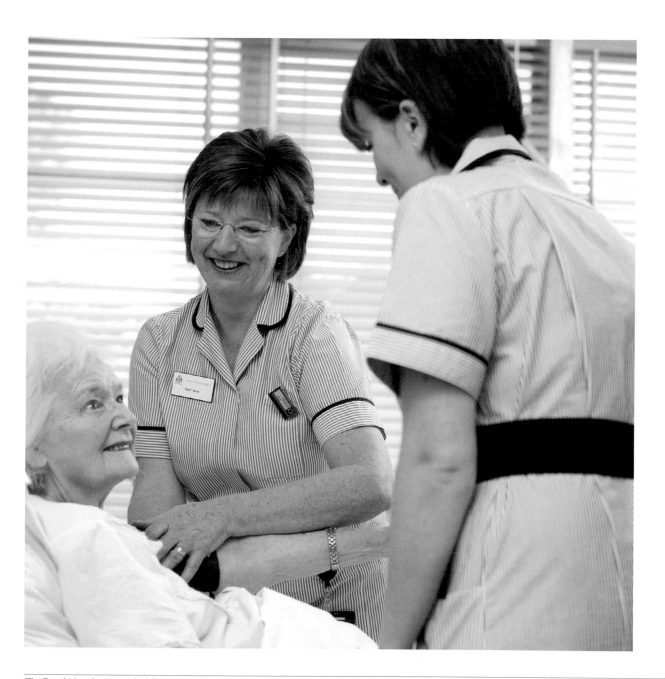

Overview

The following information relates to the patient with cancer who is entering the end of life phase of their illness, however it is recognized that many of the principles are applicable in other diseases. Definitions in palliative care are not always clear, however for the purpose of this chapter we will consider those patients who have weeks, days or hours to live while considering some of the issues that should be addressed before this period such as advance care planning and co-ordination of care. To offer some clarity, definitions have been provided, as follows.

Definitions

End of life care is recognized in much of the literature as care delivered to those patients who are deemed to be in the last year of life. Prognosis in some diseases is not always straightforward, however it is important to afford patients and their families the opportunity to plan for the future when advanced incurable disease has been diagnosed (DH 2008).

Palliative care

Palliative care is the term used for care, wherever and by whomever provided, which seeks to improve quality of life through the prevention and relief of suffering in the time leading up to death (Higgins 2010). Palliative care is applicable from early in the course of an illness, in conjunction with other therapies that aim to prolong life (WHO 2002: www.who.int/cancer/palliative/en).

Anatomy and physiology

In the days and hours leading up to an expected death, the following are common (Fürst 2004, NICE 2015):

- a weaker pulse (but regular unless previously arrhythmic)
- a gradual drop in blood pressure (though at this stage it should not be routinely taken)
- shallower, slower breathing which varies in depth, often in a Cheyne–Stokes pattern
- a decreasing level of consciousness leading eventually to coma, except in those few patients who remain awake until a few minutes before they die
- cooling and clamminess of the skin from the periphery towards the main trunk
- cyanosis of the skin on the extremities and around the mouth
- eventual loss of all signs of cardiorespiratory function and the corneal reflex – death is said to occur at this point.

Related theory

Care of the person who has reached the final stage of their life is a key aspect of maintaining human dignity and is enormously important for relatives and friends who will remember this period perhaps better than any other during the cancer journey. Unrelieved suffering of patients at the end of life is associated with increased relative distress and can unnecessarily complicate the already difficult period of bereavement. Nursing care during this period does not simply represent a continuation of previously given care, nor necessarily the complete cessation of all 'active treatment' measures that may previously have been undertaken. As with all aspects of nursing care, assessment of the individual patient and their relatives, exceptional communication and good multiprofessional working will help to determine the appropriate next steps for each individual.

Cancer has a well-defined trajectory (illustrated in Figure 9.1) and it is usual for physical deterioration to take place over several weeks, with a terminal phase lasting hours to days at the end of life. However, sometimes patients can experience sudden death, either as a result of treatment and its side-effects or from complications of the disease itself, including bleeding, infection, pulmonary embolism or a cardiac event (see Chapter 7 for Acute oncology). Those deaths that follow the former pattern will be discussed here.

Care of the dying patient starts with a recognition from the multiprofessional team that the terminal phase has begun. It is perhaps the single most important factor in enabling the achievement of all the factors associated with a 'good death' (Faull and Nyatanga 2005). The last days/hours of life can be difficult to identify, and often there are barriers from healthcare professionals reluctant to make a diagnosis of dying.

Much of the current literature advocates identification as early as possible of patients who may be reaching the end of their life to help plan their ongoing care and to ensure they and their families have the opportunity to discuss what is of importance to them; in some cases this includes preferences regarding who they want to be with them when they die and preferences around place of care and death (DH 2008, NICE 2015). Considerations such as the surprise question 'Would you be surprised if this patient were to die in the next 12 months?' can be a useful starting point for clinicians (DH 2008). The use of tools such as the Supportive and Palliative Care Indicator Tool (SPICT) supports a more in-depth flow diagram to aid clinicians in the identification process (Boyd and Murray 2010). For patients, cancer booklets such as *Your Life, and Your Choices, Plan Ahead* can help steer them through issues that may need to be considered when faced with a life-limiting illness (Macmillan Cancer Support 2015).

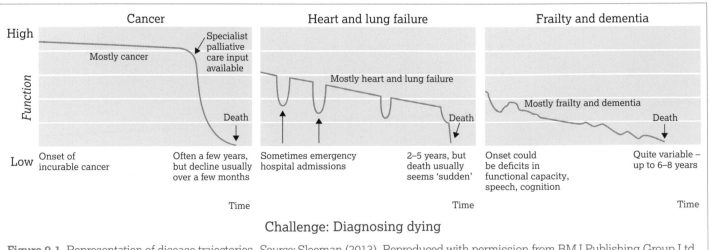

Figure 9.1 Representation of disease trajectories. *Source:* Sleeman (2013). Reproduced with permission from BMJ Publishing Group Ltd.

Recognizing dying in the last days to hours of life in patients with cancer is not easy and is a skill that develops over time. In a patient who is approaching the end of their life, clinical signs that may help us know the patient's prognosis is hours to days include reduced consciousness level and respiratory changes such as Cheyne–Stokes breathing. In the majority of cases there is a progressive physical decline, frailty and a deterioration in mobility coupled with reduced oral intake including food, fluid and oral medications (Sleeman 2013).

Following on from recognizing that a patient may be dying it is important to consider several issues (Collis 2013):

1 Was the patient's condition expected to deteriorate?
2 Is further life-prolonging treatment appropriate/inappropriate?
3 Have potentially reversible causes of deterioration been excluded?

Evidence-based approaches

Palliative care is relatively new as a specialty in nursing and medicine and its evidence base is therefore comparatively small, though growing. Nursing care of the dying patient should have as its main priority meeting personal needs that will allow the patient to have a 'good' death. It has been suggested that the following characteristics are central to a 'good' death from medical, nursing and patient perspectives: (1) control, (2) comfort, (3) closure, (4) trust in healthcare providers, (5) recognition of impending death, and (6) an honouring of personal beliefs and values (Kehl 2006).

The WHO (2002) suggests that palliative care:

- provides relief from pain and other distressing symptoms
- affirms life and regards dying as a normal process
- intends neither to hasten nor postpone death
- integrates the psychological and spiritual aspects of patient care
- offers a support system to help patients live as actively as possible until death
- offers a support system to help the family cope during the patient's illness and in their own bereavement
- uses a team approach to address the needs of patients and their families, including bereavement counselling if indicated
- enhances quality of life and may also positively influence the course of an illness
- is applicable early in the course of illness, in conjunction with other therapies that are intended to prolong life, such as chemotherapy and radiation therapy, and includes those investigations needed to better understand and manage distressing clinical complications.

Legal and professional issues

Advance directives

Advance directives, formerly known as 'living wills', allow people to make a legal decision to refuse, in advance, a proposed treatment, or the continuation of that treatment, if at the necessary time the person lacks the capacity to consent to it. Advance directives can only be made by those who are deemed to have the mental capacity to do so, and allow only for the refusal of treatments – they cannot enforce the provision of specified treatments in the same circumstances (Mental Capacity Act 2005, sections 24–26).

Decisions to refuse life-sustaining treatments must be made in writing, be signed and witnessed, and must expressly state that the decision stands even if the person's life is at risk. Advance directives can be withdrawn verbally or in writing and are not considered valid if the person has conferred lasting power of attorney on another person. Furthermore, advance directives are invalidated if the person has done anything that is clearly inconsistent with the original advance decision made, for example, any change in religious faith.

The Mental Health Capacity Act 2005 (sections 24–26) forms the legal basis for advance directives.

Assisted suicide and euthanasia

Euthanasia is the intentional killing, by act or omission, of a person whose life is thought not to be worth living. Assisted suicide is similar in intentionality but differs in that it involves one person (whether a healthcare professional or not) providing the means for another to end his or her own life, whilst not participating in the act itself (Wyatt 2009). At present, both are illegal in the UK, despite current campaigns to change the law, and it is, therefore, unlawful for any registered nurse to participate in this process.

It must be remembered, however, that those who approach healthcare professionals with a request for assisted suicide or euthanasia will be doing so from a position of significant vulnerability and deserve compassion and respect. Commonly, requests for assisted suicide or euthanasia stem from a fear of pain, indignity and dependence (Wyatt 2009) and it is imperative to ensure that patients are offered adequate opportunities to express these fears, and the specialist physical, psychosocial and spiritual support necessary to minimize their distress.

Artificial hydration

One of the most contentious issues in day-to-day palliative care practice is that of hydration at the end of life, and clear, compassionate communication with patients and their relatives about this aspect of care is therefore essential as many will be concerned about the impact of poor oral hydration on themselves or their loved one. There is currently no conclusive research in favour of either giving or withholding artificial hydration in end of life care, especially in terms of its impact on the length of remaining life. However, studies of the experiences of hospice nurses suggest that artificial hydration has no benefit and, at worst, may contribute to increased respiratory secretions (see Table 9.1) and oedema elsewhere in the body (Watson et al. 2009), therefore most palliative care practitioners usually favour stopping artificial hydration on the grounds of preventing increased symptomatology. It is important that the distress of (most often) the relatives is acknowledged in these situations, and their concerns explored. Once the rationale for discontinuing artificial hydration is offered and the patient and/or relatives have been reassured, it is important to support a decision which serves the best interests of the patient first, and their relatives as well. It may be necessary to negotiate a contract whereby a small amount of artificial hydration is given for an agreed period, on the understanding that this will be discontinued if it is causing distress to the patient. As ever, complex situations require skilled and experienced communication. For all patients the question of fluids and the continuation of nutritional support must be considered on an individualized basis and regularly reviewed (Leadership Alliance for the Care of Dying People 2014).

Pre-procedural considerations

Communication

Excellent communication is paramount in all areas of nursing practice, but perhaps most emphatically so in dealing with dying patients and their relatives. Skillful, truthful communication at the end of life affords people the dignity of making educated decisions about the management of their condition and how and where they want to spend their remaining time. Although each individual's information needs will be different and require careful assessment, healthcare professionals tend to underestimate patients' desire for information and preferences about decision-making (Oostendorp et al. 2011). A large UK study showed that the vast majority of cancer patients want all possible information, though the timing of such information and the depth of detail desired were variable (Jenkins et al. 2001). Cultural and spiritual influences must be taken into account when assessing the information needs of patients in the terminal phase of life.

It is critical that nurses have the necessary training and skills for effective therapeutic communication with terminally ill patients and their relatives.

Prognosis

Prognostication simply means predicting an outcome (Glare et al. 2004); in the care of those who are dying, patients and their families may want information about the likely time remaining before death occurs. This can be difficult to know with much certainty but is generally easier to gauge the closer death is to occurring. Although studies show that patients and their relatives tend to have different information needs regarding prognosis (relatives generally wanting more detailed information than patients, Clayton et al. 2005), it is important that these are carefully assessed to ensure that the needs of all those involved with the patient can be met. Discussions surrounding prognosis should be undertaken by professionals confident in advanced communication skills and with the appropriate experience to offer an approximation on the grounds of their clinical knowledge and experience. The principles of breaking significant news should be adhered to in undertaking discussions about prognosis.

The style and manner in which news is delivered can affect people's understanding of information, the relationship with health professionals and subsequent psychological and emotional outcomes (Street et al. 2009). Delivering news in an insensitive, rushed or otherwise unsatisfactory way is likely to be detrimental and runs the risk of longer-term harm. The overall aim of breaking significant news should be to impart clear information that enables people to become suitably involved in decisions, whilst minimizing distress (Schofield and Butow 2004).

Girgis and Sanson-Fisher (1995) identified a consensus in the key aspects of the process; these included the patient's right to decide how much to know and to receive timely, accurate, clear and honest information. People should be prepared for receiving news, taking into consideration language and cultural barriers. News should ideally be given by one person in an appropriate physical environment, but involvement of other health professionals like the key nurse can be crucial to ensuring that information is clarified and emotional support maintained. People identified by the patient's preference should be invited to attend and the person delivering the news should be warm and have excellent communication skills. Finally, but crucially, the emotional impact on everyone involved should be acknowledged and managed appropriately. Delivering significant news can be both complex and stressful for health professionals (Bousquet et al. 2015).

The process can be summarized as one involving:

- preparation (the health professional, the environment, time, information and the patient)
- delivery – following a model, for example SPIKES (Baile et al. 2000)
- planning and follow-up (what happens now, what does the patient want?)
- documentation and inter-professional communication (informing all involved in care, GP, etc.).

Self-care and debriefing is also necessary – the stress and burden of the process is well documented and health professionals must take responsibility to attend to their own emotional needs.

Procedure

Following the removal of the Liverpool Care of the Dying Patient Pathway in 2014, five priorities for care (Box 9.1) were recommended to encourage patient-centred personalized individual plans of care for patients and those closest to them (Leadership Alliance for the Care of Dying People 2014).

Box 9.1 Priorities of care

Priority 1	The possibility that a person may die within the next few days/hours is recognized and communicated clearly, decisions are made and actions are taken in accordance with the person's needs and wishes, are reviewed regularly and decisions recorded
Priority 2	Sensitive communication takes place between staff and the dying person and those identified as important to them
Priority 3	The dying person and those identified as important to them are involved in decisions about treatment and care to the extent the dying person wants
Priority 4	The needs of families and others identified as important to the dying person are actively explored, respected and met as far as possible
Priority 5	An individual plan of care which includes food and drink, symptom control and psychological, social and spiritual support is agreed, co-ordinated and delivered with compassion

Prescribing of medications for patients who have hours/days to live

The aim of the prescribing of medications in the terminal phase of life is to ensure they are prescribed in advance to avoid uncontrolled symptoms and distress for the patient. For those patients who may be at home, the prescribing of anticipatory medications can often prevent unnecessary admissions to hospital.

Principles of prescribing at this time include (Sleeman 2013):

1 stopping of non-essential medications
2 converting oral medications to the subcutaneous route if the patient is no longer able to tolerate medications by mouth
3 considering having anticipatory medications prescribed.

Physical care

Table 9.1 lists the most common physical symptoms present during the terminal phase of life and any management changes specific to the care of the patient who is dying. The first four symptoms are the most common.

Psychosocial care

Ongoing psychosocial assessment and support and care of the patient and their relatives are extremely important as death approaches. However, provision may need to be adjusted according to the changing needs of the patient – many will experience increasing anxiety and distress, increased feelings of social isolation and, alongside this, a decrease in physical energy available to them for dealing with these concerns. Relatives will naturally be distressed by the increasing illness of the patient and may exhibit signs of grief even before death occurs. Nurses should ensure that, wherever possible, the physical environment is conducive to patients and relatives being able to express their thoughts and emotions, and that appropriately trained staff are available to listen and support them.

Spiritual and religious care

As death approaches, many people will be seeking answers to life's big questions: its nature, meaning and purpose and what, if any, form it takes after death. Some may find these answers in religion, others in their own philosophy or that of others. Many

Table 9.1 Common symptoms observed in the terminal phase of life

Symptom	Management changes
Pain	Levels of pain may increase, decrease or remain stable. Analgesics may need to be rationalized and/or administered via a different route (e.g. via a subcutaneous syringe pump) as the patient may no longer be able to swallow (for further information, see Chapter 3)
	Levels of consciousness, lucidity and respiratory rate will all commonly be altered during the terminal phase. It is important to bear this in mind when assessing the effect and side-effects of analgesic medications
	Some discomfort can be caused by immobility and pressure on the skin. If appropriate (i.e. if it will not cause patient or relative distress), the patient should be moved to a pressure-relieving mattress. Otherwise regular skin care should be carried out as tolerated
Nausea/vomiting	Nausea and vomiting may increase, decrease or remain stable. Antiemetics may need to be rationalized and/or administered via a different route (e.g. via a subcutaneous syringe pump) as the patient may no longer be able to swallow
	Because the insertion of a nasogastric tube is considered a fairly invasive and uncomfortable procedure, it is unlikely to be appropriate for the management of nausea and vomiting in the terminal care setting. Those nasogastric tubes already *in situ* should remain unless causing distress to the patient
	Injectable hyoscine hydrobromide (Buscopan) or octreotide should be considered to dry gastric secretions in those patients with mechanical vomiting secondary to bowel obstruction
Respiratory secretions	'Noisy', 'bubbly' breathing or 'death rattle' in the terminal phase of life affects approximately 50% of dying patients (O'Donnell 1998) and is the result of fluid pooling in the hypopharynx
	Changing the position of the patient in the bed may reduce the noisiness of breathing. It is important to reassure the family that the patient is not drowning or choking, and is unlikely to be distressed by the symptom themselves
	Antimuscarinic (hyoscine butylbromide) or anticholinergic drugs (glycopyrronium or hyoscine hydrobromide) are often used in this setting and can be administered subcutaneously via a syringe pump
Agitation/restlessness	Confusion, delirium, agitation and restlessness are all terms used to describe patient distress in the last 48 hours of life. The symptom is fairly common, with up to 88% of patients experiencing symptoms in the last days or hours of life (Haig 2009). Careful assessment should include consideration of any precipitating factors including: medications, reversible metabolic causes, constipation, urinary retention, hypoxia, withdrawal from drugs or alcohol, uncontrolled symptoms and existential distress
	Clear, concise communication, continuity of carers if possible, the presence of familiar objects and people and a safe immediate environment can all be helpful nursing interventions
	Where the cause of the symptoms cannot be established or reversed, anxiolytics, antipsychotics or sedation may need to be considered. This may need to be discussed with relatives instead of the patient. It is important that the nurse is present for these conversations in order to facilitate reassurance of the relatives throughout
Breathlessness	Breathlessness may be a new symptom in the terminal phase or may worsen from its pre-existing state. Careful assessment is important as this symptom will usually involve physiological, psychological and environmental factors
	Low-dose opioids and anxiolytics can be of use for breathlessness, though as with other medications, the route of administration may need to be altered. Nebulized bronchodilators and oxygen may also be of benefit. Where the symptom is causing severe distress and is intractable, sedation may need to be considered in discussion with the patient and relatives
	Relaxation exercises, open windows or electric fans and massage may also be of benefit if the patient can tolerate these
Constipation	The focus of care with regard to constipation should remain on patient comfort. Oral laxatives are inappropriate if the patient cannot swallow, and rectal interventions should only be undertaken if the patient is clearly distressed by this symptom

407

nurses acknowledge the struggle to provide spiritual or religious support because they feel inadequately skilled or knowledgeable (Kissane and Yates 2003). However, assessment, even if simple, communication and onward referral will ensure that appropriate care can be given without compromising the integrity of the healthcare professional or denying the patient the opportunity to explore these central life issues.

Those with specific religious beliefs may have certain religious practices that need to be undertaken before or after death. It is important to try to discuss these with the patient,

as even where relatives share a common faith there may be differences in the way each person practises. It is, as always, vital that assumptions are not made on the basis of a previously disclosed religious preference – for example, not all Catholic believers will want to be given the sacrament of the sick. Each patient and their relatives should have the opportunity to express their needs and nurses should ensure that, wherever possible, these are met. Further information about religious/cultural perspectives and practices is available (NHS Education for Scotland 2006).

Post-procedural considerations

Nursing care does not end when the death of the patient occurs. Last Offices should be performed with as much attention to detail and respect for the individual as any other procedure.

Last Offices

Definition

The term 'Last Offices' is historically related to the Latin *officium*, meaning service or duty. It is used to refer to the final act performed on a person's body. Last Offices, sometimes referred to as 'laying out', is the term for the nursing care given to a deceased patient, which demonstrates continued respect for the patient as an individual (NMC 2015). Nursing care continues even after death. Last Offices includes health, safety and legal requirements, making the person's body safe to handle, respecting religious, cultural and spiritual requirements, and making the person who has died as pleasant as possible for others to see.

Patients, even though they have died, are still referred to as patients or people throughout this section.

Related theory

After-death care is the final act a nurse will carry out for the patient and remains associated with ritual (Pattison 2008b). Nursing care for a patient who has died has historical roots dating back to the 19th century (Wolf 1988). However, contemporary nursing has moved away from the ritualistic practices of cleansing, plugging, packing and tying the patient's orifices to prevent the leakage of body fluids to encompass much more than simply dealing with a dead body (Pattison 2008b, Pearce 1963). Consideration now has to be given to legal issues surrounding death, the removal (or non-removal) of equipment, washing and grooming, and ensuring correct identification of the patient (Costello 2004). Several national documents allude to the importance of care before death including bereavement care for those closest to the patient (DH 2008, National Nurse Consultant Group, Palliative Care 2011, National Palliative and End of Life Care Partnership 2015). This corresponds to the theory of a 'good death' in which being treated with dignity is an underlying premise (Kehl 2006, Smith 2000), and good death encompasses all stages of dying and death (Pattison 2008b). This principle, therefore, continues after death.

Carrying out such an intimate act, which in many cultures would be carried out only by certain family or community members, requires careful consideration by nurses and adequate preparation of procedures that include family members where possible. Since 60.6% of all men and women who die in England and Wales will die in an institution (hospice, hospital or care home) (ONS 2009), it is predominantly nurses who will have to carry out after-death care prior to patients being moved to mortuaries or funeral homes. Quested and Rudge (2001) suggested that this aspect of care is largely invisible to other healthcare workers.

Death threatens the orderly continuation of social life, according to Seale (1998). Last Offices can mark the social transition of the person as well as the biological death of the patient, and begins the process of handing over care to the family and funeral director. Last Offices can be considered as an important act in the rite of passage in moving the deceased person into the world of the dead (Van Gennep 1972) and is a procedure that people in all cultures recognize.

Evidence-based approaches

Rationale

Last Offices has its foundation in traditional cultures and is a nursing routine that does not have a large amount of research-based evidence (Cooke 2000). The administration of Last Offices can have symbolic meaning for nurses, often providing a sense

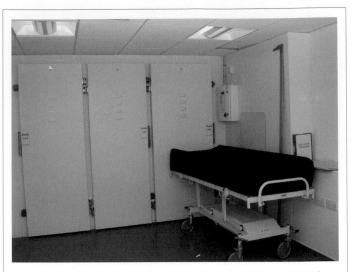

Figure 9.2 Mortuary. *Source:* Dougherty and Lister (2011).

of closure. It can be a fulfilling experience as it is the final demonstration of respectful, sensitive care given to a patient (Nearney 1998) and also the family (Speck 1992).

Many parts of this nursing procedure are based on general principles of infection prevention and control, and safe working. Furthermore, there is a cultural requirement to continue with the practice of Last Offices, as 'rituals serve to express symbolic meanings important to groups of people functioning within a subculture' (Wolf 1988, p. 59). This is particularly important with something as profound as death. Rituals have a role in providing comfort and structure at a traumatic time, which Neuberger (2004) suggests can be valuable for families. Nurses approaching this act of care with compassion might enable families to see that their family member was respected and cared for, even after death. Nurses demonstrate the respect they have for a person who has died and the family, who may now 'own' the body, through rituals associated with Last Offices (Pattison 2008b).

Last Offices can be considered a ritualistic practice that is irrational and unscientific (Philpin 2002). However, this is not to say that nurses carrying out Last Offices do it 'without thinking about it in a problem-solving way' (Walsh and Ford 1989, p. 9) or in a way that does not recognize the individual needs of deceased patients and their carers. Instead, Last Offices is carried out with insight into the meanings attached to the accomplishment of this aspect of nursing care (Philpin 2002).

This aspect of care is usually carried out on the ward. When a mortuary technician is not available nurses may be asked to prepare a body when a family request to view a patient in either a mortuary (Figure 9.2) or a designated viewing room (Figure 9.3).

National guidance for staff responsible for care after death has been developed over the last few years to help and support nurses and healthcare professionals through this procedure (National Nurse Consultant Group, Palliative Care 2011). National guidance on infection prevention and control in relation to people who have died is also available. Care of the patient who has died must take into account health and safety guidelines to ensure families, healthcare workers, mortuary staff and undertakers are not put at risk (National Nurse Consultant Group, Palliative Care 2011). This chapter incorporates this guidance into broader national guidance where appropriate. It aims to ensure that patients who have died are treated with respect and dignity even after death, that legalities are adhered to, and that appropriate infection prevention and control measures are taken.

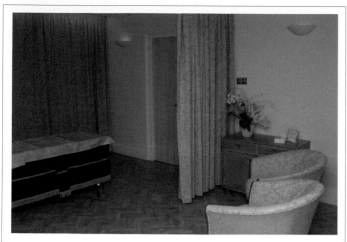

Figure 9.3 Viewing room. *Source:* Dougherty and Lister (2011).

Indications
- When a patient's death has been verified and documented.
- Adult patients who have died in hospital or in a hospice.

Contraindications
Further guidance should be sought before undertaking procedures:

- if a patient who has died is indicated for a post mortem
- if a patient who has died is a candidate for organ donation.

Legal and professional issues
In administering Last Offices, nurses need to know the legal requirements for care of patients after death, and it is essential that correct procedures are followed. Every effort should be made to accommodate the wishes of the patient's relatives (National Nurse Consultant Group, Palliative Care 2011). The UK is an increasingly multicultural and multifaith society, which presents a challenge to nurses who need to be aware of the different religious and cultural rituals that may accompany the death of a patient. There are notable cultural variations within and between people of different faiths, ethnic backgrounds and national origins. This can affect approaches to death and dying (Neuberger 2004) and needs to be remembered when administering Last Offices in order to avoid presumptions. Although those who have settled in a society where there is a dominant faith or culture other than their own might appear to increasingly adopt that dominant culture, they may choose to retain their different practices at times of birth, marriage or death (Neuberger 1999).

Practices relating to Last Offices will vary depending on the patient's cultural background and religious practices (National Nurse Consultant Group, Palliative Care 2011). The following sections provide a guide to cultural and religious variations in attitudes to death and how individuals may wish to be treated. The information that follows is not designed to be a 'fact file' (Gilliat-Ray 2001, Gunaratnam 1997, Smaje and Field 1997) of information on culture and religion that seeks to give concrete information. Such a 'fact file' would not be appropriate as we need to be aware that although death and death-related beliefs, rituals and traditions can vary widely between specific cultural groups, within any given religious or cultural group there may be varying degrees of observance of these issues (Green and Green 2006), from orthodox to agnostic and atheist. Categorizing individuals into groups with clearly defined norms can lead to a lack of understanding of the complexities of religious and cultural practice and can depersonalize care for individuals and their families (Neuberger 1999, Smaje and Field 1997).

Last Offices for an expected death may be very different to those given to a patient who has died suddenly or unexpectedly (Docherty 2000) or in a critical care setting, so these issues will be dealt with later in this chapter. In certain cases the patient's death may need to be referred to the coroner or medical examiner for further investigation and possible post mortem. If those caring for the deceased are unsure about this then the person in charge of the patient's care should be consulted before Last Offices are commenced.

Prior to the patient's death, whenever possible, it is good practice to ascertain if the patient wishes to donate organs or tissue following their death. For further information on this, visit www.organdonation.nhs.uk.

Pre-procedural considerations
Before undertaking Last Offices, several other events must take place.

Confirmation of death
Death should be confirmed or verified by appropriate healthcare staff. Verification of death is usually completed by a medical doctor but it can be undertaken by nurses in certain healthcare settings who have had the necessary training if death is *expected* and local policy permits this (Laverty et al. 2018). Certification of death occurs by the medical practitioner (National Nurse Consultant Group, Palliative Care 2011). Unexpected deaths must be confirmed by a medical doctor (and usually a senior medical doctor). Confirmation of death must be recorded in the medical and nursing notes certification process stipulates that it is mandatory for the certifying doctor to both identify the deceased and confirm the presence of any implants/devices (DH 2010).

A registered medical doctor who has attended the deceased person during their last illness is required to give a medical certificate of the cause of death (Home Office 1971). The certificate requires the doctor to state on which date they last saw the deceased alive and whether or not they have seen the body after death (this may mean that the certificate is completed by a different doctor from the one who confirmed death). Out-of-hours medical examiners can now certify death where there is a cultural/religious requirement to bury, cremate or repatriate patients quickly (DH 2008). Medical examiners can also certify for reportable deaths where a post mortem is not deemed necessary (DH 2008). The medical examiner (ME) is a primary care trust-appointed but independent healthcare professional who determines the need for coroner referral. For those who need a quick burial within 24 hours, this remains at the discretion of the local births and deaths registrar in each council and depends on the individual opening hours and on-call facilities. Local hospital policy should outline procedures for out-of-hours death registration and certification, and burial is usually easier to accommodate than cremation within 24 hours.

Repatriation to another country needs further documentation, alongside the death certification and registration documents, and this varies according to which country the body is being repatriated. Only a coroner or ME is authorized to permit the body to be moved out of England or Wales. A 'Form of Notice to a Coroner of Intention to Remove a Body Out of England' (Form 104) is required and can be obtained from coroners or registrars. This form needs to be given to the coroner along with any certificate for burial or cremation already issued. The coroner's office will acknowledge receipt of notice and inform when repatriation can occur. Coroner authorization normally takes up to 4 working days so that necessary enquiries can be made. In urgent situations, this can sometimes be expedited. The coroner's office and relevant High Commission will have further information. In terms of infection control, packing may be required by different countries and those involved with repatriation must be informed if there is a danger of infection (HSAC 2003). Funeral directors would assist with transportation issues.

409

Referral to a coroner

If the patient's death is to be referred to a coroner or ME, this will affect how their body is prepared. The need for referral to a coroner or ME should be ascertained with the person verifying the death (DH 2008). Preparation in this situation differs according to how the patient died. Broadly, two types of death are referred to the coroner:

- those from a list of cases where the coroner must be informed (which includes deaths within 24 hours of an operation, for example)
- cases where the treating doctor is unable to certify the cause of death (www.gov.uk/after-a-death/when-a-death-is-reported-to-a-coronereferral to a coroner).

The Department of Health website (www.dh.gov.uk) gives more information about when to refer to the coroner or ME and when post mortems are indicated.

Requirement for a post mortem

Post mortems can affect preparation after death, depending on whether this is a coroner's post mortem (sometimes referred to as a legal post mortem because it cannot be refused) or a post mortem requested by the consultant doctor-in-charge to answer a specific query on the cause of death (also referred to as a hospital or non-legal post mortem). A coroner's post mortem might require specific preparation but the coroner or ME will advise on this and should be contacted as soon as possible after death to ascertain any specific issues. Individual hospitals, institutions and NHS trusts should provide further guidance on these issues. If the patient is to be referred to the coroner, cap off catheters and ensure there is no possibility of leakage. Do not remove any invasive devices until this has been discussed with the coroner.

If the patient is *not* to be referred to the coroner, invasive and non-invasive attachments, such as central venous access catheters, peripheral venous access cannulas, Swan–Ganz catheters, tracheal tubes (tracheostomy/endotracheal) and drains, can be removed prior to Last Offices.

Organ donation

Consider whether the patient is a candidate for organ or tissue donation. Patients who previously expressed a wish to be a donor (or carry a donor card), or whose family has expressed such a wish, might need specific preparation (see further resources at the end of the chapter and contact local or regional transplant co-ordinators). Patients with cancer under some circumstances can continue to donate tissue such as cornea in the event of their death but this will need to be discussed with the national transplant co-ordinator in advance of the death.

Organ donation is an important consideration at the end of life. Current law is an opt-in system for donation, therefore express wishes must be made by families (next of kin) or patients. Further information can be sourced from the organ donation website www.organdonation.nhs.uk.

Infectious patient

If the patient was infectious, it needs to be established whether the infection is notifiable, for example hepatitis B, C or tuberculosis, or non-notifiable (Healing et al. 1995). There are additional requirements for patients with bloodborne infections, so the senior nurse on duty should be consulted and local infection control policy adhered to. In the UK, notifiable infections must be reported via a local authority 'proper officer', which is the attending doctor's duty. Infection prevention and control contacts in local trusts or services can provide more help and guidance around notification. Placing the patient who has died in a body bag is advised for all notifiable diseases and a number of non-notifiable infectious diseases (i.e. HIV and transmissible spongiform encephalopathies, e.g. Creutzfeldt–Jakob disease).

A label identifying the infection must also be attached to the patient's body.

Certain extra precautions are required when handling a patient who has died from an infectious disease. However, the deceased will pose no greater threat of infection than when they were alive. It is assumed that staff will have practised universal precautions when caring for all patients, and this practice must be continued when caring for the deceased patient (HSAC 2003).

Porters, mortuary staff, undertakers and those involved with Last Offices must also be informed if there is a danger of infection (HSAC 2003) or radiation.

Informing the next of kin

Inform and offer support to relatives and/or next of kin to ensure that the relevant individuals are aware of the patient's death and any specific care or practices can be carried out (National Nurse Consultant Group, Palliative Care 2011). The support of a hospital chaplain or other religious leader or other appropriate person should be offered. If the relative(s) or next of kin are not contactable by telephone or by the GP, it may be necessary to inform the police of the death.

Some families and carers may wish to assist with Last Offices, and within certain cultures it may be unacceptable for anyone but a family member or religious leader to wash the patient (National Nurse Consultant Group, Palliative Care 2011). It is necessary to prepare them sensitively for any changes to the body that occur after death and be aware of manual handling and infection control issues (National Nurse Consultant Group, Palliative Care 2011). It may also be required that somebody of the same sex as the patient undertakes Last Offices (Neuberger 2004).

There are occasions when it may not be possible for families to assist with last offices:

- certain infectious diseases
- when the case is to be referred to the coroner
- when the patient has been treated with radioactive substances (further advice from an expert in radiation protection should be sought).

Patient considerations

Ascertain any social, cultural, spiritual and/or religious considerations that should be observed during the procedure. Spiritual needs involved in preparation of the patient who has died can be diverse but the final sections offer current guidance; the patient's previous wishes should be established where possible and should always take precedence (Pattison 2008a). If these have not been documented, try to determine the patient's previous wishes from family or carers. The patient's last will and testament might have instruction on this, or an advance directive might have information. Families, carers or members of the patient's community or faith may wish to participate in Last Offices (with consent of the next of kin or as expressed in the patient's wishes when they were alive). If this is the case, they must be adequately prepared for this with careful and sensitive explanation of the procedure to be undertaken.

Considerations before undertaking last offices:

1 Respect any particular wishes of the patient.
2 Respect the family's preference to participate in Last Offices.
3 Consider any infectious diseases that require particular consideration.
4 Remember to let the family/friends sit with their relative/friend if they wish to do this.
5 If the death is being referred to the coroner then Last Offices must not begin and all lines must be left *in situ*. Do not wash the body or undertake mouth care (National Nurse Consultant Group, Palliative Care 2011).

Information required by mortuary staff and funeral directors is listed in Box 9.2.

Box 9.2 Information required by the mortuary staff and funeral directors (National Nurse Consultant Group, Palliative Care 2011)

1 Identifying information including the patient's name, date of birth, address and NHS number
2 Date and time of death
3 Implantable devices that are present
4 Any current radioactive treatments
5 Notifiable infections
6 Any jewellery or religious mementoes left on the deceased
7 Name and signature of registered nurse responsible for the care after death
8 Name and signature of any second healthcare professional who assisted with the care

Additional considerations

It is important to inform other patients, particularly if the person has died in an area where other people are present (such as a bay or open ward) and might know the patient. Senior staff should offer guidance in the event of uncertainty about how to deal with the situation.

Personal care after death needs to be carried out within 2–4 hours of the person dying to preserve their appearance, condition and dignity. The body's core temperature will take time to lower, therefore transfer to the mortuary within 4 hours of the death is optimal (National Nurse Consultant Group, Palliative Care 2011).

411

Procedure guideline 9.1   Last Offices

Essential equipment

- Disposable plastic apron
- Disposable plastic gloves
- Bowl of warm water, soap, patient's own toilet articles. Disposable wash cloths and two towels
- Comb and equipment for nail care
- Equipment for mouth care including equipment for cleaning dentures
- Identification labels × 2
- Documents required by law and by organization/institution policy, for example Notification of Death cards
- Shroud or patient's personal clothing: night-dress, pyjamas, clothes previously requested by patient, or clothes that comply with deceased patient/family/cultural wishes
- Body bag if required (if there is actual or potential leakage of bodily fluids and/or if there is infectious disease) (National Nurse Consultant Group, Palliative Care 2011, **C**)
- Gauze, tape, dressings and bandages if there are wounds, puncture sites or intravenous/arterial devices

- Valuables/property book
- Plastic bags for clinical and domestic (household) waste
- Laundry skip and appropriate bags for soiled linen
- Clean bedlinen
- Documentation for personal belongings
- Bags for the patient's personal possessions
- Disposable receptacle for collecting urine, if appropriate
- Sharps bin, if appropriate

Optional equipment

- Caps/spigots for urinary catheters (if catheters are to be left *in situ*)
- Additional equipment as needed for infectious diseases based on organizational policy
- Suction equipment and absorbent pads (where there is the potential for leakage) (National Nurse Consultant Group, Palliative Care 2011, **C**)

Pre-procedure

Action	Rationale
1 Apply gloves and apron.	To ensure staff are protected from soiled sheets/body fluids.
2 If the patient has an infectious disease additional equipment such as gowns/masks/goggles may be required.	All regular infection control principles should be applied (National Nurse Consultant Group, Palliative Care 2011, **C**).
3 If the patient is on a pressure-relieving mattress or device, consult the manufacturer's instructions before switching off.	If the mattress deflates too quickly, it may cause a manual handling challenge to the nurses carrying out Last Offices.

Procedure

Action	Rationale
4 Lay the patient on their back with their arms lying by their side. Straighten any limbs as far as possible (adhering to your own organization's manual handling policy). This should ideally be undertaken with two nurses.	To maintain the patient's privacy and dignity (NMC 2015) and for ongoing nursing care of the body. Stiff, flexed limbs can be difficult to fit easily into a mortuary trolley, mortuary fridge or coffin and can cause additional distress to any carers who wish to view the body. If there is a problem in being able to straighten limbs then the mortuary staff should be notified (National Nurse Consultant Group, Palliative Care 2011).
5 Remove all but one pillow. Close the mouth and support the jaw by placing a pillow or rolled-up towel on the chest or underneath the jaw. Do not bind the patient's jaw with bandages.	To avoid leaving pressure marks on the face which can be difficult to remove (National Nurse Consultant Group, Palliative Care 2011, **C**).
6 When the death is not being referred to the coroner remove mechanical aids such as syringe drivers, apply gauze and tape to syringe pump sites and document disposal of medication.	To try and ensure the person looks as normal as possible as the family may want to see them again.

(continued)

Procedure guideline 9.1 Last Offices *(continued)*

7 Do not tie the penis. Spigot any urinary catheters.	Pads and pants can be used to absorb any leakage from the urethra, vagina or rectum (National Nurse Consultant Group, Palliative Care 2011, **C**).
8 Close the patient's eyes by applying light pressure to the eyelids for 30 seconds. (If corneal or eye donation is to take place close the eyes with gauze moistened with normal saline to prevent them drying out. If this is unsuccessful explain to the carers that the funeral director will be able to rectify this.)	To maintain the patient's dignity (NMC 2015) and for aesthetic reasons. Closure of the eyelids will also provide tissue protection in case of corneal donation (National Nurse Consultant Group, Palliative Care 2011, **C**).
9 Contain leakages from the oral cavity or tracheostomy sites by suctioning and positioning. Suction and spigot nasogastric tubes. Cover exuding wounds or unhealed surgical incisions with a clean absorbent dressing and secure with an occlusive dressing. Leave stitches and clips intact. Cover stomas with a clean bag. Clamp drains (remove the bottles), pad around wounds and seal with an occlusive dressing. Avoid waterproof, strongly adhesive tape as this can be difficult to remove at the funeral directors and can leave a permanent mark. Cap intravenous lines and leave them *in situ*. If the body is leaking profusely then take time, prior to transfer to the mortuary, to address the problem.	Leaking orifices pose a health hazard to staff coming into contact with the patient's body (National Nurse Consultant Group, Palliative Care 2011). Ensuring that the patient's body is clean will demonstrate continued respect for the patient's dignity (NMC 2015, **C**). It is the role of the mortuary staff to pack orifices, not the nurse. If the body continues to leak, place it on absorbent pads in a body bag and advise the mortuary or funeral director (National Nurse Consultant Group, Palliative Care 2011, **C**).
10 Exuding wounds or unhealed surgical scars should be covered with a clean absorbent dressing and secured with an occlusive dressing (e.g. Tegaderm). Stitches and clips should be left intact. Consider leaving intact recent surgical dressings for wounds that could potentially leak, for example large amputation wounds. Reinforcement of the dressing should be sufficient.	The dressing will absorb any leakage from the wound site (National Nurse Consultant Group, Palliative Care 2011, **C**).
11 Stomas should be covered with a clean bag.	To contain any leakage from the stoma site.
12 It is the responsibility of mortuary staff to discuss with the funeral director collecting the body their capacity to remove intravenous lines, drains, indwelling catheters, etc. If they are unable to remove these then the mortuary technician needs to attend to this before releasing the body. When a family member collects the deceased then mortuary staff must remove all intravenous lines, drains, indwelling catheters, etc. When release to a funeral director is prompt in order to ensure same-day burial the funeral director needs to ensure all lines are removed in case family members wish to bathe or dress the body. This practice in some areas may be the responsibility of the nurse if the organization has no mortuary staff.	When a death is being referred to the coroner or ME or for post mortem, all lines, devices and tubes should be left in place (National Nurse Consultant Group 2011, **C**).
13 Wash the patient, unless requested not to do so for religious/cultural reasons or carer's preference.	To ensure dignity and respect for the deceased (National Nurse Consultant Group Palliative Care 2011, **C**).
14 The deceased should not be shaved when still warm; this can be undertaken by the funeral director and it may be necessary to discuss this sensitively with the family.	Shaving when the deceased is still warm can cause bruising to the skin (National Nurse Consultant Group, Palliative Care 2011, **C**).
15 It may be important to family and carers to assist with washing, thereby continuing to provide the care given in the period before death. It is important to have a conversation with the family before undertaking this to prepare them for how the body will look and feel.	It is an expression of respect and affection, part of the process of adjusting to loss and expressing grief (National Nurse Consultant Group, Palliative Care 2011, **C**).
16 Clean the mouth to remove debris and secretions. Clean and replace dentures as soon as possible after death. If they cannot be replaced send them with the body in a clearly identified receptacle.	To ensure dignity and respect is demonstrated (National Nurse Consultant Group, Palliative Care 2011, **C**).
17 Tidy the hair as soon as possible after death and arrange in the preferred style (if known) to guide the funeral director for final presentation.	This will guide the funeral director for final presentation (National Nurse Consultant Group, Palliative Care 2011, **C**).

18 Remove jewellery (apart from the wedding ring) in the presence of another member of staff, unless specifically requested by the family to do otherwise, and document this according to local policy. Be aware of religious ornaments that need to remain with the deceased. Secure any rings left on with minimal tape, documented according to local policy. Provide a signature if any jewellery is removed.	To ensure culture and personal wishes are respected (National Nurse Consultant Group Palliative Care 2011, **C**). Procedures are needed to provide this information to caregivers.
19 Clean and dress the deceased person appropriately (use of shrouds is common practice in many acute hospitals) before they go to the mortuary. They should never go to the mortuary naked or be released naked to a funeral director from an organization without a mortuary. Be aware that soiling can occur. The funeral director will dress them in their own clothes.	For aesthetic reasons for family and carers viewing the patient's body or religious or cultural reasons and to meet the family's or carers' wishes (National Nurse Consultant Group, Palliative Care, **C**).
20 Clearly identify the deceased person with a name band on their wrist or ankle (avoid toe tags). As a minimum this needs to identify their name, date of birth, address, ward (if a hospital inpatient) and ideally their NHS number. The person responsible for identification is the person that verifies the death. Nurses should refer to local policies for the identification of deceased patients within their organization.	To ensure correct and easy identification of the patient's body in the mortuary (National Nurse Consultant Group Palliative Care 2011, **C**).
21 Provided no leakage is expected and there is no notifiable disease present, the body can be wrapped in a sheet and taped lightly to ensure it can be moved safely. Do not bind the sheet or tape too tightly as this can cause disfigurement. If there is significant leakage or a notifiable infection is present, put the deceased into a body bag.	To avoid possible damage to the patient's body during transfer (National Nurse Consultant Group, Palliative Care 2011, **C**).
22 Secure the sheet with tape loosely.	To ensure the sheet is not too tight and causes any disfigurement (National Nurse Consultant Group, Palliative Care 2011, **C**).
23 Place the patient's body in a body bag if leakage of body fluids may be anticipated or if the patient has a known infectious disease.	To avoid actual or potential leakage of fluid, whether infection is present or not, as this poses a health hazard to all those who come into contact with the deceased patient (National Nurse Consultant Group, Palliative Care 2011, **C**).

Post-procedure

24 Request the portering staff to remove the patient's body from the ward and transport it to the mortuary.	This should be completed within 4 hours of death to allow refrigeration to take place (National Nurse Consultant Group, Palliative Care 2011, **C**).
25 In hospital, screen off the beds/area that will be passed as the patient's body is removed. The privacy and dignity of the deceased on transfer from the place of death is paramount Each organization involved is responsible for ensuring that the procedures adopted to transfer bodies respect the values of personal dignity and that these are incorporated in the design of the concealment trolley and the way the body is covered.	To ensure the transfer remains as respectful as possible (Kings Fund 2008) and to avoid causing unnecessary distress to other patients, relatives and staff.
26 Remove gloves and apron. Dispose of equipment according to local policy and wash hands.	To minimize risk of cross-infection and contamination (Fraise and Bradley 2009, **C**).
27 Record all aspects of care after death in nursing and medical documentation and identify the professionals involved. Update and organize the medical and nursing records as quickly as possible so they are available to the bereavement team and other relevant professionals, such as pathologists.	To record the time of death, names of those present, and names of those informed (NMC 2015, **C**).
28 Transfer property and patient records to the appropriate administrative department.	To allow the administrative formalities needed to complete the medical certification of death and to return the personal property of the patient to the nominated person.
It is important to remember to give the patient's property to the family/friends in a sensitive way. If there is soiled clothing to return, try and discuss this sensitively with families/friends to ascertain if they want it returned.	To avoid unnecessary further distress to families and friends (National Nurse Consultant Group, Palliative Care 2011, **C**).

Problem-solving table 9.1 Prevention and resolution (Procedure guideline 9.1)

Problem	Cause	Prevention	Action
Relatives not present at the time of the patient's death.	Possible unexpected death; non-contactable family.	Preparation of family for event of death where appropriate.	Inform the relatives as soon as possible of the death. Consider also that they may want to view the patient's body before Last Offices are completed. Ensure the family are prepared for how the body will look and feel.
Relatives or next of kin not contactable by telephone or by the general practitioner.	Out-of-date or missing contact information.	Ensure next of kin contact information is documented and up to date.	If within the UK, local police will go to next of kin's house. If abroad, the British Embassy will assist.
Death occurring within 24 hours of an operation.	n/a	In relation to documentation, ensure information around circumstance of death is documented and handed over to relevant healthcare staff.	All tubes and/or drains must be left in position. Spigot or cap off any cannulas or catheters. Treat stomas as open wounds. Leave any endotracheal or tracheostomy tubes in place. Machinery can be disconnected (discuss with coroner) but settings must be left alone. Post mortem examination will be required to establish the cause of death. Any tubes, drains, and so on may have been a major contributing factor to the death.
Unexpected death.	n/a	As above.	As above. Post mortem examination of the patient's body will be required to establish the cause of death.
Unknown cause of death.	n/a	As above.	As above.
Patient brought into hospital who is already deceased.	n/a	Not preventable but where possible ensure patients' families are prepared for all eventualities, particularly if palliative care patients whose death is expected, and that family know who to call and what to do in the event of death.	As above, unless patient seen by a medical practitioner within 14 days before death. In this instance, the attending medical officer may complete the death certificate if they are clear as to the cause of death.
Patient who dies after receiving systemic radioactive iodine.	There is a potential risk of exposure to radiation (IPEM 2002).	Radiation protection should be undertaken (see Chapter 5).	Ensure those in contact with the patient's body are aware. Pregnant nurses should not carry out Last Offices for these patients.
Patient who dies after insertion of gold grains, colloidal radioactive solution, caesium needles, caesium applicators, iridium wires or iridium hair pins.	There is a potential risk of exposure to radiation (IPEM 2002).	Radiation protection should be undertaken (see Chapter 5) when removing wires. The physicist may remove radioactive wires/needles, and so on, themselves, depending on source.	Inform the physics department as well as appropriate medical staff. Once a doctor has verified death, the sources are removed and placed in a lead container. A Geiger counter is used to check that all sources have been removed. This reduces the radiation risk when completing the Last Offices procedures. Record the time and date of removal of the sources. Ensure those in contact with the patient's body are aware. Pregnant nurses should not carry out Last Offices for these patients. For further information see Chapter 5.
Patient and/or relative wishes to donate organs/tissues for transplantation.	n/a	Discussion around transplantation should occur with families/next of kin wherever appropriate (as deemed by clinical team). Exceptions apply.	As stated in the Human Tissue Act 1961, patients with malignancies can only donate corneas and heart valves (and, more recently, tracheas). Contact local transplant co-ordinator as soon as decision is made to donate organs/tissue and before Last Offices is attempted. Obtain verbal and written consent from the next of kin, as per local policy. Prepare the patient who has died as per transplant co-ordinator's instructions. For further guidance see: www.uktransplant.org.uk
Patient to be moved straight from ward to undertakers.	n/a	n/a	Contact senior nurse for hospital as stipulated in local policy. Contact local registry office and ensure permission to remove body form is completed. Local guidelines/policies should be applied thereafter.

Problem	Cause	Prevention	Action
Relatives want to see the person who has died after removal from the ward.	n/a	n/a	Inform the mortuary staff in order to allow time for them to prepare the body. Occasionally nurses might be required to undertake this in institutions where there are no mortuary staff. The patient's body will normally be placed in the hospital viewing room. Ask relatives if they wish for a chaplain or other religious leader or appropriate person to accompany them. As required, religious artefacts should be removed from or added to the viewing room. The nurse should check that the patient's body and environment are presentable before accompanying the relatives into the viewing room. The relatives may want to be alone with the deceased but the nurse should wait outside the viewing room in order that support may be provided should the relatives become distressed. After the relatives have left, the nurse should contact the portering service who will return the deceased patient to the mortuary.
Patient has an implantable cardiac device. Deactivation of implantable cardiac defibrillators needs to be considered when the patient is recognized as entering the end of life phase.	n/a	Knowledge of device *in situ* prior to death.	Nurses must inform funeral directors and mortuary staff about patients with an implantable cardiac device and ensure it is clearly documented (National Nurse Consultant Group, Palliative Care 2011).

n/a, not applicable.

Families may request other items to accompany the patient who has died to the mortuary and funeral home. This might be an item of sentimental value, for instance, and in this case it should be at the discretion of those caring for the patient and the nurse-in-charge (local policy might also specify). It may also be possible for certain religious artefacts to remain with the patient. This should be ascertained with those closest to the patient. Further information can be found at NHS Education for Scotland (2006).

Varying degrees of adherence and orthodoxy exist within all the world's faiths. The given religion of a patient may occasionally be offered to indicate an association with particular cultural and national roots, rather than to indicate a significant degree of adherence to the tenets of a particular faith. If in doubt, consult the family members concerned.

Regardless of the faith that the patient's record states they hold, wishes for Last Offices may differ from the conventions of their stated faith. Sensitive discussion is needed by nurses to establish what is wanted at this time. If patients hold no religious beliefs, ask the relatives to outline the patient's previously expressed wishes, if any, or establish the family's wishes. Furthermore, the patient may be non-denominational and/or the family members may be multidenominational so all possibilities must be taken into account.

Post-procedural considerations

Immediate care

Relatives' time with patient after death
As there is a limit to the time a patient should remain in the heat of a ward, the senior nurse will have to exercise discretion over when to send the patient to the mortuary. This will vary according to family circumstances (there could be a short delay in a relative travelling to the ward/area) and the ward situation (side rooms are obviously easier for the family/other patients).

Viewing the patient in the viewing room
Families may wish to view the patient in the viewing room again (Figure 9.3). It is important to ensure that the patient is in a presentable state before taking the family to see them.

Spiritual, emotional and bereavement support
The bereaved family may find it difficult to comprehend the death of their family member and it can take great sensitivity and skill to support them at this time. Explaining all procedures as fully as possible can help understanding of the practices at the end of life. Offering bereavement care services may be useful to families for that difficult period immediately after death and in the future. National services such as Cruse (www.cruse.org.uk) can be useful if local services are not available.

Relatives may express extreme distress; this is a difficult situation to handle and other family members are likely to be of most comfort and support at this point. The family member may wish for their GP to be contacted.

Maintain a high degree of sensitivity when outlining the process after a patient has died because families frequently have to attend the hospital in the very near future in order to collect the documentation for registering the death.

Education of patient and relevant others
Helping the family to understand procedures after death is the role of many people in hospital but primarily it falls upon those who first meet with the family after their relative has died. Information for relatives/friends on what to do after someone dies can be found at www.gov.uk/after-a-death/

If the family states that they feel the death was unnatural or that it was interfered with, we have a responsibility to explore these feelings and even outline their legal entitlement to a post mortem.

- Prepare the family for what they might see.
- Invite the family into the bed space/room.

- Accompany the family but respect their need for privacy should they require it.
- Anticipate questions.
- Offer the family the opportunity to discuss care (at that time or in the future).
- Offer to contact other relatives on behalf of the family.
- Advise about the bereavement support services that can be accessed. Arrange an appointment if requested.
- Provide them with a point of contact with the hospital.

Some families may wish for a memento of the patient, such as a lock of hair. Try to anticipate and accommodate these wishes as much as possible.

416

Websites and useful addresses

For further information about organ donation, contact the following website or your local transplant co-ordinator: www.organdonation.nhs.uk

For further information about bereavement and bereavement advice: Cruse Bereavement Care: www.cruse.org.uk

For additional practical advice such as with Wills or financial advice following a death contact: Citizens Advice Bureau: www.citizensadvice.org.uk

Online resources

SPIKES model: http://theoncologist.alphamedpress.org/content/5/4/302.full

http://www.skillscascade.com/badnews.htm

http://www.kevinmd.com/blog/2013/01/deliver-bad-news-patients-9-tips.html

References

Baile, W.F., Buckman, R., Lenzi, R., Glober, G., Beale, E.A. & Kudelka, A.P. (2000) SPIKES – A six-step protocol for delivering bad news: application to the patient with cancer. *The Oncologist*, 5(4), 302–311.

Bousquet, G., Orri, M., Winterman, S., Brugière, C., Verneuil, L. & Revah-Levy, A. (2015) Breaking bad news in oncology: a metasynthesis. *Journal of Clinical Oncology*, 33(22), 2437–2443.

Boyd K. & Murray S.A. (2010) Recognising and managing key transitions in end of life care. *British Medical Journal*, 341:c4863.

Clayton, J.M., Butow, P.N., Arnold, R.M. & Tattersall, M.H.N. (2005) Discussing end-of-life issues with terminally ill cancer patients and their carers: a qualitative study. *Support Care Cancer*, 13(8), 589–599.

Collis E. (2013) Care of the dying patient in the community. *British Medical Journal*, 347, f4085.

Cooke, H. (2000) *A Practical Guide to Holistic Care at the End of Life*. Oxford: Butterworth Heinemann.

Costello, J. (2004) *Nursing the Dying Patient: Caring in Different Contexts*. Basingstoke: Palgrave Macmillan.

DH (2008) *End-of-Life Care Strategy*. London: Department of Health.

DH (2010) *Improving the Process of Death Certification in England and Wales: Overview of Programme*. London: Department of Health.

Docherty, B. (2000) Care of the dying patient. *Professional Nurse*, 15(12), 752.

Dougherty, L. & Lister, S. (eds) (2011) *The Royal Marsden Manual of Clinical Nursing Procedures: Professional Edition*. 8th edn. Oxford: Wiley-Blackwell.

Faull, C. & Nyatanga, B. (2005) Terminal care and dying. In: Faull, C., Carter, Y. & Daniels L. (eds) *Handbook of Palliative Care*. Oxford: Wiley-Blackwell.

Fraise, A.P. & Bradley, T. (eds) (2009) *Ayliffe's Control of Healthcare-Associated Infection: A Practical Handbook*, 5th edn. London: Hodder Arnold.

Fürst, C.J. (2004) The terminal phase. In: Doyle, D., Hanks, G., Cherny, N. & Calman, K. (eds) *Oxford Textbook of Palliative Medicine*. Oxford: Oxford University Press.

Gilliat-Ray, S. (2001) Sociological perspectives on the pastoral care of minority faiths in hospital. In: Orchard, H. (ed.) *Spirituality in Health Care Contexts*. London: Jessica Kingsley Publishers, pp. 135–146.

Girgis, A. & Sanson-Fisher, R. W. (1995). Breaking bad news: consensus guidelines for medical practitioners. *Journal of Clinical Oncology*, 13, 2449–2456.

Glare, P. & Christakis, N. (2004) Predicting survival in patients with advanced disease. In: Doyle, D., Hanks, G., Cherny, N. & Calman, K. (eds) *Oxford Textbook of Palliative Medicine*, 3rd edn. Oxford: Oxford University Press.

Green, J. & Green, M. (2006) *Dealing with Death: A Handbook of Practices, Procedures and Law*, 2nd edn. London: Jessica Kingsley Publishers.

Gunaratnam, Y. (1997) Culture is not enough: a critique of multiculturalism in palliative care. In: Field, D., Hockley, J. & Small, N. (eds) *Death, Gender and Ethnicity*. London: Routledge, pp. 166–186.

Haig S. (2009) Diagnosing dying: symptoms and signs of end-stage disease. *End of Life Care*, 3(4), 8–13.

Healing, T.D., Hoffman, P.N. & Young, S.E.J. (1995) The infection hazards of human cadavers. *Communicable Disease Report*, 5(5), R61–R68.

Health and Safety Advisory Committee (HSAC) (2003) *Safe Working and the Prevention of Infection in the Mortuary and Postmortem Room*. London: Health and Safety Advisory Committee/HSE.

Higgins, D. (2010) Care of the dying patient: a guide for nurses. In: Jevon, P. (ed.) *Care of the Dying and Deceased Patient*. Oxford: Wiley-Blackwell.

Home Office (1971) *Report of the Committee on Death Certification and Coroners*. CMND 4810. London: HMSO.

Institute of Physics and Engineering in Medicine (IPEM) (2002) *Medical and Dental Guidance Notes. A Good Practice Guide on All Aspects of Ionising Radiation Protection in the Clinical Environment*. York: Institute of Physics and Engineering in Medicine.

Jenkins, V., Fallowfield, L. & Saul, J. (2001) Information needs of patients with cancer: results from a large study in UK cancer centres. *British Journal of Cancer*, 84(1), 48–51.

Kehl, K.A. (2006) Moving toward peace: an analysis of the concept of a good death. *American Journal of Hospice Palliative Care*, 23(4), 277–286.

King's Fund (2008) *Improving Environments for Care at End of Life*. London: King's Fund.

Kissane, D. & Yates, P. (2003) Psychological and existential distress. In: O'Connor, M. & Aranda, S. (eds) *Palliative Nursing: A Guide to Practice*. Oxford: Radcliffe Medical Press.

Laverty, D., Wilson, J. & Cooper, M. (2018) Registered nurse verification of expected adult death: new guidance provides direction. *Int J Palliat Nurs*, 24(4), 178–183. doi: 10.12968/ijpn.2018.24.4.178.

Leadership Alliance for the Care of Dying People (2014) *One Chance to get it Right*. London: Leadership Alliance.

Macmillan Cancer Support (2015) *Your Life and Your Choices: Plan Ahead*. London: Macmillan Cancer Support. Available at: www.macmillan.org.uk (Accessed: 27/3/2018)

Mental Capacity Act (2005), [online] Available at: http://www.legislation.gov.uk/ukpga/2005/9/pdfs/ukpga_20050009_en.pdf (Accessed 15/6/2018)

National Nurse Consultant Group, Palliative Care (2011) Guidance for staff responsible for care after death (last offices). London: National End of Life Care Programme.

National Palliative and End of Life Care Partnership (2015) *Ambitions for Palliative and End of Life Care: A National Framework for Local Action 2015-2020*. Available at: http://endoflifecareambitions.org.uk/ (Accessed: 27/3/2018)

Nearney, L. (1998) Practical procedures for nurses part 1 last offices. *Nursing Times*, 94(26), Insert.

Neuberger, J. (1999) Cultural issues in palliative care. In: Doyle, D., Hanks, G. & MacDonald, N. (eds) *Oxford Textbook of Palliative Medicine*, 2nd edn. Oxford: Oxford University Press, pp. 777–780.

Neuberger, J. (2004) *Caring for People of Different Faiths*. Abingdon: Radcliffe Medical Press.

NHS Education for Scotland (2006) A Multi Source Resource for Healthcare Staff. Glasgow: NHS Education.

NICE (2015) Care of dying adults in the last days of life. London: National Institute for Health and Care Excellence.

NMC (2015) *The Code: Professional standards of practice and behaviour for nurses and midwives*. London: Nursing and Midwifery Council.

O'Donnell, V. (1998) The pharmacological management of respiratory secretions. *Journal of Palliative Nursing*, 4, 199–203.

Office for National Statistics (ONS) (2009) *Mortality Statistics Deaths Registered in 2008.* Kew: OPSI.

Oostendorp, L., Ottevanger, P., Van der Graaf, W. & Stalmeie, P. (2011) Assessing the information desire of patients with advanced cancer by providing information with a decision aid, which is evaluated in a randomized trial: a study protocol. *BMC Medical Informatics and Decision Making*, 11, 9.

Pattison, N. (2008a) Care of patients who have died. *Nursing Standard*, 22(28), 42–48.

Pattison, N. (2008b) Caring for patients after death. *Nursing Standard*, 22(51), 48–56.

Pearce, E. (1963) *A General Textbook of Nursing.* London: Faber and Faber.

Philpin, S. (2002) Rituals and nursing: a critical commentary. *Journal of Advanced Nursing*, 38(2), 144–151.

Quested, B. & Rudge, T. (2001) Procedure manuals and textually mediated death. *Nursing Inquiry*, 8(4), 264–272.

Schofield, P.E. & Butow, P.N. (2004). Towards better communication in cancer care: a framework for developing evidence-based interventions. *Patient Education and Counseling*, 55, 32–39.

Seale, C. (1998) *Constructing Death. The Sociology of Dying and Bereavement.* Cambridge: Cambridge University Press.

Sleeman K. (2013) Caring for a dying patient in hospital. *British Medical Journal*, 346, f2174.

Smaje, C. & Field, D. (1997) Absent minorities? Ethnicity and the use of palliative care services. In: Field, D., Hockley, J. & Small, N. (eds) *Death, Gender and Ethnicity.* London: Routledge, pp. 142–165.

Smith, R. (2000) A good death. An important aim for health services and for us all. *BMJ*, 320, 129–130.

Speck, P. (1992) Care after death. *Nursing Times*, 88(6), 20.

Street, R.L., Makoul, G., Arora, N.K. & Epstein, R.M. (2009) How does communication heal? Pathways linking clinician-patient communication to health outcomes. *Patient Education and Counselling*, 74, 295–301.

Travis, S. (2002) *Procedure for the Care of Patients Who Die in Hospital.* London: Royal Marsden NHS Foundation Trust.

Van Gennep A. (1972) *The Rites of Passage.* Chicago: Chicago University Press.

Walsh, M. & Ford, P. (1989) *Nursing Rituals: Research and Rational Actions.* Oxford: Butterworth Heinemann.

Watson, M., Lucas, C., Hoy, A. & Wells, J. (eds) (2009) Ethical issues. In: Watson, M., Lucas, C., Hoy, A. & Back, I. (eds) *Oxford Handbook of Palliative Care.* 2nd edn. Oxford: Oxford University Press.

WHO (2002) Palliative care. Available at: www.who.int/cancer/palliative/en (Accessed: 28/3/2018)

Wolf, Z. (1988) *Nurses' Work: The Sacred and the Profane.* Philadelphia: University of Pennsylvania Press.

Wyatt, J. (2009) *Matters of Life and Death.* Nottingham: Inter-Varsity Press.

Index

The Royal Marsden Manual of Cancer Nursing Procedures. Edited by Sara Lister and Lisa Dougherty, with Assistant Editor Louise McNamara.
© 2019 The Royal Marsden NHS Foundation Trust. Published 2019 by John Wiley & Sons, Ltd.

Index